Human Occupation

This comprehensive textbook provides occupational therapy and science students and practitioners with a complete overview of the key human occupation concepts, as well as a range of perspectives through which occupational therapy and occupational science can be viewed and understood.

Comprising 40 chapters, the book is divided into five sections:

- **Section 1: Overview of Human Occupation.** Introducing the occupational therapy field and its conceptual landscape, including different models of therapeutic practice and practice reasoning.
- **Section 2: Contemporary Perspectives on Human Occupation.** Including critical perspectives on disability and race and the philosophical foundations of occupational science.
- **Section 3: Principal Concepts.** Explaining the conceptual language of human occupation across key person, social, psychological, physical, performance, and environmental issues.
- **Section 4: Human Occupation across the Lifespan and Life Course.** Covers human occupation from infancy to later adulthood.
- **Section 5: Domains/Types of Human Occupation.** From sleep to play, sexuality to social participation, and education to work.

Uniquely international in scope, each chapter in this edited book includes learning objectives, key terms, summary dot points, review questions, and a list of additional online resources for readers to refer to. This is a complete resource for anyone beginning an occupational therapy course, clinicians seeking an accessible reference work to support their practice, or occupational scientists needing to refer to contemporary occupation-related concepts.

Ted Brown is Professor of Occupational Therapy and Undergraduate Course Director in the Department of Occupational Therapy at Monash University – Peninsula Campus, Australia. Prior to this, he worked as an occupational therapy clinician for 16 years in Canada and Australia, primarily in the area of pediatrics.

Stephen Isbel is Professor of Occupational Therapy at the University of Canberra, Australia. He has worked in the USA, the UK, and Australia, primarily in the areas of aged care, community care, and adult neurological rehabilitation.

Louise Gustafsson is Professor and Lead of the Occupational Therapy Program at Griffith University, Australia. Her research aims to address occupational issues of older adults and individuals with neurological conditions.

Sharon Gutman is a professor at Rutgers University in the Occupational Therapy Doctorate Program. Her body of work has primarily addressed the development and assessment of interventions designed to help sheltered homeless people transition from homelessness to supported housing.

Diane Powers Dirette is a professor in the Interdisciplinary Health Sciences PhD Program at Western Michigan University, and her research interests are focused on treatments for people with acquired brain injuries.

Bethan Collins is the Head of Occupational Therapy at the University of Salford, UK. Bethan completed her primary degree in Occupational Therapy and her PhD at Trinity College Dublin, Ireland.

Tim Barlott is an assistant professor in the Department of Occupational Therapy at the University of Alberta. His work pursues theory, practices, and collective processes that can be liberating for psychiatrized and other marginalized people.

Human Occupation

Contemporary Concepts and Lifespan Perspectives

*Edited by Ted Brown, Stephen Isbel,
Louise Gustafsson, Sharon Gutman,
Diane Powers Dirette, Bethan Collins,
and Tim Barlott*

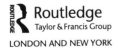

LONDON AND NEW YORK

Designed cover image: Getty

First published 2025
by Routledge
4 Park Square, Milton Park, Abingdon, Oxon, OX14 4RN

and by Routledge
605 Third Avenue, New York, NY 10158

Routledge is an imprint of the Taylor & Francis Group, an informa business

© 2025 selection and editorial matter, Ted Brown, Stephen Isbel, Louise Gustafsson, Sharon Gutman, Diane Powers Dirette, Bethan Collins, and Tim Barlott; individual chapters, the contributors

The right of Ted Brown, Stephen Isbel, Louise Gustafsson, Sharon Gutman, Diane Powers Dirette, Bethan Collins, and Tim Barlott to be identified as the authors of the editorial material, and of the authors for their individual chapters, has been asserted in accordance with sections 77 and 78 of the Copyright, Designs and Patents Act 1988.

All rights reserved. No part of this book may be reprinted or reproduced or utilised in any form or by any electronic, mechanical, or other means, now known or hereafter invented, including photocopying and recording, or in any information storage or retrieval system, without permission in writing from the publishers.

Trademark notice: Product or corporate names may be trademarks or registered trademarks, and are used only for identification and explanation without intent to infringe.

British Library Cataloguing-in-Publication Data
A catalogue record for this book is available from the British Library

Library of Congress Cataloging-in-Publication Data
Names: Brown, Ted, editor.
Title: Human occupation: contemporary concepts and lifespan perspectives / edited by Ted Brown, Stephen Isbel, Louise Gustafsson, Sharon Gutman, Diane Powers Dirette, Bethan Collins, and Tim Barlott.
Description: Abingdon, Oxon; New York, NY: Routledge, 2025. | Includes bibliographical references and index. |
Identifiers: LCCN 2024009881 (print) | LCCN 2024009882 (ebook) | ISBN 9781032790732 (hardback) | ISBN 9781032214566 (paperback) | ISBN 9781003490388 (ebook)
Subjects: LCSH: Occupational therapy.
Classification: LCC RM735 .H86 2024 (print) |
LCC RM735 (ebook) | DDC 615.8/515—dc23/eng/20240516
LC record available at https://lccn.loc.gov/2024009881
LC ebook record available at https://lccn.loc.gov/2024009882

ISBN: 978-1-032-82464-2 (hbk)
ISBN: 978-1-032-21456-6 (pbk)
ISBN: 978-1-003-50461-0 (ebk)

DOI: 10.4324/9781003504610

Typeset in Sabon
by codeMantra

Access the Support Material: www.routledge.com/9781032214566

Editors' Personal Dedications

Ted Brown
- David Stevens, life partner and constant source of support and patience for the time my academic pursuits take up.
- Archer and Oscar, our two Burmese cats, who are constant sources of occupational engagement, intrigue, companionship, and playfulness.
- John Waugh and Colin Martin, dear friends who have listened and laughed with me along the way.
- Professor Sylvia Rodger, Professor Jane Case-Smith, Professor Jim Hinojosa, and Professor Gary Kielhofner, four occupational therapy scholars, educators, researchers, champions, and visionaries whose contributions to the profession were exceptional and enduring.

Stephen Isbel
- I dedicate this book to my family, my work colleagues, and academic mentors who allowed me the opportunity, time, and space to be an Editor on this important book.

Louise Gustafsson
- To Dr Kryss McKenna and Professor Sylvia Rodger who were pivotal in my development as an early career academic and researcher, and who are missed.

Sharon Gutman
- I dedicate this book to Cake, Snow White, Chestnut, Colie, and Sandy who taught me more about unconditional love than any human being.

Diane Powers Dirette
- To my wonderful daughters, Madeleine and Claire, for the joy and meaning you bring to my life. I am eternally grateful that I get to be your mom.

Bethan Collins
- With thanks to wonderful colleagues, friends and family who support me to engage in all the meaningful occupations in my life.
- To Michael, Peter, and Cian for reminding me to engage in family occupations as well as work occupations, and in loving memory of Dad.

Tim Barlott
- To my students – I think I have learned more from you than you from me.

Contents

List of Figures	xi
List of Tables	xv
About the Editors	xvii
List of Contributors	xxi
Acknowledgments	xxix
Foreword I: Unravelling the Tapestry of Human Occupation	xxxi
Foreword II: "What Is Occupation?"	xxxiii
Foreword III: Hope, Utopia, and Solidarity	xxxvii
Foreword IV: Occupation and Occupational Engagement – The Things That People *Do*, Unites Us All	xli
List of Acronyms	xliii

SECTION ONE
Overview of Human Occupation   1

1 Introduction to Human Occupation: Contemporary Concepts and Lifespan Perspectives   3
TED BROWN, STEPHEN ISBEL, LOUISE GUSTAFSSON, SHARON GUTMAN, DIANE POWERS DIRETTE, BETHAN COLLINS, AND TIM BARLOTT

2 Overview of Human Occupation: Concepts and Principles   29
MATTHEW MOLINEUX

3 Overview of Occupation-centered Practice   47
LOUISE GUSTAFSSON AND MATTHEW MOLINEUX

CONTENTS

4 Person-centered Care in Occupation-based Practice — 61
DIANE POWERS DIRETTE AND SHARON GUTMAN

5 Models of Practice that Focus on Human Occupation — 75
ELLIE FOSSEY, GAYLE RESTALL, MARY EGAN, AND SANDRA MOLL

6 Participation and (Human) Occupation — 101
DANIELA CASTRO DE JONG, WILSON VERDUGO HUENUMÁN, ANDREA YUPANQUI-CONCHA, CAROLINA VÁSQUEZ OYARZÚN, AND CRISTIAN ARANDA-FARÍAS

7 Practice Reasoning in Occupational Therapy: Introducing the Model of Occupational Therapy Reasoning — 113
CRAIG GREBER, STEPHEN ISBEL, JUSTIN SCANLAN, AND JENNIFFER GARCIA-ROJAS

SECTION TWO
Contemporary Perspectives on Human Occupation — 141

8 Bringing Critical Perspectives into Occupation-based Practices — 143
LISETTE FARIAS, GAIL TEACHMAN, REBECCA M. ALDRICH, ROSHAN GALVAAN, AND DEBBIE LALIBERTE RUDMAN

9 The Situated Nature of Human Occupation — 157
REBECCA M. ALDRICH, LISETTE FARIAS, ROSHAN GALVAAN, DEBBIE LALIBERTE RUDMAN, AND GAIL TEACHMAN

10 Equity, Disadvantage, Justice, and Human Occupation — 171
SHARON GUTMAN

11 Undoing Coloniality: An Indigenous Occupation-based Perspective — 191
ISLA G. EMERY-WHITTINGTON

12 Critical Disability Studies Perspectives on Human Occupation — 209
MARJORIE DÉSORMEAUX-MOREAU, BETHAN COLLINS, LAURA YVONNE BULK, SUSAN MAHIPAUL, STEPHANIE LEBLANC-OMSTEAD, AND TAL JARUS

13 Occupation and Social Sanctioning — 229
NIKI KIEPEK, CRISTIAN MAURICIO VALDERRAMA NÚÑEZ, TANYA ELIZABETH BENJAMIN-THOMAS, MICHAEL PALAPAL SY, AND MARCEL NAZABAL AMORES

14 Creativity, Hope, and Collective Emancipatory Experimentation: Tools for Social Transformation through Occupational Therapy — 249
VAGNER DOS SANTOS AND GELYA FRANK

15 Social Occupational Therapy: Contributions to Design a Field of Knowledge and Practices — 267
ROSELI ESQUERDO LOPES, DENISE DIAS BARROS, AND ANA PAULA SERRATA MALFITANO

CONTENTS

16 Pragmatism: Current and Future Influence on Occupational Therapy and Occupational Science — **283**
JACOB ØSTERGAARD MADSEN, RODOLFO MORRISON, VAGNER DOS SANTOS, AND TIM BARLOTT

17 Gender and Human Occupation — **299**
JENS SCHNEIDER, AIKO HOSHINO, DANIEL SWIATEK, GUNILLA M. LIEDBERG, MATHILDA BJÖRK, HEATHER BAGLEE, GUSTAVO ARTUR MONZELI, AND TED BROWN

18 Technology and Human Occupation — **315**
EMMA M. SMITH, CHRISTOPHER TRUJILLO, STEPHANIE LANCASTER, CAROLINE FISCHL, ROSALIE H. WANG, AND TED BROWN

19 Human Occupation and Environmental Sustainability — **335**
LISA C. LIEB, TENELLE HODSON, AND CAMILLE DIETERLE

SECTION THREE
Principal Concepts — **349**

20 Key Occupational Concepts: Occupational Engagement, Occupational Balance, Occupational Adaptation, and Participation — **351**
JANE A. DAVIS, CARITA HÅKANSSON, AND KIM WALDER

21 Person Factors: Values, Beliefs, Spirituality, Body Functions, and Body Structures — **369**
BARBARA M. DOUCET AND CARRIE A. CIRO

22 Performance Skills: Motor, Process, and Social Interaction — **397**
KARINA M. DANCZA, ANITA VOLKERT, KAREN P. Y. LIU, AND LOUISE GUSTAFSSON

23 Performance Patterns: Habits, Routines, Rituals, and Roles — **413**
HEATHER FRITZ

24 Evolving and Pluralistic: Understanding the Environment in Occupational Therapy — **431**
TAMMY APLIN, ANA PAULA SERRATA-MALFITANO, AND TIM BARLOTT

SECTION FOUR
Human Occupation across the Lifespan and Life Course — **451**

25 Human Occupations of Infants, Toddlers, and Preschoolers — **453**
RONDALYN V. WHITNEY

26 Human Occupations of School-aged Children — **473**
EVGUENIA S. POPOVA, JANE C. O'BRIEN, MONG-LIN YU, JARRETT WOLSKE, ADAM DEPRIMO, AND TED BROWN

27 Human Occupations of Adolescence and Youth — **511**
SANDRA L. ROGERS

CONTENTS

28 Human Occupations of Early Adulthood — 537
LOUISE GUSTAFSSON

29 Human Occupations of Middle Adulthood (Ages 40–65) — 553
ROSANNE DIZAZZO-MILLER, LOUISE GUSTAFSSON, AND TOMOMI MCAULIFFE

30 Human Occupations of Late Adulthood — 567
EMILY J. BALOG

31 Future Considerations and Conclusion — 593
SHARON GUTMAN AND TED BROWN

Index for Chapters 1–40 — 607

SECTION FIVE (CHAPTERS AVAILABLE ONLINE ONLY; ***
LINK TO ACCESS ONLINE CHAPTERS BELOW)
Domains/Types of Human Occupation

32 Activities of Daily Living and Self-Care as Human Occupation *** — 609
BETHAN COLLINS, KAREN WHALLEY HAMMELL, AND VICKY MCQUILLAN

33 Instrumental Activities of Daily Living and Health Management as Human Occupation *** — 633
CLAIRE PEARCE, STEPHEN ISBEL, AND SUSANNE GUIDETTI

34 Work, Productivity, and Volunteering as Human Occupation *** — 651
MARY W. HILDEBRAND

35 Education as Human Occupation *** — 669
LORRY LIOTTA-KLEINFELD, MARGARET NEWSHAM BECKLEY, SHELLEY WRIGHT, BRYAN GEE, AND TED BROWN

36 Play as Human Occupation *** — 711
HELEN LYNCH, ANN KENNEDY-BEHR, SYLVIE RAY-KAESER, LAURETTE OLSON, AND TED BROWN

37 Leisure and Recreation as Human Occupation *** — 745
BENITA POWRIE, SZU-WEI CHEN, BARBARA PRUDHOMME WHITE, AND TED BROWN

38 Social Participation as Human Occupation *** — 785
LUKE ROBINSON AND LISA O'BRIEN

39 Sleep and Rest as Human Occupation *** — 805
WHITNEY LUCAS MOLITOR, LORENA LEIVE, BEN SELLAR, BELKIS LANDA-GONZALEZ, AND TED BROWN

40 Sexuality as Human Occupation *** — 835
BREANNE GRASSO

*** Readers should visit www.routledge.com/9781032214566 to access the online material

Figures

1.1	The wheel of power and privilege	7
1.2	The coin model of privilege and critical allyship	8
1.3	Human occupation: The connecting element between occupational therapy and occupational science	11
1.4	International classification of functioning, health and disability	14
1.5	Occupational therapy domain and process based on the OTPF-4	15
4.1	The occupational therapist creates a partnership with the individual to tailor therapeutic interventions that are best suited to the characteristics, needs, values, environment, and occupational preferences of the individual	63
4.2	The occupational therapist uses compassion, collaboration, teaching-learning, and nurturing integrated with clinical reasoning and decision making	65
4.3	The occupational therapist achieves intentionality by managing their own communication style, vocal tone, body language, and facial expression and using therapeutic approaches that assist the client to feel at ease	67
5.1	Steps to guide therapeutic reasoning using the Model of Human Occupation	82
5.2	Graphic representation of the Canadian Model of Occupational Participation	85
5.3	The Canadian Occupational Therapy Inter-relational Practice Process (COTIPP) Framework	89
7.1	The Model of Occupational Therapy Reasoning	115
7.2	Biomedical versus occupational diagnosis	128
10.1	Impoverished communities are commonly characterized by lack of livable wage employment opportunities, crime, drug use, and proximity to environmental pollutants	175
10.2	Children who are a product of disadvantaged homes, communities, and school systems may not have the support needed to create daily routines to participate in educational activities such as homework and school assignments	178

FIGURES

10.3	Community and school systems in disadvantaged areas may not be able to provide safe spaces and activities in which adolescents can socialize with each other and engage in enjoyable occupations. If deprived of these occupational environments, adolescents may turn to nonsanctioned, adverse occupations such as substance use, crime, and violence	180
10.4	Homelessness is a severe form of societal exclusion where people are often denied the basic necessities of shelter, consistent and nutritious meals, sanitary toileting and bathing, as well as the opportunity to sleep without fear of harm	185
14.1	All elements and the seven principles of Occupational Reconstruction Theory	255
14.2	The elements and phases of Occupational Reconstruction as a practice framework	260
21.1	A client limited by a diagnosis of multiple sclerosis has a family ritual where her children and grandchildren congregate at her home for a family meal on Sundays	379
21.2	A 16-year-old female volleyball player who sustained a mild TBI may have difficulty with headaches (pain), appreciating the location of the volleyball (visual), knowing where she is in space to position her body correctly (vestibular), and choosing the appropriate pressure to hit the ball (touch)	386
21.3	Mrs. Lyons is a 55-year-old female who was recently diagnosed with a left frontal lobe brain tumor and has undergone a craniotomy to remove the tumor. She is currently receiving chemotherapy and is referred to occupational therapy for evaluation and treatment	393
22.1	Example of observation notes	408
23.1	Disparities in infrastructure and living environments that can impact habits of thought and action of individuals	417
25.1	Infant playing with toy	457
25.2	Toddler swimming with parent	458
25.3	Child pretending to drive a sports car while being pushed by sibling	459
25.4	Maslow's hierarchy of needs (Maslow, 1987)	467
25.5	Zone of proximal development (Vyotsky, 1078)	469
26.1	Depiction of Bronfenbrenner's Ecological Theory	478
26.2	Factors influencing school-aged children's performance patterns	484
27.1	Adolescents gain musculoskeletal strength that allow engagement in competitive sports, improved fine motor precision for tool use, and heightened mental focus to achieve personal goals	514
27.2	In adolescence, youth begin to explore ways of being independent from their family both socially and emotionally and begin to form friendships and share private thoughts with their friends instead of family members	516
27.3	Maslow's hierarchy of needs	521
28.1	Emerging Adulthood Vignettes	542
28.2	Established Adulthood Vignettes	543
30.1	Navy veteran, Rosa, powerwalking through her community to manage her health	581
30.2	Jane knitting on Brigantine Beach, NJ, as a way to keep her mind and hands occupied	583
30.3	Army Veteran, Frank (left), discusses plans for remembering fallen service members with a friend from his Veterans' Club	584
31.1	Protestors of systemic racism and the murder of George Floyd in police custody, New York City	596

31.2	Women faired far worse during the pandemic, both sustaining greater job losses and having to leave the workforce because of childcare and child education responsibilities	599
31.3	Protesters fighting for women's reproductive rights	601
33.1	What is the Global North?	637
33.2	Maslow's Hierarchy of Needs (1943)	638
34.1	Farmer with a mobility impairment on a tractor lift	656
34.2	Work-hardening client performing work task	660
34.3	A former physical therapist volunteers at Spaulding Rehabilitation Hospital after retirement	663
35.1	Education as human occupation throughout the lifespan	675
35.2	Interactions and intersections: Factors that impact educational participation	684
36.1	Two boys wrestling with each other in a playful way	715
36.2	Children playing at the beach	720
36.3	Play is a sociocultural-spatial occupation that takes place in available spaces, and with available objects	721
37.1	Skiing as an occupation	748
37.2	The tree of leisure	749
37.3	Meaningful outcomes from leisure	751
37.4	Playing musical instrument as a leisure occupation	753
37.5	Calligraphy as a leisure occupation	755
37.6	Melissa skiing with friends	777
37.7	Matthew working DJ control system	778
38.1	Social participation assessment selection	793
39.1	Need, ability, and opportunity model with occupational elements	810
39.2	Bedtime in the sociocultural context	814
39.3	Child resting	814
40.1	Interpretation of the Circles of Sexuality	838
40.2	The ex-PLISSIT model	841

Tables

1.1	Occupations Included in the OTPF-4 Domain	17
1.2	Contexts and Performance Patterns Included in the OTPF-4 Domain	18
1.3	Performance Skills and Client Factors Included in the OTPF-4 Domain	19
2.1	Comparison of Two Different Taxonomies of Types of Occupation	35
2.2	A Combined Taxonomy of Occupation	36
2.3	Comparison of Occupation, Person, and Environment across Four Models	42
3.1	Definitions of Terms from Fisher (2013)	50
4.1	Continuum of Client Behaviors Indicating Their Ability to Engage in the Therapeutic Relationship	69
4.2	Range of Therapist Behaviors Indicating Ability to Facilitate and Engage in Therapeutic Relationship	69
5.1	MOHO Key Concepts	78
7.1	The Influence of Guiding Factors for John and Max	117
7.2	The Practice Reasoning Process for John and Max	134
12.1	Definitions and Resources	211
18.1	Classes of Assistive Products Based on Functions, from ISO 9999:2022(E)	319
18.2	Technology-related Terms and Applications in Occupational Therapy	320
18.3	Human Occupation and Technology across the Lifespan	326
21.1	Non-Inclusive List of Client Factors Assessment	372
22.1	Steps and Actions When Buying Noodles and Juice from a Street Stall	399
22.2	Motor Skills	400
22.3	Process Skills	402
22.4	Social Interaction Skills	404
22.5	Performance Skill Observations of Note for Eva	409

TABLES

24.1	Example of an Interactional Approach to Understanding the Environment – OTPF-4 Environmental Factors	444
25.1	Observing Normal Development	456
25.2	Using Routines for Development	460
25.3	Occupational Profile of Case	462
26.1	Occupations of School-aged Children	476
26.2	Developmental Progression of Independence during IADL within Home Context	486
26.3	Developmental Expectations for Occupational Participation of School-aged Children	487
26.4	Occupation-centered Assessments for School-aged Children	495
27.1	Changes During Adolescent Development	517
27.2	Health Conditions, Prevalence, and Occupational Risk in Adolescence	519
27.3	Highlighted Occupations for Youth in Young-Middle and Middle-Late Adolescence	522
27.4	Typical Western Society Rites of Passage	528
27.5	Developmental Goals of Adolescence	528
28.1	Developmental Tasks of Early Adulthood	539
28.2	An Occupational Profile of Early Adulthood	546
29.1	Middle Adulthood Occupational Profile	558
32.1	ADL Assessment Tools	614
32.2	Summary of Strategies to Enable Self-Care Performance	620
35.1	Selected Psychoeducation and Occupational Therapy Theories, Models, and Frames of Reference to Enable Optimal Educational Engagement	677
35.2	Summary of Areas for Intersectoral Collaboration between Health and Education	684
35.3	Assessments of Education as an Occupation with Mapping onto the ICF Components	687
36.1	Commonly Used Categories and Taxonomies of Play	717
36.2	Play Assessments	726
36.3	Play Characteristics of Children Based on Different Diagnostic Groups	736
36.4	Continuum from Therapist-initiated to Child-initiated Play	739
37.1	Leisure Assessments that Occupational Therapists Use with Clients and Their Families	759
38.1	Levasseur et al.'s (2022) Taxonomy of Six Levels of Involvement of the Individual with Others in Social Activities	790
38.2	Assessment Tools used in Occupational Therapy Practice that Evaluate Social Participation	794
39.1	Assessment of Sleep for Children and Adolescents	815
39.2	Assessment of Sleep for Adults	821
39.3	Occupational Therapy Interventions Categorized by Intervention Principle	826
40.1	Examples of Treatment Ideas Based on Circles of Sexuality and AOTA Intervention Focus Recommendations	846

About the Editors

Ted Brown, PhD, MSc, MPA, BScOT(Hons), GCHPE, OT(C), OTR, MRCOT, FOTARA, FAOTA completed his undergraduate occupational therapy education in Canada in 1986 and his doctoral education in occupational therapy at the University of Queensland in 2003. He worked as an occupational therapy clinician for 16 years in Canada and Australia primarily in the area of pediatrics. In 2005, he then moved into the higher education sector taking up an academic position in the Department of Occupational Therapy at Monash University – Peninsula Campus in Australia. Professor Brown has published three edited books, 30 book chapters, and over 390 journal manuscripts. He has supervised 65 honors, 25 masters, and 15 doctoral students to completion. He was made an inaugural Fellow of the Occupational Therapy Australia Research Academy in 2017 and was inducted into the American Occupational Therapy Association Roster of Fellows in 2019. Professor Brown has served as an associate editor of the *American Journal of Occupational Therapy* for 11 years (2010–2021) and the *Australian Occupational Therapy Journal* for 16 years (2005–2021).

Stephen Isbel HScD, MOT, MHA, GCTE, BAppSc(OccTher) completed his undergraduate and doctoral qualifications at Sydney University. He has worked in the USA, the UK, and Australia as an occupational therapist, primarily in the areas of aged care, community care, and adult neurological rehabilitation. Stephen has research interests in aged care, post-stroke rehabilitation, driver rehabilitation, public health, and occupational therapy education. He is a Professor of Occupational Therapy at the University of Canberra where he teaches into the bachelor and masters programs and supervises masters and doctoral candidates. Stephen lives and works on Ngunnawal country in Canberra, the federal capital of Australia.

ABOUT THE EDITORS

Louise Gustafsson, PhD, BOccThy(Hons), FOTARA, SFHEA is an occupational therapy teaching and research academic at Griffith University in Queensland. She has a clinical background of predominantly hospital-based rehabilitation, commencing her PhD as a clinician researcher and transitioning to a full-time academic career at the University of Queensland in 2002. Professor Gustafsson has received over $6 million in research funding and has published over 150 papers and supported over 60 undergraduate and 12 postgraduate research students to completion. Her research is predominantly in collaboration with older adults and people living with neurological conditions and injury. She is most interested in how to better support and empower people to engage in their occupations long after the acute event, injury, or diagnosis. Her commitment and contribution to research and teaching have been recognized by a range of awards, most recently being named as a Fellow of the Occupational Therapy Australia Research Academy (2019) and a Senior Fellow of the Higher Education Academy (2021).

Sharon Gutman, PhD, OTR/L, FAOTA is a professor at Rutgers University in the Occupational Therapy Doctorate Program. Her body of work has primarily addressed the development and assessment of interventions designed to help sheltered homeless people learn the needed daily life skills to transition from homelessness to supported housing. Between 2008 and 2014, Professor Gutman served as the Editor-in-Chief of the *American Journal of Occupational Therapy* (AJOT). The AJOT is one of the leading core Q1 occupational therapy peer-reviewed journals in the world. Professor Gutman was awarded the Cordelia Myers Best Paper in AJOT in 2021. In the areas of research, Professor Gutman has authored 73 journal articles, 18 book chapters, and 12 books, and was nominated and inducted into the American Occupational Therapy Association Roster of Fellows in 2009 and awarded the Eleanor Clarke Slagle Lectureship in 2020. The Slagle Lectureship is one of the highest and most prestigious awards given by the American Occupational Therapy Association.

Diane Powers Dirette, PhD, OTL, FAOTA is a professor in the Interdisciplinary Health Sciences PhD Program at Western Michigan University. She earned her bachelor's degree at Eastern Michigan University and her masters and doctorate degrees at New York University, studying occupational therapy at all levels. She has published in national and international journals and has presented at local, regional, national, and international conferences. Dr Dirette's main research interests are focused on treatments for people with acquired brain injuries, for whom she developed a frame of reference titled Self-awareness Enhancement through Learning and Function (SELF). Other areas of research include evidence-based practice, the use of compensatory strategies for cognitive deficits, and occupational therapy service provision in post-secondary settings. She has served on the editorial boards of numerous journals in the health professions and is the co-editor of the textbooks, *Occupational therapy for physical dysfunction* (8th ed.) and *Conditions in occupational therapy: Effect on occupational performance*. She is the co-founder and Editor-in-Chief of *The Open Journal of Occupational Therapy*. Dr Dirette was inducted into the American Occupational Therapy Association Roster of Fellows in 2016. She was the recipient of the fourth annual Jim Hinojosa Distinguished Alumni Award from New York University in 2020.

ABOUT THE EDITORS

Bethan Collins (she/her) is the Head of Occupational Therapy in the University of Salford, UK. Bethan completed her primary degree in Occupational Therapy and her PhD in Trinity College Dublin, Ireland. Her clinical practice included working with adults with physical disability, older adults in rehabilitation services, services for people with dementia, and in post-acute stroke rehabilitation. She also worked as an occupational therapist in a University Disability Service. Her career as an occupational therapy academic began in 2002, and she taught at Trinity College Dublin, Bournemouth University, and the University of Liverpool before moving to Salford in March 2020. Bethan is blind and identifies as a disabled occupational therapist and academic. Her particular interests are in disability studies and lifestyle, particularly the factors that enable and limit human occupation for disabled people.

Tim Barlott, PhD, MScRS, Grad Cert CBRE, BScOT is an assistant professor in the Department of Occupational Therapy at the University of Alberta. Tim completed his undergraduate (occupational therapy) and masters (rehabilitation science) degrees at the University of Alberta, and his doctorate (sociology) at the University of Queensland. Tim's research is at the interface of occupational science and the sociology of health, exploring the sociopolitical aspects of everyday life and pursuing transformative change. His work pursues theory, practices, and collective processes that can be liberating for psychiatrized and other marginalized people. Tim has worked as a community practitioner (occupational therapist, addictions counsellor, and youth worker), educator, and participatory researcher in Canada, Australia, and internationally. Currently, he lives and works on Treaty 6 territory in Edmonton, Alberta, Canada.

Contributors

Rebecca M. Aldrich Professor of Clinical Occupational Therapy, USC Chan Division of Occupational Science and Occupational Therapy, University of Southern California, Los Angeles, California, United States.

Marcel Nazabal Amores Research Assistant, Dalhousie University, Halifax, Nova Scotia, Canada.

Tammy Aplin Conjoint Research Fellow, School of Health and Rehabilitation Sciences, Faculty of Health and Behavioural Sciences, University of Queensland, Brisbane, Queensland, Australia.

Cristian Aranda Farías Associate Professor and Researcher, Occupational Therapy Department, University of Magallanes, Punta Arenas, Magallanes and Chilean Antarctic Region, Chile.

Heather Baglee Course Director, Occupational Therapy, School of Health, Leeds Beckett University, United Kingdom.

Emily J. Balog Assistant Professor and Doctoral Capstone Coordinator, Rutgers, The State University of New Jersey, Department of Rehabilitation and Movement Sciences, Occupational Therapy Doctorate Program, Newark, New Jersey, United States.

Tim Barlott Assistant Professor, Department of Occupational Therapy, Faculty of Rehabilitation Sciences University of Alberta, Edmonton, Alberta, Canada.

Tanya Elizabeth Benjamin-Thomas Assistant Professor, School of Occupational Therapy, College of Health Sciences, Texas Woman's University, Houston, Texas, United States.

CONTRIBUTORS

Mathilda Björk Deputy Head of Department & Professor, Department of Health, Medicine and Caring Sciences, Division of Prevention, Rehabilitation and Community Medicine, Faculty of Medicine and Health Sciences, Linköping University, Sweden.

Ted Brown Professor of Occupational Therapy & Undergraduate Course Director, Department of Occupational Therapy, School of Primary and Allied Health Care, Faculty of Medicine, Nursing and Health Sciences, Monash University – Peninsula Campus, Frankston, Victoria, Australia.

Laura Yvonne Bulk Assistant Professor of Teaching, Department of Occupational Science and Occupational Therapy, Faculty of Medicine, University of British Columbia, Vancouver, British Columbia, Canada.

Daniela Castro de Jong Assistant Professor in Occupational Therapy, Faculty of Health, University of Canberra Hospital, University of Canberra, Canberra, Australian Capital Territory, Australia.

Szu-Wei Chen Postdoctoral Research Associate, Program in Occupational Therapy, Washington University School of Medicine in St. Louis, St. Louis, Missouri, United States.

Carrie A. Ciro Associate Professor, Occupational Therapy, Chair, OU Department of Rehabilitation Sciences, University of Oklahoma College of Allied Health, Oklahoma City, Oklahoma, United States.

Bethan Collins Head of Occupational Therapy, School of Health and Society, University of Salford, Manchester, United Kingdom.

Karina M. Dancza Associate Professor, Discipline of Occupational Therapy, Health and Social Sciences, Singapore Institute of Technology, Singapore.

Jane A. Davis Assistant Professor, Teaching Stream, Department of Occupational Science and Occupational Therapy, Temerty Faculty of Medicine, University of Toronto, Toronto, Ontario, Canada.

Adam DePrimo Assistant Professor, Occupational Therapy Department, Westbrook College of Health Professions, University of New England, Portland, Maine, United States.

Marjorie Désormeaux-Moreau Professor, School of Rehabilitation, Faculty of Medicine and Health Sciences, Université de Sherbrooke, Sherbrooke, Quebec, Canada.

Denise Dias Barros Professor, Postgraduate Program in Esthetic and Art History, School of Arts, Sciences and Humanities, University of São Paulo, São Paulo, Brazil.

Camille Dieterle Associate Professor of Clinical Occupational Therapy, Director of the Graduate Certificate Program in Foundations of Lifestyle Redesign®, USC Chan Division of Occupational Science and Occupational Therapy, USC Independent Health Professions at the Herman Ostrow School of Dentistry, University of Southern California, Los Angeles, California, United States.

Rosanne DiZazzo-Miller Associate Professor Occupational Therapy, Department of Occupational Therapy, Eugene Applebaum College of Pharmacy and Health

Sciences, Director of Mentoring Division of Health Care Sciences, Wayne State University, Detroit, Michigan, United States.

Vagner Dos Santos Senior Lecturer & Head of Discipline for Occupational Therapy, School of Allied Health, Exercise and Sports Sciences, Charles Sturt University, Port Macquarie, New South Wales, Australia.

Barbara M. Doucet Associate Clinical Professor, Director of Doctoral Capstone & Scholarship, Baylor University, Occupational Therapy Program, Waco, Texas, United States.

Mary Egan Professor and Director, School of Rehabilitation Sciences, University of Ottawa, Ottawa, Ontario, Canada.

Isla G. Emery-Whittington SHORE Whāriki Research Centre, Massey University, Auckland, New Zealand & Occupational Therapist at Emery-Whittington Consultants Ltd.

Roseli Esquerdo Lopes Professor, Department of Occupational Therapy, Postgraduate Program in Occupational Therapy and Postgraduate Program in Education, Federal University of São Carlos, São Carlos, São Paulo, Brazil.

Lisette Farias Assistant Professor, Division of Occupational Therapy, Department of Neurobiology, Care Sciences and Society, Karolinska Institute, Stockholm, Sweden.

Caroline Fischl Assistant Professor in Occupational Therapy, Department of Rehabilitation, School of Health and Welfare, Jönköping University, Jönköping, Sweden.

Ellie Fossey Professor and Head, Department of Occupational Therapy, School of Primary and Allied Health Care, Faculty of Medicine, Nursing and Health Sciences, Monash University, Victoria, Australia.

Gelya Frank Professor Emerita, Mrs. T. H. Chan Division of Occupational Science & Occupational Therapy, and Department of Anthropology, University of Southern California, United States.

Heather Fritz Association Professor and Founding Director, School of Occupational Therapy, Pacific Northwest University of the Health Sciences, Yakima, Washington, United States.

Roshan Galvaan Professor, Division of Occupational Therapy, Department of Health and Rehabilitation Sciences, Faculty of Health Sciences, University of Cape Town, Cape Town, South Africa.

Jenniffer Garcia-Rojas Head of Evidence-based Medicine Department, COANIQUEM, Chilean Rehabilitation Center for Children with Burns & Lecturer of Occupational Therapy, Faculty of Medicine, Universidad del Desarrollo, Santiago, Chile.

Bryan Gee Professor, Chair, and Program Director, Department of Occupational Therapy, College of Rehabilitation Sciences, Rocky Mountain University of Health Professions, Provo, Utah, United States.

CONTRIBUTORS

Breanne Grasso Private occupational therapy practitioner and consultant, Toms River, New Jersey, United States.

Craig Greber Associate Professor of Occupational Therapy, School of Health and Medical Sciences, University of Southern Queensland – Ipswich Campus, Ipswich, Queensland, Australia.

Susanne Guidetti Professor in Occupational Therapy, Department of Neurobiology, Care Sciences and Society (NVS), Division of Occupational Therapy, Karolinska Institutet, Stockholm, Sweden.

Louise Gustafsson Professor, Discipline of Occupational Therapy, School of Health Sciences and Social Work, Griffith University – Nathan Campus, Nathan, Queensland, Australia.

Sharon Gutman Professor, Occupational Therapy Doctorate Program, Department of Rehabilitation & Movement Sciences, School of Health Professions, Rutgers University, Newark, New Jersey, United States.

Carita Håkansson Senior Lecturer, Division of Occupational and Environmental Medicine, Lund University, Lund, Sweden.

Karen Whalley Hammell Honorary Professor, Department of Occupational Science and Occupational Therapy, Faculty of Medicine, University of British Columbia, Vancouver, British Columbia, Canada.

Mary W. Hildebrand Associate Professor, Department of Occupational Therapy, MGH Institute of Health Professions, Boston, Massachusetts, United States.

Tenelle Hodson Lecturer, Discipline of Occupational Therapy, School of Health Sciences and Social Work, Griffith University – Nathan Campus, Nathan, Queensland, Australia.

Aiko Hoshino Lecturer, Graduate School of Medicine & School of Health Sciences, Nagoya University, Japan.

Stephen Isbel Professor of Occupational Therapy, Faculty of Health, University of Canberra Hospital, University of Canberra, Canberra, Australian Capital Territory, Australia.

Tal Jarus Professor, Department of Occupational Science and Occupational Therapy, Faculty of Medicine, University of British Columbia, Vancouver, British Columbia, Canada.

Ann Kennedy-Behr Occupational Therapist, Noosa Heads, Queensland, Australia & Adjunct Senior Lecturer, Allied Health & Human Performance, University of South Australia, South Australia, Australia.

Niki Kiepek Associate Professor, School of Occupational Therapy, Faculty of Health, Dalhousie University, Halifax, Nova Scotia, Canada.

Debbie Laliberte Rudman Distinguished University Professor, School of Occupational Therapy, Faculty of Health Sciences, University of Western Ontario, London, Ontario, Canada.

CONTRIBUTORS

Stephanie Lancaster Associate Professor, Department of Occupational Therapy, University of Tennessee Health Science Center, Memphis, Tennessee, United States.

Belkis Landa-Gonzalez Professor and Program Director of Occupational Therapy Programs, College of Health and Wellness, Barry University, Miami, Florida, United States.

Stephanie LeBlanc-Omstead Health Professional Education, Faculty of Health Sciences, Western University, London, Ontario, Canada.

Lorena Leive Occupational Therapist, AATO (Asociación Argentina de Terapistas Ocupacionales), Assistant Professor, Medicine, Universidad Nacional de Rio Negro, Bariloche, Provincia de Río Negro, Argentina.

Lisa C. Lieb Occupational Therapist & Independent Scholar, Beaver, Pennsylvania, United States.

Gunilla M. Liedberg Principal for Postgraduate Studies, Department of Health, Medicine and Caring Sciences Division of Prevention, Rehabilitation and Community Medicine, Faculty of Medicine and Health Sciences, Linköping University, Sweden.

Lorry Liotta-Kleinfeld Professor, School of Occupational Therapy, Belmont University, Nashville, Tennessee, United States.

Karen P. Y. Liu Professor, Discipline of Occupational Therapy, School of Health Sciences, Translational Health Research Institute, Western Sydney University, New South Wales, Australia.

Whitney Lucas Molitor Assistant Professor, Department of Occupational Therapy, University of South Dakota, Vermillion, South Dakota, United States.

Helen Lynch Senior Lecturer & Graduate Studies Coordinator, Department of Occupational Science & Occupational Therapy, Brookfield Health Sciences Complex, University College Cork, Cork, Ireland.

Jacob Østergaard Madsen Senior Lecturer, Department of Occupational Therapy, Division of Health Studies, Professionshøjskolen University College of Northern Denmark, Aalborg, Denmark.

Susan Mahipaul Disability and Health Navigator, Occupational Therapist & Advocate, Disability and Health Navigation, London, Ontario, Canada.

Ana Paula Serrata-Malfitano Associate Professor, Postgraduate Program in Occupational Therapy, Department of Occupational Therapy, Federal University of São Carlos, São Carlos, São Paulo, Brazil.

Tomomi McAuliffe Lecturer in Occupational Therapy, School of Health and Rehabilitation Sciences, Faculty of Health and Behavioural Sciences, University of Queensland, St Lucia, Queensland, Australia.

Vicky McQuillan Lecturer, Discipline of Occupational Therapy, School of Health Sciences, University of Liverpool, Liverpool, United Kingdom.

CONTRIBUTORS

Matthew Molineux Professor and Head, Discipline of Occupational Therapy, School of Health Sciences and Social Work, Griffith University, Gold Coast, Queensland, Australia.

Sandra Moll Associate Professor, School of Rehabilitation Sciences, McMaster University, Hamilton, Ontario, Canada.

Gustavo Artur Monzeli Associate Professor, Department of Occupational Therapy, Federal University of Paraiba, Brazil.

Rodolfo Morrison Department of Occupational Therapy and Occupational Science, Faculty of Medicine University of Chile, Santiago, Chile.

Margaret Newsham Beckley Clinical & Educational Consultants, St. Louis, Missouri, United States.

Jane C. O'Brien Professor, Occupational Therapy Department, Westbrook College of Health Professions University of New England, Portland, Maine, United States.

Lisa O'Brien Professor & Discipline Lead and Course Director, Occupational Therapy Department of Nursing and Allied Health, School of Health Sciences, Swinburne University of Technology, Hawthorn, Victoria, Australia.

Laurette Olson Professor and Program Director, Graduate Occupational Therapy Program, New York-Presbyterian Iona School of Health Sciences, Iona College, New Rochelle, New York, United States.

Claire Pearce Assistant Professor of Occupational Therapy, Faculty of Health, University of Canberra Hospital, University of Canberra, Canberra, Australian Capital Territory, Australia.

Evguenia S. Popova Assistant Professor, Department of Occupational Therapy, College of Health Sciences Rush University, Chicago, Illinois, United States.

Diane Powers Dirette Professor, Interdisciplinary Health Sciences PhD Program, College of Health and Human Services, Western Michigan University, Kalamazoo, Michigan, United States.

Benita Powrie Senior Lecturer, Occupational Therapy, School of Allied Health, Faculty of Health Sciences, Australian Catholic University, Brisbane, Queensland, Australia.

Barbara Prudhomme White Professor, Occupational Therapy, College of Health and Human Services, University of New Hampshire, Durham, New Hampshire, United States.

Sylvie Ray-Kaeser Professor, Department of Occupational Therapy, School of Social Work and Health Sciences, EESP, University of Applied Sciences and Arts of Western Switzerland, Lausanne, Switzerland.

Gayle Restall Senior Scholar, Department of Occupational Therapy, College of Rehabilitation Sciences, University of Manitoba, Winnipeg, Manitoba, Canada.

Luke Robinson Senior Lecturer & Fourth Year Undergraduate Coordinator, Department of Occupational Therapy, School of Primary & Allied Health Care,

Faculty of Medicine, Nursing and Health Sciences, Monash University – Peninsula Campus, Frankston, Victoria, Australia.

Sandra L. Rogers Program Director and Associate Professor, Occupational Therapy Doctorate Program Rehabilitation and Movement Sciences, Rutgers, State University of New Jersey, Newark, New Jersey, United States.

Justin Scanlan Associate Professor in Occupational Therapy, Sydney School of Health Sciences, Faculty of Medicine and Health, University of Sydney – Camperdown Campus, Sydney, New South Wales, Australia.

Jens Schneider Freelance Occupational Therapist & Lecturer at Ergotherapie Jens Schneider, Frankfurt am Main, Germany.

Ben Sellar Lecturer in Occupational Therapy, Allied Health & Human Performance, University of South Australia, Adelaide, South Australia, Australia.

Emma M. Smith Postdoctoral Research Fellow, Assisting Living and Learning (ALL) Institute, Maynooth University, Maynooth, Ireland.

Daniel Swiatek Assistant Professor, Department of Occupational Therapy, College of Health, Human Services and Nursing, California State University, Dominguez Hills, California, United States.

Michael Palapal Sy Senior Researcher, Institute of Occupational Therapy, School of Health Sciences Zurich University of Applied Sciences, Winterthur, Switzerland.

Gail Teachman Assistant Professor, School of Occupational Therapy, Faculty of Health Sciences, University of Western Ontario, London, Ontario, Canada.

Christopher Trujillo Assistant Professor, Occupational Therapy Program, College of Health Sciences – AZ Midwestern University, Glendale, Arizona, United States.

Cristian Mauricio Valderrama Núñez Master in Occupational Therapy, Associate Professor, Faculty of Rehabilitation Sciences, Andrés Bello University, Concepción, Chile.

Carolina Vásquez Oyarzún Assistant Professor and Director, Occupational Therapy Department, University of Magallanes, Punta Arenas, Magallanes and Chilean Antarctic Region, Chile.

Wilson Verdugo Huenumán Associate Academic and Researcher, Occupational Therapy Department, University of Magallanes, Punta Arenas, Magallanes and Chilean Antarctic Region, Chile.

Anita Volkert Lecturer and Practice Placements Lead for the Allied Health Professions, Department of Occupational Therapy and Human Nutrition & Dietetics, School of Health and Life Sciences, Glasgow Caledonian University, Glasgow, United Kingdom.

Kim Walder Lecturer, Discipline of Occupational Therapy, School of Health Sciences and Social Work Griffith University – Nathan Campus, Brisbane, Queensland, Australia.

CONTRIBUTORS

Rosalie H. Wang Associate Professor, Intelligent Assistive Technology and Systems Lab, Department of Occupational Science and Occupational Therapy, Temerty Faculty of Medicine, University of Toronto, Toronto, Ontario, Canada.

Rondalyn V. Whitney Chair & Professor of Occupational Therapy, School of Health Sciences, Quinnipiac University, Hamden, Connecticut, United States.

Jarrett Wolske Coordinator of Accommodations and Adjunct Clinical Instructor, McHenry County College Crystal Lake, Illinois, United States.

Shelley Wright Lecturer, Occupational Therapy Program, Allied Health and Human Performance, University of South Australia – City East Campus, Adelaide, South Australia, Australia.

Mong-Lin Yu Senior Lecturer & Fieldwork Coordinator, Department of Occupational Therapy, School of Primary and Allied Health Care, Faculty of Medicine, Nursing and Health Sciences, Monash University – Peninsula Campus, Frankston, Victoria, Australia.

Andrea Yupanqui Concha Associate Professor and Researcher, Occupational Therapy Department, University of Magallanes, Punta Arenas, Magallanes and Chilean Antarctic Region, Chile.

Acknowledgments

As the seven book editors, we want to extend our sincere gratitude and thanks to the contributing chapter authors. Without their generosity, tenacity, good will, enthusiasm, teamwork, creativity, occupational engagement, constructive feedback, exceptional conceptual thinking, and visionary forethought, the scope, breadth, depth, and critical commentary included in this book would not have been possible. Thanks are also extended to Karen Jacobs, Liat Gafni-Lachter, Nick Pollard, Mandy Stanley, and Lilian Magalhães who agreed to write Forewords for the book. In addition, we extend our acknowledgments to Mr Jamie Etherington whose attention to detail in his pre-submission copy-editor role ensured that the 40 chapter manuscripts were consistent in their presentation, format, referencing style, and English language use despite the diversity of contributing authors. Mr David Stevens is acknowledged for his formatting of the PowerPoint slides that accompany each of the chapters and his creation of the list of figures, pictures, and tables located within the book's 40 chapters. Finally, we as editors would like to extend our thanks to Mr Russell George, Senior Commissioning Editor, Health & Social, Routledge Publishers for his support and guidance throughout the publishing process.

Foreword I: Unravelling the Tapestry of Human Occupation

Karen Jacobs and Liat Gafni-Lachter

In the ever-evolving tapestry of human existence, a phenomenon has captivated thinkers, scholars, and curious minds for centuries: human occupation. It is a subject that not only delves into the intricacies of our daily lives but also unravels the threads of power, privilege, diversity, and inclusion that weave through the fabric of society. In this comprehensive work, the authors embark on a journey to illuminate the paths of understanding, shedding light on the sources of privilege and power and offering invaluable insights into how we can foster a world of true diversity and inclusivity.

Drawing on authoritative models and contemporary wisdom, this book transcends the boundaries of conventional discourse. It offers a panoramic view of human occupation, enriching the knowledge of both novices and experts alike. Within its pages lies a meticulous exploration of the diverse forms of human engagement, underpinned by the fundamental elements that comprise the essence of occupation: personal factors, performance skills and patterns, and the contextual milieu in which they unfold. Through the authors' lens, we discern how these elements combine to shape the multifaceted landscape of human occupation across the expanse of a lifespan.

What sets this work apart is its fusion of groups of authors, using classical foundational knowledge with the currents of modernity, seamlessly blending tradition with our time's urgent concerns and evolving theories. The authors, trailblazers in this endeavor, deftly navigate this intersection, offering readers a compass to navigate the complexities of human occupation in today's world.

As we navigate the pages of this work, we find ourselves immersed in a symphony of perspectives that deepen our understanding of equity, disadvantage, justice, and the complexities of human occupation. It is a testament to the authors' dedication to presenting a comprehensive view, acknowledging the myriad voices that shape our discourse. Moreover, each chapter demonstrates a commitment to the art of adult learning, thoughtfully structured to facilitate comprehension and retention, providing an abstract followed by clearly defined learning objectives and key terms that anchor the reader in the subject matter. The main text reveals a wealth of knowledge and insights, leading to a conclusion that encapsulates the key takeaways. A summary crystallizes the chapter's essence, while review questions prompt reflection and reinforce understanding. References provide a robust foundation for further exploration. The authors' positionality and reflexivity statements are a commendable practice, exemplary of transparency in a landscape that often demands scrutiny. We were inspired to include our statements and encourage readers to develop their own.

This book is not merely a scholarly and professional read; it is a call to action. It invites readers to look beyond the surface, to challenge preconceptions, and to engage with the profound implications of privilege, power, and the pursuit of equity. It confronts the disparities that pervade our society and advocates for a world where everyone can flourish.

It is a joy to read this book, which extends an invitation to explore the depths of human occupation and a roadmap towards a more inclusive and equitable world. It is a valuable resource for all who seek to broaden their understanding of human experience, from the eager novice to the seasoned expert. Through its pages, we embark on a journey that unfolds the intricacies of occupation actively and its contribution to a world where diversity and inclusion are celebrated as the cornerstone of our shared humanity.

Positionality Statement: Karen Jacobs
As a scholar-practitioner, my approach to research and practice is influenced by my background and experiences. I identify as a white cisgender female and was fortunate to grow up in a middle-class household, which provided me with stability and access to higher education to become an occupational therapist. From a young age, I took on employment responsibilities which instilled in me a strong work ethic and a sense of self-reliance in funding my own education. As a mother and grandmother, I bring a generational perspective to my work, valuing intergenerational dynamics and the impact of health care and wellness practices on families. I am aware that my privileges, including access to higher education, financial stability, and the opportunities afforded by residing in an affluent urban center, have played a substantial role in shaping my worldview. I acknowledge that these privileges may inadvertently influence my interpretations and interactions with people. I commit to remaining vigilant and self-aware, seeking to recognize and mitigate any potential biases that may arise due to my positionality. I value transparency and will be forthright about how my background may influence my perceptions.

Positionality Statement: Liat Gafni-Lachter
I am a white, middle-aged cisgender female from a middle-class background with a safe and supportive upbringing and privileged higher education, living in a country deeply influenced by colonialism. I acknowledge that my privileges and life experiences often limit my perspective and influence my interpretations and interactions. I am committed to ongoing reflexivity in my personal and professional life to enhance awareness of biases due to my positionality. I believe that to foster compassion and understanding among diverse groups, we must also recognize that our similarities are greater than our differences – we are all one, arrived from, and will return to the same place.

Foreword II: "What Is Occupation?"

Nick Pollard

When I was a student at Derby School of Occupational Therapy in the late 1980s, our lecturers asked us "what is human occupation?" several times in each year of our diploma training. It seemed to me then that the occupational therapy notion of occupation might connote something different to the occupation that was part of the life narratives taking place outside the hospital doors; perhaps our educators were challenging us to reflect about this. The mantra "doing, being, becoming and belonging" (Wilcock & Hocking, 2015) had not yet evolved and Cheryl Mattingly had just begun to publish her work on the relationship between narrative and clinical practice as a means for the professional to unravel complex issues (Mattingly, 2007). As Mattingly related, those narratives are impacted by experiences which come from beyond the direct clinical context, the ongoing issues of homelife, the experiences of relatives and family, and of giving care.

These occupational experiences are often the stuff of everyday conversation, and perhaps overlooked as a cultural force outside academic studies. The collective impact of working-class writing and community publishing groups exchanging many such stories and the worlds of literature and historical legacies that they related to influenced my approach to occupation. The Federation of Worker Writers and Community Publishers (FWWCP) was a diverse network mostly formed of informal groups, often former adult education classes, activists who developed print or bookshop collectives, community artist, or oral history projects which had somehow continued to survive through their members (Woodin, 2018). It was important to these groups to make their own publications and define themselves through both print and their performances, because they were otherwise not visible, not included, and as far as the dominant culture was concerned, not interesting. We, as worker writers and community publishers, confronted this marginalization (Woodin, 2018).

FOREWORD II: "WHAT IS OCCUPATION?"

Around the time of my occupational therapy graduation, the FWWCP was joined by the Survivors Poetry movement, formed of people with experiences of mental distress (Woodin, 2018). Talking and working with people in this group exposed many contradictions between our worker writer/community publishing membership and my professional role as a practitioner in mental health. I could see that most people on the caseload of the teams I worked with had a real need for social change. I found myself questioning whether I worked in a system of psychiatric care or oppression. Individual narratives of experience could be more telling than clinical notes and diagnostic assessments.

One Boxing Day I took a service user shopping. Boxing Day in the United Kingdom is the day of the opening of the winter sales; an hour's expedition became a five-hour nose and tail traffic grind. Stuck in the car's confines, we talked about all kinds of experiences and life in general. It was a turning point in our rapport. I could see how the various events of his life dropped into place in the way he now lived. I had never had that extended opportunity to talk with any of my service users under the usual constraints of practice or occupational assessments.

The chapters in *Human Occupation: Contemporary Concepts and Lifespan Perspectives* offer a really imaginative and refreshed view of the profession and occupational therapy practices that are based on contemporary realities of occupation. They explore diversity and are centered on participation in human occupation in the context of the barriers that impact a shared and communal everyday life, viewed through inclusive tools such as the Coin Model of Privilege and Critical Allyship (Nixon, 2019) alongside well-established occupational frameworks. Nixon (2019) introduces her model through an illustration of the invisibility of oppression and privilege within occupation, things that are so embedded in daily life that people do not recognize them until they are confronted with them. The ordinariness of everyday narratives puts them into sharper focus when they are performed or in print and then critically discussed, or perhaps when a space for narrative opens up instead of a situation of practice in which the focus might have been assessment or some functional task. The narrative of doing, being, becoming, and belonging expressed in the vernacular experience of people constrained by everyday injustices, limiting their access to doing the things that have meaning to them, may not dovetail neatly with the occupational narrative defined by the professional occupational therapist.

The occupational therapist has an array of tools for classifying occupation and categorizing its elements, and this book has the aim of enabling therapists to engage – or re-engage – with those key-defining professional skills and concepts. The chapters of *Human Occupation: Contemporary Concepts and Lifespan Perspectives* are produced by international teams of progressive authors working from different perspectives across the global north and south. The reader is constantly minded of positionality as a feature of this writing which includes explorations of gender, sex, sleep, and non-sanctioned occupations that are overdue, alongside other recent areas of interest such as the impact of environmental change and technology. These are written in ways that encourage the professional to use their occupational lenses to unpick their privilege and power, and recognize the wider and intersectional features of the structures that produce health problems and affect occupational engagement and performance.

This edited text comes at a significant time with unprecedented scaling up of the influences on the evolution of occupation both as a field of professional knowledge and in terms of the nature of occupation itself. It is doing the dual tasks of catching up and taking forward concepts to address the question "What is occupation?" in the light of future changes in how humans do, be, become, and belong.

Positionality Statement: Nick Pollard

The author of this foreword has worked with people experiencing mental distress in acute and enduring services in the UK and has also worked for over two decades in higher education. I grew up in the UK during the last stages of its colonial power. Consequently, my knowledge and perspectives are privileged through my Western, English-speaking, university-educated, professionally qualified, social class, cisgendered, heterosexual, and white ethnic experiences, as well as the economic advantages of Britain's long extractive relationship with the global south. However, I have also been influenced by some personally challenging experiences during the course of my life, including mental health issues and long-term unemployment.

References

Mattingly, C. F. (2007). Acted narratives. In D. J. Clandinin (Ed.), *Handbook of narrative inquiry: Mapping a methodology* (pp. 405–425). Sage Publications, Inc. https://doi.org/10.4135/9781452226552.n16

Nixon, S. A. (2019). The coin model of privilege and critical allyship: Implications for health. *BMC Public Health*, 19(1), 1–13. https://doi.org/10.1186/s12889-019-7884-9

Wilcock, A. A., & Hocking, C. (2015). *An occupational perspective of health* (3rd ed.). Slack.

Woodin, T. (2018). *Working-class writing and publishing in the late twentieth century: Literature, culture and community*. Manchester University Press.

Foreword III: Hope, Utopia, and Solidarity

Lilian Magalhães

A book is a recollection artifact with many meanings and cultural values. A book can create memories, provide hope, disseminate new knowledge, and initiate a public dialogue and deliberation. It also might offer answers to daunting questions posed by individuals; the list is endless. Individuals who love books know all too well how exciting it is to open a new book as well as to read an old, familiar, appreciated one for a second time. Reading is a much-loved occupation, as much as the meaningful activity of crafting and writing a new one. And yet, my intent here is neither one of these. I am here as a foreword writer, which places me somewhere between the occupation of writing a book and the pleasure of reading it. Of course, I am cognizant that the main topic of this book is occupation itself. As we may concede, occupation is an intimidating, complex, constantly evolving phenomenon that has been giving meaning to most of the scholarship conducted in occupational therapy and occupational science fields. However, despite our continuous efforts, the term "occupation" creates opposing views and debates more often than we like to admit. As such, one should not expect homogeneity from a book on human occupation, which seems obvious. So, again, I wonder what I should recommend to the reader as part of this foreword.

As such, despite being very humbled and honored by the invitation, but unable to grasp the usefulness of my comments here, I am inclined to offer my insights on the context in which this book has been written, wondering about the type of expectation that might have motivated its seven editors, while highlighting some of their impressive accomplishments. As I investigated the decisions they made, I was amazed by the tremendous challenges the seven editors and numerous contributing chapter authors likely faced, while also being impressed by their persistence and gracefulness.

Let us put in perspective the creation of the book, within its context. This book was probably planned in the last three or four years, while the planet faced a health crisis that is yet to be fully described. As someone who spent the whole ordeal in Brazil, a country that had just over 705,000 deaths due to the pandemic, not to mention the uncountable cases of long COVID, financial losses, disruption of collective projects, a surge of emotional distress with persistent consequences, and so on, I can testify to the dire contexts that we all faced. Going back to the task of designing a book, the seven editors were probably puzzled by their personal hurdles and acted to look ahead to better times post-COVID-19 pandemic through engagement in a collective, audacious, creative, inspiring project.

Well, let me explain how it came to fruition. At first glance, consider 40 chapters, and 98 authors, situated within 16 distinct countries where the chapter writing took place. Scholars, educators, and practitioners from Japan, Argentina, South Africa, Ireland, Denmark, the United Kingdom, Singapore, Brazil, and Chile worked together with Canadians, Americans, New Zealanders, and Australians, among others, to deliver a contemporary global account of human occupation, occupational therapy, and occupational science. Then, we must focus on the wide scope of topics that range from the traditional and much-needed discussion on the challenges of defining occupation within a pluriverse frame of reference (Chapter 1), to some cutting-edge conversations about volunteering as occupation (Chapter 27), or the underpinnings of occupation and social sanctioning (Chapter 13).

Furthermore, a range of accomplished scholars, from different parts of the planet and from very different fields of practice and research, all candidly stated their positionalities. This will allow prospective readers to access another layer of context, besides the traditional professional information. So, one must consider that amid the greatest occupational disaster that the planet has endured in recent centuries (Magalhães, 2024), a group of like-minded people kept working to bring information, contextual analysis, and technical expertise in the form of an edited book that focused on the many varied facets of human occupation that are front of mind for occupational therapists and occupational scientists. I would like to emphasize, essentially bringing hope through planning and creating better conditions to grasp the contemporary landscape of human occupation, that will be vital when the pandemic turmoil recedes.

Among the many layers of the study of occupation, the concept that interests me the most is co-occupation. It refers to the "occupation in which two or more people engage together, although there may be individual differences in the way the occupation is active, purposeful, meaningful, contextualized, and impacting on health" (Molineux, 2017). While the concept is yet to be further explored, co-occupations, as Lawlor reminds us, are mostly meant to promote togetherness (2003), which brings us back to the context in which those 98 writers meant to engage in the occupation of writing, that would later afford us the opportunity of reading it, and profiting from their insights and ideas, consolidating a full circle of co-occupation and promoting what Paulo Freire enunciated as the future as a collective project, not as an unavoidable destiny (Freire, 2021).

In short, applying an underdeveloped notion of untested feasible, also suggested by Freire, we could say that the unprecedented dystopia in which the authors found themselves probably prompted them to act, together, moved by hope, utopia, and courage. While they did not know what to expect, they worked through critical issues and in solidarity to achieve diverse layers of conceptual interpretations and actions about one of the essential axes of the very idea of community: doing together, as occupational beings. Furthermore, throughout the book, this collective occupation accomplished an intent, first announced by Molineux in his excellent chapter, *Overview of Human Occupation: Concepts and Principles*, to deliberately commit to and embrace our ethical responsibilities as professionals and fellow beings, in the pursuit of a praxis that addresses "who and what has been silenced, and who and what has been privileged" (Molineux, 2024). Collective healing scholarship, for collective healing times.

Positionality Statement: Lilian Magalhães

My professional background relates to occupational therapy and occupational science, especially from decolonial and critical perspectives. I was born in Rio de Janeiro, Brazil, 68 years ago, but I have been living elsewhere, in and out of Brazil, for the last four decades. I present myself as a woman of African descent, cisgender, and heterosexual, being the first in my extended family to achieve postgraduate education. I am the mother of two sons and have a wonderful family and circle of friends. I am extremely privileged, as I am contemporary and work with and have strong alliances with remarkable warriors for social change, who shape my worldview and set examples that I try to pursue in my sphere.

References

Freire, P. (2021). *Pedagogy of hope: Reliving pedagogy of the oppressed*. Bloomsbury Publishing.

Lawlor, M. C. (2003). The significance of being occupied: The social construction of childhood occupations. *American Journal of Occupational Therapy, 57*(4), 424–434. https://doi.org/10.5014/ajot.57.4.424

Magalhães, L. (2024). Building knowledge of occupation from the ground up: A field in search of epistemic fairness and social relevance. *Journal of Occupational Science, 31*(1), 21–31. https://doi.org/10.1080/14427591.2023.2271484

Molineux, M. (2017). *Oxford dictionary of occupational science and occupational therapy*. Oxford University Press.

Molineux, M. (2024). Overview of human occupation: Concepts and principles. In T. Brown, S. Isbel, L. Gustafsson, S. Gutman, D. Powers Dirette, B. Collins, & T. Barlott (Eds.), *Human occupation: Contemporary concepts and lifespan perspectives* (Chapter 2). Routledge.

Foreword IV: Occupation and Occupational Engagement – The Things That People *Do*, Unites Us All

Mandy Stanley

What a pleasure to be asked to write a foreword for a book on Occupation. This text comes from an esteemed group of experienced editors and comprises chapters written by contributors from across the globe. I commend the editors for their foresight and vision to bring such a wide range of authors from no less than 16 countries together to contribute to this important text. The word occupation does not translate well into all languages as there is always a word that provides an exact equivalent. An exploration of the etymology of the word occupation (https://www.etymonline.com/word/occupation) reveals that it derives from about the mid-12th century from the Latin root word "*occupare*" (v) which referred to the action of seizing or taking control (Reed et al., 2013). In this text, the word is used to refer to those activities that engage or occupy a person's time that are orchestrated into daily life. Despite these issues of language, the concept of occupation and occupational engagement, the things that people *do*, unites us all.

It is a delight to see a text written which foregrounds the topic of occupation for occupational therapists. Occupation and its therapeutic application are the core domain of occupational therapy. I come from a standpoint, heavily influenced by Wilcock, that occupational science provides the knowledge base that informs occupational therapy, and that occupational therapy is the profession that implements that knowledge in practice with individuals, groups, communities, and populations. This text provides a comprehensive source of information about occupational science concepts as well as occupation-based practice with Section 1 providing an overview of occupation. Included chapters present models of practice that focus on human occupation, participation, and practice reasoning. In Section 2, with a theme of contemporary perspectives on human occupation, the chapters present critical perspectives and discuss the intersections of occupation and issues such as equity, disadvantage, decolonization, gender, and environmental sustainability. Section 3 presents principal concepts, including occupational adaptation and occupational balance as well as the domains of human occupation, including play, work, sleep and rest, leisure, and sexuality. The final section is a comprehensive examination of current knowledge with attention paid to occupation across the lifespan from infancy through childhood, adolescence to young, middle, and older adulthood.

This text is a valuable contribution to advancing knowledge about occupation. Wilcock argued, and indeed had the t-shirts printed, that not all occupational scientists were occupational therapists, but that all occupational therapists needed to be occupational scientists. Her views on that were not shared by all internationally; however, this text is testament to her work and that of other early occupational scientists. It honors all those who have contributed to the writing and to those who have contributed to knowledge about occupation that have brought us to this point. I recommend to the reader to *seize* the opportunity to take up this knowledge and allow it to *occupy* your thoughts and ideas, and to influence your *doing*.

Positionality Statement: Mandy Stanley

One of the defining features of this text is the inclusion of an author positionality statement at the beginning of each chapter which I will echo here at the beginning of the foreword. I am an Australian female, currently living and working on Whadjuk Noongar Boodjar (Perth, Western Australia) having grown up and lived the first almost 60 years of my life on Kaurna land (Adelaide, South Australia). I acknowledge that I live a privileged life having had the privilege of a free education both for my undergraduate degree and for my doctoral studies, as I doubt that I would have been able to participate in that education if I had had to have the finances to pay for it. I have also had the very great privilege to be part of the occupational therapy profession and to have worked alongside internationally renowned occupational therapists and occupational scientists, including Ann Wilcock. What a privilege it is to be able to indulge my curiosity in the study of humans as occupational beings, and to harness the power of engagement in occupation to positively influence health and well-being. I also acknowledge the privilege of being brought up in a country where the first language is English when the majority of science communication occurs in English. Whilst I enjoy learning languages, I am not able to write in any other language and I applaud my colleagues who write academic papers in English when that is not their first language.

Reference

Reed, K., Smythe, L., & Hocking, C. (2013). The meaning of occupation: A hermeneutic (re)view of historical understandings. *Journal of Occupational Science*, 20(3), 253–226 https://doi.org/10.1080/14427591.2012.729487

Acronyms

AAA	American Anthropological Association
AAB	Academic Achievement Battery
AAC	alternative and augmentative communication technology
AAP	American Academy of Pediatrics
ABAS-II	Adaptive Behavior Assessment System, Second Edition
ABI	acquired brain injury
ABIM	American Board of Internal Medicine
ACPQ	Australian Community Participation Questionnaire
ADA	Americans with Disabilities Act
ADHD	Attention Deficit Hyperactivity Disorder
ADL	activities of daily living
AFDD	Agrupación de Familiares de Detenidos Desaparecidos
ALIP	Adolescent Leisure Interest Profile
ALS	amyotrophic lateral sclerosis
AMPS	Assessment of Motor and Process Skills
AOTA	American Occupational Therapy Association
AOTI	Association of Occupational Therapists of Ireland
APS	Affect in Play Scale
APS-P	Affect in Play Scale – Preschool version
ARC	ARC Self-Determination Scale
ASCA	Academic Self Concept for Adolescents
ASI	Ayres Sensory Integration
AWP	Assessment of Work Performance
BEARS	Bedtime issues, Excessive daytime sleepiness, night Awakenings, Regularity and duration of sleep, Snoring
BIPOC	Black and Indigenous People Of Color

ACRONYMS

BRCA-1	breast cancer gene mutation
BRQ	Bedtime Routines Questionnaire
CADL	Client-Centered Activities in Daily Living Intervention
CAIMI	Children's Academic Intrinsic Motivation Inventory
CANMOP	Canadian Model of Occupational Performance
CAPABLE	Community Aging in Place, Advancing Better Living for Elders
CAPE/PAC	Children's Assessment of Participation and Enjoyment/Preferences for Activities
CAPIQ	Children's Active Play Imagery Questionnaire
CAS	critical autism studies
CASP	Child and Adolescent Scale of Participation
CBI	Child Behaviors Inventory of Playfulness
CBI	Career Beliefs Inventory
CDC	Centers for Disease Control and Prevention
CDPI	Children's Developmental Play Instrument
CDS	critical disability studies
CEMA	Centro de Madres para Artesanía
CES	Classroom Environment Scale
CHIME	Connectedness, Hope and optimism, Identity, Meaning, and Empowerment
CHIPPA	Child-Initiated Pretend Play Assessment
CHORES	Child Helping Out: Responsibilities, Expectations, and Supports
CIM	Community Integration Measure
CIQ-R	Community Integration Questionnaire – Revised
CISS	Campbell Interest and Skill Survey
CLASS	Children's Leisure Assessment Scale
CMI FORM C	Career Maturity Inventory – Form C
CMOP-E	Canadian Model of Occupational Performance and Engagement
CO-OP	Cognitive Orientation to daily *Occupational* Performance
COP26	UN Climate Change Conference
COPD	chronic obstructive pulmonary disease
COPM	Canadian Occupational Performance Measure
COSA	Child Occupational Self Assessment
COTAD	Coalition of Occupational Therapy Advocates for Diversity
COTIPP	Canadian Occupational Therapy Inter-relational Practice Process Framework
CPQ	Children Participation Questionnaire
CPQ-S	Children Participation Questionnaire – School
CPS	Children's Playfulness Scale
CR	conditioned response
CRSP	Children's Report of Sleep Patterns
CS	conditioned stimulus
CSH	Centre for Sustainable Healthcare
CSHQ	Children's Sleep Habit Questionnaire
CTI	Career Transitions Inventory
CVA	cerebral vascular accident

DEI	diversity, equity, and inclusion
DJ	disc jockey
DOT	Dictionary of Occupational Titles
EASY-OT	Educational Assessment of School Youth for Occupational Therapists
EBP	evidence-based practice
EHP	Ecology of Human Performance
ESI	Evaluation of Social Interaction
ESL	English as a Second Language
ex-PLISSIT	Extended Permission, Limited Information, Specific Suggestions, and Intensive Therapy
FCE	Functional Capacity Evaluation
FIM	Functional Independence Measure
FOR	frames of reference
HAAT	Human Activity Assistive Technology Model
HSIO	Human Subsystems that Influence Occupation
HWPQ	Health and Work Performance Questionnaire
IADL	instrumental activities of daily living
ICF	International Classification of Functioning, Disability and Health
ICF-CY	International Classification of Functioning, Disability and Health Children and Youth Version
ICMOP-E	Integrated Canadian Model of Occupational Performance and Engagement
IOM	Institute of Medicine
IPA	Impact on Participation and Autonomy
I-PAS	Infant – Preschool Play Assessment Scale
IPCC	Intergovernmental Panel on Climate Change
JAN	Job Accommodations Network
KAP	Keele Assessment of Participation
KIPP	Kid Play Profile
LGBTQIA2S+	lesbian, gay, bisexual, transgender, queer and/or questioning, intersex, asexual, two-spirit, and the countless affirmative ways in which people choose to self-identify
LIFE-H	Assessment of Life Habits
LR	Lifestyle Redesign
LSVT	Lee Silverman Voice Treatment
MAPP	Motivational Appraisal of Personal Potential Career Test
MBTI	Myers-Briggs Type Indicator
MCP	My Child's Play Questionnaire
MOHO	Model of Human Occupation
MPAI	McDonald Play Activity Inventory
MPI	McDonald Play Inventory
MPSI	McDonald Play Style Inventory
NAO	Need Ability Opportunity Model
NAP	National AgrAbility Project
NARCH	Navajo Native American Research Center for Health Partnership

ACRONYMS

NEADL	*Nottingham Extended Activities of Daily Living*
NGO	non-governmental organization
NHS	National Health System
OBQ11	Occupational Balance Questionnaire
OCWFOT	Occupation, Capability and Wellbeing Framework for Occupational Therapy
OECD	Organisation for Economic Co-operation and Development
O*NET	Occupational Information Network
OPC	Occupational Performance Coaching
OPHI-II	Occupational Performance History Interview-II
OPISI	Occupational Performance Inventory of Sexuality and Intimacy
OPPUS	Observed Peer Play in Unfamiliar Settings
OT	occupational therapist or occupational therapy
OTPAL	Occupational Therapy Psychosocial Assessment of Learning
OTPF-4	Occupational Therapy Practice Framework – 4th edition
PACS	Paediatric Activity Card Sort
PADL	personal activities of daily living
PAGS	Play Assessment for Group Settings
PALS	Principles of Adult Learning Scale
PAR-PRO	Participation Profile
PAS	Play Assessment Scale
PASS	Performance Assessment of Self-care Skills
PD	Parkinson's disease
PEDI	Pediatric Evaluation of Disability Inventory
PedsQL	Pediatric Quality of Life Inventory
PEM-CY	Participation and Environment Measure for Children and Youth
PEOP	Person-Environment-Occupation-Performance model
PIECES	Play in Early Childhood Evaluation System
PIP	Pediatric Interest Profiles
PIPPS	Penn Interactive Peer Play Scale
POEMS	Preschool Outdoor Environment Measurement Scale
POPS	Participation Objective, Participation Subjective
POS	Play Observation Scale
P-SCALE	Participation Scale
PSQI	Pittsburgh Sleep Quality Index
PSSRQ	Play Skills Self-Report Questionnaire
PTSD	post-traumatic stress disorder
PVQ	Pediatric Volitional Questionnaire
REAL	Roll Evaluation of Activities of Life
RIASEC	Realistic; Investigative; Artistic; Social; Enterprising; Conventional
RTI	Routine Task Inventory
School AMPS	School Assessment of Motor and Process Skills
SCMS	Self-Control and Self-Management Scale
SCOPE	Short Child Occupational Profile

SCOPE-IT	Synthesis of Child, Occupational Performance and Environment – In Time
SDH	social determinants of health
SDT	self-determination theory
SES	socioeconomic status
SELF	Self-awareness Enhancement through Learning and Function
SESQ	Student Engagement in Schools Questionnaire
SETT	Student Environment Tasks and Tools Framework
SexGen-OTOS	International Network on Sexualities and Genders within Occupational Therapy and Occupational Science
SFA	School Function Assessment
SMLSI	School Motivation and Learning Strategies Inventory
SP	Social Profile
SPC	Social Play Continuum
SSCS	Student Self-Concept Scale
SSEDSP	Smilansky Scale for Evaluation of Dramatic and Sociodramatic Play
SSI	School Setting Interview
STEM	science, technology, engineering, mathematics
TAM	Technology Acceptance Model
TBI	traumatic brain injury
ToP	Test of Playfulness
TPBA-2	Transdisciplinary Play-Based Assessment, 2nd edition
TPI-3	Transition Planning Inventory – third edition
TPI-UV	Transition Planning Inventory – Updated Version
WFOT	World Federation of Occupational Therapists
WHO	World Health Organization
UCS	unconditioned stimulus
UDHR	Universal Declaration of Human Rights
UN	United Nations
US	United States
UNCRC	United Nations Convention of the Rights of the Child
UNICEF	United Nations Children's Fund
UPIAS	*Union of the Physically Impaired Against Segregation*
USBLS	US Bureau of Labor Statistics
USC	University of Southern California
USDOL	US Department of Labor Employment and Training
USDVA	US Military Vocational Rehabilitation and Employment divisions
USP	University of São Paulo
VABS-II	Vineland Adaptive Behavior Scales, Second Edition
VABS-3	Vineland Adaptive Behavior Scales – 3rd edition
VFI	Volunteer Functions Inventory
WEEFIM	Functional Independence Measure for Children
WRAT5	Wide Range Achievement Test – Fifth Edition
Y-SPET	Yonsei-Social Play Evaluation Tool
ZPD	Zone of Proximal Development

SECTION ONE

Overview of Human Occupation

CHAPTER 1

Introduction to Human Occupation
Contemporary Concepts and Lifespan Perspectives

Ted Brown, Stephen Isbel, Louise Gustafsson, Sharon Gutman, Diane Powers Dirette, Bethan Collins, and Tim Barlott

Abstract

This chapter introduces the overall structure and intent of the current edited book on human occupation. It provides a brief overview of the realm of human occupation, internal and external factors that impact human occupation, and the relationship between the disciplines of occupational therapy and occupational science. The Wheel of Power and Privilege graphic and the Coin Model of Privilege and Critical Allyship are mentioned to contextualize the types of inequalities that can exist in the daily lives of clients and families with whom therapists interact. The Decolonising the Curriculum Wheel – a Reflection Framework is presented as one way that occupational therapy educators and students can decolonize curriculum using a collaborative codesign process. In addition, this chapter provides an overview of the chapter structure of the edited book as well as summaries of the two overarching frameworks that influence how human occupations are viewed and considered: those frameworks being the International Classification of Functioning, Disability and Health (ICF) and the main components of the Occupational Therapy Practice Framework – 4th edition (OTPF-4). The chapter ends with individual positionality and reflexivity statements from each of the seven co-editors.

Objectives

This chapter will allow the reader to:

- Achieve an overview of the structure and intent of the chapters in the edited book titled *Human Occupation: Contemporary concepts and lifespan perspectives*.
- Have an appreciation of the relationship between occupational science and occupational therapy.

- Become familiar with the Wheel of Power and Privilege graphic, the Coin Model of Privilege and Critical Allyship, and the Decolonising the Curriculum Wheel – a Reflection Framework.
- Be knowledgeable about the International Classification of Functioning, Disability and Health (ICF) and the main components of the Occupational Therapy Practice Framework – 4th edition (OTPF-4).
- Gain an overview of the reflexivity and positionality of the seven co-editors in relation to the book.

Key terms

- occupation
- participation
- activity
- personal factors
- environmental factors
- occupational therapy
- occupational science
- performance skills
- performance patterns
- client factors
- contexts
- domain
- process
- occupational equilibrium and occupational alignment
- human occupational homeostasis

1.1 Introduction

This chapter introduces the general topic of human occupation as well as provides an overview of the structure and rationale for the current edited book. The relationship between the occupational therapy profession and the academic discipline of occupational science is discussed. The Wheel of Power and Privilege graphic (Duckworth, 2020) and the Coin Model of Privilege and Critical Allyship (Nixon, 2019) are used to contextualize the key inequities that clients and families who seek occupational therapy services may experience as part of their daily occupational lives. The Decolonising the Curriculum Wheel – a Reflection Framework (Ahmed-Landeryou, 2023c) is presented as one way that occupational therapy educators and students can decolonize curriculum using a collaborative codesign process. The two key frameworks that inform the contents of the book chapters are summarized: those being the International Classification of Functioning, Disability and Health (World Health Organization, 2001) and the

Occupational Therapy Practice Framework – 4th edition (American Occupational Therapy Association [AOTA], 2020). The positionality statements of the seven co-editors then conclude the chapter.

The structure of the chapters in this edited book will follow a similar format where they include an abstract, learning objectives, key words, positionality statement of the chapter authors, introduction, main text that focuses on the chapter topic, conclusion, summary, review questions, and references. The editors have made a concerted effort to bring authorship teams together to write chapters who have diverse backgrounds, broad content knowledge, and wide-ranging occupational experiences. We, as co-editors, do acknowledge that in places there is a bias toward westernized, First World views of human occupation and that not all perspectives, life experiences, and diversity viewpoints may be represented in this edited book. However, where feasible, we, as co-editors, have attempted to include contributing authors from different countries, cultural backgrounds, occupational perspectives, content knowledge areas of expertise, and occupational lived experiences. We have also included author positionality and reflexivity statements as part of the chapter formats to make potentially biasing factors and perspectives transparent for prospective readers.

1.2 Human Occupation

Human occupation is present at all times of our lives, from birth through to end of life. Being born and dying as well as all the other occupations in which we engage in-between, those two life events are significant, meaningful, and sustaining. We all perform daily self-care occupations often intermingled with work, leisure, play, and education occupations. To restore, regenerate, and recuperate our physical and mental selves, we then engage in sleep and rest occupations (Leive & Morrison, 2020). All human beings also benefit from daily social participation occupations where we socialize and interact with family, friends, co-workers, neighbors, clients, and others. Engaging in human occupations is as essential as the air we breathe, the water we drink, the food we eat, the shelter we create for ourselves, and the social connectedness we actively seek out with others.

There are many internal and external factors that influence and impact our daily repertoire of occupations in which we engage. External factors include the physical landscape where we live, the season or time of year, the cultural norms, traditions and expectations, and the laws of the society in which we live. Personality traits, resilience, emotional intelligence, cultural beliefs, personal values and habits, locus of control, self-concept, physical and mental abilities, level of educational attainment, and socioeconomic status are all internal elements that impact a person's daily occupational performance (AOTA, 2020; Gallagher et al., 2015). As human beings engaging in human occupations, we are in a constant occupational push-pull relationship between internal human factors that *pull* and external environmental pressing agents that *push*. We try to maintain and sustain a state of *occupational equilibrium* and occupational alignment within ourselves, trying to safeguard our state of *human occupational homeostasis*.

1.3 Issues and Events Impacting Human Occupation

Currently, there are many issues and events at the local, national, and international stages that also impact human occupation. The Occupy Wall Street protest, #Metoo

Movement, the Black Lives Matter campaign, the LGBTIA+ rights movement, the focus on gender equality and women's rights, the ongoing issue of climate change and environmental activism, the increasing recognition of the negative impacts that colonization has had on traditional Indigenous first nations peoples, and the political jousting between the Western democracies and authoritarian regimes in other parts of the world. The exponential development and uptake of the World Wide Web and the large degree of instantaneous, over-connectedness, and over-reliance on online social media platforms have created a whole set of social, economic, legal, health, ethical, and moral issues that impact many aspects of our everyday occupational lives. For instance, cyber-addiction, online stalking, cyber-bullying, internet gaming disorders, repetitive musculoskeletal strain injuries, digital eye strain, social isolation, divulging of personal information, sleep problems, depression, and anxiety can all result from too much screen time. There are also issues of privacy breaches, collection of megadata, and increasing use of facial recognition software and webcams to record our daily transactions, comings, and goings.

We are now more aware of white privilege, social inequality, colonial impacts on Indigenous populations, racism, discrimination, classism, ableism, ageism, mentalism/sanism, religious intolerance, sexism, cisgenderism, heterosexism, and lack of awareness of gender diversity (Trentham et al., 2022). We are starting to acknowledge the impacts of each of these systems of inequality and inequity on society, marginalized communities, the clients, families, communities, and organizations to whom we provide services, and our own profession.

The Wheel of Power and Privilege graphic created by Ms Sylvia Duckworth (2020) represents 12 identity categories related to power, privilege, and marginalization. In the center of the wheel graphic is the word "power" (and privilege), and on the outside is the word "marginalize" (see Figure 1.1). It provides occupational therapists with a visual overview on the issues of inequality and inequity that their clients may present with. The identity category slices that make up the Wheel of Power and Privilege include body size, mental health, neurodiversity, sexuality, ability, formal education, skin color, citizenship, gender, language, wealth, and housing (Duckworth, 2020). These identity types are shown as circles connected to three concentric rings (outer, middle, and inner) of "identity" categories with power and privilege increasing toward the center. The impact of the concentric rings in Duckworth's Wheel of Power and Privilege (2020) makes it appear like a cone or funnel – the individuals that hold the most power and privilege in society are located at the center of the funnel, while the individuals that possess the least power in a population are on the outer borders of the graphic.

The Coin Model of Privilege and Critical Allyship developed by Nixon (2019) (see Figure 1.2) depicts several of the key inequality and inequity polar dichotomies that exist throughout the world. She states that the Coin Model of Privilege and Critical Allyship "embraces an intersectional approach to understand how systems of inequality, such as sexism, racism, and ableism, interact with each other to produce complex patterns of privilege and oppression" (Nixon, 2019, p. 1). It is essential that occupational therapy practitioners with power and privilege engage in serious discussions about injustice, marginalization, and oppressive systems and structures that promulgate those inequalities. Part of the intent of this book is to spark constructive debate of this type about historical and current occupational inequities, oppression, discrimination, and injustices.

INTRODUCTION TO HUMAN OCCUPATION

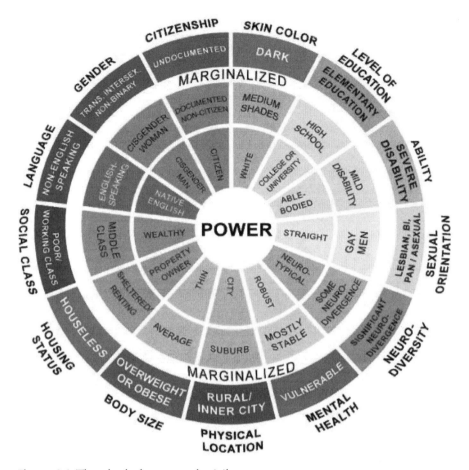

Figure 1.1 The wheel of power and privilege.

Source: Reproduced with the permission of Duckworth, S. (2020, October 18). Wheel of power/privilege [Infographic]. Flickr. CC BY-NC-ND 2.0. https://www.flickr.com/photos/sylviaduckworth/50500299716. The educational version of the graphic was created by T. Dugdale from the Center for Teaching, Learning & Mentoring, Division for Teaching & Learning, University of Wisconsin-Madison, Madison, WI (https://kb.wisc.edu/instructional-resources/page.php?id=119380). Licensed under the Creative Commons Attribution 4.0 International License (http://creativecommons.org/licenses/by/4.0/).

Occupational therapy as a profession originated largely in the Global North regions of the world and with that came a dominant perspective of how we engage in daily occupations (Andersen & Reed, 2017; Paterson, 2010; Trentham et al., 2022). This has arisen at the expense of the beliefs, values and lived experiences of individuals, and communities from the Global South in addition to the traditional culture, identity, and human rights of Indigenous and First Nations groups residing in the Global North areas largely not being taken into consideration (Hammell, 2023; Pollard & Sakellariou, 2017; Simaan, 2020). The Global North dominant view has also influenced the theories, frameworks, and scopes of practice that have been formulated within the occupational therapy discipline (Hammell, 2015; Turcotte & Holmes, 2023a, 2023b).

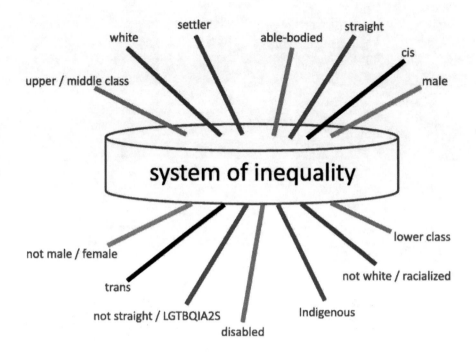

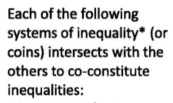

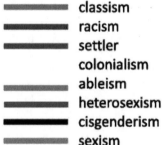

Figure 1.2 The coin model of privilege and critical allyship.

Source: Reproduced with permission from Nixon, S. A. (2019). The Coin Model of Privilege and Critical Allyship: Implications for health. *BMC Public Health*, *19*, Article number 1637. https://doi.org/10.1186/s12889-019-7884-9. Licensed under the Creative Commons Attribution 4.0 International License (http://creativecommons.org/licenses/by/4.0/).

Through this biased Global North occupational worldview lens, a traditionalist colonial view of occupational therapy practice and how we work with clients and their families has evolved (Emery-Whittington, 2021; Rudman et al., 2021). In response to this, there has been an emerging social justice movement within the occupational therapy field for it to actively examine its historical and present colonial stance (Emery-Whittington & Te Maro, 2018; Gibson, 2020; Ivlev, 2023). This can take the form of occupational justice that acknowledges racism, oppression, discrimination, social isolation, and stigmatization of traditionally marginalized groups and communities (Ahmed-Landeryou, 2023a; Beagan et al., 2022; Pooley & Beagan, 2021); taking an inclusive, dynamic decolonial praxis approach to human occupation and occupational therapy practice (Galvaan et al., 2022; Peters et al., 2023); and decolonization of the curricula taught in entry-to-practice occupational therapy courses (Ahmed-Landeryou, 2023b, 2023c; Ahmed-Landeryou et al., 2022; Mahoney & Kiraly-Alvarez, 2019; Simaan, 2020; Sterman et al., 2022).

Ahmed-Landeryou (2023c), an occupational therapy educator from London South Bank University in the United Kingdom, has developed an evidence-based "decolonising the curriculum wheel – a reflection framework" (p. 176). Since the decolonization of university-based curriculum is an ongoing, dynamic process to ensure equity and justice, Ahmed-Landeryou (2023c) incorporated the wheel-like design. The center of the wheel includes collaborating with students from marginalized groups to seek their views for curriculum codesign. The spokes of the decolonization curriculum wheel include decolonizing pedagogies, decolonizing teaching and learning content, decolonizing assessments, institutional responsibility in decolonizing curricula, decolonizing assessment feedback given to students, and outcome measures of impact decolonizing curricula (Ahmed-Landeryou, 2023c). According to Ahmed-Landeryou (2023c), the "wheel is not a prescription of how to transform, but a guidance regarding the components to review and explore" (p. 178) and that "marginalised and minoritised students have to be central in the decolonising work" (p. 178). Using the decolonization curriculum wheel can be one way to promote decolonialized occupational therapy curriculum and decolonization praxis among educators and students going forward.

One of the most recent events that has impacted the economies and health care systems on a worldwide scale is the COVID-19 pandemic. It affected the way we conduct our home, personal, work, leisure, and educational lives. For example, most of us adapted our daily occupations to include things like wearing masks, socially distancing ourselves, getting vaccinated, working remotely at home, or going to school online. It also meant that occupational therapy practitioners had to quickly pivot in how they provided service to clients and their families with a rapid and extensive increase in the use of tele-health and tele-rehabilitation services (Robinson et al., 2021). We had to swiftly adapt and modify our daily occupational routines, roles, habits, and rituals almost overnight. The global and societal response to the COVID-19 pandemic is an example of humanity's occupational adaptation to an occupational challenge (Grajo et al., 2018; Hoel et al., 2021). The world's population had to quickly re-calibrate and transform its collective state of *occupational equilibrium* to preserve our shared and communal *human occupational homeostasis*. This world event also highlights the ongoing importance of the occupational therapy-occupational science nexus.

1.4 Relationship between Occupational Therapy and Occupational Science

Historically, the occupational therapy profession emerged from the increasing recognition of people as occupational beings responding to the daily demands the environment placed on them, when occupational disruption occurred due to physical, social, psychological, or developmental problems and the impact these had on their health and well-being. Examples of this from the past included injured soldiers returning from war, children contracting polio, people being infected with tuberculosis and being placed in sanatoriums, and people with mental illness being institutionalized (Woodside, 1971). At the start of our profession, occupational therapy focused on the occupational needs of people and their related health benefits, often referred to as moral treatment (Andersen & Reed, 2017). Then, in the 1930s through to the 1960s, therapists relied on the medical, mechanistic, and biomechanical models of practice (Colman, 1990). From the 1980s onward, there was a renaissance in the occupational therapy discipline where we went back and claimed our human occupation origins (Shannon, 1977; Whiteford et al., 2000).

Later, occupational science was proposed as an emerging discipline that would underpin the occupational therapy discipline and grow its body of empirical knowledge (Clark, 1993; Yerxa, 1990). However, an ongoing distance appears to exist between occupational therapy as a profession and occupational science as an academic discipline (Lunt, 1997; Molke et al., 2004; Morley et al., 2011; Mosey, 1992; Pollard et al., 2010). Whether this schism is intentional or merely an artifact of factors, the two fields in theory should complement and underpin one another (Clark et al., 1991; Lunt, 1997; Yerxa, 1993). Ideally, the work of occupational scientists should in part contribute to the evidence base of occupational therapy (Clark et al., 1993; Eklund et al., 2017; Kristensen & Petersen, 2016; Laliberte Rudman, 2018). Likewise, occupational therapy practice should provide a rich source of ideas for occupational scientists to research and investigate (Blanche & Henny-Kohler, 2000; Hocking & Wright-St Claire, 2011; Hocking et al., 2015; Riley, 2012).

This edited book is an attempt to bring the professional and academic discipline camps closer together by having *human occupation* as its primary focus and including chapters related to the impact of a range of contemporary societal factors on human occupation, the range of types of human occupation, and how human occupation evolves over the lifespan. One aim of this book is to bring the fields of occupational therapy and occupational science into closer alignment with each other. We are not suggesting that they are at odds with each other but in many instances, there could be many more strategic collegial alliances between the two disciplines. The common bonding agent between the two disciplines should be growing the body of evidence and knowledge about human occupation (see Figure 1.3). As mentioned by Laliberte Rudman (2018), there is the "potential for occupational therapy and science to form productive, critically-informed alliances that support occupation-based socially transformative work" (p. 241).

1.5 Types of Human Occupation

There are several different types of human occupation and levels of occupational engagement that occur throughout the lifespan (O'Brien & Kuhaneck, 2019). For example, a child starting primary school learns to print, hold a pencil, socialize with other children, and pay attention within a classroom environment. A young parent may need to manage running a household, raising children, and working to pay for living expenses. An older adult who has retired from full-time employment has to adjust to new ways of managing their time, socializing with friends and family, and engaging in leisure activities that provide enjoyment and satisfaction. These are all types of daily occupations

INTRODUCTION TO HUMAN OCCUPATION

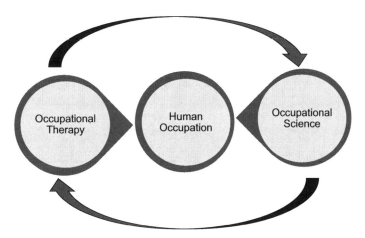

Figure 1.3 Human occupation: The connecting element between occupational therapy and occupational science.
Source: © T. Brown, 2023.

that individuals engage in at different times in their life. Occupational therapists focus on human occupation and assist clients and families when occupational performance challenges and dysfunction arise. Occupational science can provide significant insights about the who, what, when, where, how, and why of human occupation, both in individuals, families, groups, and communities, and in those who present with physical, mental, or developmental problems.

Currently, there is no comprehensive source of information about human occupation available for students studying to be occupational therapists. There are several books that focus on one type of human occupation (such as play, sleep, work, or education) or specific aspects of lifespan development of human occupation. However, at present there is no book that brings the many diverse features of human occupation together as one accessible, inclusive reference from the perspective of the primary concepts related to occupation (Section 1: *Overview of human occupation*), current viewpoints of human occupation (Section 2: *Contemporary perspectives on human occupation*), principal concepts of human occupation (Section 3: *Principal concepts*), its specific types (Section 4: *Domains and types of human occupation*), and its development across the lifespan (Section 5: *Human occupation across the lifespan*). Therefore, the aim of this edited compendium is to provide an overview of human occupation from occupational therapy and occupational science viewpoints.

1.6 Book Structure

Human Occupation: Contemporary concepts and lifespan perspectives is divided into five main sections: (i) overview of human occupation, (ii) contemporary perspectives on human occupation, (iii) principal concepts of human occupation, (iv) domains and types of human occupation, and (v) human occupation across the lifespan. Each of the five sections has 5–12 chapters written by individual authors or small teams of occupational therapy and occupational science authors. Woven throughout the edited book are sections of chapters that will highlight the unique features of human occupation, occupational performance and participation, occupational science, and occupational therapy practice. The target audience for the book are occupational therapy students enrolled in entry-to-practice undergraduate courses, graduate-entry masters and clinical doctorate courses, postgraduate students, and newly graduated occupational therapists. It is also a reference that experienced occupational therapists can refer to update their skills or to refocus their professional practice through a human occupation lens. A further target audience are occupational therapists trained in one country migrating to another and who need to become more conversant with the topic of human occupation. For example, occupational therapists educated in a country where occupation-based practice is not emphasized, but who are moving to a practice context where it is. Finally, occupational scientists will find a comprehensive overview of how human occupation is viewed in the contemporary world.

The first section of the book introduces human occupation. The link between human occupation and occupational science will also be discussed. This section of the book covers core concepts and principles related to human occupation as well as factors that impact it. Topics covered in this section of the book include the following:

- Concepts and principles of human occupation
- Person-centered and client-centered occupation-based practice
- Models of practice that focus on human occupation
- Participation and human occupation
- Professional and clinical reasoning underpinning human occupation

The second section of the book covers a range of contemporary viewpoints on human occupation. This section will examine the link between occupational science and human occupation with chapters focusing on:

- Critical perspectives in occupational science
- The situated nature of human occupation
- Equity, disadvantage, justice, and human occupation
- An Indigenous occupation-based perspective on coloniality
- Non-sanctioned occupations
- Inclusion, participation, and reconstruction
- Social occupational therapy
- Pragmatism
- Gender and human occupation
- Technology and human occupation
- Human occupation and sustainability

The third section of the book covers a range of the primary views, beliefs, constructs, and factors that underpin human occupation. Most of these concepts are drawn from the International Classification of Functioning, Disability and Health (ICF) (World Health Organization, 2001), Model of Human Occupation (MOHO) (Taylor, 2017), Canadian Model of Occupational Performance & Engagement (CMOP-E) (Townsend & Polatajko, 2007), and the Occupational Therapy Practice Framework – 4th edition (OTPF-4) (AOTA, 2020). Chapters for this section include the following:

- Key occupational concepts: Occupational balance, occupational engagement, and occupational adaptation
- Person Factors: Values, beliefs, spirituality, body functions, and body structures (physical, physiological, sensory, cognitive, social, psychological, emotional)
- Performance skills: Motor, process, and social interaction
- Performance patterns: Habits, routines, rituals, and roles
- Context and environment: Cultural, personal, physical, social, temporal, and virtual

The fourth section provides overviews of the specific types of human occupation: Activities of Daily Living (ADLs)/self-care, Instrumental Activities of Daily Living (IADLs), health management, work/productivity/volunteering, education, play, leisure/recreation, social participation, and sleep and rest. These specific types of occupation are derived from the OTPF-4 published by AOTA (2020). Human sexuality as an occupation that individuals engage in is also discussed. Each chapter provides a descriptive, practical, and theoretical overview of one of the types of human occupation listed above.

The fifth and final section of the book deals with human occupation across the lifespan course. Each chapter reviews the types of human occupation (e.g., ADL/self-care; IADL; health Management/self-determination/self-management; work/productivity/volunteering; education; play; leisure/recreation; social participation; sleep and rest; and sexuality) at each of the following life stages: infants, toddlers, and pre-schoolers; school age; adolescence/youth; early adulthood; middle adulthood; and later adulthood. The human occupation domains are viewed from a developmental and occupational life course perspective at each of the six life stages.

1.7 International Classification of Functioning, Disability, and Health (ICF)

The ICF (World Health Organization [WHO], 2001) is one of the key frameworks that will influence how this edited book is structured. The ICF was designed as a universal framework to view the impacts of disability and disease on a person's health and daily occupational performance. Each component of the ICF has a specific meaning and the inter-relationships demonstrate the connections of each of the ICF components (see Figure 1.4). *Body functions and structures* refer to the physiological and psychological systems in a person (WHO, 2001). Physiological body functions include the musculoskeletal, cardiovascular, respiratory, reproductive, hematological, immunological, neurological, digestive, lymphatic, endocrine, movement, dermatological, sensory, and urinary systems (WHO, 2001). Psychological body functions include mental functions, attention, concentration, cognitive skills, problem solving, memory, and perceptual skills (WHO, 2001). Body structures are the anatomical components of the body such as limbs, organs, nerves, skin, muscles, blood vessels, and bones (WHO, 2001). Impairments at the body functions and structures level can cause notable health and well-being challenges and dysfunction. Examples of an impairment would be a broken femur, a spinal cord injury, a diagnosis of dementia, the onset of osteoarthritis, or experiencing panic attacks related to anxiety.

Activity occurs at the individual level and refers to the completion of a task or an action taken by a person, while *activity limitations* are problems a person may

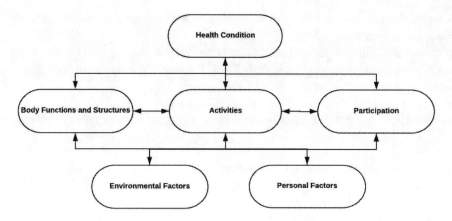

Figure 1.4 International classification of functioning, health and disability.

Source: Reproduced with permission from World Health Organization (2001). *International Classification of Functioning, Health and Disability*, p. 18.

experience in completing daily life activities (WHO, 2001). Examples of activity include working at a job, attending school, preparing a meal, socializing with family members, or playing on a sports team. *Participation* is involvement and engagement in a daily life circumstance or context at the societal level (WHO, 2001) (see Figure 1.4). Likewise, *participation restrictions* refer to difficulties and obstructions that a person may encounter when engaged in daily life situations. Types of participation restriction can include attitudinal, legal, social, or economic constraints or controls that inhibit a person's taking part in daily life to its fullest.

Personal and environmental factors occur at the contextual level (see Figure 1.4). *Personal factors* relate to elements of a person's life and living situation, including gender identity, age, socioeconomic status, ethnicity, sexual orientation, education, fitness, lifestyle, habits, social background, and coping styles (WHO, 2001). These factors delineate a person as a unique individual. *Environmental factors* constitute the physical, social, economic, legal, political, and attitudinal environment where people live their lives (WHO, 2001). Personal and environmental factors can have a positive or negative impact on a person's activities, participation, and body functions and structures.

1.8 Occupational Therapy Practice Framework – 4th Edition (OTPF-4)

The Occupational Therapy Practice Framework was first published in 2002 by the AOTA and has been revised on three occasions, in 2008, 2014, and 2020 (AOTA, 2020). In the context of the OTPF-4, occupational therapy clients fall into three categories: (i) *persons* (individuals, including family member, caregiver, teacher, or relevant other), (ii) *group* (group of individuals who have common characteristics or a shared purpose), and (iii) *population* (that includes aggregates of people with common traits, attributes, beliefs, or experiences) (AOTA, 2020). Within the OTPF-4, there are four main *cornerstones* that assist to distinguish the occupational therapy profession from other health care disciplines: (i) core values and beliefs embedded in occupation,

INTRODUCTION TO HUMAN OCCUPATION

(ii) knowledge and expertise in the therapeutic application of occupation, (iii) professional behaviors and dispositions, and (iv) therapeutic use of self (AOTA, 2020). The cornerstones are not hierarchical in nature, each influences the other, they are ever evolving, and develop over time in occupational therapy practitioners through education, mentorship, and professional experience.

Figure 1.5 provides a visual representation of the aspects of the OTPF-4's Domain and Process for the occupational therapy profession and its overarching goal of "achieving health, well-being, and participation in life through engagement in occupation" (AOTA, 2020, p. 7412410010p5). The Domain and Process interact in complex ways throughout the provision of occupational therapy services to clients. The Domain "outlines the profession's purview and the areas in which its members have an established body of knowledge and expertise," while the Process "describes the actions practitioners take when providing services that are client centered and focused on engagement in occupations" (AOTA, 2020, p. 7412410010p4). The Domain comprises the outer ring of Figure 1.5 and is made up of five parts: *Occupations, Contexts, Performance*

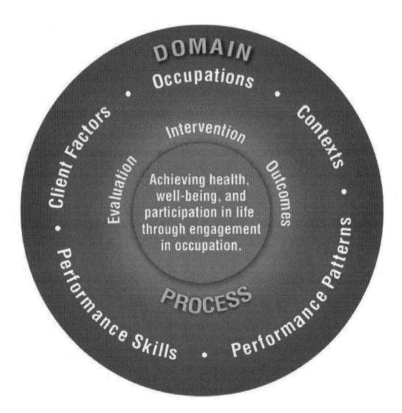

Figure 1.5 Occupational therapy domain and process based on the OTPF-4.

Source: Reproduced with permission from American Occupational Therapy Association. (2020). Occupational therapy practice framework: Domain and process (4th ed.). *American Journal of Occupational Therapy*, 74(Suppl. 2), Article 7412410010, p. 5. https://doi.org/10.5014/ajot.2020.74S2001. Copyright Clearance Center License Number:1409974-1. License Date: 25-10-2023.

patterns, *Performance skills*, and *Client factors* (AOTA, 2020). The inner ring of Figure 1.5 is the *Process* section of the OTPF-4 and has three elements: *Evaluation*, *Intervention*, and *Outcomes* (AOTA, 2020).

1.8.1 OTPF-4 Domain

The first part of the OTPF-4 *Domain* includes nine categories of *Occupation*: (i) *ADLs*, (ii) *IADLs*, (iii) *Health management*, (iv) *Rest and sleep*, (v) *Education*, (vi) *Work*, (vii) *Play*, (viii) *Leisure*, and (ix) *Social participation* (AOTA, 2020) (see Table 1.1). Meanings and beliefs related to occupations are based on cultural, social, psychological, economic, legal, and political factors. Occupations that involve two or more individuals are called *co-occupations*. Co-occupations are socially interactive and can be parallel (e.g., different occupations completed near each other) and shared (e.g., same occupation but different activity) (AOTA, 2020).

The next component of the Domain refers to *Context* and consists of *Environmental factors* (that make up the physical, social, and attitudinal environment where people live and conduct their lives) and *Personal factors* (that refer to the unique, enduring background elements of an individual's internal life) (AOTA, 2020) (see Table 1.2). "Context affects clients' access to occupations and the quality of and satisfaction with performance" (AOTA, 2020, p. 7412410010p9). It is an important part of occupational services since it informs the provision of assessment, intervention planning, and implementation of services.

The next part of the Domain refers to *Performance patterns*. They are the acquired *Habits*, *Routines*, *Roles*, and *Rituals* used in the process of engaging regularly in occupations that can support or impede occupational performance (AOTA, 2020) (see Table 1.2). *Performance patterns* assist to establish a person's lifestyle and daily routines, occupational balance in an individual day, and are shaped by context such as cultural norms, social calendars, or work hours. *Habits* refer to specific behaviors that are automatic, adaptive or maladaptive, healthy or unhealthy, efficient or inefficient, or supportive or unsafe (AOTA, 2020). Occupational balance is the amount of time we spend engaging in productive, restorative, and leisure occupations (AOTA, 2020). It is shaped by cultural norms, social calendars, a person's work hours, group, or population. We need to understand an individual's meaning of time and how it impacts their performance patterns. Time provides an organizational structure and rhythm for performance patterns to occur. *Routines* are sets of repetitive, consistent, and observable behaviors that provide structure to daily life patterns (AOTA, 2020). *Roles* are facets of a person's life that are influenced by culture and context. Likewise, roles are frequently linked with specific activities and occupations, while *Rituals* are predictable patterns of behavior that are influenced by culture, values, and habits (AOTA, 2020) (see Table 1.2). Some rituals are linked with different seasons, times of the year, days of the week, and times of the day.

The next component of the OTPF-4 Domain is *Performance skills* which are goal-directed actions observable as small units of daily life occupations. There are three categories of *Performance skills*: *Motor skills*, *Process skills*, and *Social interaction skills* (AOTA, 2020). Motor, process, and social interaction skills each include several subskill categories (see Table 1.3).

Table 1.1 Occupations Included in the OTPF-4 Domain

Occupation	Examples
Activities of daily living (ADLs)	<ul><li>Bathing and showering</li><li>Toileting</li><li>Dressing</li><li>Eating and swallowing</li><li>Feeding</li><li>Functional mobility</li><li>Grooming</li><li>Sexual activity</li></ul>
Instrumental activities of daily living (IADLs)	<ul><li>Care of pets and animals</li><li>Communication management</li><li>Driving and community mobility</li><li>Financial management</li><li>Home establishment and management</li><li>Meal preparation and clean-up</li><li>Religious and spiritual expression</li><li>Safety and emergency maintenance</li><li>Shopping</li></ul>
Health management	<ul><li>Social and emotional health promotion and maintenance</li><li>Symptom and condition management</li><li>Communication with the health care system</li><li>Medication management</li><li>Physical activity</li><li>Nutrition management</li><li>Personal care device management</li></ul>
Rest and sleep	<ul><li>Rest</li><li>Sleep preparation</li><li>Sleep participation</li></ul>
Education	<ul><li>Formal educational participation</li><li>Informal personal educational needs or exploration</li><li>Informal educational participation</li></ul>
Work	<ul><li>Employment interests and pursuits</li><li>Employment seeking and acquisition</li><li>Job performance and maintenance</li><li>Retirement preparation and adjustment</li><li>Volunteer exploration</li><li>Volunteer participation</li></ul>
Play	<ul><li>Play exploration</li><li>Play participation</li></ul>
Leisure	<ul><li>Play exploration</li><li>Play participation</li></ul>
Social Participation	<ul><li>Community participation</li><li>Family participation</li><li>Friendships</li><li>Intimate partner relationships</li><li>Peer group participation</li></ul>

Source: American Occupational Therapy Association. (2020). Occupational Therapy Practice Framework: Domain and process (4th ed.). *American Journal of Occupational Therapy,* 74(Suppl. 2), Article 7412410010, p. 7. https://doi.org/10.5014/ajot.2020.74S2001

Table 1.2 Contexts and Performance Patterns Included in the OTPF-4 Domain

Contexts	Performance patterns
Environmental factors	**Habits – examples**
- Natural environment and human-made changes to the environment - Products and technology - Support and relationships - Attitudes - Services, systems, and policies	- Looking both ways before crossing road - Checking mobile phone for emails and texts - Locking door before leaving home - Saving email document after writing it - Using passwords to access online accounts - Stopping car at red traffic light - Saying hello and shaking hands with a person when you greet them
Personal factors	**Routines – examples**
- Chronological age - Sexual orientation; gender identity - Race and ethnicity - Cultural identification and attitudes - Social background, social status, and socioeconomic status - Upbringing and life experiences - Habits - Psychological assets, temperament, unique character traits, and coping styles - Education - Profession and professional identity - Lifestyle - Health conditions and fitness status	- Engaging in morning self-care routine - Dressing oneself in a certain order - Following steps to prepare breakfast - Following a sequence of steps to log onto a computer account - Going through a set of sets to start a car - Sequence of events when putting children to bed - Getting ready to go out for an evening meal at a restaurant - Taking an umbrella with you when it is raining outside - Going to the doctor for a flu shot - Having a dental check-up once a year
	Roles – examples
	- Family member - Worker/employee - Student - Citizen - Volunteer - Community member - Religious participant - Caregiver or receiver - Organizational member
	Rituals – examples
	- Saying prayer before bed - Observing special holidays or family traditions - Bowing when meeting someone - Waving goodbye to someone leaving - Hugging a person who you care for

(Continued)

Table 1.2 (Continued)

	■ Clapping after attending a speech ■ Saying thank you when you receive a gift ■ Wearing a certain color or type of clothing to recognize a cultural event

Source: American Occupational Therapy Association. (2020). Occupational Therapy Practice Framework: Domain and process (4th ed.). *American Journal of Occupational Therapy, 74*(Suppl. 2), Article 7412410010, p. 7. https://doi.org/10.5014/ajot.2020.74S2001

Table 1.3 Performance Skills and Client Factors Included in the OTPF-4 Domain

Performance skills	*Client factors*
Motor skills	**Values, beliefs, and spirituality**
■ Positioning the body: stabilizes, aligns, and positions ■ Obtaining and holding objects: reaches, bends, grips, and manipulates ■ Moving self and objects: coordinates, moves, lifts, walks, transports, calibrates, and flows ■ Sustaining performance: endures and paces	
Process skills	**Body functions**
■ Sustaining performance: paces, attends, and heeds ■ Applying knowledge: chooses, uses, handles, and inquires ■ Organizing timing: initiates, continues, sequences, and terminates ■ Organizing time and objects: searches/locates, gathers, organizes, restores, and navigates ■ Adapting performance: notices/responds, adjusts, accommodates, and benefits	■ Specific mental functions: cognitive level, attention, memory, perception, thought, sequencing movements, emotional, experience of self and time ■ Global mental functions: consciousness, orientation, psychosocial, temperament and personality, energy, and sleep ■ Sensory functions: visual, hearing, vestibular, taste, smell, proprioceptive, touch, interoception, pain, temperature, and pressure sensitivity ■ Neuromusculoskeletal and movement-related functions: joint mobility and joint stability, muscle power, tone and endurance, movement functions (reflexes, involuntary, and voluntary movements), and gait patterns ■ Cardiovascular, hematological, immune, and respiratory system functions ■ Voice and speech functions: digestive, metabolic, and endocrine system functions; genitourinary and reproductive functions ■ Skin and related structure functions

(Continued)

Table 1.3 (Continued)

Social interaction skills	Body structures
■ Initiating and terminating social interaction: approaches/starts, and concludes/disengages ■ Producing social interaction: produces speech, gesticulates, and speaks fluently ■ Physically supporting social interaction: turns toward, looks, places self, touches, and regulates ■ Shaping content of social interaction: questions, replies, discloses, expresses emotions, disagrees, and thanks ■ Maintaining flow of social interaction: transitions, times response, times duration, and takes turns ■ Verbally supporting social interaction: matches language, clarifies, acknowledges and encourages, and empathizes ■ Adapting social interaction: heeds, accommodates, and benefits	■ Nervous system ■ Eyes and ears ■ Voice and speech ■ Cardiovascular, immunological, and respiratory systems ■ Digestive, metabolic, and endocrine systems ■ Genitourinary and reproductive systems ■ Movement

Source: American Occupational Therapy Association. (2020). Occupational Therapy Practice Framework: Domain and process (4th ed.). *American Journal of Occupational Therapy,* 74(Suppl. 2), Article 7412410010, p. 7. https://doi.org/10.5014/ajot.2020.74S2001

The final part of the OTPF-4 Domain is *Client factors* which includes *Values, beliefs, and spirituality; Body functions;* and *Body structures* (AOTA, 2020) (see Table 1.3). Client factors are specific capacities, characteristics, or beliefs that reside within the person and influence occupational performance. Client factors influence performance skills and need to be present for a person to successfully complete an occupation.

1.8.2 OTPF-4 Process

The OTPF-4 *Process* is fluid and dynamic as well as responsive to any changes that are needed. It involves a three-part process: (i) evaluation, (ii) intervention, and (iii) outcomes (AOTA, 2020) (see Figure 1.5). The *Evaluation* portion of the Process involves the completion of the Occupational Profile and Analysis of Occupational Performance sections (AOTA, 2020). Synthesizing the evaluation results allows for an intervention plan to be created.

The *Intervention* component of the Process is now viewed as a dynamic process versus a linear process where the use of best evidence is emphasized. It includes an Intervention Plan, Intervention Implementation, and Intervention Review (AOTA, 2020). Specific types of interventions can include occupations and activities, interventions to support occupations (physical agent modalities and mechanical modalities, orthotics and prosthetics, assistive technology, environmental modifications, wheeled mobility, self-regulation), education and training, self-advocacy, group interventions, and virtual interventions (AOTA, 2020). Approaches to intervention can include create and promote (health promotion), establish, and restore (remediation and restoration), maintain, modify (compensation and adaptation), and prevent (disability prevention) (AOTA, 2020).

The *Outcomes* section of the OTPF-4 describes the results that clients can achieve from occupational therapy interventions. This involves discharge, transitions, and outcomes. Outcome categories can include occupational performance, improvement, enhancement, prevention, health and wellness, quality of life, participation, role competence, well-being, and occupational justice (AOTA, 2020).

1.9 Book Editors' Positionality and Reflexivity Statements

1.9.1 Ted Brown

I am a Western-trained occupational therapist who was raised, educated, and worked in Ontario, Canada, until the age of 39. I am the eighth generation of Irish, Scottish, and English colonists who originally settled on the traditional, ancestral, and unceded lands of the Algonquin Anishinabe nation. These lands are known colonially as the settler regions of the Ottawa valley in the province of Ontario. In 2002, I emigrated from Canada to Australia as an independent migrant where I settled on the traditional lands of the Bunurong Boon Wurrung and Wurundjeri Woi Wurrung peoples of the Eastern Kulin Nation. I identify as a white cisgender gay left-handed able-bodied English-speaking male. I acknowledge my white male privilege, my Global North outlook, and the impacts of colonial hegemony on the First Nation peoples of Canada and Australia. I support decolonization, racial equality, queer inclusivity, cultural sensitivity, social and occupational justice, and gender-affirmative and culturally inclusive health care and education. This impacts my worldview, how I understand the perspectives of others, and my scholarly writing.

1.9.2 Steven Isbel

I strive to recognize how my own positionality shapes the way I view the world and how I interpret the experience of other people. I acknowledge that my positionality influences the way I create scholarly work and in the way I critique and understand the work of others. For this reason, I acknowledge my own positionality as an Australian, English-speaking, cisgendered, heterosexual, and privileged occupational therapist. I have spent most of my life on Ngunnawal country and am committed to incorporating Indigenous ways of doing and knowing into my writing, teaching, and research.

1.9.3 Louise Gustafsson

I am a cisgender, heterosexual, white female who was afforded a privileged education at an all-girls school and entry into a female-dominated profession as an occupational therapist. My clinical background was predominantly hospital-based rehabilitation, partnering with adults and older adults living with a range of medical and neurological conditions. I had formative experiences, personal and professional, that shaped my early understanding of bias, exclusion, and injustice. However, I continue to learn and understand how systems and services disadvantage. I actively partner with First Australians to explore and expand my understanding of our true history and to decolonize the occupational therapy curriculum. I prioritize the contributions of people with lived experience as equal members in research teams and I am a proud ally for the LGTBQIA+ community.

1.9.4 Sharon Gutman

From the time I can remember, I have rejected most institutions and labels that have been placed upon me by the larger Western society in which I was born. Labels are constructs of the larger society that serve to separate and emphasize differences. Most Eastern and First Nation philosophies tell us that we are all one and emerge from one creative source. We appear separate from our source and from each other because of being in separate physical bodies. But we are connected through an energetic matrix. We return to the collective source upon death of the physical body. Labels such as religion, race, ethnicity, gender, gender orientation, disability, and socioeconomic status are just that – labels that are illusions to which we give credence. It's time that as a global community, we recognize that we are interconnected with each other, the planet, and all life forms; that we are more than the labels society has imposed upon us; and that collaboration and compassion are the only path that will heal us and the global problems we have created.

1.9.5 Diane Powers Dirette

I was born and raised on a farm in a small town in the Midwestern United States with a relatively low socioeconomic status and learned from an early age that occupation in the form of work was the way forward for me. As young as I can remember, I rode my bike to work jobs like selling newspapers, picking strawberries, babysitting, and supervising children at YMCA playgrounds so that I could buy clothes for school. In high school, I lived with and cared for my grandmother and my great aunt. My grandmother once said to me, "if you are going to do everything for me, then I may as well die." With that lesson, I bought what I would learn to call "adaptive equipment" such as a reacher and shower bench so that she could be more independent. To pay for college, I always worked at least two jobs and I consider myself fortunate to have found my way to a career in occupational therapy that reaffirmed the words of my grandmother. Fostering participation in occupation so that people have meaning in their lives became apparent to me as a young girl and will always be at the core of my values as an occupational therapist.

1.9.6 Bethan Collins

I am an Irish-educated white female mid-career occupational therapy academic who is currently the Head of Occupational Therapy in a British university. I currently live and work in the United Kingdom. I have lived in Southeast Asia and most of my formative years, including my occupational therapy degree and doctorate, were undertaken in Ireland. My clinical experience as an occupational therapist primarily took place in Ireland and focused on working with adults and older people with physical and sensory disability. I identify as disabled and blind; I use a guide dog and access information through non-visual means, such as screen reading software and braille. I argue for critical disability perspectives to be further integrated into occupational therapy theory and practice and for the experiential knowledge of disabled people to further inform our theory and practice. I have been involved in the disability movement and critique some ableist assumptions that remain within some aspects of occupational therapy practice. My experience as a disabled person and as an occupational therapist influences my practice. My aspiration for occupational therapy is for a profession that can focus on occupation and enable any individual to achieve their own occupational goals.

1.9.7 Tim Barlott

I am a white, male, English-speaking, heterosexual, cisgendered, currently able-bodied settler (of both Canada and Australia). I currently live, work, and play in Amiskwacîwâskahikan (also known as Edmonton, Canada), which is part of Treaty 6 and the traditional and ancestral territory of the Nehiyawak (Cree), Dene, Blackfoot, Saulteaux, Nakota Sioux, a diversity First Nations, and also the home to the Métis people. My grandparents settled in Treaty 6 territory in the early 1900s and benefited from settler farming policies, something that was not available to First Peoples (rather, there were policies to prevent First Peoples from earning a comparable livelihood in farming). I have benefited from settler colonialism and my social location has afforded me and my family opportunities to thrive. I also acknowledge that social forces of settler colonialism, heteronormativity, ableism, and sanism that benefit me simultaneously harm others. These social forces are also woven through the fabric of our profession. I desire for my teaching and research to be affirming for marginalized people, center-lived experience knowledge, and the unsettling of dominant social forces. This involves an ongoing process of checking and re-checking, resisting, and re-resisting the entangled privilege I carry with me.

1.10 Conclusion

This chapter has presented an overview and rationale for the edited book, *Human Occupation: Contemporary concepts and lifespan perspectives*. Each chapter is presented in a similar format that includes an abstract, learning objectives, key words, the chapter authors' group positionality statement, introduction, main text that focuses on the chapter topic, conclusion, summary, review questions, and references. The primary focus of this edited book is threefold: first, it is an attempt to bring together aspects of the occupational therapy profession and the academic discipline of occupational science; second, the discussion of several contemporary topics related to human occupation; and third, the presentation of human occupation relative to different phases of the lifespan. The two key frameworks that inform the focus of the book are the ICF and the OTPF-4. The team of co-editors hope that you find the book informative and, in places, challenging in relation to viewing the world through an occupational lens.

1.11 Summary

- Human occupation is present at all times of our lives, from birth through to end of life.
- People try to maintain and sustain a state of *occupational equilibrium* within themselves to maintain and protect their state of *human occupational homeostasis*.

- Both the Wheel of Power and Privilege graphic and the Coin Model of Privilege and Critical Allyship outline several systems of inequality which can assist occupational therapists when working with clients and their families.
- Both occupational therapy and occupational science focus on human occupation but from slightly differing perspectives; however, the common goal between the two disciplines is growing the body of evidence and knowledge about human occupation through strategic collaborations.
- The ICF is one of the two key frameworks that inform aspects of this book; the ICF includes several relevant concepts, including body functions and structures, activity, participation, personal factors, and environmental factors.
- The OTPF-4 is the second framework that contributes to the human occupation stance of the book and includes the Domain and Process of the occupational therapy standpoint.
- The OTPF-4 Domain includes Occupations, Contexts, Performance Patterns, Performance Skills, and Client Factors, while the OTPF-4 Process has three elements: Evaluation, Intervention, and Outcomes.
- Human occupation is a complex, dynamic, life-sustaining phenomenon that is influenced by external and internal factors. As occupational therapists and occupational science experts, we try to understand these processes and make sense of our complex and dynamic occupational world.

1.12 Review Questions
- What is the relationship between the occupational therapy profession and the academic discipline of occupational science?
- Based on the Wheel of Power and Privilege, what are six identity categories related to power, privilege, and marginalization?
- According to the Coin Model of Privilege and Critical Allyship, what are four systems of inequality that can intersect with each other?
- What are the two contextual components of the ICF?
- Describe activity limitations and participation restrictions in the context of the ICF.
- Name five types of occupations that are included in the OTPF-4.
- The OTPF-4 Process involves a three-part process. Name those three Process steps.
- In the OTPF-4, identify and define the four types of performance patterns?

References

Ahmed-Landeryou, M. J., Emery-Whittington, I., Ivlev, S., & Elder, R. (2022). Pause, reflect, reframe: Deep discussions on co-creating a decolonial approach for an antiracist framework in occupational therapy. *Occupational Therapy Now, 25*(March-April), 14–16.

Ahmed-Landeryou, M. J. (2023a). *Antiracist occupational therapy: Unsettling the status quo.* Jessica Kingsley Publishers.

Ahmed-Landeryou, M. (2023b). A critical reflection from inside, looking back and forward: Theorising perspectives on decolonising occupational science theory and practice. *Journal of Occupational Science*, in press. https://doi.org/10.1080/14427591.2023.2246986

Ahmed-Landeryou, M. (2023c). Developing an evidence-informed decolonising curriculum wheel – A reflective piece. *Equity in Education & Society, 2*(2), 157–180. https://doi.org/10.1177/27526461231154014

American Occupational Therapy Association. (2020). Occupational therapy practice framework: Domain and process (4th ed.). *American Journal of Occupational Therapy, 74*(Suppl. 2), 7412410010p1–7412410010p87. https://doi.org/10.5014/ajot.2020.74S2001

Andersen, L. T., & Reed, K. L. (2017). *History of occupational therapy.* Slack Incorporated.

Beagan, B. L., Sibbald, K. R., Bizzeth, S. R., & Pride, T. M. (2022). Systemic racism in Canadian occupational therapy: A qualitative study with therapists. *Canadian Journal of Occupational Therapy, 89*(1), 51–61. https://doi.org/10.1177/00084174211066676

Blanche, E. I., & Henny-Kohler, E. (2000). Philosophy, science and ideology: A proposed relationship for occupational science and occupational therapy. *Occupational Therapy International, 7*(2), 99–110. https://doi.org/10.1002/oti.110

Clark, F. (1993). Occupation embedded in a real life: Occupational science and occupational therapy. *American Journal of Occupational Therapy, 47*(12), 1067–1078. https://doi.org/10.5014/ajot.47.12.1067

Clark, F., Parham, D., Carlson, M. E., Frank, G., Jackson, J., Pierce, D., Wolfe, R. J., & Zemke, R. (1991). Occupational science: Academic innovation in the service of occupational therapy's future. *American Journal of Occupational Therapy, 45*(4), 300–310. https://doi.org/10.5014/ajot.45.4.300

Clark, F., Zemke, R., Frank, G., Parham, D., Neville-Jan, A., Hedricks, C., Carson, M., Fazio, L., & Abreu, B. (1993). Dangers inherent in the partition of occupational therapy and occupational science. *American Journal of Occupational Therapy, 47*(2), 184–186. https://doi.org/10.5014/ajot.47.2.184

Colman, W. (1990). Evolving educational practices in occupational therapy: The war emergency courses, 1936–1954. *American Journal of Occupational Therapy, 44,* 1028–1036.

Duckworth, S. (2020, October 18). Wheel of power/privilege [Infographic]. Flickr. CC BY-NC-ND 2.0. https://www.flickr.com/photos/sylviaduckworth/50500299716

Eklund, M., Orban, K., Argentzell, E., Bejerholm, U., Tjörnstrand, C., Erlandsson, L.-K., & Håkansson, C. (2017). The linkage between patterns of daily occupations and occupational balance: Applications within occupational science and occupational therapy practice. *Scandinavian Journal of Occupational Therapy, 24*(1), 41–56. https://doi.org/10.1080/11038128.2016.1224271

Emery-Whittington, I. (2021). Occupational justice–Colonial business as usual? *Canadian Journal of Occupational Therapy, 88*(2), 153–162. https://doi.org/10.1177/00084174211005891

Emery-Whittington, I., & Te Maro, B. (2018). Decolonising occupation: Causing social change to help our ancestors rest and our descendants thrive. *New Zealand Journal of Occupational Therapy, 65*(1), 12–19.

Gallagher, M., Muldoon, O. T., & Pettigrew, J. (2015). An integrative review of social and occupational factors influencing health and wellbeing. *Frontiers in Psychology, 6,* Article number 1281. https://doi.org/10.3389/fpsyg.2015.01281

Galvaan, R., Peters, L., Richards, L. A., Francke, M., & Krenzer, M. (2022). Pedagogies within occupational therapy curriculum: centering a decolonial praxis in community development practice. *Cadernos Brasileiros de Terapia Ocupacional, 30,* e3133. https://doi.org/10.1590/2526-8910.ctoAO24023133

Gibson, C. (2020). When the river runs dry: Leadership, decolonisation and healing in occupational therapy. *New Zealand Journal of Occupational Therapy, 67*(1), 11–20.

Grajo, L., Boisselle, A., & DaLomba, E. (2018). Occupational adaptation as a construct: A scoping review of literature. *The Open Journal of Occupational Therapy, 6*(1). https://doi.org/10.15453/2168-6408.1400

Hammell, K. W. (2015). Respecting global wisdom: Enhancing the cultural relevance of occupational therapy's theoretical base. *British Journal of Occupational Therapy, 78*(11), 718–721. https://doi.org/10.1177/0308022614564170

Hammell, K. W. (2023). Focusing on "what matters": The occupation, capability and wellbeing framework for occupational therapy. *Cadernos Brasileiros de Terapia Ocupacional, 31,* e3509. https://doi.org/10.1590/2526-8910.ctoAO269035092

Hocking, C., Jones, M., & Reed, K. (2015). Occupational science informing occupational therapy interventions. In I. Söderback (Ed.), *International handbook of occupational therapy interventions* (pp. 127–134). Springer. https://doi.org/10.1007/978-3-319-08141-0_9

Hocking, C., & Wright-St Claire, V. (2011). Occupational science: Adding value to occupational therapy. *New Zealand Journal of Occupational Therapy, 58*(1), 29–35.

Hoel, V., von Zweck, C., Ledgerd, R., & World Federation of Occupational Therapists. (2021). The impact of Covid-19 for occupational therapy: Findings and recommendations of a global survey. *World Federation of Occupational Therapists Bulletin, 77*(2), 69–76. https://doi.org/10.1080/14473828.2020.1855044

Ivlev, S. R. (2023). *Occupational therapy disruptors: What global OT practice can teach us about innovation, culture, and community*. Jessica Kingsley Publishers.

Kristensen, H. K., & Petersen, K. S. (2016). Occupational science: An important contributor to occupational therapists' clinical reasoning. *Scandinavian Journal of Occupational Therapy, 23*(3), 240–243. https://doi.org/10.3109/11038128.2015.1083054

Laliberte Rudman, D. (2018). Occupational therapy and occupational science: Building crucial and transformative alliances. *Brazilian Journal of Occupational Therapy, 26*(1), 241–249. https://doi.org/10.4322/2526-8910.ctoEN1246

Leive, L., & Morrison, R. (2020). Essential characteristics of sleep from the occupational science perspective. *Cadernos Brasileiros de Terapia Ocupacional, 28*(3), 1072–1092. https://doi.org/10.4322/2526-8910.ctoARF1954

Lunt, A. (1997). Occupational science and occupational therapy: Negotiating the boundary between a discipline and a profession. *Journal of Occupational Science, 4*(2), 56–61. https://doi.org/10.1080/14427591.1997.9686421

Mahoney, W. J., & Kiraly-Alvarez, A. F. (2019). Challenging the status quo: Infusing non-western ideas into occupational therapy education and practice. *The Open Journal of Occupational Therapy, 7*(3), 1–10. https://doi.org/10.15453/2168-6408.1592

Molke, D. K., Laliberte Rudman, D., & Polatajko, H. J. (2004). The promise of occupational science: A developmental assessment of an emerging academic discipline. *Canadian Journal of Occupational Therapy, 71*(5), 269–281. https://doi.org/10.1177/000841740407100505

Morley, M., Atwal, A., & Spiliotopoulou, G. (2011). Has occupational science taken away the occupational therapy evidence base? A debate. *British Journal of Occupational Therapy, 74*(10), 494–497. https://doi.org/10.4276/030802211X13182481842065

Mosey, A. C. (1992). Partition of occupational science and occupational therapy. *American Journal of Occupational Therapy, 46*(9), 851–853. https://doi.org/10.5014/ajot.46.9.851

Nixon, S. A. (2019). The coin model of privilege and critical allyship: Implications for health. *BMC Public Health, 19*, Article number 1637. https://doi.org/10.1186/s12889-019-7884-9

O'Brien, J. C., & Kuhaneck, H. (2019). *Case-Smith's occupational therapy for children and adolescents*. Elsevier.

Paterson, C. F. (2010). *Opportunities not prescriptions: The development of occupational therapy in Scotland 1900–1960*. Aberdeen History of Medicine Publications.

Peters, L., Abrahams, K., Francke, M., Rustin, L., & Minen, G. (2023). Towards developing a decolonial transdisciplinary praxis that supports a socially-transformative occupational science: Emergent insights from an educational project in South Africa. *Journal of Occupational Science*, in press. https://doi.org/10.1080/14427591.2023.2233970

Pollard, N., & Sakellariou, D. (2017). Occupational therapy on the margins. *World Federation of Occupational Therapists Bulletin, 17*(2), 71–75. https://doi.org/10.1080/14473828.2017.1361698

Pollard, N., Sakellariou, D., & Porter, A. (2010). Will occupational science facilitate or divide the practice of occupational therapy? *International Journal of Therapy and Rehabilitation, 17*, 648–654. https://doi.org/10.12968/ijtr.2010.17.1.45992Pooley, E. A., & Beagan, B. L. (2021). The concept of oppression and occupational therapy: A critical interpretive synthesis. *Canadian Journal of Occupational Therapy, 88*(4), 407–417. https://doi.org/10.1177/00084174211051168

Riley, J. (2012). Occupational science and occupational therapy: A contemporary relationship. In G. Boniface & A. Seymour (Eds.), *Using occupational therapy theory in practice* (pp. 165–179). Wiley Blackwell. https://doi.org/10.1002/9781118709634.ch14

Robinson, M. R., Koverman, B., Becker, C., Ciancio, K. E., Fisher, G., & Saake, S. (2021). Lessons learned from the COVID-19 pandemic: Occupational therapy on the front line. *American Journal of Occupational Therapy, 75*(2), 7502090010p1–7502090010p7. https://doi.org/10.5014/ajot.2021.047654

Rudman, M. T., Flavell, H., Harris, C., & Wright, M. (2021). How prepared is Australian occupational therapy to decolonise its practice?. *Australian Occupational Therapy Journal, 68*(4), 287–297. https://doi.org/10.1111/1440-1630.12725

Shannon, P. (1977). The derailment of occupational therapy. *American Journal of Occupational Therapy, 31*(4), 229–234.

Simaan, J. (2020). Decolonising occupational science education through learning activities based on a study from the Global South. *Journal of Occupational Science, 27*(3), 432–442. https://doi.org/10.1080/14427591.2020.1780937

Sterman, J., Njelesani, J., & Carr, S. (2022). Anti-racism and occupational therapy education: Beyond diversity and inclusion. *Journal of Occupational Therapy Education, 6*(1). https://doi.org/10.26681/jote.2022.060103

Taylor, R. E. (2017). *Kielhofner's Model of Human Occupation*. Wolters Kluwer.

Townsend, E. A., & Polatajko, H. J. (2007). *Enabling occupation II: Advancing an occupational therapy vision for health, well-being, & justice through occupation*. CAOT Publications ACE.

Trentham, B., Laliberte Rudman, D., Smith, H., & Phenix, H. (2022). The socio-political and historical context of occupational therapy in Canada. In E. Egan & G. Restall (Eds.), *Promoting occupational participation: Collaborative relationship-focused occupational therapy* (pp. 31–56). Canadian Occupational Therapy Association.

Turcotte, P. L., & Holmes, D. (2023a). From domestication to imperial patronage: Deconstructing the biomedicalisation of occupational therapy. *Health (London), 27*(5), 719–737. https://doi.org/10.1177/13634593211067891

Turcotte, P. L., & Holmes, D. (2023b). The shadow side of occupational therapy: Necropower, state racism and colonialism. *Scandinavian Journal of Occupational Therapy*, in press. https://doi.org/10.1080/11038128.2023.2264330

Whiteford, G., Townsend, E., & Hocking, C. (2000). Reflections on a renaissance of occupation. *Canadian Journal of Occupational Therapy, 67*(1), 61–69. https://doi.org/10.1177/000841740006700109

Woodside, H. H. (1971). Occupational therapy: A historical perspective. The development of occupational therapy 1910–1929. *American Journal of Occupational Therapy, 25*(5), 226–230.

World Health Organization. (2001). *International Classification of Functioning, Disability and Health: ICF*. World Health Organization. https://apps.who.int/iris/bitstream/handle/10665/42407/9241545429-eng.pdf?sequence=1&isAllowed=y

Yerxa, E. J. (1990). An Introduction to occupational science: A foundation for occupational therapy in the 21st century. *Occupational Therapy in Health Care, 6*(4), 1–17. https://doi.org/10.1080/J003v06n04_04

Yerxa, E. J. (1993). Occupational science: A new source of power for participants in occupational therapy. *Journal of Occupational Science, 1*(1), 3–9. https://doi.org/10.1080/14427591.1993.9686373

CHAPTER 2

Overview of Human Occupation
Concepts and Principles

Matthew Molineux

Abstract
Although occupation is the central concept in occupational therapy, there is no universally agreed definition. In fact, there are several different ways that occupation is conceptualized in the occupational therapy and occupational science literature. This leads to confusion and impacts on communication because each way of representing occupation is slightly different, although there are some similarities. This chapter provides an overview of four ways in which occupation is presented in the literature: definitions, taxonomies, occupation and other terms, and models. The intention is to provide readers with a structure that can be used when they are engaging with the literature and to encourage greater precision in communicating about occupation. The chapter acknowledges that most of the literature on occupation has been presented from a colonized perspective, and therefore all occupational therapists and students must be critical of how that has shaped the concept of occupation.

Author's Positionality Statement
The author of this chapter has experiences of working with clients and their families in acute and rehabilitation services in hospitals and the community, as well as extensive experience working within higher education in Australia and the United Kingdom. I therefore acknowledge that my perspective has been influenced by my Western, English-speaking, university-educated, professionally qualified, cisgendered, and privileged experiences. I also acknowledge that I have experience of being a member of minority groups that are discriminated against, and that has also shaped my perspective.

> **Objectives**
> This chapter will allow the reader to:
>
> - Understand the range of ways occupation is represented in the professional literature.
> - Recognize some of the strengths and weaknesses of different ways of conceptualizing occupation.
> - Use the term "occupation" more deliberately and precisely.
> - Navigate the professional literature about occupation more confidently.

> **Key terms**
> - occupation
> - model
> - taxonomy
> - activity
> - purposeful activity
> - role
> - task
> - action

2.1 Introduction

Occupation is the central organizing concept within occupational therapy. It is the concept that defines our expertise as professionals and so it must be deeply understood by all occupational therapists. It must therefore be an important aspect of entry-level education for students studying to become an occupational therapist. Occupation is, however, immensely complex because that one word encompasses many ideas such as: what is, and what is not, an occupation; what is the relationship between occupation and health and well-being; what are the factors that give rise to occupation; how can occupation be used therapeutically with individuals, groups, and communities? To be skilled in the use of occupation, occupational therapists must receive a strong grounding in occupation in their entry-level education, but they must also continue to deepen their knowledge of occupation and strengthen their skills in using occupation.

Given its centrality in the profession, occupation has been, and continues to be, the focus of extensive theorizing and research. While this means that we now have multiple ways of understanding occupation, it also reinforces the need for occupational therapists to continue to develop their understanding by reading, thinking, and talking about occupation. This chapter aims to provide a high-level overview of the different ways in which occupation is conceptualized in the professional literature. It is not intended to provide a comprehensive exposition of occupation; rather, the aim of this chapter is to provide a map to assist in navigating the many and varied ways occupation is written about. In doing so, it will enable readers to become more focused in their use of the professional literature and be precise in their use of language about the profession's core concept.

2.2 Occupation in Occupational Therapy

Many authors have written about the place of occupation in occupational therapy throughout the profession's history. Probably the most useful was the history provided by Kielhofner (2009) because he used the paradigm as a way to distinguish between different periods in the history of the profession (Kuhn, 1996): the pre-paradigm era; the paradigm of occupation; the mechanistic paradigm; and the contemporary paradigm. Kielhofner's analysis is particularly interesting because it very clearly shows that occupation has been more or less central in the thinking and practice of the profession depending on the dominant paradigm.

According to Kielhofner (2009), the profession is currently in the contemporary paradigm, and in fact has been for several decades now. The basic assumptions of this paradigm place occupation front and center: humans are viewed as occupational beings; their challenges are viewed as occupational challenges; and occupational therapists provide occupation-based interventions to address those challenges (Kielhofner, 2009). While there are examples of occupational therapists around the world who are embracing the contemporary paradigm and practicing in ways that are deeply rooted in a concern for occupation, this approach is not universal. Of course, practice varies from place to place, but a paradigmatic approach would suggest that all occupational therapists are committed to, knowledgeable about, and skilled in using occupation. This is not the case and has been the topic of much research (see, for example, Burley et al., 2018; Di Tommaso et al., 2019; Murray et al., 2020).

One possible reason for this lack of a universal acceptance of an occupation-centered approach to occupational therapy practice may, paradoxically, be occupation itself. As discussed earlier, occupation is inherently complex and one way of supporting people to learn and think about it, and to use it in practice, is to simplify it. However, Yerxa (1988) warned the profession 35 years ago that oversimplification is dangerous for occupational therapy. To make occupation more accessible to students, occupational therapists, as well as clients and the other staff we work with, we have created short one-line definitions or simplistic models to try and capture occupation. While this has brought benefits, it has also been problematic. Over-reliance on simplistic representations of occupation has reduced our familiarity and comfort with the complexity of occupation.

All occupational therapists and students must therefore be cognizant of this paradox; that occupation is inherently complex and yet occupational therapy has sought to simplify it for ourselves and others. Members of the profession must become knowledgeable and skilled in, and perhaps more importantly become comfortable with, the complexity of occupation. This is vital if we are to live up to our responsibility as a recognized professional group (Sullivan, 1995) to enable individuals, groups, and communities to engage in occupations in order to achieve and maintain health and well-being. The remainder of this chapter will provide an overview of some of the key ways in which occupation is conceptualized in the occupational therapy and occupational science peer-reviewed literature. The aim of this chapter is not to provide a comprehensive overview of all the ways occupation has been conceptualized, nor is it intended to cover those presented in great depth, but to provide a map for understanding the existing literature on occupation. In this way, it is hoped that readers will be better prepared to negotiate and engage with the many ways occupation has been written about.

2.3 Conceptualizing Occupation

This section includes an introduction to several ways that occupation is, and has been, conceptualized in occupational therapy and occupational science. It will present four broad ways this has been done:

- by providing distinct definitions of occupation
- by creating taxonomies of occupation
- in relation to other concepts, particularly activity
- by creating models that include occupation directly or indirectly.

2.3.1 Adopting a Critical Lens

It is important at this point to remind readers of what many see as a significant problem in occupational therapy and occupational science, including our conceptualizations of occupation. Namely, that most of the work in these fields has been produced from a Western perspective because most theorists and researchers have come from the Global North. The dominant voice in occupational therapy and occupational science has therefore been a white, Western, First World one. Depending on the specific context being considered, that voice has also been predominantly female, middle to upper class, individualistic, Christian, imperialist, neoliberal, and industrialized (see Hammell (2009) and Kantartzis and Molineux (2012) for an exploration of some of these influences). In his seminal work, Iwama (2003) challenged occupational therapists "to explore the relevance of our ideas and how culture-bound occupational therapy might actually be" (p. 582), while Hammell (2009) argued that the assumptions which underpin occupational therapy are in fact culturally specific. More recently, scholars have highlighted the ways in which health disparities are caused by racism (Grenier, 2020) and that engaging in occupation is racialized (Lavalley & Johnson, 2020).

Despite the greater attention drawn to these issues and scholars' exploration of them, more work needs to be done. For example, one study in Jordan revealed the general acceptance of traditional folk medicine; yet, the idea of occupation, and therefore the occupational therapy discipline, was not well accepted because of the dominance of the medical model (Malkawi et al., 2020). In Australia, Ryan et al. (2020) explored occupation from the perspective of Aboriginal and Torres Strait Islander people and identified a range of issues, including how fears of safety and the impact of racism stopped people from engaging in advocacy occupations, the importance of collective occupations for health and well-being, and how occupations of Indigenous people "are not always valued, promoted, or recognized" (p. 10).

What follows then is an overview of several ways that occupation has been conceptualized. We acknowledge that this presents, and perhaps perpetuates, white, Western, middle to upper class, individualistic, Christian, imperialist, neoliberal, and industrialized perspectives. Indeed, the word occupation can have very different associations in different contexts. In some contexts, for example, occupation refers to occupation of country by an invading force. However, readers are encouraged to first be mindful of how these are potentially problematic and, second, to be critical of what Hammell (2009) has referred to as the "sacred texts" (p. 7) of occupational therapy. She exhorts all occupational therapists to be skeptical of the assumptions, theories, and practices of the profession – which includes those presented in the remainder of this chapter – so that we can produce more relevant and inclusive theory and practice (Hammell, 2009).

2.4 Definitions of Occupation

To say that the word occupation is contentious is an understatement. The term is not easily translated into some languages, and even in the English language its meaning is at best ambiguous. While some have argued that the term's ambiguity and all-encompassing nature is a strength (Breines, 1995), many occupational therapists would disagree. For this reason, scholars have proposed innumerable definitions of occupation in an attempt to bring clarity to the term, develop a shared understanding, and facilitate communication. Unfortunately, there is no single truly universal definition of occupation that has been agreed upon except for the one from the World Federation of Occupational Therapists (WFOT) (2012, para 2): "the everyday activities that people do as individuals, in families and with communities to occupy time and bring meaning and purpose to life. Occupations include things people need to, want to and are expected to do". This definition is echoed in the *Occupational Therapy Practice Framework: Domain and Process – 4th Edition* (OTPF-4) (AOTA, 2020, p. 79): "everyday personalized activities that people do as individuals, in families, and with communities to occupy time and bring meaning and purpose to life". These definitions are easily understood and include important concepts such as everyday activities, individual and collective engagement, meaning, and purpose. While they are suitable for use with clients and the general public, they do not recognize the complexity of occupation and so are probably inadequate for occupational therapy students and practitioners.

There are innumerable other definitions that we can choose from depending on why we need to define occupation and who will be on the receiving end of the definition.

- "specific chunks of activity within the ongoing stream of human behaviors which are named in the lexicon of the culture" (Yerxa et al., 1990, p. 5)
- "a specific individual's personally constructed, nonrepeatable experience" (Pierce, 2001, p. 139)
- "the things people do" (Hocking, 2009, p. 142)
- "what people do alone and together in particular times, places, and cultures" (Dickie, 2016, p. 523).

As much as some members of the profession might long for a single definition that we can all agree on and use, that is unlikely, and some might say unrealistic. Occupation is the central concept in both occupational therapy and occupational science and is under continual scrutiny; this develops our understanding and, therefore, definitions of the concept (Pierce, 2001; Wood, 1996).

Some authors, however, have rejected attempts to write a single definition of occupation (Laliberte Rudman et al., 2022; Molineux, 2009) and instead proposed characteristics or features of occupation that can be used to interrogate human experiences to determine if they are occupations or not. For example, Laliberte Rudman and Aldrich (2017) proposed that occupations, matter for individual and collective health and well-being, can lead to individual and societal changes; take place in time, space, and place; are given meaning according to individual and collective values; and are influenced by various contexts. However, Molineux (2009) argued that occupations are those experiences which are active, purposeful, meaningful, contextualized, uniquely human, and impact health.

Definitions are just one way that occupation has been conceptualized in the occupational therapy and occupational science literature. Not only do scholars disagree on what the definition should be, resulting in many, there is disagreement about whether definition is even possible and desirable. Students, occupational therapists, and occupational scientists will find definitions in the literature and in informal communications, and while they can be a helpful starting point, they are unlikely to represent the actual complexity of occupation.

2.5 Taxonomies

One way to address the inherent complexity of occupation is the use of taxonomies. A taxonomy is a structured approach to classifying an object or phenomenon so that the relationship between related phenomena can be demonstrated. Occupational therapy has several taxonomies. Perhaps most common in some settings are taxonomies of occupational therapy intervention which are created to allow accurate specification of what occupational therapists do or what clients experience, for the purpose of documentation in research, to determine billing in fee-based health care, or to understand staff workload and workforce requirements (see, for example, Ozelie et al., 2009; Soderback & Magill, 2015; Tornquist & Sonn, 2014). These do not always classify occupation per se, but these taxonomies do exist. There are two types of taxonomies that classify occupation. The simpler ones categorize types of occupations. The second, slightly more complex, type of taxonomy includes higher and lower order concepts to demonstrate relationships between occupation and other concepts.

2.5.1 Taxonomies of Types of Occupation

The simplest taxonomies are those that classify occupations into different categories and these taxonomies are commonly understood in occupational therapy. One example is the three categories of occupations named by Canadian occupational therapists: self-care, productivity, and leisure (Polatajko et al., 2013). Another example from Australia has four categories: self-maintenance, rest, leisure, and productivity (Chapparo et al., 2017). While there are others, the final example is from the OTPF-4 (AOTA, 2020), which includes nine types of occupations: activities of daily living, instrumental activities of daily living, health management, rest and sleep, education, work, play, leisure, and social participation. There are other taxonomies of types of occupation and students and practitioners should not be unduly concerned with the differences and a seeming lack of consistency. As shown in Table 2.1, what looks like inconsistency is just a variation in the level of classification: some are specific and detailed, while others are broader. There are an almost innumerable number of occupations that humans around the world engage in and it is no surprise that there are slight differences in the way different authors classify them. When using these taxonomies,

Table 2.1 Comparison of Two Different Taxonomies of Types of Occupation

Broad categorization Polatajko et al. (2013)	Specific categorization American Occupational Therapy Association (2020)
Self-care	Activities of daily living, rest and sleep, health management
Productivity	Instrumental activities of daily living, education, work, health management
Leisure	Play, leisure, social participation

the key task is not to try and choose the best or most accurate; it is to choose one and be explicit about your use of it.

The value of categorizing types of occupations is that they can be used as a useful shorthand when explaining the scope of occupation therapy to others. The public often think that the profession is concerned only with work, but by explaining that we focus on self-care, productivity, and leisure (with examples of each), we can relatively quickly and easily describe the profession's concerns. Another use for these taxonomies is to remind practitioners of our scope of practice. For example, when working in an acute, fast-moving institution, it is easy for occupational therapists to focus on the organizational priorities of self-care occupations such as showering, dressing, and using the toilet. These taxonomies can be used as prompts in initial interviews, for example, to remind therapists that we can, and perhaps should, ask about all types of occupations to understand the client as an occupational being. Even if the practice setting might not permit therapists to address issues in all areas of occupations, knowing clients more fully as occupational beings will enhance the therapeutic relationship.

2.5.2 Taxonomies of Occupation and Other Concepts

The second type of taxonomies categorizes occupation in relation to other concepts, such as roles and activities. Once again, different taxonomies have been proposed by different authors and so students and practitioners should critically appraise each one and choose one that serves the required purpose. One example of this type of taxonomy was provided by Harvey and Pentland (2010). They proposed that "daily life consists of engaging in tasks to perform activities required by occupations" (p. 102) in the pursuit of fulfilling roles. In this way, those items lower in the taxonomy are smaller and are required in order to complete the slightly larger or more significant items the next step up the hierarchy. For example, if you combine multiple tasks such as turning on a burner on a stove, filling a pan with water, getting an egg out of the refrigerator, placing the egg in the pan, placing the pan on the lit burner, then you are completing the activity of boiling eggs. If you combine multiple activities such as boiling eggs, making toast, making a pot of tea, then you are completing the occupation of cooking breakfast. If you combine multiple occupations such as cooking breakfast, doing the family laundry, cleaning the house, helping children with homework, then you are performing the role of parent. Consideration of this taxonomy will reveal a gap or at least a question – are there units smaller than tasks?

Polatajko and her colleagues also published a taxonomy that provided greater detail at the lower end of the taxonomy (Polatajko et al., 2004, 2013). They proposed that tasks comprised actions, that actions comprised movement patterns, and that movement patterns comprised voluntary movements (Polatajko et al., 2004). Despite this increased detail at the lower end of the taxonomy, there was a lack of precision at the upper levels of the taxonomy. For example, the first iteration suggested that the upper level of the taxonomy was "occupational grouping" such as self-care, productivity, and leisure (Polatajko et al., 2004), whereas a later version ended at occupation (Polatajko et al., 2013). Furthermore, the later version suggests that accountancy is an example of occupation (Polatajko et al., 2013), but that is in fact the name of a profession or type of work.

While there is no single taxonomy that is robust and widely accepted, it is possible to combine the two taxonomies presented above to create a powerful tool for understanding occupation: roles comprise multiple occupations, occupations comprise multiple activities, activities comprise multiple tasks, tasks comprise multiple actions, and actions comprise multiple voluntary movements (see Table 2.2).

It should be noted that only one example has been provided at each level of the taxonomy in Table 2.2. Consider identifying and recording all the voluntary movements required to form a grip around a panhandle, all of the movement patterns in the entire body to carry the pan to the sink, all of the actions required to fill the pan with water, and so on. This highlights the complexity of occupation. This is in fact one of the benefits of taxonomies of occupation and other concepts: they remind us of the complexity of occupation and, in particular, the ways different levels support (or inhibit) people to engage in occupations. This is particularly useful when conducting occupation analyses. Another benefit is that these taxonomies remind occupational therapists that the domain of concern is at the level of occupation. Our concern is with enabling individuals, groups, and communities to engage in occupations. We are not interested in joint range of movement per se; we are only interested in it in so much as it contributes to an action, which contributes to a task, which contributes to an activity, which contributes to an occupation.

There are two potential problems with taxonomies of occupation and other concepts. First, they can encourage dissection of occupation into smaller and smaller components, which might then become the focus of attention. As in the example provided, if a therapist was to focus on all the joint movements required for an occupation, they might lose sight of the occupation and their assessment and intervention could stray

Table 2.2 A Combined Taxonomy of Occupation

Level	Example
Role	Parent of a young child
Occupation	Cooking breakfast... *and others*
Activity	Boiling eggs... *and others*
Task	Filling a pan with water... *and others*
Action	Carrying the pan to the sink... *and others*
Voluntary movement	Flexion of finger joints to form a grip... *and others*

Source: Harvey & Pentland (2010); Polatajko et al. (2004, 2013).

from occupation. Second, a cursory glance at the taxonomies presented reveal that the other components and factors that enable or inhibit occupations are not explicit. For example, the combined taxonomy lacks any mention of cognitive and affective aspects. Similarly, there is no reference to contextual factors that impact occupations such as legal restrictions, cultural expectations, and the non-human environment. While some of these were acknowledged in the original work by Polatajko et al. (2004), they were not included in a comprehensive way and could still be easily overlooked if the taxonomies were not used with a critical eye.

2.6 Occupation and Activity

Throughout the history of occupational therapy, the term "activity" has been often used synonymously with occupation. While the term might be more accessible to clients, colleagues, and the public, it may not actually mean the same as occupation – in fact, there continues to be confusion in the professional discourse regarding terms such as "occupation" and "activity".

Confusion regarding terminology is not new. Golledge (1998) examined what was even then a long-standing lack of consistency in the literature and identified three terms in usage: "occupation", "purposeful activity", and "activity". In her view, which focused on what occupational therapists did with clients, occupations were "daily living tasks that are part of an individual's lifestyle" (p. 102). Despite that wording, she went on to elaborate that occupations are not necessarily limited to those daily living tasks that are *currently* part of the person's lifestyle. They can also include "occupations that the individual has an interest in, or perhaps needs or wants to develop or relearn" (p. 102). Examples of occupations in this sense include shopping, driving, playing sport, and cooking. These are distinct from activities which "do not have meaning or relevance to an individual's life" (p. 103) such as stacking cones, using peg boards, and joint ranging. With her focus on occupational therapy practice, Golledge (1998) argued that occupations should be used in therapy with clients and that the use of activities should be minimal.

In her paper, Golledge (1998) highlights an intermediate type of experience that sits between occupation and activity. She called these experiences "purposeful activity" and identified two types. The first type are those experiences which resemble occupations, but which demonstrate a lack of attention to the importance of context. For example, engaging clients in simple cooking tasks or showering after an illness or injury seems reasonable because it could be assumed that those are important to all people. However, without considering the contexts of the specific person, that is merely an assumption. The client may not want or need to focus on cooking because they have a partner who will do that when they leave hospital and, instead, they would rather focus on ten-pin bowling. The second type are arts and crafts that are used without considering whether or not they have a place within the person's lifestyle. For example, the use of pottery with a group of clients in an outpatient group, when none of them have ever done nor want to do pottery, is an example of this type of purposeful activity. Looking at the group, it could be assumed that pottery is an occupation because for many people, pottery is an occupation, but for this particular group of people, it is not.

Golledge's (1998) specification of activity, purposeful activity, and occupation starts to tease out the differences between these experiences, and draws attention to both the appropriateness of some approaches in occupational therapy and the variable therapeutic value of these experiences. While Golledge (1998) had a particular focus on what occupational therapists did in practice with clients, Pierce (2001) focused on a more theoretical distinction between activity and occupation, although there are clearly practice implications of her work. Pierce proposed that "an activity is an idea held in the minds of persons and shared in their cultural language" (p. 139). The important terms here are "idea" and "in their cultural language". In this view, an activity is not something a person (or group of persons) can experience except as an idea. A person can think about cooking or swimming in the ocean, but they are merely ideas. Additionally, an activity is something that is named and shared within the minds of people who belong to a particular culture. This aspect of her distinction harks back to the first occupational science definition of occupation: "specific chunks of activity within the ongoing stream of human behaviors which are *named in the lexicon of the culture* [emphasis added]" (Yerxa et al., 1990, p. 5).

According to Pierce (2001, p. 139), an occupation, however, "is a specific individual's personally constructed, nonrepeatable experience". It is not until a person "does the thing" that it becomes an occupation. Pierce makes it clear in her definition of occupation that it is unique – it is a specific individual, it is personally constructed, and it is nonrepeatable. This is because for her, occupations occur in "temporal, spatial, and sociocultural conditions that are unique to that one-time occurrence" (p. 139). A person may cook dinner on both Monday and Tuesday but there will be differences between those two occurrences that make each one unique. For example, one night the person might be cooking for themselves and another night for someone else; one night they may have had a busy day at work and the other night they might have had the day off work; one night they might be aching after a strenuous workout at the gym and the other day they may be feeling relaxed after a massage.

Pierce's (2001) distinction between activity and occupation is useful because it reminds us that occupations are experiences humans engage in; humans do occupations. They are not merely theoretical constructs. Furthermore, she reminds us that while people in a particular cultural group might all share an understanding of what a specific activity is (such as making breakfast), the uniqueness of humans and human experience means that we cannot fully understand how an individual, group, or community engages in that occupation until they engage in it.

These distinctions might seem pedantic and unnecessary to some, but they serve a valuable purpose if we engage with them. Reflecting on these distinctions and applying them in relation to our own experiences as occupational beings and in relation to our practice as occupational therapists encourage us to think more deeply about occupation and become more sophisticated in our understanding. However, there is an important caveat in relation to this work. These distinctions and definitions should not be used to justify occupational therapy practice that is not as occupational as it can or should be. For example, just because Golledge (1998) has identified activity and purposeful activity as types of human experience that take place in occupational therapy practice, does not mean they should necessarily be used in practice. In fact, she stated that "occupational therapists should most notably be using occupations and purposeful activity in their interventions. Activities should form a minimal and adjunctive element…" (Golledge, 1998, p. 104). Contemporary views of occupation-centered practice might therefore be much more critical of the use of activity, and probably purposeful activity too.

Similarly, using Pierce's (2001) definition of occupation, it would be possible to explain almost any human experience as an occupation. For example, one could engage a client who has never engaged in any type of art or craft in macramé during occupational therapy and potentially justify that as an occupation because it would be "a specific individual's personally constructed, nonrepeatable experience" (Pierce, 2001, p. 139). Not only would this justification be at odds with Pierce (2001) because it doesn't recognize the importance of personal meaning (e.g., if we asked the client engaged in macramé about their occupational history and their preferences and interests, we would realize that it is not meaningful to them), it would also run counter to a deeper understanding of occupation suggested by definitions and models of occupation.

2.7 Models of Occupation

The final way that occupation is conceptualized and presented in occupational therapy and occupational science literature is in the form of models. As already discussed, occupation is complex and models, by definition, represent something complex in simplified form (Steward, 1995). Therefore, the professional literature contains many models, and while some have garnered significant attention, others are less well known. It should be noted that readers will also encounter many terms that are sometimes presented as distinct from models and sometimes used interchangeably with the term "model"; these include "theory", "frame of reference", "paradigm", "conceptual practice model", "practice model". In this chapter, the term "model" is used deliberately and quite broadly to avoid unnecessary confusion.

2.7.1 Canadian Model of Occupational Performance and Engagement

While the Canadian Model of Occupational Performance and Engagement (CMOPE) (Polatajko et al., 2013) has a long history in occupational therapy, it has recently been replaced with the Canadian Model of Occupational Participation (CanMOP) (Egan & Restall, 2022). In light of the recent introduction of the CanMOP, this section will focus on the CMOPE which is currently in wider use and has a longer record of use within the occupational therapy discipline.

The CMOPE uses the Canadian Association of Occupational Therapists' (1997) definition of occupation: "Occupation is everything people do to occupy themselves, including looking after themselves (self-care), enjoying life (leisure), and contributing to the social and economic fabric of their communities (productivity)" (p. 34). In its clear use of the three categories of occupation, it demonstrates a taxonomy of the types of occupation. The CMOPE's other key elements include person and environment, where the person is viewed as comprising spiritual, physical, cognitive, and affective capacities and environment as comprising physical, social, cultural, and institutional aspects. Interestingly, the core constructs of the model, namely occupational performance and occupational engagement, are not represented in the model's diagrammatics. Rather, occupational performance and engagement are seen as the outcome of the interaction between the person, occupation, and environment.

It could be argued that occupation is not the CMOPE's central concern because it is only one of three elements which interacts to produce occupational performance and engagement. Polatajko et al. (2013), however, point out that it is in fact where occupation overlaps/interacts with person and environment that defines the central concern of the profession. They further suggest that this means occupational therapists are only concerned with person factors (e.g., spirituality, range of motion, memory, and mood) and environments (e.g., physical accessibility, social and cultural expectations, and legal limits on humans) when they impact occupation.

2.7.2 Model of Human Occupation

The Model of Human Occupation (MOHO) (Kielhofner, 2008) was developed in the 1980s and has become one of the most widely used models in occupational therapy. Interestingly, there is no concept in the MOHO that is named "occupation" and the model instead uses a taxonomy to distinguish between three levels in which a person engages in occupation: occupational participation, occupational performance, and occupational skill. Occupational participation represents the highest level in the MOHO and is probably most closely aligned with occupation. Occupational participation is about "engaging in work, play, or activities of daily living (ADL) that are part of one's sociocultural context and that are desired and/or necessary to one's well-being" (Forsyth et al., 2019, p. 509). A taxonomy of types of occupations is used and explicit links to context and health are made clear.

The other two key concepts within the MOHO include person and environment, each with a number of elements. Person includes volition (personal causation, values, interests), habituation (habits, roles), and performance capacity (underlying mental and physical abilities). Environment is seen as "the particular physical, social, cultural, economic, and political features" (Forsyth et al., 2019, p. 508) the person exists within. The model also includes another group of concepts: occupational identity, occupational competence, and occupational adaptation.

2.7.3 Occupational Therapy Practice Framework – 4th Edition

What is now the OTPF-4 (AOTA, 2020) began as "uniform terminology" documents as long ago as the late 1970s. Although it's not a model by any definition in the literature, the OTPF-4 is used as such in some areas and compared to the other models presented here, the OTPF-4 does not focus narrowly on occupation. Although occupation and related concepts are included in the document, it goes further to present an occupational therapy process. Nonetheless, occupation is defined in the OTPF-4 using the definition from the WFOT (2012, para 2): "occupations refer to the everyday activities that people do as individuals, in families and with communities to occupy time and bring meaning and purpose to life. Occupations include things people need to, want to and are expected to do".

Another key difference between the OTPF-4 and other models is that it is not grounded in a single theoretical perspective or body of research. Instead, it draws on a wide range of occupational therapy and occupational science theories and research. For example, the document includes concepts from the MOHO (Kielhofner, 2008), the Assessment of Motor and Process Skills (Fisher & Bray Jones, 2011), and the International Classification of Functioning, Disability and Health (World Health Organization, 2001).

2.7.4 Human Subsystems that Influence Occupation

The final model presented here is the Human Subsystems that Influence Occupation (HSIO) (Clark et al., 1991). The HSIO is not well known but is presented as an example of a model that was developed within occupational science, and as such it was not concerned with occupational therapy practice (not initially at least), unlike the other models presented in this section. In fact, because it was developed as part of the process of establishing both occupational science and obtaining approval for a PhD program in occupational science at the University of Southern California, it was envisioned as a "blueprint from which the research activities of the faculty and students flow" (Clark et al., 1991, p. 303).

The HSIO was developed using general systems theory and presents the person "as an open system in interaction with his or her environment over the entire life span" (Clark et al., 1991, p. 302). Occupation is seen as the output of the human system in response to environmental circumstances and is defined as "chunks of culturally and personally meaningful activity in which humans engage that can be named in the lexicon of our culture" (USC Department of Occupational Therapy, 1989, as cited in Clark et al., 1991, p. 301). The environmental circumstances identified in the HSIO include sociocultural and historical contexts as well as environmental challenges. The internal human subsystems are transcendental, symbolic-evaluative, sociocultural, information processing, biological, and physical.

2.7.5 Different but Similar

The purpose of this section was not to provide a solid grounding in different models, but to identify that one of the ways occupation has been conceptualized in the professional literature is either as a focus of, or part of, a model. A second purpose was to encourage readers not to be overwhelmed by the multitude of models in the profession, but to recognize instead that each model is merely the perspective of one person or group of people. Furthermore, because the models all essentially focus on occupation or humans as occupational beings, there are perhaps more similarities than differences. Each of the models presented here, and many others, can be viewed as different ways of viewing persons, environments, and occupation, as demonstrated in Table 2.3.

2.8 Conclusion

This chapter has presented several ways occupation is conceptualized within occupational therapy and occupational science. The aim was to support readers in navigating the different ways occupation is presented in the literature and in professional conversations – sometimes as seemingly succinct and clear definitions, sometimes as one location in a taxonomy, sometimes in contrast to the term "activity", and at other times within models. While all are useful, it is important that readers are mindful of how the term "occupation" is being used and to also become more precise in their own use of the term. Greater precision in our use of terminology will enable a more robust engagement with occupation as the central idea within occupational therapy and occupational science.

Readers are also reminded that the ideas presented in this chapter are from largely white, Western, middle to upper class, individualistic, Christian, imperialist, neoliberal, and industrialized perspectives. Readers are therefore prompted to be critical of what

Table 2.3 Comparison of Occupation, Person, and Environment across Four Models

	CMOPE	MOHO	OTPF-4	HSIO
Occupation	Self-care, productivity, leisure	Occupational participation, occupational performance, occupational skills	Activities of daily living, instrumental activities of daily living, health management, rest and sleep, education, work, play, leisure, social participation	Occupation
Person	Spirituality, physical, cognitive, affective	Volition (personal causation, values, interests), habituation (habits, roles), performance capacity (physical and mental abilities)	Context – person factors; performance patterns – habits, routines, roles, rituals; performance skills – motor, process, social interaction; client factors – values, beliefs, spirituality, body functions, body structures	Transcendental, symbolic-evaluative, sociocultural, information processing, biological, physical
Environment	Physical, social, cultural, institutional	Physical, social, cultural, economic, political	Context – environmental factors	Sociocultural and historical context, environmental challenges

Note: CMOPE: Canadian Model of Occupational Performance and Engagement; HSIO: Human Subsystems that Influence Occupation; MOHO: Model of Human Occupation; OTPF-4: Occupational Therapy Practice Framework – 4th Edition.

has been presented in this chapter, as well as in other literature they read and in ideas presented during any professional communication. In recent years, the profession has begun to recognize that some groups of people have been silenced in our theory development. It is important, therefore, that part of our critical engagement with the profession's concepts must be consideration of who and what has been silenced, and who and what has been privileged.

2.9 Summary
- Occupation is the core concept in occupational therapy and occupational science.
- Due to its complexity, numerous ways of conceptualizing occupation have been presented in the literature.

- Specificity of language is important for effective communication in practice, education, and research.
- Most theories and conceptualizations of occupation have developed in largely white, Western, middle to upper class, individualistic, Christian, imperialist, neoliberal, and industrialized contexts.
- There are four ways that occupation has been presented in the literature: definitions, taxonomies, occupation and other terms, and models.
- Understanding the ways occupation is presented will enable a more sophisticated use of the literature and language related to occupation.

2.10 Review Questions
1. Why is the oversimplification of occupation problematic?
2. What are the different perspectives that have shaped how occupation is conceptualized?
3. What are the four ways that occupation has been conceptualized?
4. How are activity and occupation used in the literature?
5. What are the similarities and differences between the models presented in this chapter?

References

American Occupational Therapy Association. (2020). Occupational therapy practice framework: Domain and process (4th ed.). *American Journal of Occupational Therapy, 74*(Suppl. 2), 7412410010p1–7412410010p87. https://doi.org/10.5014/ajot.2020.74S2001

Breines, E. (1995). Understanding 'occupation' as the founders did. *British Journal of Occupational Therapy, 58*(11), 458–460. https://doi.org/10.1177/030802269505801102

Burley, S., Di Tommaso, A., Cox, R., & Molineux, M. (2018). An occupational perspective in hand therapy: A scoping review. *British Journal of Occupational Therapy, 81*(6), 299–318. https://doi.org/10.1177/0308022617752110

Canadian Association of Occupational Therapists. (1997). *Enabling occupation: An occupational therapy perspective*. CAOT.

Chapparo, C., Ranka, J., & Nott, M. (2017). Occupational Performance Model (Australia): A description of constructs, structure and propositions. In M. Curtin, M. Egan, & J. Adams (Eds.), *Occupational therapy for people experiencing illness, inury or impairment: Promoting occupation and participation* (7th ed., pp. 134–147). Elsevier.

Clark, F., Parham, D., Carlson, M., Frank, G., Jackson, J., Pierce, D., Wolfe, R., & Zemke, R. (1991). Occupational science: Academic innovation in the service of occupational therapy's future. *American Journal of Occupational Therapy, 45*(4), 300–310. https://doi.org/10.5014/ajot.45.4.300

Dickie, V. (2016). A course in occupational science for occupational therapy students. *Journal of Occupational Science, 23*(4), 519–524. https://doi.org/10.1080/14427591.2016.1230929

Di Tommaso, A., Wicks, A., Scarvell, J., & Isbel, S. (2019). Experiences of occupation-based practice: An Australian phenomenological study of recently graduated occupational therapists. *British Journal of Occupational Therapy, 82*(7), 412–421. https://doi.org/10.1177/0308022618823656

Egan, M., & Restall, G. (2022). The Canadian model of occupational participation. In M. Egan & G. Restall (Eds.), *Promoting occupational participation: Collaborative relationship-focused occupational therapy* (pp. 73–95). CAOT.

Fisher, A., & Bray Jones, K. (2011). *Assessment of motor and process skills: Volume 1 – Development, standardisation, and administration manual* (7th ed.). Three Stars Press.

Forsyth, K., Taylor, R. E., Kramer, J., Prior, S., Richie, L., Whitehead, J., Owen, C., & Melton, J. (2019). The model of human occupation. In B. B. Schell, G. Gillen, M. Scaffa, & E. Cohn (Eds.), *Willard and Spackman's occupational therapy* (12th ed., pp. 505–526). Lippincott Williams & Wilkins.

Golledge, J. (1998). Distinguishing between occupation, purposeful activity and activity, Part 1: Review and explanation. *British Journal of Occupational Therapy, 61*(3), 100–105. https://doi.org/10.1177/030802269806100301

Grenier, M.-L. (2020). Cultural competency and the reproduction of White supremacy in occupational therapy education. *Health Education Journal, 79*(6), 633–644. https://doi.org/10.1177/0017896920902515

Hammell, K. (2009). Sacred texts: A sceptical exploration of the assumptions underpinning theories of occupation. *Canadian Journal of Occupational Therapy, 76*, 6–13. https://doi.org/10.1177/000841740907600105

Harvey, A., & Pentland, W. (2010). What do people do? In C. Christiansen & E. Townsend (Eds.), *Introduction to occupation: The art and science of living* (2nd ed., pp. 101–133). Prentice Hall.

Hocking, C. (2009). The challenge of occupation: Describing the things people do. *Journal of Occupational Science, 16*(3), 140–150. https://doi.org/10.1080/14427591.2009.9686655

Iwama, M. (2003). Towards culturally relevant epistemologies in occupational therapy. *American Journal of Occupational Therapy, 57*(5), 582–588. https://doi.org/10.5014/ajot.57.5.582

Kantartzis, S., & Molineux, M. (2012). Understanding the discursive development of occupation: Historico-political perspectives. In G. Whiteford & C. Hocking (Eds.), *Occupational science: Society, inclusion, participation* (pp. 38–53). Blackwell. https://doi.org/10.1002/9781118281581.ch4

Kielhofner, G. (Ed.). (2008). *Model of human occupation: Theory and application* (4th ed.). Lippincott Williams & Wilkins.

Kielhofner, G. (2009). *Conceptual foundations of occupational therapy practice* (4th ed.). F. A. Davis.

Kuhn, T. (1996). *The structure of scientific revolutions* (3rd ed.). University of Chicago Press.

Laliberte Rudman, D., & Aldrich, R. (2017). Occupational science. In M. Curtin, J. Adams, & M. Egan (Eds.), *Occupational therapy for people experiencing illness, injury or impairment* (7th ed., pp. 17–27). Elsevier.

Laliberte Rudman, D., Aldrich, R., & Kiepek, N. (2022). Evolving understandings of occupation. In M. Egan & G. Restall (Eds.), *Promoting occupational participation: Collaborative relationship-focused occupational therapy* (pp. 11–30). CAOT.

Lavalley, R., & Johnson, K. R. (2020). Occupation, injustice, and anti-Black racism in the United States of America. *Journal of Occupational Science, 29*(4), 487–499. https://doi.org/10.1080/14427591.2020.1810111

Malkawi, S. H., Alqatarneh, N. S., & Fehringer, E. K. (2020). The influence of culture on occupational therapy practice in Jordan. *Occupational Therapy International, 1092805*. https://doi.org/10.1155/2020/1092805

Molineux, M. (2009). The nature of occupation. In M. Curtin, M. Molineux, & J. Supyk-Mellson (Eds.), *Occupational therapy and physical dysfunction: Enabling occupation* (6th ed., pp. 17–26). Elsevier.

Murray, A., Di Tommaso, A., Molineux, M., Young, A., & Power, P. (2020). Contemporary occupational therapy philosophy and practice in hospital settings. *Scandinavian Journal of Occupational Therapy, 28*(3), 213–224. https://doi.org/10.1080/11038128.2020.1750691

Ozelie, R., Sipple, C., Foy, T., Cantoni, K., Kellogg, K., Lookingbill, J., Backus, D., & Gassaway, J. (2009). SCIRehab Project series: The occupational therapy taxonomy. *Journal of Spinal Cord Medicine, 32*(3), 283–297. https://doi.org/10.1080/10790268.2009.11760782

Pierce, D. (2001). Untangling occupation and activity. *American Journal of Occupational Therapy, 55*(2), 138–146. https://doi.org/10.5014/ajot.55.2.138

Polatajko, H., Davis, J., Hobson, S., Landry, J., Mandich, A., Street, S., Whippey, E., & Yee, S. (2004). Meeting the responsibility that comes with the privilege: Introducing a taxonomic code for understanding occupation. *Canadian Journal of Occupational Therapy, 71*(5), 261–264. https://doi.org/10.1177/000841740407100503

Polatajko, H., Davis, J., Stewart, D., Cantin, N., Amoroso, B., Purdie, L., & Zimmerman, D. (2013). Specifying the domain of concern: Occupation as core. In E. Townsend & H. Polatajko (Eds.), *Enabling occupation II: Advancing an occupational therapy vision for health, well-being, & justice through occupation* (2nd ed., pp. 13–36). CAOT.

Ryan, A., Gilroy, J., & Gibson, C. (2020). #Changethedate: Advocacy as an on-line and decolonising occupation. *Journal of Occupational Science, 27*(3), 405–416. https://doi.org/10.1080/14427591.2020.1759448

Soderback, I., & Magill, K. (2015). Towards a taxonomy of occupational therapy interventions: A comparative literature analysis of scientific review publications published 2008–2013. In I. Soderback (Ed.), *International handbook of occupational therapy interventions* (2nd ed., pp. 27–52). Springer. https://doi.org/10.1007/978-3-319-08141-0

Steward, B. (1995). Maps and models. *British Journal of Therapy and Rehabilitation, 2*(7), 359–363. https://doi.org/10.12968/bjtr.1995.2.7.359

Sullivan, W. (1995). *Work and integrity: The crisis and promise of professionalism in America.* Jossey-Bass.

Tornquist, K., & Sonn, U. (2014). Towards an ADL taxonomy for occupational therapists. Previously published in *Scandinavian Journal of Occupational Therapy* 1994; 1:69–76. *Scandinavian Journal of Occupational Therapy, 21*(Suppl 1), 20–27. https://doi.org/10.3109/11038128.2014.952885

Wood, W. (1996). Legitimizing occupational therapy's knowledge. *American Journal of Occupational Therapy, 50*(3), 626–634. https://doi.org/10.5014/ajot.50.8.626

World Federation of Occupational Therapists. (2012). *About occupational therapy.* https://www.wfot.org/about/about-occupational-therapy

World Health Organization. (2001). *International classification of functioning, disability and health: ICF.* WHO.

Yerxa, E. (1988). Oversimplification: The hobgoblin of theory and practice in occupational therapy. *Canadian Journal of Occupational Therapy, 55*(1), 5–6. https://doi.org/10.1177/000841748805500101

Yerxa, E., Clark, F., Jackson, J., Parham, D., Pierce, D., Stein, C., & Zemke, R. (1990). An introduction to occupational science, A foundation for occupational therapy in the 21st century. *Occupational Therapy in Health Care, 6*(4), 1–17. https://doi.org/10.1080/J003v06n04_04

CHAPTER 3

Overview of Occupation-centered Practice

Louise Gustafsson and Matthew Molineux

Abstract
Occupation is at the core of the profession's philosophy and occupation-centered practice is the term applied when occupation is at the core of occupational therapy practice. This chapter will critically explore the terms occupation-centered, occupation-based, and occupation-focused which are often used in literature and practice. Theoretical and research-based evidence will be discussed to demonstrate how occupational therapy can be made more occupation-centered. This will include changes that can be made by individual occupational therapists, workplaces, and professional bodies. Strategies for enhancing occupation-centered practice and clinical scenarios and vignettes are included to enhance understanding.

Authors' Positionality Statement
The authors of this chapter have experiences of working with clients and their families in acute and rehabilitation services in hospitals and the community, as well as extensive experience working with students as occupational therapy educators and researchers in higher education, in Australia, and in the United Kingdom. We therefore acknowledge our perspective as influenced by our Western, English-speaking, university-educated, professionally qualified, cisgendered, and privileged experiences. We also acknowledge that we have experience of being members of minority groups or groups that are discriminated against, and that has also shaped our perspective.

Objectives
This chapter will allow the reader to:

- Recognize the key characteristics of occupation-centered practice.
- Recognize the value of occupation-centered practice.

DOI: 10.4324/9781003504610-4

- Understand that change is required at multiple levels of the profession to support occupation-centered practice.
- Identify strategies to enhance occupation-centered practice.

Key terms
- occupation-centered
- occupation-based
- occupation-focused
- occupational science

3.1 Introduction

Occupation-centered practice should be the defining feature of occupational therapy, as it signifies the unique contribution of occupational therapists to clients, colleagues, funders, and policymakers. However, despite the espoused focus of the profession on people as occupational beings who experience occupational issues, not all occupational therapy practice is occupation-centered. This chapter describes the historical and current paradigms of the profession and recognizes that the profession has been working for over 20 years to reconnect to occupation as the core of all that we do. The terminology introduced by Anne Fisher (2013) is defined and described with examples to clarify what occupation-centered, occupation-based, and occupation-focused practice might look like. The complexity of occupation-centered practice is then explored, before strategies for enacting occupation-centered practice are presented.

3.2 Occupation and Occupational Therapy

Occupational therapy was founded on the assumption that engaging in occupations was beneficial for health. The initial evidence for the relationship between occupation and health came from the personal experiences of the founders of the profession. Founders in the United States, e.g., included George Edward Barton who had first-hand experience of receiving occupation as therapy after hysterical paralysis on one side of his body, and the nurse Susan Elizabeth Tracy who observed that patients who were occupied appeared to cope better with their situation than those who were not (Peloquin, 1991). In the United Kingdom, Elizabeth Casson noticed a change in the mood of patients at a hospital for people with mental health issues on the day they started hanging the Christmas decorations (Hilton, 2022). Since those early days, occupation has held a place in occupational therapy, but it has not always been as prominent as it was in the time of the profession's founders.

Kielhofner (2009) provided a useful history of the profession which showed that occupation held a central place in the philosophy and practice of the profession during the initial Paradigm of Occupation. However, occupation fell out of favor when the profession was forced to become more scientific to align itself more closely with the medical profession, and so the Mechanistic Paradigm emerged. During that paradigm, occupational therapists began to view humans as systems with constituent parts. Problems arose when those parts did not work correctly due to injury or illness and so the role of the occupational therapist was to either fix the faulty aspect or create a way for the person to still engage in their daily activities. Eventually, occupational therapists began to see that the mechanistic approach was not particularly effective, especially for people with chronic ill health, and so there was a renewed interest in occupation which gave rise to the Contemporary Paradigm (Kielhofner, 2009). This current paradigm of occupational therapy focuses on humans as occupational beings and views the problems people face as occupational problems and the interventions occupational therapists provide as occupation-based (Kielhofner, 2009).

For over 20 years, since what some have called the renaissance of occupation (Whiteford et al., 2000), occupational therapists around the world have been trying to reconnect with occupation. This is because occupational therapists have realized that it is an occupational perspective of humans and health that distinguishes them from other professions and enables their contribution to society. Despite these attempts, many (but not all) occupational therapists continue to find it difficult to work in ways that are clearly and explicitly concerned with occupation (Britton et al., 2016; Di Tommaso et al., 2016; Molineux, 2004). Fisher (2013) summarized the issue clearly when she said that "we do not always respond to our mandate and use interventions and evaluation methods that reflect the central power of occupation" (p. 163).

Occupation is what makes the profession unique – no other profession has the same knowledge and skills in occupation and its relationship with health. Yet, it proves challenging for occupational therapists and students to talk about occupation with confidence and authority, to understand their clients as occupational beings with occupational challenges, and to devise intervention programs that involve engaging clients in occupations. A significant change since the founding of the profession is that while practice was based on assumption and personal experience in the early days, there is now a growing evidence base to support occupational therapy practice that is grounded in occupation (see, e.g., Ciro et al., 2014; Pellegrini et al., 2018; Pillastrini et al., 2008).

3.3 Terminology

In this chapter, we have adopted the definitions articulated by Fisher (2013) to assist occupational therapists to think about the place of occupation in occupational therapy practice. We have purposefully adopted occupation-centered practice as the chapter title to emphasize the importance of occupation at the core of all that we do as occupational therapists. This contrasts with occupation-based which places emphasis on evaluation and intervention only (Fisher, 2013). Table 3.1 presents the terms as differentiated by Fisher.

While the terms are clear at first reading, consideration of their use in practice highlights that these are in fact difficult concepts to grasp, and it can seem that the boundaries between them are sometimes blurred. It is very clear that adopting an occupation-centered approach during assessment requires an occupational therapist and client to identify challenges with occupational performance and engagement, and agree upon goals to address the occupational challenges or issues. Purists might argue that if an occupational therapist is truly occupation-centered, then intervention would

Table 3.1 Definitions of Terms from Fisher (2013)

- Occupation-centered: "to adopt a profession-specific perspective… where occupation is placed in the centre and ensures that what we do is linked to the core paradigm of occupational therapy" (p. 167).
- Occupation-based: "to use occupation as the foundation – to engage the person in occupation… as the method used for evaluation and/or intervention" (p. 167).
- Occupation-focused: "to focus one's attention on occupation – to have occupation as the proximal (i.e., immediate) focus of the evaluation or the proximal intent of the intervention" (p. 167).

engage the client in occupations (Molineux, 2010). However, this is not the case in Fisher's (2013) original paper. She proposed that an intervention that involved client attendance at an educational seminar, although not occupation-based, may be occupation-focused and therefore an appropriate occupational therapy intervention. This point was clarified further by Fisher and Marterella (2019) who explained that an educational group is only occupation-focused if the attendees are learning about or discussing occupations. If the focus of the group is on strategies for managing changes to body structures and functions, these groups would not be considered occupation-focused.

Given the complexity of these terms, some illustrative examples follow to support your understanding of the terms within practice.

3.4 Occupation-centered

Practice is occupation-centered when the therapist views every aspect of their work from an occupational lens and so the client is viewed as an occupational being and occupation is at the center of our professional reasoning. Consider when you first meet a client, where does your professional reasoning start? Is your focus on the diagnosis and the impact on the person's body structure and functions? Or is your focus on the occupational issues the person is experiencing? If your focus is on the latter, you likely place occupation at the center and your practice is more likely to include evaluations and interventions that are designed to understand the occupational issues experienced by the person, and to devise interventions that engage the person in occupation. An example of occupation at the core is provided in the brief vignette about Remy.

> Remy (33 years old) is a violinist in a well-regarded symphony orchestra and is in hospital following a left hemisphere stroke. Remy is experiencing low mood and the occupational therapist recognizes that engaging with music and playing the violin are important occupations for Remy. Remy is encouraged to ask someone to bring recordings of the orchestra and the violin into the hospital. The occupational therapist and Remy incorporate the recordings and the violin into their work together. With some adaptation, Remy can hold the bow in their right hand, and although they are initially unable to draw the bow across the strings, they spend time each day listening to the recordings and working towards their goal of playing the violin by handling the violin and bow.

In this vignette, the occupational therapist is occupation-centered because they considered Remy as an occupational being and identified occupations that impact on

OVERVIEW OF OCCUPATION-CENTERED PRACTICE

Remy's health and well-being. This resulted in the occupational therapist being both occupation-based (engaging the client in an occupation by using the recording and the violin in therapy) and occupation-focused (the occupation of playing the violin is the proximal focus of intervention).

3.5 Occupation-based

Practice is occupation-based when there is direct engagement in occupation during evaluation and intervention. That is, evaluation is occupation-based when clients are observed while engaging in occupation. Similarly, intervention is occupation-based when the client is engaged in occupation. In the following vignette, both the evaluation and intervention involve engagement in occupation, and so practice is occupation-based.

> Aisha is 12 years old, lives with her family, attends school, and spends time with friends. Aisha has a visual impairment and wants to learn to independently don (put on) their hijab. Firstly, the occupational therapist who was unfamiliar with the steps involved in putting on a hijab observed Aisha's older sister during the occupation. The occupational therapist then observed Aisha and completed an occupation analysis. The occupational therapist and Aisha discussed the observations from the occupation analysis and worked collaboratively to identify the steps in preparing the hijab, placing the hijab onto Aisha's head, and adjusting and securing the hijab into position on Aisha's head and upper body. Aisha and the occupational therapist used part-practice to successfully learn to complete each step, prior to whole-practice towards the end of each session.

In this vignette, the occupational therapist demonstrates occupation-based practice because Aisha is engaged in the occupation of putting on the hijab as part of assessment, when the occupational therapist completes an occupation analysis, and then again during intervention when different stages of putting on the hijab are practiced before the whole occupation is attempted.

3.6 Occupation-focused

Fisher and Marterella (2019) identified that there is a continuum along which we can evaluate the extent to which practice is occupation-focused. At one end of the continuum, occupation has the proximal focus, while the other end of the continuum identifies that practice may have body functions, the environment, or other contextual factors as the proximal focus. In the following vignette, we introduce how practice may have an initial proximal focus on environment (in this case assistive technology).

> Alex (73 years old) lives in a third level apartment block with his spouse. Alex enjoyed being able to walk across the road to a supermarket to collect groceries and join a regular social group at the coffee shop. However, Alex is no longer able to engage in those occupations because he can no longer walk the distances required due to a medical condition and frequent falls. Alex and his occupational therapist discuss a motorized scooter as a solution and assessment for the motorized scooter is an initial focus of their work together. While assessment is focused on the practicalities of the motorized scooter (e.g., does it fit Alex's body, can Alex use the controls, can Alex store the scooter?) practice is not occupation-focused.

Next, the occupational therapist completes an occupation analysis of Alex completing the shopping while using the motorized scooter. The focus is on the occupation of grocery shopping.

The focus of practice may at one point be on the person (body functions or structure) or the environment (assistive devices or home modification) and so it does not have a proximal focus on occupation. However, once the person or environmental factors are addressed, the focus can then shift toward occupation. Fisher and Marterella (2019) highlight that the best way to identify when practice is occupation-focused is to consider where the client's attention is focused. When their attention is directed by the occupational therapist toward occupation, then practice is likely to be occupation-focused. Alternatively, if the client's attention is focused toward increasing grip strength or choosing an assistive product, occupation is a distal focus and therefore practice has a body function or environmental focus.

3.7 The Complexity of Occupation-centered Practice

Fisher and Marterella (2019) identified that evaluations and interventions can be occupation-based but not occupation-focused. This may initially sound impossible, but there are circumstances where it is possible. For example, when conducting a home evaluation, the occupational therapist may ask the client to complete occupations within the home and so the practice is occupation-based. However, the proximal focus of the occupational therapist and the client is toward the identification of environmental enablers and barriers, and not the occupational performance and engagement. At this point, the proximal focus or purpose of the evaluation is to direct environmental modifications and their attention is directed toward the environment and not the occupational performance and engagement. Similarly, occupational therapy practice can be occupation-focused but not occupation-based (Fisher & Marterella, 2019). We previously provided the example of an educational group when the focus of the discussion is occupation. This group is considered occupation-focused but not occupation-based because there is no direct engagement in the occupation during the session. However, if the group were to include direct engagement in the occupations discussed, then the practice would be both occupation-based and occupation-focused.

Occupational therapy conceptual practice models place occupation at the core of our practice, but they also encourage us to think about person, environment, and other contextual elements or influences. As a result, occupational therapy practice may at times move away from occupation to address person, environmental, or contextual influences. It is the responsibility of occupational therapy students and practitioners to deliberately reflect on their practice, identify when their practice is moving along the continuum toward or away from occupation, and make deliberate decisions that ensure we are able to articulate how occupation is positioned in our evaluation and intervention.

Given the complexity of occupation-centered practice, a recent scoping review sought to understand the extent to which Fisher's (2013) terms had been adopted in the literature. Ford et al. (2021) found that only some papers had used the terms as defined by Fisher, many papers used the terms but did not define them at all, and that occupation-based and occupation-focused were used interchangeably. A subsequent Delphi study with a panel of international experts aimed to further understand how the term occupation-centered was understood and operationalized (Ford et al., 2022). Participants included academics and clinicians from many countries who were asked about occupation-centered practice over a three-round Delphi process. Participants suggested that the following ideas were characteristic of occupation-centered practice (Ford et al., 2022, p. 31):

1. Occupation-centered practice is grounded in theory and philosophy which recognizes the importance of occupation to health and well-being.
2. In occupation-centered practice, occupation and occupational terminology are prioritized in verbal and written communication.
3. Occupation-centered practice requires occupational therapists to understand and consider the contextual aspects that influence occupations. The "gold standard" is that people engage in occupations, as part of occupational therapy, in the natural context.
4. Occupation-centered practice has occupation at the core of assessment, goal setting, and intervention.

It therefore appears that the panel of international experts probably agreed with Fisher's (2013) definition of occupation-centered practice. Furthermore, it appears that they rolled up occupation-based and occupation-focused into occupation-centered, or at the very least confirmed that occupation-centered is the overarching concept. The findings support the definition of occupation-centered practice as having occupation at the core of occupational therapy practice, and that it should be readily visible in occupational therapists' work with clients, as well as how they speak and write about their work.

It is worth noting a challenge that Ford et al. (2022) experienced when analyzing data from the Delphi rounds. They had difficulty "trying to distinguish between characteristics of occupation-centered practice and what may be seen as 'standard' characteristics of occupational therapy practice" (Ford et al., 2022, p. 33). Examples of the concepts and processes that their participants identified as central to occupation-centered practice included being client-led and collaborative goal setting. Most occupational therapists would argue that both of those examples are fundamental to all occupational therapy practice, regardless of how occupation-centered that practice might be. After all, client-centeredness is well documented as key to occupational therapy (Townsend & Polatajko, 2013), as is collaborative goal setting (Costa et al., 2017). It is important for occupational therapy students and practitioners to remember that occupation-centered practice cannot be achieved by client-centeredness and collaborative goal setting alone.

3.8 Enacting Occupation-centered Practice

Throughout the profession's history, and particularly in recent times, a focus on enabling occupation and its use in therapy has not always been central to practice (Bryden & McColl, 2003; Whiteford et al., 2000; Wilding & Whiteford, 2007, 2008). The attention given to occupation by many, but not all, occupational therapists is at best not explicit and at worst is inadequate. This can be partly explained by the dominance of the medical model, the associated pressure to provide empirical justifications for practice, and the increasing specialization of healthcare systems and therefore many healthcare practitioners.

Conforming to the culture of a workplace, especially where the view of humans and health is biomedical, can be very limiting for occupational therapists' profession-specific reasoning. Wilding and Whiteford's (2009) collaborative action research study of occupational therapy practice in an acute hospital setting found that occupational therapists conformed to the dominant medical culture of prioritizing physical and impairment-based intervention, and that this adversely affected therapists' ability to think and talk about occupational therapy-specific values.

Some occupational therapists feel undervalued by their team members because the occupational perspective of humans and health was not understood by their colleagues (Murray et al., 2020). As a result, occupational therapists feel less able to implement practice which is grounded in occupation, which likely perpetuates misunderstanding by members of the multidisciplinary team. Other research has suggested that occupational therapists may have a knowledge gap in relation to occupation-centered practice. Murray et al. (2019) conducted interviews with occupational therapists working in a highly specialized acute hospital setting and found that some participants struggled to describe the core of occupational therapy. Other studies have also documented that some occupational therapists recognize that they lack knowledge and skills to deliver occupation-centered practice (Murray et al., 2020). It is likely therefore that occupational therapists who do not have current knowledge about, and skills in, occupation-centered practice will be unable to implement occupation-centered practice in their work.

3.8.1 Strategies to Support Occupation-centered Practice

Although there are barriers to implementing occupation-centered practice, there is a large amount of advice available to support occupational therapists to be more occupation-centered in their work with clients.

1. *Know about occupation and the relationship between occupation and health.*

    In order to deliver occupation-centered practice, occupational therapists must be knowledgeable about occupation and the relationship between occupation and health, and to have the skills to use that knowledge in practice. It is therefore important that time is devoted to re-engaging with the core philosophy and paradigm of the profession to build and refresh knowledge and skills as understanding develops.

    This chapter has provided you with definitions and introductory information that assists you to start to interrogate your practice and understand what is, or isn't, occupation-centered, -based, or -focused. You could explore the references included in this chapter, or other occupational therapy or occupational science literature that examines occupation and the relationship between occupation and health. You could also:

    - Use occupational therapy theory and conceptual practice models to guide and justify your practice.
    - Have regular team meetings that focus on exploration of the theory and skills of occupation-centered practice.
    - Seek out people with expertise in and experience of being occupation-centered and discuss your practice with them.

2. *Prioritize occupation-centered practice.*
   It is possible to work in ways that are occupation-centered if there is a commitment to do so – either individually or collectively. Some of our unpublished research shows that prioritizing time to engage in practice development programs was pivotal to occupational therapists changing their practice. Some illustrative examples of successful strategies include the following:

   - Including occupation-centered practice in the vision and/or mission of the service.
   - Supervisors or managers who support the allocation of time for individuals to prioritize occupation-centered practice in their professional development.
   - Supervisors and managers who include discussions about occupation-centered practice in supervision sessions and provide professional development opportunities about occupation-centered practice.
   - All occupational therapy staff agreeing to articulate their contribution to the service/organization using occupation as the key feature.

3. *Use tools that support occupation-centered practice.*
   There are a number of tools that can be used to support or enhance occupation-centered practice and these can be used either by individual occupational therapists or by whole departments which might agree to incorporate them as part of their standard practice.

   - The Assessment of Motor and Process Skills (AMPS) (Fisher & Bray Jones, 2011) is a standardized well-researched assessment tool that not only focuses on occupation as the medium for assessment, but provides detailed insights into the person and environmental factors that impact occupational performance and engagement.
   - The Canadian Occupational Performance Measure (COPM) (Law et al., 2014) is another assessment tool that engages the client in a discussion about occupations in order to identify current occupational issues. While it does not include engaging the client in occupation, the focus of the discussion is clearly on the occupations the client wants, needs, and has to do.
   - Occupation analysis is a fundamental skill that occupational therapists learn in their education. The value of occupation analysis is that it can be used anywhere, with any client, with any occupation. The outcome of a full occupation analysis is a better understanding of the client as an occupational being, as well as the person, environment, and occupation factors that are enabling and inhibiting their occupational performance and engagement.
   - The Cognitive Orientation to daily Occupational Performance (CO-OP) (Dawson et al., 2017) is an intervention approach that provides support to clients to improve their ability to engage in their occupations. The approach has been used successfully with children and adults by providing them with strategies they can use to be successful in their chosen occupations.
   - Group-based interventions that engage group members in occupations, rather than body structures and functions like some occupational therapy groups, can result in significant changes in self-efficacy, performance, and satisfaction (Spalding et al., 2023).

4. *Use occupational language.*

   The language of occupation is uniquely understood by the profession and evidences the unique contribution of occupational therapy to our colleagues and clients. It is therefore vital that occupational therapists use that language to describe what we do in formal and informal, written and verbal communications. Some therapists have reported that as they become more knowledgeable about occupation, then their language changes, while others have found that using occupational language in the first instance caused them to expand their knowledge and skills. We must be clear with ourselves and our colleagues that occupation does not equate function, a term commonly used in many practice settings. Related strategies that support occupation-centered practice include the following:

   - Explaining our contribution to clients and colleagues with occupation as the proximal concern.
   - Changing the template for reporting or recording progress to include headings such as "Occupational Issue" and reporting under headings such as occupation, environment, and person.
   - Providing explanations of occupational therapy to the fullest extent of your role to open conversations about occupation.
   - When providing a handover of a client, start with a description of the person as an occupational being and not the diagnosis, e.g., "Mr Arrow is a pastry chef and a volunteer at the local homeless shelter. He is experiencing occupational issues in [insert relevant occupations here] due to a recent diagnosis of [insert relevant diagnosis here]".

5. *Conversations about occupation are powerful, but engaging is better.*

   It is one thing to say that occupation is at the core of occupational therapy and to use occupational language, but we must prioritize the incorporation of occupation into assessment, goal setting, intervention, and evaluation. Occupational therapists have a stronger professional identity when their practice is occupation-centered (Estes & Pierce, 2012; Murray et al., 2020). More importantly, client outcomes are greater when therapy is meaningful and individualized to the specific occupational issues of the client (Estes & Pierce, 2012). Examples of strategies to support engagement in occupations include the following:

   - Ensuring that documented goals are occupation-centered.
   - Commencing assessment with occupation-based assessment tools (e.g., AMPS and occupation analysis), or occupation-focused tools (e.g., COPM).
   - Including occupation-based interventions in your practice (e.g., CO-OP).
   - Adapting the environment to support opportunities for clients to discover/engage in occupations.
   - Looking for other places to meet that are more natural such as hospital coffee shops or outdoor gardens, rather than bedside on the ward.

3.9 Conclusion

Occupation is the concept that defines occupational therapy as a profession and so it should define occupational therapy practice. The profession and individual occupational therapists have struggled for many decades to embrace and enact an occupational approach to practice. Occupation-centered practice is the term given to occupational therapy practice which adopts an occupational perspective at all stages of the occupational therapy process. It can be challenging to enact occupation-centered practice as an individual due to lack of knowledge and skills, lack of confidence, and/or because of the power of workplace paradigms and approaches that are not concerned with occupation. This chapter has explored occupation-centered practice and related terms, and acknowledged some of the challenges occupational therapists face in working in that way. The chapter also included an overview of some key strategies that occupational therapists can use to enact occupation-centered practice. While it may not always be easy, it is important that all occupational therapists embrace and deliver occupation-centered practice so that clients can reap maximum benefits, and so we can demonstrate our value to colleagues, funders, and policymakers.

3.10 Summary

- Occupational therapy was founded on the belief in the power of occupation to influence health.
- The place of occupation in the practice of occupational therapists has varied greatly over the 20th and 21st centuries.
- The terms occupation-centered, occupation-based, and occupation-focused provide some help in reflecting on practice.
- Enacting occupation-centered practice can be challenging for several reasons, but it is imperative that occupational therapists deliver practice grounded in occupation.
- There are several strategies that can be used to support occupational therapists, individually and collectively, to enact occupation-centered practice.

3.11 Review Questions

1. Explain why it is important for occupational therapists to work in an occupation-centered way.
2. Describe the relationship between occupation-centered, occupation-based, and occupation-focused.
3. Describe one strategy that you can apply as an individual to enable you to make your practice more occupation-centered.
4. Describe one strategy that you could implement as part of a team to make your practice more occupation-centered.
5. Reflect on the assessment tools identified in this chapter and how they might be useful in your practice.

References

Britton, L., Rosenwax, L., & McNamara, B. (2016). Occupational therapy in Australian acute hospitals: A modified practice. *Australian Occupational Therapy Journal*, 63(4), 257–265. https://doi.org/10.1111/1440-1630.12298

Bryden, P., & McColl, M. A. (2003). The concept of occupation: 1900 to 1974. In M. McColl, M. Law, D. Stewart, L. Doubt, N. Pollock, & T. Krupa (Eds.), *Theoretical basis of occupational therapy* (pp. 27–38). Slack.

Ciro, C., Dung Dao, H., Anderson, M., Robinson, C., Hamilton, T., & Hershey, L. (2014). Improving daily life skills in people with dementia: Testing the STOMP Intervention

Model. *Journal of Alzheimers Disease & Parkinsonism, 4*, 165. https://doi.org/10.4172/2161-0460.1000165

Costa, U. M., Brauchle, G., & Kennedy-Behr, A. (2017). Collaborative goal setting with and for children as part of therapeutic intervention. *Disability and Rehabilitation, 39*(16), 1589–1600. https://doi.org/10.1080/09638288.2016.1202334

Dawson, D., McEwen, S., & Polatajko, H. (2017). *Cognitive orientation to daily performance in occupational therapy*. AOTA Press.

Di Tommaso, A., Isbel, S., Scarvell, J., & Wicks, A. (2016). Occupational therapists' perceptions of occupation in practice: An exploratory study. *Australian Occupational Therapy Journal, 63*(3), 206–213. https://doi.org/10.1111/1440-1630.12289

Estes, J., & Pierce, D. (2012). Paediatric therapists' perspectives on occupation-based practice. *Scandinavian Journal of Occupational Therapy, 19*(1), 17–25. https://doi.org/10.3109/11038128.2010.547598

Fisher, A. (2013). Occupation-centred, occupation-based, occupation-focused: Same, same or different? *Scandinavian Journal of Occupational Therapy, 20*(3), 162–173. https://doi.org/10.3109/11038128.2012.754492

Fisher, A., & Bray Jones, K. (2011). *Assessment of motor and process skills: Volume I - Development, standardisation, and administration manual* (7th ed.). Three Stars Press.

Fisher, A. G., & Marterella, A. (2019). *Powerful practice: A model for authentic occupational therapy*. Center for Innovative OT solutions.

Ford, E., Di Tommaso, A., Gustafsson, L., & Molineux, M. (2021). Describing the occupational nature of practice: A scoping review. *Scandinavian Journal of Occupational Therapy, 29*(5), 353–362. https://doi.org/10.1080/11038128.2021.1968949

Ford, E., Di Tommaso, A., Molineux, M., & Gustafsson, L. (2022). Identifying the characteristics of occupation-centred practice: A Delphi study. *Australian Occupational Therapy Journal, 69*(1), 25–37. https://doi.org/10.1111/1440-1630.12765

Hilton, C. (2022, March 2). International Women's Day: Dr Elizabeth Casson, 100 years on. *Royal College of Psychiatrists History, Archives and Library Blog*. https://www.rcpsych.ac.uk/news-and-features/blogs/detail/history-archives-and-library-blog/2022/03/07/elizabeth-casson

Kielhofner, G. (2009). *Conceptual foundations of occupational therapy practice* (4th ed.). F. A. Davis.

Law, M., Baptiste, S., Carswell, A., McColl, M., Polatajko, H., & Pollock, N. (2014). *The Canadian occupational performance measure* (5th ed.). CAOT Publications ACE.

Molineux, M. (2004). Occupation in occupational therapy: A labour in vain? In M. Molineux (Ed.), *Occupation for occupational therapists* (pp. 1–14). Blackwell Publishing.

Molineux, M. (2010). Occupational science and occupational therapy: Occupation at centre stage. In C. Christiansen & E. Townsend (Eds.), *Introduction to occupation: The art and science of living* (2nd ed., pp. 359–383). Prentice Hall.

Murray, A., Di Tommaso, A., Molineux, M., Young, A., & Power, P. (2019). Occupational therapists' perceptions of service transformation towards contemporary philosophy and practice in an acute specialist paediatric hospital. *British Journal of Occupational Therapy, 18*(12), 759–769. https://doi.org/10.1177/0308022619876836

Murray, A., Di Tommaso, A., Molineux, M., Young, A., & Power, P. (2020). Contemporary occupational therapy philosophy and practice in hospital settings. *Scandinavian Journal of Occupational Therapy, 28*(3), 213–224. https://doi.org/10.1080/11038128.2020.1750691

Pellegrini, M., Formisano, D., Bucciarelli, V., Schiavi, M., Fugazzaro, S., & Costi, S. (2018). Occupational therapy in complex patients: A pilot randomized controlled trial. *Occupational Therapy International, 2018*, 3081094. https://doi.org/10.1155/2018/3081094

Peloquin, S. (1991). Occupational therapy service: Individual and collective understandings of the founders, Part 1. *American Journal of Occupational Therapy, 45*(4), 352–360.

Pillastrini, P., Mugnai, R., Bonfiglioli, R., Curti, S., Mattioli, S., Maioli, M., Bazzocchi, G., Menarini, M., Vannini, R., & Violante, F. (2008). Evaluation of an occupational therapy program for patients with spinal cord injury. *Spinal Cord, 46*(1), 78–81. https://doi.org/10.1038/sj.sc.3102072

Spalding, K., Di Tommaso, A., & Gustafsson, L. (2023). Uncovering the experiences of engaging in an inpatient occupation-based group program: The LifeSkills group. *Scandinavian Journal of Occupational Therapy, 30*(2), 251–260. https://doi.org/10.1080/11038128.2022.2081604

Townsend, E. A., & Polatajko H. J. (2013). *Enabling occupation II: Advancing an occupational therapy vision for health, well-being, and justice through occupation* (2nd ed.). Canadian Association of Occupational Therapists.

Whiteford, G., Townsend, E., & Hocking, C. (2000). Reflections on a renaissance of occupation. *Canadian Journal of Occupational Therapy, 67*(1), 61–69. https://doi.org/10.1177/000841740006700109

Wilding, C., & Whiteford, G. (2007). Occupation and occupational therapy: Knowledge paradigms and everyday practice. *Australian Occupational Therapy Journal, 54*(3), 185–193. https://doi.org/10.1111/j.1440-1630.2006.00621.x

Wilding, C., & Whiteford, G. (2008). Language, identity and representation: Occupation and occupational therapy in acute settings. *Australian Occupational Therapy Journal, 55*(3), 180–187. https://doi.org/10.1111/j.1440-1630.2007.00678.x

Wilding, C., & Whiteford, G. (2009). From practice to praxis: Reconnecting moral vision with philosphical underpinnings. *British Journal of Occupational Therapy, 72*(10), 434–441. https://doi.org/10.1177/030802260907201004

CHAPTER 4

Person-centered Care in Occupation-based Practice

Diane Powers Dirette and Sharon Gutman

Abstract
This chapter defines, describes, and provides the historical context of person-centered occupational therapy practice. The philosophical assumptions and core values that form the foundation for person-centered care and the need to integrate the art and science of the profession are discussed. To provide direct application for therapists, this chapter presents a specific frame of reference to guide person-centered care in the profession of occupational therapy and discusses the implications for occupation-based practice.

Authors' Positionality Statement: See Chapter 1, Section 1.9

Objectives
This chapter will allow the reader to:

- Understand the term "person-centered care" and differentiate it from "patient-centered care," "client-centered care," and "personalized medicine."
- Understand the historical events that shaped person-centered care and distinguish it from laboratory-based medicine.
- Understand how the core values of the occupational therapy profession (altruism, dignity, equality, freedom, justice, truth, and prudence) align with and support person-centered care.
- Understand how person-centered, occupational therapy practice is based on a consideration of both evidence (evidence-based practice) and the unique needs of persons regarding physical and emotional health, personal goals, and environmental demands.

- Understand how occupational therapy frames of reference are constructed based on theoretical information about human physical, cognitive, and psychosocial mechanisms.
- Understand Taylor's Intentional Relationship Approach (2020) as an example of a person-centered frame of reference.
- Understand how person-centered, occupation-based therapy consists of activities that clients identify as most authentic, meaningful, and desirable to maintain, regain, or newly learn despite disability.

Key terms

- art of practice
- core values
- evidence-based practice
- frames of reference
- Intentional Relationship Approach
- occupation-based practice
- philosophical assumptions

4.1 Introduction

Person-centered treatment is the bedrock of occupational therapy practice. The profession was developed during a person-centered movement and the foundations of person-centered care are reflected in the philosophical basis and core values of the occupational therapy profession. Through merging the art and science of the profession, occupational therapists are able to provide evidence-based care that is focused on the individual characteristics, values, needs, and preferences of the people with whom we work. Based in person-centered theories, the Intentional Relationship Approach provides specific guidelines for occupational therapy practice. In conclusion, the implications for occupation-based practice are outlined, including occupational goals and occupation-based treatment merged with person-centered care.

4.2 Definitions

Several terms have been used related to the necessity for occupational therapy practice to center on the individuals with whom we work. Some of these terms include patient-centered, client-centered, person-centered, and more recently, personalized medicine. While all these terms have similar meanings and intent, the terms patient-centered, client-centered, and personalized medicine seem limited to settings with a medical focus and therefore in this chapter we will use the term person-centered care. Person-centered care is a partnership between the therapist and the individual formed to tailor therapeutic interventions that are best suited to the characteristics, needs, values, environment, and occupational preferences of the individual (Burke et al., 2014; Topol, 2014) (see Figure 4.1).

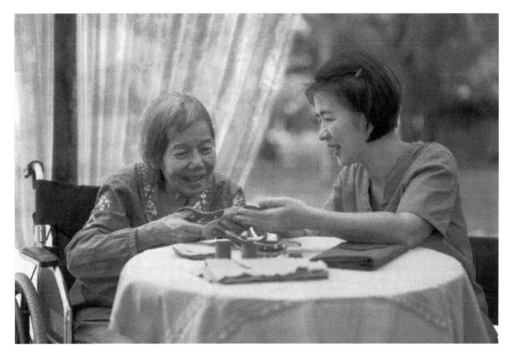

Figure 4.1 The occupational therapist creates a partnership with the individual to tailor therapeutic interventions that are best suited to the characteristics, needs, values, environment, and occupational preferences of the individual.

Source: Image used under license from Shutterstock.com.

4.3 Historical Basis of Person-centered Occupational Therapy

The health professions, in general, were born from biographical medicine that consisted of a bedside visit during which the physician considered the entire body and mind of the person in relation to the surrounding environment. According to Tutton,

> physicians understood that each patient had their own unique equilibrium and drew on their detailed understanding of the biography of the individual – their gender, their age, their family background, and occupation – in order to customize their treatment of their disease. (2012, p. 1723)

Before the advent of laboratory-based medicine,

> Doctors could not assume that a therapeutic intervention to alleviate one person's suffering in a particular place and time could be used again in different circumstances with a different individual. Therefore, treatment was very much directed at the person and not the disease. (Tutton, 2012, p. 1723)

In the 1800s, laboratory-based medical practice, which is founded on the concept that pharmaceuticals can be used to treat disease universally, replaced biographical medicine as physicians aligned themselves with laboratory science based on its promise to transform medical practice. During this movement, the interest in the unique qualities of the individual and treatment of the whole person evaporated and was replaced by universal guidelines for treatment developed by the laboratory sciences (Tutton, 2012).

In the early 1900s, laboratory-based medical practice was challenged by the patient-as-a-person movement which emphasized the unique nature of the doctor–patient relationship and the understanding of the whole person. The patient-as-a-person movement acknowledged the universality of scientific knowledge to assist with the diagnosis and treatment of diseases and embraced the status of medicine as a science-based profession, but pushed to balance that information with an understanding of the unique nature of the individual. Disease was conceptualized as a scientific construct that could be defined by its biological processes, but illness included the psychological and emotional reactions of the individual in the specific social and physical environment (Tutton, 2012). The profession of occupational therapy developed during this patient-as-a-person paradigm shift (Gordon, 2009).

4.4 Person-centered Philosophy in Occupational Therapy

The fact that the occupational therapy profession was founded during the patient-as-a-person initiative of the early 1900s is evident in our philosophical assumptions. These philosophical assumptions include eight statements distilled from the occupational therapy literature to summarize the profession's basic beliefs about the nature of the individual and the environment, the relationship between the individual and the environment, and the purpose of the occupational therapy profession in meeting the needs of the individual and society (Mosey, 1996). Of the eight philosophical statements listed, six begin with the phrase "each individual." These six statements summarize the occupational therapy philosophy as focusing on the rights and preferences of individuals relative to their biological and social environment. The seventh statement discusses functional interdependence and the eighth statement concludes that the focus of the occupational therapy intervention depends on the individual's needs (Mosey, 1996).

In addition to our core philosophical assumptions, the core values of the occupational therapy profession, as set forth in the article titled, "Core values and attitudes of occupational therapy practice" (Kanny, 1993), are altruism, dignity, equality, freedom, justice, truth, and prudence. These core values, especially dignity, equality, and freedom, are the profession's moral guide to person-centered care. They guide us to value differences, to treat people equally despite those differences, and to encourage individuals to make their own choices based on differing perspectives and preferences.

4.5 Art and Science Integration in Person-centered Care

In the late 1800s, the famous physician William Osler observed that, "If it were not for the great variability among individuals, medicine might as well be a science and not an art" (quoted in Tutton, 2012, p. 1721). The art of practice in occupational therapy is the therapeutic skill of interacting with the client and using clinical reasoning to plan and carry out treatment based on the uniqueness of the individual and the individual's circumstances (Mosey, 1996). Most recently, the science of the occupational therapy profession has been driven by the push for evidence-based practice (EBP). EBP is the "conscientious, explicit, and judicious use of current best evidence in making decisions about the care of individual patients" (Sackett et al., 1996, p. 71).

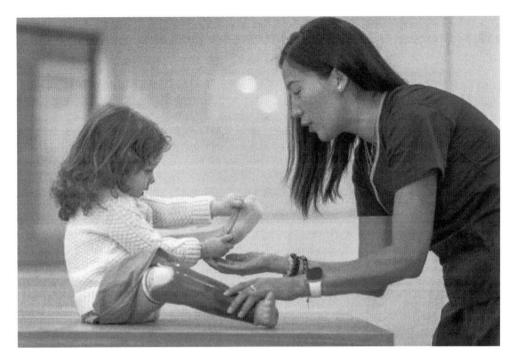

Figure 4.2 The occupational therapist uses compassion, collaboration, teaching-learning, and nurturing integrated with clinical reasoning and decision making.

Source: Image used under license from Shutterstock.com.

The science of the profession in the form of EBP is focused on the universal application of evidence to support treatment choices and has, at times, been regarded as conflicting with the art of practice which is focused on individualized treatments tailored to the variable needs of the person. Instead of promoting a conflict between the art and the science of practice, occupational therapists should merge these two concepts for person-centered care. Treatments should be chosen based on the best available evidence with consideration for a person's varied characteristics, values, needs, and preferences along with the tasks that the person performs and the environment in which the person must function. The art of practice, which includes therapeutic interactions using compassion, collaboration, teaching-learning, and nurturing, should not be separated from the use of evidence, but rather integrated with scientific knowledge as part of the clinical reasoning and decision-making process. Using person-centered care, the therapist modifies the treatment for the individual based on individual variances deciphered by the art of practice and the best available scientific information (see Figure 4.2).

4.6 Person-centered Theory in Occupational Therapy

To achieve person-centered therapy that addresses the unique health needs of individuals, occupational therapy frames of reference must be sufficiently flexible to address both (a) general concerns associated with a diagnosis at a population level and (b) specific needs unique to an individual's personal values, goals, identity, and cultural background. A frame of reference is a written set of guidelines that provides direction for intervention with a specific diagnostic population, the members of which are experiencing similar problems in the performance of desired occupational roles and daily activities (Mosey, 1996). Frames of reference identify:

1. The clinical population for which intervention is intended.
2. The theoretical base of information from which the intervention was developed.
3. The function-dysfunction continuum, which identifies the spectrum of behaviors characteristic of a specific area of human experience and extending from desired performance to atypical, undesired performance.
4. Directions for the therapist and person to work together to facilitate desired change in human experience addressed by the frame of reference, otherwise known as the postulates regarding change.

Occupational therapy frames of reference are based on theoretical information about how humans function biologically, psychologically, emotionally, socially, and developmentally. Many of the profession's frames of reference are drawn from theories about the:

- anatomy and physiology of the human body
- neurological and social mechanisms that support human learning
- physiological and environmental processes underlying how humans develop and maintain skills such as motor control and communication skills throughout the lifespan
- roles that humans assume and lose as they interact with each other in families and social groups at different life stages
- ways through which the primary occupations of play, education, work, and leisure reflect human goals throughout a lifetime
- ways that culture, historical era, race, ethnicity, and gender shape and modify human self-identity over a life course.

In occupational therapy, person-centered theories form the basis for the development of many of the profession's frames of reference. Person-centered theories describe how an individual's unique interaction with the human and nonhuman environments serves to shape a person's self-identity, values, goals, and expectations. In turn, one's self-identity, values, goals, and expectations influence the social and occupational roles that people seek, as well as the habits, routines, and occupations that support or impede participation in those roles.

Person-centered theories suggest that each client who attends therapy has a unique set of individual personality characteristics, cultural norms, beliefs, values, and goals that must be understood and addressed to make therapy optimally meaningful. Each client also has a unique constellation of past experiences, family background, relationship/interactional style, comfort level, fears, and way of relating to authority that must be understood and addressed on a conscious level by the therapist, or such characteristics can inadvertently interfere with therapy. Each client can also be triggered indirectly or directly by their reactions to the therapist and the therapeutic setting and display behaviors that interfere with desired therapeutic outcomes. Clients can be unconsciously triggered by the therapist's appearance, verbalizations, tone of voice, and body language; the level of noise and odors in the clinical setting; and the behaviors of other clients and health care professionals. Therapists must understand these dynamics to make the therapeutic setting a safe place where clients experiencing illness, disability, anxiety, and pain can feel safe to express emotions, make mistakes as part of the learning process, ask uncomfortable questions, and request help.

4.6.1 Using Person-centered Theories in the Development of Practice Guidelines: The Intentional Relationship Approach

One example of the use of person-centered theories in the development of practice guidelines is Taylor's (2020) Intentional Relationship Approach. Taylor defines intentionality as the ability of the therapist to be consciously aware of and manage all aspects of the client–therapist relationship so that difficult client behaviors and interpersonal conflicts can be prevented or quickly resolved. To achieve intentionality, therapists must have an acute understanding of, and be consciously able to manage, their own communication style, vocal tone, body language, and facial expression. Therapists must be able to understand the types of client behaviors that are triggering for them, recognize triggering behaviors in the moment, and respond by using therapeutic approaches that assist clients to feel at ease (see Figure 4.3).

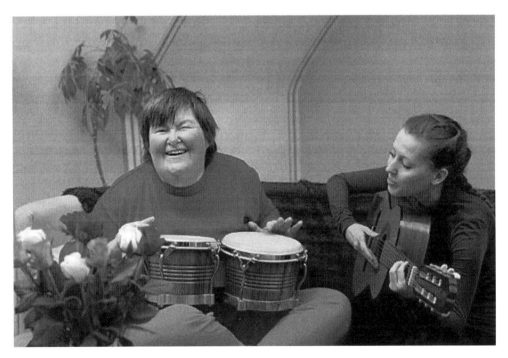

Figure 4.3 The occupational therapist achieves intentionality by managing their own communication style, vocal tone, body language, and facial expression and using therapeutic approaches that assist the client to feel at ease.

Source: Image used under license from Shutterstock.com.

Similarly, intentionality also requires therapists to consciously understand and manage client interactions and behaviors with regard to client communication styles, vocal tone, body language, and facial expression. Therapists must be able to understand how the following client characteristics can impact the therapeutic relationship: response to change and challenge, level of trust, need for control, ability to make needs known and ask for help, ability to give and receive feedback, ability to tolerate human diversity, and ability to tolerate human touch. Intentional therapists are able to use a set of professional therapeutic behaviors to create a nonthreatening, nonjudgmental environment where clients can feel safe to make mistakes as they learn new skills and have confidence that the therapist will always act in their best interest and prioritize their therapeutic needs.

4.6.2 Theoretical Base

Much of the theoretical information from which Taylor's Intentional Relationship Approach has been drawn emerged from psychodynamic theories that suggest human behavior is embedded within conscious and unconscious beliefs and perceptions that impact all daily events. Both therapists and clients also hold conscious and unconscious beliefs and perceptions that can adversely affect the therapeutic relationship if left unexamined. Clients will transfer their unconscious beliefs, emotions, and fears about themselves and others onto the therapist – a process called transference. A well-trained therapist will be able to recognize transferred client behaviors, refrain from being triggered and responding inappropriately, and gently help clients understand that their beliefs and fears are not reality-based. Therapists who have not examined their own unconscious motivations and beliefs are at a risk of transferring their own unconscious emotions to their clients – a process called countertransference.

When either transference or countertransference occurs in a therapeutic relationship, conflicts and empathic breaks between the therapist and client are inevitable. Taylor suggests that intentional therapists are able to manage difficult client behaviors and the complexities within client–therapist relationships because they are able to (a) refrain from personalizing difficult client behaviors and (b) understand that such behaviors are often rooted in fears about loss triggered by the client's current health situation. Instead of inappropriately responding defensively to difficult behaviors, intentional therapists are able to allow clients to express their emotions in a safe environment and consciously explore feelings of loss.

4.6.3 Function-Dysfunction Continuum

Taylor suggests that there is a continuum of client behaviors indicating their ability to engage in the therapeutic relationship, with behaviors ranging from healthy to conflicted. To facilitate a healthy therapeutic relationship that can assist the client to enhance self-awareness and eventual adoption of functional behaviors, therapists must be able to identify a client's current behavioral status. Taylor identifies the following continuum (see Table 4.1):

Taylor also suggests that there is a range of therapist behaviors from optimal to suboptimal and that suboptimal behaviors can adversely affect the client–therapist relationship (see Table 4.2):

Table 4.1 Continuum of Client Behaviors Indicating Their Ability to Engage in the Therapeutic Relationship

Healthy behavior	Difficult behavior
Clients:	
■ are able to express emotions about their current situation without blaming the therapist or expressing anger with the therapist	■ express strong emotion in a way that blames the therapist or identifies the therapist as the source of the client's anger
■ are able to disclose personal information that is relevant to their current emotions	■ withhold information and emotionally close off from therapeutic engagement
■ are able to see the therapist as someone who has knowledge that can help their current situation and allow the therapist to guide therapy	■ display power struggles and argue with the therapist about the direction therapy should take
■ communicate clearly and directly with the therapist about concerns and needs	■ use nonverbal cues, verbal innuendos, and/or resistance to indicate disappointment or disagreement with the therapist
■ are able to maintain appropriate boundaries set by the therapist	■ continuously test boundaries with the therapist
■ appropriately discuss desired outcomes with the therapist	■ use manipulative behavior with the therapist to attain desired outcomes
■ rely on the therapist for guidance but increase their independence as therapy progresses	■ are excessively dependent on the therapist
■ are aware of their symptoms but can focus on therapeutic activities	■ focus on symptoms to such an extent that they are unable to engage in therapeutic activities

Table 4.2 Range of Therapist Behaviors Indicating Ability to Facilitate and Engage in Therapeutic Relationship

Optimal behavior	Suboptimal behavior
Therapists:	
■ engage clients in a collaborative way to set goals and select therapeutic activities	■ dominate clients in all therapeutic decisions
■ respectfully treat 18+-year-old clients as autonomous adults	■ act in a parental way with adult clients and limit autonomous decisions
■ respond to client questions about therapy with respect and thoroughness	■ respond to client questions about therapy defensively, dismissively, or patronizingly
■ encourage client communication by deeply listening and responding with respect and full attention	■ close off communication by responding to client emotion with inappropriate humor, clichés, and/or minimizing statements
■ encourage clients to feel that their emotional expression is important by responding with empathy and compassion	■ convey that client emotions are not important through culturally insensitive behaviors, socially embarrassing responses, and comparisons between clients
■ respond to client intimate disclosures with full attention, empathy, and appropriate affect	■ convey disinterest in client intimate disclosures by failing to listen and instead over-disclosing information about themselves

4.6.4 Postulates Regarding Change

Taylor identifies three key therapeutic skills that should be mastered by therapists to build rapport with clients, set clients at ease, and empower them to engage in therapeutic activities to attain identified goals. The first of these skills is mode use. Taylor suggests that occupational therapists use six therapeutic modes to facilitate client engagement and desired outcomes:

i) Empathizing mode: Therapists use empathy to build rapport, deeply listen to client concerns, and demonstrate that client emotions and experiences are important to them. In the empathizing mode, therapists allow clients to demonstrate their emotions and talk about their experience of disability without interrupting, forming judgments, or rushing to intervene. Intentional therapists use body language, vocal tone, and facial expressions that demonstrate compassion and understanding. While the empathizing mode is often initially used to get to know clients and demonstrate an appreciation for their experience of disability, it can also be used at any time during therapy in response to clients' displays of fear, anxiety, depression, grief, and anger.

ii) Encouraging mode: The encouraging mode is used to provide hope to clients who express fear that they will not be able to attain a desired goal. Often, the encouraging mode is used to help clients engage in activities they believe are too difficult. The encouraging mode is often used sequentially after the empathizing mode.

iii) Instructing mode: Therapists provide instructions to clients to help them understand the steps needed to complete specific activities. Often, this involves helping clients understand what they need to do motorically, cognitively, and psychosocially. Therapists must provide instructions at a level that matches the cognitive ability of clients. Instructions must also be paced to prevent clients from feeling overwhelmed, anxious, and resistant. The instructing mode is used whenever clients need direction because they have not yet attained the necessary knowledge to complete an activity independently or through their own attempts at problem-solving.

iv) Problem-solving mode: In the problem-solving mode, clients and carers are encouraged to become partners with the therapist in the steps of problem identification, strategy generation, strategy execution, and strategy evaluation. Therapists guide clients and carers through the steps of problem-solving and help them consider a variety of options and the likely consequences of those options.

v) Collaborating mode: In the collaborating mode, therapists act more as a consultant and allow clients and carers to develop strategies and resolutions with a high level of independence. Therapists may provide information but allow clients and carers to direct the course of therapy. To participate in collaboration, clients and carers must be at an emotional and cognitive level sufficient to identify areas of concern and develop effective strategies.

vi) Advocating mode: Therapists use the advocating mode when they provide information to client and carers that is needed to secure entitled resources, funds, and rights. Therapists also use the advocating mode when they independently act on the client's behalf to secure resources, funds, and rights for them.

In addition to mode use, Taylor also identifies mode matching and mode shifting as key therapeutic skills of intentional therapists. Mode matching occurs when therapists intentionally mirror the effect of clients to demonstrate empathy, compassion, and understanding. Mode shifting occurs when therapists consciously realize that a change has occurred in the client or clinical situation that calls for a different mode to be implemented to best address client needs in the moment. Taylor emphasizes that in order to implement mode use, mode matching, and mode shifting consciously and intentionally, therapists must be acutely aware of their own and their client's current emotions, trait-based and situationally based interpersonal characteristics, and responses to the inevitable interpersonal events that occur in therapy.

4.7 Implications for Occupation-based Practice
4.7.1 Goals of the Therapeutic Relationship
The goals of a therapeutic relationship require therapists to provide a physically and emotionally safe environment where clients can:

- feel comfortable expressing their emotions regarding loss, anxiety, fear, and depression
- have faith that they will be treated respectfully and compassionately
- have confidence that service will be provided non-discriminatively despite any form of human diversity
- practice new skills without fear of making mistakes, being judged, or being shamed
- be challenged at a pace that does not overwhelm or erode their confidence or hope
- feel assured that their needs are prioritized and that the therapist will always act in their best interest
- have confidence that personal disclosures and information will be maintained confidentially.

To promote therapeutic relationships, occupational therapists must:

- understand how to facilitate open and reciprocal communication with clients
- have tolerance for and be able to manage clients' strong emotions
- refrain from personalizing client behaviors and emotions that are rooted in feelings of loss resulting from disability
- be able to identify client cues that indicate the occurrence of an empathic break or conflict within the therapeutic relationship
- be able to successfully implement conflict resolution strategies when an empathic break has occurred within the therapeutic relationship.

4.7.2 Occupational Goals in Person-centered Care
Occupational goals in person-centered care are founded on the idea that clients must be respected as autonomous beings and that goal setting is a collaborative experience between clients and therapists. Occupational goals are selected based on the activities and roles that clients prioritize as most meaningful and desired as they rebuild their lives after illness, disability, or injury. Although it is important for clients to select their own goals in person-centered therapy, it is the therapist's responsibility to (a) guide the client to set realistic and attainable goals, (b) break goals into manageable components with feasible timelines, and (c) provide intervention that supports the attainment of client-selected goals.

4.7.3 Occupation as Treatment in Person-centered Care

The act of relearning or newly learning to participate in meaningful occupations that may have been lost or disrupted by disability is therapeutic in itself. Learning to participate in highly prioritized occupations and occupational roles that were disrupted by disability commonly gives clients hope that their ability to meaningfully reconstruct their lives after trauma can be successful in ways they had not previously envisioned. For clients to be optimally engaged in therapy, they must perceive therapeutic activities to be directly meaningful to their lives. Research has shown that the most meaningful and engaging therapeutic activities are authentic occupations that clients wish to maintain, regain, or newly learn despite disability (Ikiugu et al., 2019). Simulated occupations or contrived activities that mirror the motor actions of authentic occupations (e.g., using pegs and cones to simulate the act of reaching into a cabinet to retrieve a cooking pot) are often misunderstood by clients, perceived as meaningless, and erode client confidence in therapy effectiveness.

4.8 Conclusion

Person-centered occupational therapy emerged during the 1900s when laboratory-based medicine was challenged to integrate a person's unique set of social, emotional, and environmental factors as contributors to human disease and disability (Gordon, 2009; Tutton, 2012). Although the occupational therapy profession was initially founded on the patient-as-a-person paradigm, it departed from this clinical ideology for several decades after WWII to more closely align with the medical model and gain professional respect (Andersen & Reed, 2017). Push-back against a medical model paradigm re-emerged in the 1990s and early 2000s, characterized by a call for occupational therapists to resume person-centered, occupation-based practice using authentic daily life activities that clients desired to regain despite illness, disability, or injury.

Taylor' Intentional Relationship Approach (2020) is one of the first occupational therapy frames of reference designed to help therapists understand how to address the potential impact of client and therapist personal factors on therapy outcomes. According to Taylor, person-centered occupational therapy encompasses the idea that each client comes to therapy with a specific history, family background, and personality style, which may impact the therapeutic relationship positively or adversely depending on the therapist's use of intentionality.

Intentionality involves the therapist's ability to consciously be aware of and manage all aspects of the client–therapist relationship so that difficult therapist–client interactions do not escalate into empathic breaks. Therapists must not only be consciously aware of and manage their own communication style (e.g., vocal tone, body language, and facial expression), but they must also be cognizant of the types of client behaviors that serve as personal triggers, recognize triggers when they occur, refrain from personalizing clients' difficult behaviors, and respond therapeutically to allow clients to feel safe and respected. Intentionality and person-centered therapy also encompass the idea that clients are autonomous beings who should be invited to collaborate in the therapeutic activities of goal setting and treatment planning.

Today, the profession's call for action is for therapists to provide therapy that is both person-centered and occupation-based. Research has shown that clients are most fully engaged in therapy when it provides the opportunity for them to maintain, regain, or newly assume highly prioritized daily life activities that were lost, disrupted, or never emerged because of disability (Ikiugu et al., 2019). Clients perceive therapy to be most beneficial when they can directly relate therapeutic activities to real-life, desired occupations that support the resumption or reconstruction of occupational roles that are most personally meaning. Intentional therapists invite and collaborate with clients to set realistic and attainable goals; develop treatment trajectories that challenge clients to progress, but neither overwhelm nor erode their confidence; and create safe treatment environments in which clients can practice new skills without fear of making mistakes, being judged, or being shamed.

4.9 Summary

- Person-centered care is a partnership formed between the therapist and the individual to tailor therapeutic interventions that are best suited to the characteristics, needs, values, environment, and occupational preferences of the individual.
- In the 1800s, laboratory-based medical practice was founded on the concept that pharmaceuticals could be used to treat disease universally. As laboratory-based medicine became the primary medical paradigm, treatment that considered the whole person evaporated and was replaced by universal treatment guidelines developed by the laboratory sciences.
- The occupational therapy profession was founded during the patient-as-a-person initiative of the early 1900s in which laboratory-based medicine was challenged to integrate a person's unique set of social, emotional, and environmental factors as contributors to human disease and disability. Despite periods in the profession's history in which therapists departed from the patient-as-a-person practice approach to align with the medical model, the profession has since returned to an appreciation of person-centered therapy, integrated with scientific evidence supporting practice.
- Taylor's Intentional Relationship Approach is one of the first occupational therapy frames of reference that was designed to help therapists address client and therapist personal factors that can impact therapy outcomes. Intentionality involves recognizing that each client has a unique constellation of past experiences, family background, relationship/interactional style, comfort level, fears, and way of relating to authority that must be understood and addressed on a conscious level by the therapist. Otherwise, such characteristics can inadvertently interfere with therapy.
- For occupational therapy to be most beneficial and meaningful to clients, it must be both person-centered and occupation-based. Research has shown that the most effective therapies allow clients to practice real-life desired occupations that became disrupted by disability, illness, or injury. Simulated activities that are inauthentic and do not relate to clients' occupational roles are commonly perceived as meaningless and erode client confidence in therapy effectiveness.

4.10 Review Questions

1. Describe the patient-as-a-person paradigm shift in the early 1900s in which the profession of occupational therapy developed. How was laboratory-based medicine challenged by this paradigm shift? Describe how the patient-as-a-person approach helped to establish the core values of the occupational therapy profession.
2. Describe how "the art of practice" and "evidence" can be merged to promote occupational therapy that is person-centered?

3. Describe the four primary component parts of a frame of reference and identify several major theories from which occupational therapy frames of reference are commonly drawn. Describe the main tenets of person-centered theories.
4. According to Taylor's Intentional Relationship Approach, what does the term "intentional" mean? Identify five behaviors on the function/dysfunction continuum that characterize difficult client interactional styles. Identify five suboptimal behaviors that therapists may display which can adversely affect the client–therapist relationship.
5. Describe each of the following therapeutic modes: empathizing, encouraging, instructing, problem-solving, collaborating, and advocating. What are the goals of a therapeutic relationship and how can occupational therapists promote these goals?

References

Andersen, L. T., & Reed, K. L. (2017). *The history of occupational therapy: The first century*. SLACK.

Burke, W., Trinidad, S. B., & Press, N. A. (2014). Essential elements of personalized medicine. *Urologic Oncology: Seminars and Original Investigations, 32*(2), 193–197. http://doi.org/10.1016/j.urolonc.2013.09.002

Gordon, D. (2009). The history of occupational therapy. In E. B. Crepeau, E. S. Cohn, & B. A. Boyt Schell (Eds.), *Willard and Spackman's occupational therapy* (11th ed., pp. 202–215). Wolters Kluwer/Lippincott Williams & Wilkins.

Ikiugu, M. N., Lucas-Molitor, W., Feldhacker, D., Gebhart, C., Spier, M., Kapels, L., Arnold, R., & Gaikowski, R. (2019). Guidelines for occupational therapy interventions based on meaningful and psychologically rewarding occupations. *Journal of Happiness Studies, 20*(7), 2027–2053. https://doi.org/10.1007/s10902-018-0030-z

Kanny, E. (1993). Core values and attitudes of occupational therapy practice. *American Journal of Occupational Therapy, 47*, 1085–1086. https://doi.org/10.5014/ajot.47.12.1085

Mosey, A. C. (1996). *Applied scientific inquiry in the health professions: An epistemological orientation* (2nd ed.). American Occupational Therapy Association.

Sackett, D. L., Rosenberg, W. M., Gray, J. A. M., Haynes, R. B., & Richardson, W. S. (1996). Evidence based medicine: What it is and what it isn't. *British Medical Journal, 312*(7023), 71–72. https://doi.org/10.1136/bmj.312.7023.71

Taylor, R. R. (2020). *The intentional relationship: Occupational therapy and use of self* (2nd ed.). F. A. Davis.

Topol, E. J. (2014). Individualized medicine from prewomb to tomb. *Cell, 157*(1), 241–253. http://doi.org/10.1016/j.cell.2014.02.012

Tutton, R. (2012). Personalizing medicine: Futures present and past. *Social Science & Medicine, 75*(10), 1721–1728. http://doi.org/10.1016/j.socscimed.2012.07.031

CHAPTER 5

Models of Practice that Focus on Human Occupation

Ellie Fossey, Gayle Restall, Mary Egan, and Sandra Moll

Abstract
This chapter provides an overview of two widely known occupational therapy practice models focused on human occupation: the Model of Human Occupation (MOHO) and the latest Canadian model of practice comprising three parts: the Canadian Model of Occupational Participation (CanMOP), the Collaborative Relationship-Focused Practice approach, and the Canadian Occupational Therapy Inter-relational Practice Process Framework (COTIPP). For each practice model, the origins and key concepts are described and illustrated using a practice scenario to highlight how practice models focused on human occupation guide occupational therapists' reasoning and actions in practice.

Authors' Positionality Statement
All the authors of this chapter are women and qualified occupational therapists who have practiced in varied settings. The authors have also completed advanced academic and research training in the form of doctorates and have worked in university settings as occupational therapy faculty. In relation to cultural backgrounds, the authors have lived and worked in the following countries: Canada, Australia, New Zealand, and the United Kingdom; they acknowledge and pay respects to the Traditional Territories, Owners, and Elders of these lands. They also acknowledge the impact of various external factors on the individuals, families, and communities with whom occupational therapists work, including, but not limited to, economic and social inequities, sex, gender and racial inequality, sexual identity discrimination, ageism, past and continuing impacts of colonization on Indigenous communities, and systemic and structural racism in societies. The authors acknowledge that the examples of occupational therapy models and practice in this chapter have origins in the Global North. They recognize the limitations of Global North perspectives and the importance of being inclusive and respectful of a spectrum of cultures, social identities, and worldviews.

DOI: 10.4324/9781003504610-6

ELLIE FOSSEY ET AL.

> **Objectives**
> This chapter will allow the reader to:
>
> - Understand the key concepts within two key practice models focused on human occupation.
> - Appreciate how these models have evolved over time.
> - Consider how the practice models focused on human occupation shape occupational therapy practice.

> **Key terms**
> - occupational participation
> - volition
> - habituation
> - performance capacity
> - occupational performance
> - occupational identity
> - micro, meso, and macro contexts
> - self-determination

5.1 Introduction

Occupational therapy is rooted in a rich understanding of "occupation" and its links to health and well-being across the life course. Conceptual models about occupation have been designed to help occupational therapists frame and explain core concepts and principles that inform practice and understand how these concepts and principles relate to people's experience of engaging in occupations that address their needs and their aspirations. This conceptual information is then integrated into practice using process frameworks. This chapter is designed to inspire readers to reflect on two prominent occupation-focused models: the Model of Human Occupation (MOHO) and the Canadian Model of Occupational Participation (CanMOP). Readers will gain an understanding of each model, through an overview that includes each model's primary aims and key concepts. They will also become aware of how selecting a model of practice influences the goals and focus of occupational therapy. First, a practice scenario is presented which is then followed by an introduction to the MOHO and the CanMOP. When each practice model is discussed, a practice scenario will be used to illustrate how each model might shape occupational therapy practice.

5.2 Practice Scenario

Sam (he/him) is the occupational therapist on the rehabilitation unit of a regional hospital that provides service to a small city and surrounding rural areas. Sam received a referral to see *Micheline Imbault* (she/her), a 53-year-old woman recently transferred to the unit from acute care after an admission related to a fall. The referral indicated that this is Micheline's fourth fall-related admission over the past two years, and the acute care team is concerned about her return home. It also noted that she was diagnosed with multiple sclerosis approximately 20 years ago, and has experienced decreased strength, endurance, and mobility over the last five years.

Sam meets initially with Micheline to welcome her to the rehabilitation unit and briefly explain its services and the role of the occupational therapist there. Sam also asks Micheline a few questions about herself and makes a time with Micheline to talk further about her situation. In their initial conversations, he learns that Micheline has been living in a rural community for much of her life. She takes pride in her 30-plus years working in the mining industry and raising her 24-year-old son as a single parent. She lives in a bungalow with her retired 84-year-old father, Jack. Her son, Travis, lives and works in a neighboring community. Sam also learns that Micheline has concerns about her father, who recently lost his driver's license due to declining eyesight. She is also currently on disability leave from her work and is worried that her position may be terminated. Sam is familiar with Micheline's local community and aware that there are fewer community services available than in the city where the hospital is located approximately 100 kilometers away.

5.3 Model of Human Occupation (MOHO)

The MOHO is an explanatory framework used by occupational therapists to explore how people choose, organize, and perform occupations within their particular contexts, and how personal and environmental factors shape our patterns of participation in occupations and capability to adapt them over time. Occupational therapists around the world use this understanding to collaborate with individuals and groups of people, such as families, to address the disruptions and challenges experienced in choosing, organizing, and orchestrating their occupations during times of life transitions and due to ill health, developmental delay, aging, or environmental restrictions.

The MOHO was developed through the scholarship of the late Professor Gary Kielhofner in collaboration with many practitioners and researchers internationally. It was initially developed in the 1980s to focus theory and practice on occupation at a time when the predominant emphasis of occupational therapy was on understanding and alleviating impairments (Kielhofner, 2009; Taylor, 2024). The emergence of new thinking, research evidence, and applications of the MOHO in diverse practice settings have contributed to the refinement and revision of the original MOHO concepts over more than four decades, as reflected in revised editions of the MOHO textbook (Kielhofner, 2008, 2009; Taylor, 2017; Taylor et al., 2024).

5.3.1 Key Concepts

The MOHO recognizes that occupational engagement, participation, and performance develop and change across the course of people's lives, and that making changes in response to life circumstances is necessary to sustain meaningful engagement in chosen occupations *(occupational adaptation)* (Bowyer et al., 2024; O'Brien & Kielhofner, 2017). The MOHO describes two key concepts as important for understanding the process of occupational adaptation: a person's sense of who they are based on their cumulative experiences of occupations *(occupational identity)* and the degree to which their *occupational competence* matches that identity (Bowyer et al., 2024; O'Brien & Kielhofner, 2017; Parkinson & Brookes, 2021). Occupational identity and occupational competence can be profoundly affected by ill health, developmental delay, aging, environmental restrictions, or life transitions.

To formulate an understanding of how an individual's occupational identity and occupational competence may be impacted, the MOHO identifies four key contributing factors: volition, habituation, performance, and environment. These four factors describe how people are motivated toward choosing and engaging in particular occupations *(volition)*, how they organize their actions into patterns and routines *(habituation)*, how they use and experience their capacities *(performance capacity)*, and the features of the immediate, local, and broader *environment* that powerfully shape engagement, participation, and performance of occupations (Taylor, 2024). By exploring how these four factors (volition, habituation, performance capacity, and environment) have shaped a person's experiences of *participation*, their *occupational skills*, and *occupational performance* over time, the MOHO provides the therapist with a way to understand a person's occupational history and occupational adaptation. Table 5.1 outlines each of these MOHO concepts in more detail.

Table 5.1 MOHO Key Concepts

Occupational adaptation: the degree to which occupational identity and occupational competence support ongoing participation in chosen occupations	▪ Occupational identity: a person's sense of who they are and wish to be based on their occupational history ▪ Occupational competence: the extent to which a person participates in occupations that reflect their occupational identity
Volition: motives and choices for engaging occupations	Volition consists of a person's thoughts and feelings about three issues: ▪ **Interests:** the activities that a person finds enjoyable and satisfying to do or that spark their curiosity to pursue ▪ **Values:** what a person considers to be important or meaningful to do ▪ **Personal causation:** a person's view of their own abilities and how capable and effective they feel
Habituation: habits and roles that anchor and organize daily life	Patterns of daily occupation are organized by: ▪ Habits: Learned ways of routinely responding and acting consistently in familiar environments and situations ▪ Roles: The socially or personally defined statuses or positions, accompanying attitudes, and behaviors that a person takes on and enacts
Performance capacity: capacities for sensing the world, moving the body, planning actions, and interacting	Performance capacity includes objective and subjective aspects: ▪ **Mental and physical capacities** that are used and experienced during performance ▪ **Lived body experience:** a person's experience of themselves and their bodies in a lived sense

(Continued)

Table 5.1 (Continued)

Environment: features of specific contexts that impact motivation, organization, performance, and participation in occupations	Specific environments have physical, social, and occupational features: - **Physical:** built and natural spaces and objects, their qualities, and availability within - **Social:** people and relationships and the quality and availability of interactions - **Occupational:** presence, qualities, cultural relevance, and availability of occupations These physical, social, and occupational features exist in environments at three levels: immediate contexts (e.g., home and work), local contexts (e.g., neighborhood and community), and societal contexts
Dimensions of doing: three levels at which participation and performance can be understood	- Occupational participation: describes what a person does in terms of broad areas/categories of activity, such as play, study, work, and so on - Occupational performance: describes performance of a specific activity, of which there may be many within a broad area of occupational participation - Occupational skills: describes observable, goal-directed actions used in occupational performance (e.g., motor skills, process skills, and communication and interaction skills)

When working with people whose participation has been disrupted or who are having difficulties in performing their occupations, the occupational therapist can use the MOHO concepts of volition, habituation, performance capacity, and environment as a guide to identify factors that are contributing to this situation and its impacts on people's occupational lives. This can be illustrated by considering how the MOHO might guide Sam, the occupational therapist in the practice scenario, to further explore Micheline and her father's situations.

Volition is about how people choose and are motivated to engage in particular occupations both on a day-to-day basis (e.g., which toys to play with and what meal to prepare) and longer term (e.g., commitment to a particular career or hobby) (Lee & Kielhofner, 2017a). Volitional thoughts and feelings have a pervasive influence throughout life on how people view their occupational choices, opportunities and challenges in their environments, and their experiences of the occupations in which they engage. Volitional thoughts and feelings shape how people *anticipate engaging* in particular occupations (e.g., looking forward to an event and worrying about difficulty doing one's work); *what they do* (e.g., making plans or practicing to be well-prepared); *their experience of doing* (e.g., enjoying the outing and feeling stressed at work); and how they *interpret the experience* (e.g., reflecting that outings are enjoyable when well planned, reflecting on poor performance, and needing to be better prepared in future) (Lee & Kielhofner, 2024).

In the practice scenario, Micheline has already told Sam that she has worked in the mining industry for many years, is not presently working, and has concerns about her position. The MOHO concept of *Volition* guides Sam to think to himself: what does Micheline find enjoyable and satisfying to do now, and when she was working (*interests*)? What is important or meaningful to Micheline to do (*values*)? What is Micheline thinking about her abilities and how confident is she feeling (*personal causation*)? Sam knows that it is important to learn more from Micheline about whether or not she has opportunities to participate in valued occupations, to feel capable, and to gain pleasure or satisfaction from what she has been doing, especially given that not working, declining physical health, and repeated falls might each potentially have undermined Micheline's motivations toward engaging in occupations. In turn, this guides Sam to select a semi-structured interview – for instance, the Occupational Performance History Interview-II or the Worker Role Interview – for talking with Micheline to understand her perspective of these issues (Morris et al., 2024).

Everyday life typically involves organizing participation in several occupations, such as taking care of oneself or others, learning, earning an income, playing, socializing, and so on. The concept of *habituation* explains that *habits* and *roles* facilitate the establishing and maintaining of routine patterns of participation in daily life and allow people to carry out multiple occupations on a regular basis (Lee & Kielhofner, 2017b; Wolske, Lee et al., 2024). Being linked to time and place, habits and roles bring temporal rhythm to daily life in familiar physical and social contexts (Clark, 2000; Wolske, Lee et al., 2024). In the practice scenario, Sam has noted that Micheline and her father live together. This prompts Sam to consider: what are Micheline's and her father's roles at home, and in their neighborhood or community? And how might their habits and routines have been changed by Micheline not working, and by her father no longer driving? Aware that the loss of valued social roles may contribute to difficulties with time use, routines, and making daily life more difficult to manage, Sam decides that in their next meeting, he will ask Micheline what her and her father's days are like, their usual roles, and routines. Sam could do this through informal conversation, or by using a semi-structured interview like the Occupational Performance History Interview-II (Kielhofner et al., 2004; Morris et al., 2024); he may also select the Role Checklist 3 (Popova et al., 2024; Scott, 2019) as a more structured way to explore Micheline's previous, present, and desired roles and satisfaction with her role participation.

Performance capacity is concerned with how mental and physical abilities are used and experienced in performance. The MOHO acknowledges that performance is affected by underlying sensory, musculoskeletal, neurological, cardiopulmonary, and other bodily capacities; it also draws a distinction between objective and subjective understandings of performance (Fisher et al., 2024). In other words, while underlying body structures and functions contribute to performance from an objective viewpoint, the MOHO also emphasizes the importance of the *lived body* experience, particularly to enhance understanding of how altered experiences impact performance. To illustrate, while the referral in the practice scenario indicated that Micheline's strength, endurance, and mobility had decreased and her speech was becoming slower, the concept of *performance capacity* guides Sam to consider: what impact might her reduced strength, endurance, and mobility be having on Micheline's ability to participate in her occupations? And how have Micheline's physical limitations and her speech difficulties altered her experiences of herself and her performance?

From a MOHO perspective, doing or performing any kind of occupation *(occupational performance)* also relies on the effective use of *skills*, so that not only limitations in performance capacities but also not having developed or gained experience in using specific skills may contribute to a person's difficulties in occupational performance (Bowyer et al., 2024). To explore these issues further, Sam decides on a combination of talking further with Micheline about her lived experience of doing her everyday activities and using an observation-based performance measure, the Assessment of Motor and Process Skills (Fisher & Jones, 2014), to understand Micheline's strengths and difficulties in performing activities of daily living.

In combination with volition, habituation, and performance-related factors, environmental conditions contribute to how a person's particular occupations are chosen, organized, and performed in daily life and how changes in their occupational engagement unfold. In the MOHO, the *environment* is conceptualized as those *physical, social, cultural, economic,* and *political features* of a person's context that impact their choices and motivation, habits and roles, and performance of occupations in daily life (Fisher et al., 2024). For instance, economic and political conditions shape individuals' resources and opportunities for doing (including the spaces and objects available for use), while cultural and social groups (e.g., family, club/team members, and co-workers) influence how occupations are done (e.g., rules, clothing, and objects used). These physical, social, cultural, economic, and political features of environments also have impacts in *immediate, local,* and *global* contexts.

In the practice scenario, Sam asks himself: what is Micheline and her father's home like? And what physical, social, or occupational features of their home create opportunities for meaningful occupational engagement, but also are there aspects of the home environment that may be barriers to safe and effective occupational performance? Hence, Sam decides to seek Micheline's permission to visit her and her father in their home to better understand their occupational engagement and participation within the *immediate* environment of their bungalow. Similarly, Sam thinks visiting Micheline's workplace with her may be useful if Micheline wishes to explore returning to work with her current employer.

Living in a rural community some distance from the nearest major center also places constraints on the resources and opportunities for participation available to Micheline and her father without transport, so Sam is thinking that he needs to explore ideas with Micheline and her father about possible social groups within their local community. These might potentially offer volunteer-run transport options or create other supports to sustain their participation within the community.

5.3.2 Using MOHO in Practice

MOHO is used by occupational therapists around the world to develop and deliver occupation-focused services for children, adults, and older adults experiencing diverse occupation-related challenges. Therapists use MOHO concepts in thinking about client situations, planning, and implementing therapy in a client-centered manner, not only through the therapist's effort to appreciate the client's perspective and circumstances but insofar as is possible also through involving the client (Wolske, Raber et al., 2024). This therapeutic reasoning process is illustrated in Figure 5.1.

The kinds of theory-driven questions that therapists ask themselves to guide their information-gathering were illustrated with examples of Sam's thinking relevant to

Step	Description
Generating theory-driven questions	• The therapist generates explicit MOHO-informed questions to guide information gathering. These MOHO-informed questions facilitate the therapist to select the types of information gathering most relevant to the issues for individuals and families with whom they are working. • For instance, using his MOHO knowledge and the initial information that he has about Micheline's situation, Sam has questions about Micheline's volition, roles, habits, immediate home, and local community environments.
Gathering information from and with the client	• The therapist gathers information using unstructured and structured methods, the choices being guided by the questions previously generated. • Based on Sam's theory-driven questions about Micheline's volition, roles, and routines he chooses a semi-structured interview to learn more about Micheline's situation from her perspective. Questions about how the physical, social, and occupational features of their home may be impacting both her and her father's occupational performance guide Sam to collaborate with Micheline to arrange a visit to their home.
Creating an occupational formulation of the client's situation	• The therapist organizes the information gathered to formulate an understanding of the client's occupational life and circumstances. This includes identifying factors contributing to the client's experiences of disruptions or challenges in occupations, and the strengths that can be built upon. • For instance, from interviewing Micheline, Sam learns about how she and her father have been looking after their home, shopping, cooking, and supporting each other, as well as about the challenges in daily living activities that they have faced, particularly since her father's declining eyesight meant he could no longer drive them to shops or visit friends.
Developing measurable goals and strategies for change	• The therapist's occupational formulation of the client's circumstances can then be used to guide identifying goals and plans for therapy in collaboration with the client. • For instance, Sam may share his understanding that their home is important to Micheline and her father; that their lack of transport seems a key obstacle to doing what is most important to them (e.g., shopping, meeting friends, and potentially working), and suggest that they work together to mobilize community resources to find a local solution to this issue.
Implementing and monitoring intervention	• Implementing the planned actions with the client(s), monitoring the intervention, and collaborating with the client(s) and adjusting actions as client feedback, new information, or unanticipated issues emerge. • For instance, Micheline and Sam together explore strategies to re-organize some objects in Micheline and her father's home so as to reduce hazards. Micheline and her father, supported by Sam, also investigate potential community transport options but a visit to the local library indicates there are few options. Micheline's father then suggests contacting retired miners in the community to explore interest in creating a volunteer transport network. Supported by Sam and Micheline, her father prepares an advertisement for a meeting which Sam then distributes to shops, the library, and a local hall where retired community members meet.
Assessing outcomes of intervention	• Collecting information through unstructured and structured means to determine with the client the extent to which their desired improvements and intervention goals were achieved. • Sam reviews progress with Micheline and her father by visiting them at home. Micheline reports that she is finding daily living activities less challenging since implementing strategies to re-organize the kitchen and bathroom, and that she feels safer around the home. Micheline and her father have yet to find an ongoing solution to their transport difficulties, although they have made contact with some other community members interested in these issues.

Figure 5.1 Steps to guide therapeutic reasoning using the Model of Human Occupation.

Source: Kielhofner (2008); Wolske, Raber et al. (2024).

using key MOHO concepts in the practice scenario. An extensive range of MOHO informed-interviews, self-report, and observational tools are available that are relevant to the concepts of volition, habits and roles, performance, environmental impact, occupational identity, and occupational competence, through which the information for formulating an understanding of clients' occupational lives and environments is gathered, and goals and strategies are formulated in collaboration with clients to facilitate desired change in their occupational engagement. Further, it provides a framework for identifying strategies to enable change in occupational engagement that is focused on creating opportunities for participation, enabling skill development, collaborative problem-solving, and making environmental adjustments (whether physical and/or social).

5.3.3 Evidence to Inform Using MOHO in Practice

Uses of the MOHO to support occupation-focused and client-centered assessment, planning, and implementation of occupational therapy within hospitals, rehabilitation services, home and long-term residential care, schools, employment services, and other community settings have been extensively documented, including in the MOHO textbooks (Kielhofner, 2008; Taylor, 2017; Taylor et al., 2024). A substantial body of research supports this use of the MOHO in guiding evidence-informed occupational therapy practice. This includes studies contributing to the development of a range of MOHO-informed and psychometrically sound assessment tools; studies seeking to understand the occupational participation of people with disabilities and factors impacting their daily lives; and research investigating practice applications of MOHO, the effectiveness of occupational therapy interventions informed by MOHO, and client perspectives of MOHO-based services (Bowyer & Kramer, 2017; Wolske, Lin et al., 2024). While it is beyond the scope of this chapter to review this evidence base in detail, substantial bibliographies of MOHO research, assessment tools, practice applications, and supporting evidence can be found in the MOHO textbook (Taylor et al., 2024) and accessed from the Model of Human Occupation Clearinghouse at https://moho-irm.uic.edu/

5.4 The Canadian Model of Occupational Participation (CanMOP), Collaborative Relationship-Focused Practice, and the Canadian Occupational Therapy Inter-relational Practice Process Framework (COTIPP)

In this section, we present the most recent Canadian occupation model, the CanMOP. In practice, this model is used concurrently with an approach – collaborative relationship-focused practice – and a process framework – the Canadian Occupational Therapy Inter-relational Practice Process Framework (COTIPP). While presented separately, they provide a set of integrated overall guidelines for occupational therapy.

5.4.1 The Canadian Model of Occupational Participation (CanMOP)

The CanMOP is the latest iteration of the occupation model developed for the Canadian Association of Occupational Therapists. Originally based on Reed and Sanderson's (1980) work, several iterations of the Canadian model have depicted a central individual, made up of physical, psychological, sociocultural, and spiritual dimensions, acting in physical, social, and cultural environments to produce productivity, self-care, and leisure occupations. Consideration of an institutional (sociopolitical) environment and the concepts of occupational engagement and enablement were later added to the model (Townsend & Polatajko, 2013). However, the fundamental conceptualization remains similar to the original model.

The CanMOP represents a significant departure from earlier versions of the Canadian model in three major ways. First, *occupational participation*, rather than an individual, is central. Second, there are no attempts to categorize occupation. Third, multiple new elements have been added with the aim of deepening the therapist's understanding of what the person (or collective) needs and wants to do and the current possibilities for such occupations. These new elements and other key concepts and principles of the model are described below.

The CanMOP guides reasoning in two ways. First, reasoning with the CanMOP points to areas for consideration in attempting to understand what individuals and collectives need to do and want to do: what are these occupations? And what does it look like when they are being done in a meaningful way as defined and valued by the individual or collective? Second, reasoning with the CanMOP indicates where substantial barriers and facilitators of access to and initiation and sustaining of valued occupations lie. This indicates the types of changes that should be most successful in promoting occupational participation.

5.4.2 Key Concepts

Occupational participation is the central focus of the CanMOP. Occupational participation is defined as "having access to, initiating, and sustaining valued occupations within meaningful relationships and contexts" (Egan & Restall, 2022, p. 76). Valued occupations can only be defined by the individual or collective involved. Therefore, in contrast to previous models, the CanMOP does not classify occupations into the predetermined categories of self-care, productivity, and leisure. Instead, it uses a broad conceptualization of occupation that includes a wide range "of everyday and extraordinary doings of individuals and groups, which have implications for individuals, societies, and the Earth" (Rudman et al., 2022, p. 15). Occupations have various meanings, values, and purposes that are done alone or as part of collectives. *Collectives* encompass the social units in which individuals are embedded and include families, groups, communities, and populations. Occupations include gathering resources for the survival of individuals, families, and communities, caring for oneself and others, connecting to people, land, ancestors, and spirituality, exerting power, resisting oppressions, expressing individual and collective identity, and promoting social change, among many other occupations.

In the graphic representation of the model (see Figure 5.2), the left half of the model presents the concepts that are critical to understanding what valued occupations in meaningful contexts look like for specific individuals and collectives. The right half directs the therapist to collaboratively consider ways to improve access to and initiate and sustain valued occupations through analyzing barriers and potential facilitators within the context of the individual or collective.

Specific occupations are valued by individuals and collectives for their *meaning and purpose*. Purpose can best be understood in connection with the needs that the occupations fulfill. Two sets of needs *as perceived by the individual or collective* are particularly important to explore. The first set relates to the individual or collective's survival and safety as it concerns personal, family, or community safety. These considerations include physical, emotional, spiritual, and cultural safety. Concerns related to safety often underlie the why and how of valued occupations. Whether occupations adequately fulfill safety considerations can only be determined by the individuals and collectives involved. In exploring with Micheline, Sam would ask about her survival and safety concerns in a broad sense and as perceived by her. He would be sensitive to and provide help addressing issues related to food security and housing and other survival and safety issues. He would appreciate that Micheline's concerns might extend to or be primarily related to people close to her or her community.

MODELS OF PRACTICE THAT FOCUS ON HUMAN OCCUPATION

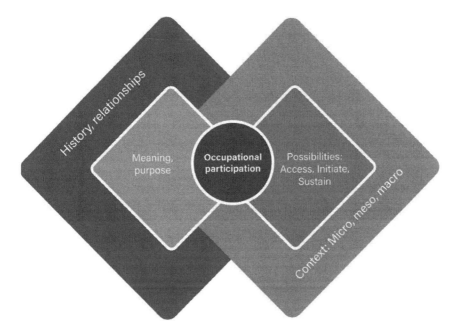

Figure 5.2 Graphic representation of the Canadian Model of Occupational Participation.
Source: Egan and Restall (2022) (CanMOP).

The second set of needs relates to universal human requirements as identified in self-determination theory: autonomy, relatedness, and competence (Ryan & Deci, 2019). Here again, the individual or collective's perception of these needs and how they can be adequately met are paramount. Sam would listen for and might ask Micheline directly how these needs are fulfilled in the occupations important to her.

Exploration of *relationships and history* further assists in identifying and determining the unique aspects of occupations valued by the individuals and collectives involved. Relationships connected with valued occupations may be close or distant, comfortable, or strained; they may belong to the past, present, or hoped for future. Exploring valued occupations from the perspective of relationship helps the therapist understand who needs to be involved in the occupation and how it needs to be done to be meaningful to the individual or collective.

Exploration of history for individuals is carried out using the concept of life course. This perspective attends to not only the person's age and life stage but also to historical forces the person has experienced that have affected their values, opportunities, and perspectives. For collectives, history is considered through the perspective of community history. This includes community experiences of unity and thriving, as well as experiences of disconnection and trauma. It also includes patterns of relationships with groups such as governments and adjacent communities. Together, relationships and history help better define the purpose, meaning, and forms of specific valued occupations. This helps the individual or collective share a clear picture of what satisfying occupational participation looks like, so that goals are relevant and plans meaningfully meet the needs and aspirations of the individual or collective.

The therapist collaboratively explores the current possibilities for *access to and initiating and sustaining the satisfying, valued occupation* as envisioned by the person or collective. The therapist looks for strengths and resources within these environments that can be tapped to improve possibilities for initiating and sustaining occupational participation. Where there are barriers to initiating and sustaining occupational participation, the therapist collaboratively identifies aspects of the micro, meso, and macro contexts that need to be changed to facilitate initiating and sustaining occupational participation.

The *micro context* relates to people and things in direct contact with the person or collective. People include family members, friends, colleagues, and service providers, while things might include tools, furniture, architecture, sidewalks, paths – any aspect of the physical environment in direct contact with the person or collective. Aspects of the individual or collective may also be considered at this time and might include aspects of body structure or function, spirituality, and social identities of individuals. For collectives, this includes family or community resources and identities.

The *meso context* is made up of socially created structures. These include health, education, and social service organizations and their programs. It also includes neighborhood and community infrastructures. The meso environment has a significant impact on access to and initiation and sustaining of valued occupations. For example, accessibility and routes of public transportation limit the degree of ease that a person who uses public transportation can get to a valued occupation.

The *macro context* is the larger sociopolitical context that produces aspects of the micro and meso contexts of valued occupations. It includes social and cultural beliefs and the political systems that sustain and enact these beliefs through governance processes. For example, implicit societal beliefs that seniors who no longer drive due to vision or cognitive concerns should move to larger centers might influence transportation planners and regional governments to not consider designing public transportation that might meet seniors' needs in small communities.

In examining the contexts of occupational participation, the therapist focuses on existing strengths and meaningful changes leading to initiation and sustaining of occupational participation. When collective access is an issue, where access to occupational participation is implicitly or explicitly barred for a group of people, the therapist looks for opportunities to work at the meso and macro levels with others who are dedicated to opening possibilities for access.

5.4.3 Evidence Supporting the CanMOP

The CanMOP builds on work carried out in the development of the original Canadian occupational model, with adaptation arising from critique and research. The central focus on occupational participation increases attention to holistic considerations of individuals and collectives. Research findings reflect that imposing categories, such as self-care, productivity, and leisure, as found in previous models prejudices how occupations are viewed and limits which occupations are considered in an occupational therapy context (Hammell, 2009). In addition, such categorizations do not encourage people characterize their occupations (Brooke et al., 2007).

Occupational therapists frequently refer to meaning and purpose when discussing people's occupations (Reed et al., 2011). The CanMOP explicitly considers meaning and purpose, and does so with reference to needs as identified in self-determination theory, with the addition of survival and safety needs. This makes use of current best evidence regarding motivation (Ryan & Deci, 2019). The CanMOP explicitly considers the life course of individuals and community history of collectives and expands beyond implicit considerations of life stage to appreciate that non-linear paths and individual and community histories affect possibilities.

Finally, the CanMOP continues to build on the original and subsequent models by expanding further on contextual factors that promote or hinder occupational participation. It explicitly describes contextual conditions that directly affect occupational participation (micro) and those that indirectly affect the person through their influence on the micro context (meso and macro). This delineation helps therapists to examine and act with others on broader issues such as attitudes, societal bias, and poverty that are increasingly understood to have major impacts on occupational possibilities.

The CanMOP assists occupational therapists to reflect on occupational participation and its meaning and value as determined by the individuals and collectives with whom they work. To promote occupational participation through occupational therapy practice, therapists use the CanMOP within a Collaborative Relationship-Focused Practice approach, guided by the COTIPP.

5.4.4 Approach: Collaborative Relationship-Focused Practice

Collaborative relationship-focused practice (Restall & Egan, 2021) is a practice approach that builds on previous conceptualizations of client-centered practice while increasing the focus on equity, justice, and rights. This practice approach explicitly acknowledges occupational therapists' imperatives to critically reflect on and address the power structures in society and therapy relationships that disproportionately enhance, constrain, or limit people's occupations and occupational participation. Collaborative relationship-focused practice is defined as:

> an approach to occupational therapy that attends to, and concentrates on, the relational aspects of the therapist self and the individuals and collectives (i.e., families, groups, communities, and populations) who use occupational therapy services. These relationships are embedded within the multilayered historical and contemporary contexts in which people live and occupational therapy occurs. The therapist continuously strives to develop a collaborative relationship with the individual or collective to jointly work toward priorities and goals that are meaningful to the individual or collective.
>
> *(Restall & Egan, 2022, p. 100)*

The approach retains the key characteristics of occupational therapy practice of respect for people and collectives, their choices and informed decisions (Sumsion, 2000), being trustworthy (Leclair et al., 2019), attending to power structures, and collaborating effectively with people using occupational therapy services (Townsend et al., 2013).

Importantly, collaborative relationship-focused practice highlights four additional descriptors. The first descriptor highlights the need for relationships to be *contextually relevant*. This requires the therapist to be critically self-aware of how their own social identities and positionalities, implicit and explicit biases, and worldviews interact with those of the people they work with. In addition, therapists become aware of practice contexts and the ways that dominant worldviews and epistemologies shape structures and decision making in these contexts. When therapists engage in collaborative relationship-focused practice they continuously seek to understand micro, meso, and macro level influences on themselves and the individuals and collectives who use their services. Contextually relevant relationships require therapists to critically reflect on how oppressions in the form of stigmas, ableism, racism, sexism, and additional discriminatory behaviors occur, how they are created and maintained, and how to take action to mitigate their effects (Krupa, 2008).

The second descriptor highlights how relationships need to be *nuanced* contextually and over time. Collaborative relationships vary depending on whether the therapist is working with an individual, family, group, or community, the purpose of therapy, and the particular needs and vulnerabilities of the people the therapist is working with. During long-term therapy, relationships vary over time as needs and priorities change. A nuanced relationship requires therapists to adjust their approach as needed through deep listening, reflection, and critical reflection.

The third descriptor emphasizes the therapist's actions to *strive for safety* in therapy relationships where the therapist continually works to create and maintain safer relationships. Safety includes physical, emotional, cultural, and spiritual dimensions as defined by the individual or collective (Curtis et al., 2019). Examples of ways that therapists take action to mitigate threats to relationship safety include the following:

- the application of universal precautions including those related to trauma-informed care
- following guidance for establishing culturally safer relationships, and
- carefully and critically attending to relational boundaries and addressing policies regarding relationships to support, rather than undermine, the emotional and spiritual well-being of people and communities.

The fourth descriptor of collaborative relationship-focused practice is the *promotion of rights-based self-determination*. Rights-based self-determination prompts occupational therapists to acknowledge that people have the right to make decisions that affect their health, well-being, survival, and participation in occupations. These choices and decision making are embedded within the rights and responsibilities that people have in relation to themselves, their families, and their communities. The relational aspects of rights-based decisions (Durocher et al., 2015) and contextual factors that facilitate or constrain choices (Hammell, 2020) are important considerations. In relationship-focused practice, therapists have a responsibility to facilitate the self-determining decisions of individuals and collectives in the therapy context, and to address the contextual factors that limit people's choices and rights.

5.4.5 Framework: The Canadian Occupational Therapy Inter-relational Practice Process Framework (COTIPP)

The COTIPP (Restall et al., 2022) is intended to guide occupational therapists through the therapy process as they promote occupational participation. As shown in Figure 5.3, the essential underlying process is building and sustaining relationships

MODELS OF PRACTICE THAT FOCUS ON HUMAN OCCUPATION

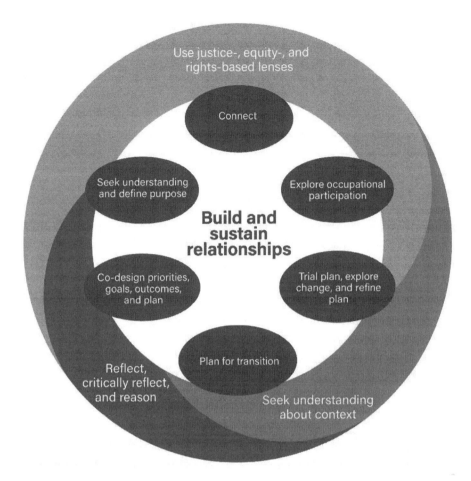

Figure 5.3 The Canadian Occupational Therapy Inter-relational Practice Process (COTIPP) Framework.
Source: Restall et al. (2022).

through collaborative relationship-focused practice (Restall & Egan, 2021) as discussed above. In addition, there are three foundational processes and six action domains. These processes integrate understanding of occupational participation through the CanMOP, the collaborative relationship-focused approach, three foundational processes, and six action domains that encompass the doing of occupational therapy.

In previous sections, we described the CanMOP and the collaborative relationship-focused approach. In the next section, we describe the three foundational processes and six action domains. Use of the practice scenario described at the beginning of this chapter provides illustrative examples of these concepts.

5.4.6 Three Foundational Processes

The three foundational processes begin prior to the therapist's first *connection with the individual or collective* and continue throughout the therapy process. The first foundational process seeks understanding about context at micro, meso, and macro levels. Understanding an individual's or collective's occupational participation and the barriers and constraints to occupations and the therapy itself is essential. Seeking to understand context begins with the therapist reflecting on their own personal contexts and that of their practice environments. These include the broader social, political, and historical contexts that shape health, education, and social care, as well as the health, well-being, and occupations of the individuals and collectives that use their services.

Thus, Sam needs to understand his own social positionality, history, and how his beliefs, learnings, and actions have been shaped by social, political, and historical contexts. Sam critically reflects on his social position and considers ways that his relative social position and identity may impact his interactions with Micheline. He also reflects on the social political context of the community that may impact how he is perceived in the community and by Micheline. Sam is an experienced therapist, secure in his employment and his skills. However, he notes his discomfort as he considers working with Micheline. Reflecting on this discomfort, he realizes that this stems from several sources. First, there is a real, but little spoken of, tension between the members of the mining community and health "professionals." There is a sense that the "miners" find the "professionals" haughty, naïve, and overpaid. He wonders how Micheline will react.

Sam also needs to seek to understand the context of his practice setting within the community in which Micheline lives. This can include the history of the community, its strengths, resources, and aspirations. To do this, Sam explores the physical environment by walking or driving through the community. He also explores the social, political, and historical contexts by reading available information and connecting with community leaders and researching business and agency resources in the community.

The second foundational process is *to reflect, critically reflect, and reason*. Therapists' reflection on practice helps them to make good, in-the-moment decisions, and to think deeply between practice events on how to improve their practice. Thus, Sam's deep reflection on how to improve his practice based on previous therapy events can help him improve his practice reasoning when he interacts with Micheline. Critical reflection builds on deep reflection to question and take action that promotes constructive change in harmful social systems and structures (Brookfield, 2009). For example, through critical reflection, Sam questions the social and political structures that are limiting occupational possibilities for Micheline and, more broadly, people with chronic health conditions, disabilities, and additional socially marginalized identities within the community. He gains greater understanding of how context has and may continue to limit the occupational possibilities for Micheline.

The third foundational process is *using justice, equity, and rights-based lenses to critically evaluate how occupational therapy practice and its contexts promote or create barriers to justice, equity, and the rights of the individuals and collectives* who use occupational therapy services. Building on critical reflection, this foundational process asserts Sam's responsibility to consider the ways that justice, equity, and rights for occupational participation are being upheld or denied within the community. Sam's responsibility extends to taking action to promote justice, equity, and rights at macro, meso, and micro levels of practice (Bailliard et al., 2020).

These three foundational processes provide essential underpinning for the six action domains of the practice process. We will first name the action domains and, using the practice scenario, then describe examples of their use in therapy.

5.4.7 Six Action Domains

The COTIPP framework describes six action domains: (1) connect; (2) seek understanding and define purpose; (3) explore occupational participation; (4) codesign priorities, goals, outcomes, and plan; (5) trial the plan, explore change, and refine the plan; and (6) plan for transition (Restall et al., 2022). These domains are not prescriptive and will not necessarily follow in a particular sequence or be appropriate in every process. Instead, the domains prompt consideration of options to achieve therapy intentions and are flexible enough to provide guidance when the therapist is working with individuals or collectives in a variety of practice contexts. Sam will need to integrate his understanding of the CanMOP, a collaborative relationship-focused approach, and the three foundational processes as he collaboratively engages with Micheline in the therapy action domains.

Sam reflects on his discomfort as he prepares for meeting with Micheline. Last year, another "miner" dismissed him from his hospital room stating, "Your kind will never understand the problems I face." Sam has always felt quite empathetic, and this left him shaken. Micheline is living with a serious, potentially progressive neurological disorder and Sam worries that he will not find a way to discuss this frankly with Micheline. Finally, he knows that Micheline has been adamant in the past about not leaving her home to live in a retirement home. He is worried that the community has few resources that could allow her to remain in her own home. Given all these considerations, he is worried that she may become angry with him.

Acknowledging the importance of creating safer relationships in Collaborative Relationship-Focused Occupational Therapy, Sam considers where they will meet in the unit, how he will position himself, and what he will do and say to initiate the conversation with Micheline that creates a situation in which Micheline feels as physically, emotionally, culturally, and spiritually safe as possible.

Sam begins his relationship with Micheline *(connect)* by asking her what her experience of occupational therapy has been. Sam's reflection has led him to consider how he can build a collaborative relationship with Micheline. Sam recognizes that while he has expertise in occupational therapy, Micheline has had 20 years' experience living with the effects of multiple sclerosis. This expertise may have been discounted by health professionals (Thorne et al., 2000) in the past and Sam does not want to reproduce that type of experience. Sam also recognizes that Micheline may have experienced many traumas in her past of which he is unaware and he must be sensitive in the relationship to potential vulnerabilities engendered by their different social positions and her possible past traumas.

He listens carefully and respectfully, while noting his discomfort when she shares her frustration with and fear of being forced to move to a retirement home. Sam recognizes his potential role and tells Micheline what occupational therapy can potentially offer. They tentatively agree that they would collaboratively focus on Micheline's occupational participation – that is, the things that she needs to do and wants to do in the places and with the people that are important to her *(seek understanding and define purpose of occupational therapy)*.

This initiates a series of discussions focused on what is important to Micheline *(co-design priorities, goals, outcomes, and plan)*. Micheline relates to Sam that she would really like to return to work, but she cannot imagine this would be possible, particularly as she is having increasing difficulty with fatigue. At this point, she states firmly that what she most wants is to be able to continue to manage at home.

To better understand Micheline's occupation of "continuing to manage at home," Sam explores related *history and relationships.* He asks Micheline to tell him more about her home and what it means to be home. Micheline relates the struggle she faced buying and paying for her home while working and raising her son, Travis. It was a lot of work, but she was proud of her home and how it was the favored location of after-school play and sleepovers for Travis's friends. She tells Sam that she was also proud to welcome her mother and father into her home when her mother's health was failing, and how she cared for her mother there until her death five years ago.

Sam asks her about the meaningful activities she carries out there now *(explore occupational participation)*. He listens and prompts her to tell him more about how she does these things, and with whom. He listens carefully for her descriptions of the purpose and meaning of these activities. Sam relates that he is struck by the importance Micheline has placed on caring for family and the attention she put into making the home a welcoming place *(meaning, purpose, life stage)*. Micheline's voice breaks as she tells him how comfortable her home is, and how her experience caring for her mother led to many changes to the home that she hoped might be useful if she herself needed them one day.

When Micheline sees that Sam is truly listening and trying to understand what is important to her, she begins to speak of how things are beginning to become more difficult for herself and her father. In the past, they shared household tasks and she relied on him to get groceries and take her to specialized appointments in the city 100 kilometers away. She is not sure how she will manage these things now that he is not able to drive.

Together, Sam and Micheline determine that their primary collaborative focus in occupational therapy will be to find ways to continue to live at home with her father *(seek understanding and define purpose)*. Sam asks Micheline if she would like her father to be included in these discussions, and she agrees that this would be good. They arrange times when Jack can join them by speaker phone to begin to discuss the activities that Micheline sees as essential to them both living comfortably at home together.

During these discussions, Micheline and Jack, supported by Sam, explore potential resources in the community *(meso environment)* that can support them to manage well at home *(co-design priorities, goals, outcomes, and plan)*. They are both reluctant to request too much of Micheline's son Travis. He has taken on extra hours at work and appears to be in line for promotion – they would like him to be able to make the best of this opportunity.

Together, Micheline, Jack, and Sam develop potential plans for dealing with maintaining the home *(co-design priorities, goals, outcomes, and plan)*. They make use of the knowledge that all three of them have about potential community resources *(meso environment)*. For example, Jack has learned from friends about a seniors' community bus to the grocery store. Sam shares information regarding a lower-cost housekeeping service for seniors that Jack can access. Jack reflects that a lot of his friends from work are facing health issues and decides to bring this up at the next "miners" breakfast (an informal monthly meeting of retired mine employees) to see how they might support one another. Sam relates that it may be worth reaching out to the provincial member of parliament about possible funding sources for initiatives in smaller communities that they could be eligible for *(meso environment)*.

Within two weeks of her stay on the unit, Micheline has become stronger; she transfers independently if unsteadily. Sam asks Micheline if she would be open to adding "falls prevention" to the things she is working on with him *(co-design priorities, goals, outcomes, and plan)*. Micheline agrees. Together, they review her activities at home and think about how falls have happened in the past, with a view to finding ways to prevent them in the future *(explore occupational participation)*. They plan a home visit to test out and revise these solutions as necessary.

Prior to her discharge from the unit, Micheline and Sam review her plans for continuing her valued activities at home and preventing the falls that take her away from her home *(plan for transition)*. They talk about how Micheline might connect with a community-based therapist for new solutions if further problems arise. At this time Micheline tells Sam that she feels hopeful that she may be able to return to her work as a bookkeeper in the company office. Micheline and Sam collaboratively discuss the option of Micheline contacting the human resources department at the company to determine what possibilities there may be for part-time or casual work. Sam asks Micheline if she would like him to reach out to her disability insurer or personnel office to explore services to help her plan a return to work. In these ways, sustainability of Micheline's occupational participation is promoted.

Using justice-, equity-, and rights-based lenses, Sam critically reflects on the disparity of the health and social service resources available to Micheline in comparison to people in similar situations in larger urban communities. Noting the lack of public transportation options both within the community and into the city that limit Micheline's choices to participate in occupations she needs and wants to do, Sam also begins to work within his circle of influence to promote service accessibility in partnership with people with disabilities in the community.

This scenario has provided an illustrative example of how the CanMOP, Collaborative Relationship-Focused Occupational Therapy, and the COTIPP can be used in practice to guide therapists reasoning and actions. Next, we briefly describe how the MOHO and CanMOP, as practice models, are linked with occupational science.

5.5 Occupational Science and Practice Models that Focus on Human Occupation

Occupational science is focused on advancing knowledge and understanding of human occupation itself (Wright St. Clair & Hocking, 2018). This knowledge is not static but, like any area of study, it is developing over time. Studies of individual and shared occupations are extending knowledge about how biological, social, cultural, temporal, political, and historical factors shape these specific occupations. Occupational science research about participation in occupations is also advancing understanding of occupational injustices and building knowledge about the relationships of occupation with health and well-being over the lifespan.

Occupational science and occupational therapy are not mutually exclusive areas of knowledge. Occupational science was envisioned as building knowledge about the nature of human occupation, its benefits and the factors restricting access to these benefits that could be used by occupational therapists working with clients to address the impacts on their lives of disrupted or restricted participation (Wright St. Clair &

Hocking, 2018). The significance of meaning in what people do, occupational balance, occupational justice are just some areas in which occupational science research is informing occupational therapy practices (Durocher et al., 2014; Eklund et al., 2017; Malfitano et al., 2019; Wright St. Clair & Hocking, 2018). Some further illustrations of links between occupational science and the occupational therapy practice models described in this chapter are outlined below.

The MOHO is used by occupational therapists to understand what their clients do in daily life, why and how to address the impacts of ill health, disability, aging, or environmental restrictions on their occupational identity, and occupational competence. Several key concepts articulated in MOHO have been the focus of research in occupational science. For example, studies of occupational choice, temporal aspects of daily life (e.g., habits and routines), and occupational identity highlight their importance in influencing participation, successful life transitions, and adaptation (Clark, 2000; Crider et al., 2015; Nizzero et al., 2017), adding to the evidence that underpins MOHO as an occupational therapy practice model.

Both the MOHO and the CanMOP draw attention to contextual factors that hinder or facilitate the initiation and sustaining of occupational participation. Studies of occupations in their sociocultural, economic, physical, geographic, political, historical contexts being undertaken by occupational scientists serve to identify contextual factors that need consideration when applying these occupational therapy practice models in differing settings globally, but also identify new possibilities for overcoming barriers to participation through occupational therapists' practice (Wright St. Clair & Hocking, 2018).

As noted earlier in the chapter, the CanMOP has moved away from attempts to classify occupation into pre-determined categories (such as self-care, productivity, leisure), in recognition of accumulating knowledge that occupations are not readily categorized and hold varied meanings, values, and purposes in differing contexts (Bailliard & Dickie, 2022; Jonsson, 2008). The CanMOP also places greater emphasis on collective aspects of occupation, noting the role of social connections and relationships in initiating and sustaining occupational participation, as well as in defining the meaning, value, and purpose of specific occupations. This is supported by recognition in occupational science that possibilities for occupational participation are constructed and negotiated by both individuals and by collectives (Laliberte Rudman, 2013). These shifts in how occupation is viewed within CanMOP also align with calls in occupational science to build more inclusive and globally relevant knowledge about the occupations of diverse populations from diverse geographic locations, and about hidden and neglected occupations that allow further examination of assumptions about the relationships of occupation, health, and well-being (Bailliard & Dickie, 2022). Further the re-conceptualisation of client-centered practice as a justice, opportunity and rights-based practice articulated in the Collaborative Relationship-Focused Practice approach links to the conceptual development of occupational justice and emerging understandings of occupational injustices within occupational science (Durocher et al., 2014; Malfitano et al., 2019).

5.6 Conclusion

Occupational therapy practice models focused on human occupation guide occupational therapists' reasoning and actions in practice. Conceptual models about occupation have been developed to frame and explain core concepts relevant to understanding people's experience of engaging in occupations, and the principles that inform and guide occupational therapy in practice. This chapter focused on two prominent models of practice: the MOHO and its accompanying therapeutic reasoning process; and the CanMOP, the Collaborative Relationship-Focused Practice approach, and the COTIPP. Occupational therapists may select either of these models focused on human occupation to guide authentic occupation-focused and client-centered occupational therapy practice. The origins and key concepts of each of these two occupational therapy practice models have been described. Their application has been illustrated in a practice scenario, showcasing the occupational therapist's use of reasoning and collaborative relationships to support their practice. These practice models emphasize various aspects of reasoning that guide therapists to consider, collaboratively with the people they are working with, the options for choosing evidence-informed courses of action.

Use of the MOHO in practice guides the occupational therapist to appreciate the personal and environmental factors shaping how a person chooses, organizes, and performs their occupations; how these factors may impact occupational identity and competence; and, in turn, how change in these factors can enable occupational engagement, skill development, and opportunities for participation in occupations of meaning and value. MOHO-informed practice is also supported by an extensive range of tools and evidence developed over more than three decades, several being referred to in the illustrative scenario.

The Canadian occupation model, practice approach, and process framework have developed over a similar period of time. As described in this chapter, the latest version conceptualizes occupation as an individual and a collective phenomenon. It leads the therapist to focus on occupations that the person or collective prioritizes, carefully considering their unique purpose and meaning developed with history, relationships, and contexts. It emphasizes a collaborative relationship-focused approach and brings a critical reflective lens to the practice of occupational therapy.

These two practice models may each be used to identify barriers and facilitators of access to valued occupations and to inform the development and delivery of occupational therapy services to promote the occupational participation of children, adults, and older adults as individuals, families, and within communities.

5.7 Summary

- Occupational therapists select practice models focused on human occupation to guide authentic occupation-focused and client-centered occupational therapy practice.
- The MOHO is widely used by occupational therapists as a framework to explore how people choose, organize, and perform occupations within their particular contexts, and how these personal and environmental factors shape their patterns of participation in occupations and capability to adapt them over time.
- MOHO-informed practice is also supported by an extensive range of tools and evidence drawing on its key concepts concerning volition, habituation, performance, and the environmental contexts in which occupational engagement and performance occur.
- The CanMOP, the Collaborative Relationship-Focused Practice approach, and the COTIPP Framework together place emphasis on people's occupational participation

individually and collectively; working through collaborative relationships; and bringing a critical reflective lens to occupational therapy practice.
- The CanMOP prompts occupational therapists to focus on occupations prioritized by individuals and collectives, to consider their purpose in meaning in light of history and relationships, and to collaboratively identify high-impact considerations in the micro, meso, and macro contexts that promote access to, initiation, and sustaining of occupational participation.
- Occupational therapists may use each of these practice models to collaborate with individuals and groups of people, such as families, to address disruptions or challenges in occupational participation experienced during times of life transitions and due to ill health, developmental delay, aging, and environmental restrictions.

5.8 Review Questions

1. How is occupation defined and conceptualized in each of the two models, the MOHO and the CanMOP?
2. The MOHO provides a framework for identifying strategies to enable change in occupational engagement. What is the relationship between a person's occupational identity and occupational competence, and how might this impact their day-to-day engagement and participation?
3. The CanMOP focuses on exploring barriers and facilitators to initiating and sustaining valued occupations. Equity and justice are emphasized as a key focus of practice. What are three ways in which a therapist could engage in critical reflection to address equity and justice issues within a collaborative relationship-focused approach?
4. How might your preparation for an initial client encounter be different depending on the model you choose to guide your practice? Consider theory-driven questions that inform the initial step in the therapeutic-reasoning process using the MOHO. How might this look different from the initial foundational process of critical reflection recommended in the COTIPP framework?
5. Both models consider how the environmental context might impact occupational participation. What aspects of the client's environment are the focus of clinical reasoning when using the MOHO? What aspects of the micro, meso, and macro contexts are the focus of clinical reasoning when using the CanMOP?

References

Bailliard, A. L., Dallman, A. R., Carroll, A., Lee, B. D., & Szendrey, S. (2020). Doing occupational justice: A central dimension of everyday occupational therapy practice. *Canadian Journal of Occupational Therapy, 87*(2), 144–152. https://doi.org/10.1177/0008417419898930

Bailliard, A. & Dickie, V. (2022). JOS Special Issue: Things people do: Toward a comprehensive understanding of human occupations. *Journal of Occupational Science, 29*(1), 1–5. https://doi.org/10.1080/14427591.2022.2057398

Brooke, K. E., Desmarais, C. D., & Forwell, S. J. (2007). Types and categories of personal projects: A revelatory means of understanding human occupation. *Occupational Therapy International, 14*(4), 281–296. https://doi.org/10.1002/oti.239

Brookfield, S. (2009). The concept of critical reflection: Promises and contradictions. *European Journal of Social Work, 12*(3), 293–304. https://doi.org/10.1080/13691450902945215

Bowyer, P., & Kramer, J. (2017). Evidence for practice from the Model of Human Occupation. In R. R. Taylor (Ed.), *Kielhofner's Model of Human Occupation* (5th ed., pp. 418–452). Lippincott, Williams & Wilkins.

Bowyer, P., Wolske, J., Cabrera, J. P., & Fisher, G. (2024). Dimensions of doing. In R. R. Taylor, P. Bowyer, & G. Fisher (Eds.), *Kielhofner's Model of Human Occupation: Theory and application* (6th ed., pp. 110–121). Wolters Kluwer.

Clark, F. A. (2000). The concepts of habit and routine: A preliminary theoretical synthesis. *Occupational Therapy Journal of Research, 20*(Supplement 2000), 123S–137S. https://doi.org/10.1177/15394492000200S114

Crider, C., Calder, C. R., Bunting, K. L., & Forwell, S. (2015). An integrative review of occupational science and theoretical literature exploring transition. *Journal of Occupational Science, 22*(3), 304–319. https://doi.org/10.1080/14427591.2014.922913

Curtis, E., Jones, R., Tipene-Leach, D., Walker, C., Loring, B., Paine, S.-J., & Reid, P. (2019). Why cultural safety rather than cultural competency is required to achieve health equity: A literature review and recommended definition. *International Journal for Equity in Health, 18*(1), 174. https://doi.org/10.1186/s12939-019-1082-3

Durocher, E., Gibson, B. E., & Rappolt, S. (2014). Occupational justice: A conceptual review. *Journal of Occupational Science, 21*(4), 418–430. https://doi.org/10.1080/14427591.2013.775692

Durocher, E., Kinsella, E. A., Ells, C., & Hunt, M. (2015). Contradictions in client-centred discharge planning: Through the lens of relational autonomy. *Scandinavian Journal of Occupational Therapy, 22*(4), 293–301. https://doi.org/10.3109/11038128.2015.1017531

Egan, M., & Restall, G. (2022). Canadian Model of Occupational Participation (CanMOP). In M. Egan & G. Restall (Eds.), *Promoting occupational participation: Collaborative relationship-focused occupational therapy* (pp. 71–95). Canadian Association of Occupational Therapists.

Eklund, M., Orban, K., Argentzell, E., Bejerholm, U., Tjörnstrand, C., Erlandsson, L. K., & Håkansson, C. (2017). The linkage between patterns of daily occupations and occupational balance: Applications within occupational science and occupational therapy practice. *Scandinavian Journal of Occupational Therapy, 24*(1), 41–56. https://doi.org/10.1080/11038128.2016.1224271

Fisher, A. G., & Jones, K. B. (2014). *Assessment of motor and process skills: Volume 2 user manual* (7th ed.). Three Star Press.

Fisher, G., Haglund, L., & Ullah, M. M. (2024). The environment and human occupation. In R. R. Taylor, P. Bowyer, & G. Fisher (Eds.), *Kielhofner's Model of Human Occupation: Theory and application* (6th ed., pp. 93–109). Wolters Kluwer.

Fisher, G., Tham, K., Erikson, A., Fallahpour, M., & Wolske, J. (2024). Performance capacity and lived body. In R. R. Taylor, P. Bowyer, & G. Fisher (Eds.), *Kielhofner's Model of Human Occupation: Theory and application* (6th ed., pp. 72–92). Wolters Kluwer.

Hammell, K. W. (2009). Self-care, productivity, and leisure, or dimensions of occupational experience? Rethinking occupational "categories." *Canadian Journal of Occupational Therapy, 76*(2), 107–114. https://doi.org/10.1177/000841740907600208

Hammell, K. W. (2020). Making choices from the choices we have: The contextual-embeddedness of occupational choice. *Canadian Journal of Occupational Therapy, 87*(5), 400–411. https://doi.org/10.1177/0008417420965741

Jonsson, H. (2008). A new direction in the conceptualization and categorization of occupation. *Journal of Occupational Science, 15*(1), 3–8. https://doi.org/10.1080/14427591.2008.9686601

Kielhofner, G. (2008). *Model of Human Occupation: Theory and application* (4th ed.). Lippincott, Williams & Wilkins.

Kielhofner, G. (2009). *Conceptual foundations of occupational therapy* (4th ed.). F. A. Davis.

Kielhofner, G., Mallinson, T., Crawford, C., Nowak, M., Rigby, M., Henry, A., & Walwns, D. (2004). *Occupational Performance History Interview – Second Version (OPHI-II).*

Assessment manual. Model of Human Occupation Clearinghouse, Department of Occupational Therapy, University of Illinois at Chicago.

Krupa, T. (2008). Part of the solution… or part of the problem? Addressing the stigma of mental illness in our midst. *Canadian Journal of Occupational Therapy, 75*(4), 198–207. https://doi.org/10.1177/000841740807500404

Laliberte Rudman, D. (2013). Enacting the critical potential of occupational science: Problematizing the 'individualizing of occupation'. *Journal of Occupational Science, 20*(4), 298–313. https://doi.org/10.1080/14427591.2013.803434

Leclair, L. L., Lauckner, H., & Yamamoto, C. (2019). An occupational therapy community development practice process. *Canadian Journal of Occupational Therapy, 86*(5), 345–356. https://doi.org/10.1177/0008417419832457

Lee, S. W., & Kielhofner, G. (posthumous) (2017a). Volition. In R. R. Taylor (Ed.), *Kielhofner's Model of Human Occupation* (5th ed., pp. 38–56). Lippincott, Williams & Wilkins.

Lee, S. W., & Kielhofner, G. (posthumous) (2017b). Habituation: Patterns of daily occupation. In R. R. Taylor (Ed.), *Kielhofner's Model of Human Occupation* (5th ed., pp. 57–73). Lippincott, Williams & Wilkins.

Lee, S. W., & Kielhofner, G. (2024). Volition: Patterns of thoughts and feelings about oneself as one anticipates, chooses, experiences, and interprets what one does. In R. R. Taylor, P. Bowyer, & G. Fisher (Eds.), *Kielhofner's Model of Human Occupation: Theory and application* (6th ed., pp. 41–60). Wolters Kluwer.

Malfitano, A. P. S., de Souza, R. G. D. M., Townsend, E. A., & Lopes, R. E. (2019). Do occupational justice concepts inform occupational therapists' practice? A scoping review. *Canadian Journal of Occupational Therapy, 86*(4), 299–312. https://doi.org/10.1177/0008417419833409

Morris, A., Haglund, L., Hemmingsson, H., Menks, L., Nygard, L., & Rosenberg, L. (2024). Talking with clients: Assessments that collect information through interviews. In R. R. Taylor, P. Bowyer, & G. Fisher (Eds.), *Kielhofner's Model of Human Occupation: Theory and application* (6th ed., pp. 283–309). Wolters Kluwer.

Nizzero, A., Cote, P. & Cramm, H. (2017). Occupational disruption: A scoping review. *Journal of Occupational Science, 24*(2), 114–127. https://doi.org/10.1080/14427591.2017.1306791

O'Brien, J., & Kielhofner, G. (posthumous) (2017). The interaction between the person and the environment. In R. R. Taylor (Ed.), *Kielhofner's Model of Human Occupation* (5th ed., pp. 25–37). Lippincott, Williams & Wilkins.

Parkinson, S., & Brookes, R. (2021). *A guide to the formulation of plans and goals in occupational therapy*. Routledge.

Popova, E. S., Kramer, J. M., Scott, P. J., Maciver, D., Linddahl, I., & Norrby, E. (2024). Eliciting clients' perspectives: Gathering information from clients, caregivers and other professionals. In R. R. Taylor, P. Bowyer, & G. Fisher (Eds.), *Kielhofner's Model of Human Occupation: Theory and application* (6th ed., pp. 256–282). Wolters Kluwer.

Reed, K. D., Hocking, C. S., & Smythe, L. A. (2011). Exploring the meaning of occupation: The case for phenomenology. *Canadian Journal of Occupational Therapy, 78*(5), 303–310. https://doi.org/10.2182/cjot.2011.78.5.5

Reed, K. L., & Sanderson, S. R. (1980). *Concepts of occupational therapy*. Williams and Wilkins.

Restall, G., & Egan, M. (2022). Collaborative relationship-focused occupational therapy. In M. Egan & G. Restall (Eds.), *Promoting occupational participation: Collaborative relationship-focused occupational therapy* (pp. 98–117). Canadian Association of Occupational Therapists.

Restall, G., Egan, M., Valavaara, K., Phenix, A., & Sack, C. (2022). Canadian occupational therapy inter-relational practice process framework. In M. Egan & G. Restall (Eds.), *Promoting occupational participation: Collaborative relationship-focused occupational therapy* (pp. 120–149). Canadian Association of Occupational Therapists.

Restall, G. J., & Egan, M. Y. (2021). Collaborative relationship-focused occupational therapy: Evolving lexicon and practice. *Canadian Journal of Occupational Therapy, 88*(3), 220–230. https://doi.org/10.1177/00084174211022889

Rudman, D. L., Aldrich, R., & Kiepek, N. (2022). Evolving understandings of occupation. In M. Egan & G. Restall (Eds.), *Promoting occupational participation: Collaborative relationship-focused occupational therapy* (pp. 12–30). Canadian Association of Occupational Therapists.

Ryan, R. M., & Deci, E. L. (2019). Brick by brick: The origins, development, and future of self-determination theory. *Advances in Motivation Science*, 6, 111–156. https://doi.org/10.1016/bs.adms.2019.01.001

Scott, P. J. (2019). *Role Checklist: Role Checklist Version 3: Participation and Satisfaction (RCv3)*. Model of Human Occupation Clearinghouse, Department of Occupational Therapy, University of Illinois at Chicago.

Sumsion, T. (2000). A revised occupational therapy definition of client-centred practice. *British Journal of Occupational Therapy*, 63(7), 304–309. https://doi.org/10.1177/030802260006300702

Taylor, R. R. (Ed.). (2017). *Kielhofner's Model of Human Occupation* (5th ed.). Lippincott, Williams & Wilkins.

Taylor, R. R. (2024). Introduction to the Model of Human Occupation. In R. R. Taylor, P. Bowyer, & G. Fisher (Eds.), *Kielhofner's Model of Human Occupation: Theory and application* (6th ed., pp. 1–8). Wolters Kluwer.

Taylor, R. R., Bowyer, P., & Fisher, G. (Eds.) (2024). *Kielhofner's Model of Human Occupation: Theory and application* (6th ed.). Wolters Kluwer.

Thorne, S. E., Ternulf Nyhlin, K., & Paterson, B. L. (2000). Attitudes toward patient expertise in chronic illness. *International Journal of Nursing Studies*, 37(4), 303–311. https://doi.org/10.1016/s0020-7489(00)00007-9

Townsend, E. A., Beagan, B., Kumas-Tan, Z., Versnel, J., Iwama, M., Landry, J., Stewart, D., & Brown, J. (2013). Enabling: Occupational therapy's core competency. In E. Townsend & H. J. Polatajko (Eds.), *Enabling occupation: Advancing an occupational therapy vision for health, well-being and justice through occupation* (2nd ed., pp. 87–133). CAOT Publication.

Townsend, E. A., & Polatajko, H. J. (Eds.). (2013). *Enabling occupation: Advancing an occupational therapy vision for health, well-being and justice through occupation* (2nd ed.). CAOT Publication.

Wolske, J., Lee, S. W., Ullah, M. M. & Anvarizadeh, A. (2024). Habituation: Patterns of daily occupation. In R. R. Taylor, P. Bowyer, & G. Fisher (Eds.), *Kielhofner's Model of Human Occupation: Theory and application* (6th ed., pp. 61–71). Wolters Kluwer.

Wolske, J., Lin, T. T., Bowyer, P., & Magasi, S. (2024). Evidence for practice from the model of human occupation. In R. R. Taylor, P. Bowyer, & G. Fisher (Eds.), *Kielhofner's Model of Human Occupation: Theory and application* (6th ed., pp. 463–479). Wolters Kluwer.

Wolske, J., Raber, C., Pépin, G., & Fisher, G. (2024). Therapeutic reasoning: Planning, implementing, and evaluating the outcomes of therapy. In R. R. Taylor, P. Bowyer, & G. Fisher (Eds.), *Kielhofner's Model of Human Occupation: Theory and application* (6th ed., pp. 161–187). Wolters Kluwer.

Wright St. Clair, V. A., & Hocking, C. (2018). Occupational science: The study of occupation. In B. Schell, G. Gillen (Eds.), *Willard and Spackman's occupational therapy* (13th ed., pp. 348–375). Wolters Kluwer Health.

CHAPTER 6

Participation and (Human) Occupation

Daniela Castro de Jong, Wilson Verdugo Huenumán, Andrea Yupanqui-Concha, Carolina Vásquez Oyarzún, and Cristian Aranda-Farías

Abstract
Occupational therapy considers occupation and participation as core constructs required to support people's engagement on what matters to them. In the first part of this chapter, we look at participation from a theoretical perspective. Over history, the profession's understanding of the notion of participation has evolved, progressively acknowledging its complex nature. Participation matters as it is the way in which we are in and connect with the world. In the second part of the chapter, we look at participation in an applied manner. Through contextualized scenarios in the Global South, we present an applied understanding of the idea of participation for different age groups and the importance of our surrounding circumstances on it. This chapter is an invitation for readers to reflect on the idea of participation from a theoretical and a situated practical perspective.

Authors' Positionality Statement
The team who co-wrote this chapter represent a diverse group of occupational therapy practitioners with more than 75 years of combined professional experience working with young and older clients, their families, and communities, as well as working as academics in the higher education sector. Geographically, we were all born, raised, and completed our bachelor's degree in occupational therapy in Chile; however, our educational, research, and work experiences have also taken us to Spain, Sweden, and Australia. As participation is as broad as human experiences can be, we do not therefore aim to provide a final response to what the phenomenon is. We see this chapter as an opportunity to explore the topic, an invitation to learn, and reflect about it. We also wish to explicitly recognize our own positionality (Latin American, multilingual, im/migrants, cisgendered, university educated, professionally qualified occupational therapists) as citizens, practitioners, educators, researchers, and scholars. We recognize that the subject matter included in this chapter may represent the social, political, cultural, and local views arising from our own experiences across the world, with a clear

influence of our initial leaning and practices in Latin America. In the process of drafting this chapter, we have made a concerted effort to include evidence-based, scholarly, inclusive, culturally sensitive, gender-affirmative material to embrace a diverse range of perspectives from both the Global South and the Global North. However, we acknowledge that the chapter contents reported below are not exhaustive, nor completely bias free or representative of every single cultural, racial, gender, economic, political, or social reality. We hope that the material included in this chapter will promote critical, inclusive, respectful, progressive debate among current and future members of the occupational therapy profession, nationally and internationally.

Objectives
This chapter will allow the reader to:

- Define participation from an occupational perspective.
- Introduce the importance of participation in occupational therapy.
- Through a case study format illustrate how social, economic, and environmental factors shape participation.
- Illuminate aspects of participation in a Global South context.

Key terms
- **community participation**
- **Global South**
- **Latin America**
- **participation across the lifespan**
- **social participation**

6.1 Introduction

Occupational therapy is devoted to support people from all walks of life, ages, and abilities to engage in what matters to them and to participate in their daily occupations. Participation then is about taking part in *something*. The *something* could be as broad as going to church, working at a local market, or celebrating a traditional festival. The *something* could happen every day, or just once in a lifetime. It could be *something* which someone has just learnt or has done many times before. The list of what we would consider as participation is as extensive as human diversity can be and, as a result, defining, understanding, and measuring participation as used in occupational therapy is a challenging and fascinating task. This chapter provides the reader with an introduction to participation from an occupational perspective, acknowledging that the topic's diversity and complexity provide further opportunity for exploration. An initial section looks at commonly used and discipline-specific definitions of participation as applied in occupational therapy. We then review how the concept has evolved and been embraced by the profession in the last few decades. Embracing the concept of participation as a core idea has allowed occupational therapy to develop in context-specific ways. To highlight this development, examples are given from Latin America and across the life span, and participation is examined through local practices and with collectives (or communities) as clients.

6.2 Definitions of Participation

Participation or the action of taking part in something is a commonly used term. Think about your own experiences of attending after-school activities, going to church, playing sports, or any activity you need to do, must do, or are expected to do. Participation involves sharing, doing with others, and different levels of active involvement. The *Cambridge Dictionary* defines participation as *"the fact that you take part or became involved in something"* (Cambridge Dictionary, 2022). The act of taking part in something, or "doing," has been at the core of occupational therapy since its inception. This can be traced back to the seminal work of Adolf Meyer, considered one of the founders of the profession, who recognized that people with mental illness benefitted from "doing" something that was meaningful to them (Meyer, 1922). The definition of participation appears to be straightforward from a semantic perspective, but occupational therapists take a more nuanced view of the concept when applying an occupational perspective in theory and practice. Describing how occupational therapy conceptualizes participation is important as it is closely tied to the concepts that contribute to "occupation," health, and well-being, which are at the core of our profession (WFOT, 2012). It also links closely with the World Health Organization position on participation which is that it is an essential element of individual and collective health (WHO, 2019).

Participation must not be confused or equated with performance in occupation. While performance relates to the objective and observable components of the occupation, participation also adds a subjective side which can be seen through engagement and reflection (Larsson-Lund & Nyman, 2017). For example, think about two teenagers attending a driving lesson. While *performance* can be similar for both (movements required to drive a car), their *participation* will be different according to their personal learning experiences. This is in line with the ground-breaking ideas of Ann Wilcock and the understanding of an occupational perspective in health through her vision on doing, being, becoming, and belonging (Wilcock, 1998, 2006). The dynamic and fluid integration of the four dimensions outlined by Wilcock allows participation to embrace objective and subjective components. The most current definition of occupational therapy proposed by the World Federation of Occupational Therapists (WFOT, 2012) includes enabling participation in daily occupations as the profession's main goal.

The Occupational Therapy Practice Framework IV (OTPF-IV) (AOTA, 2020) explains that participation, in conjunction with health and well-being through our engagement in occupation, is the best way to explain our domain and process in its fullest sense. According to the OTPF-IV: "Participation occurs naturally when clients are actively involved in carrying out occupations or daily life activities they find purposeful and meaningful. More specific outcomes of occupational therapy intervention are multidimensional and support the end result of participation" (AOTA, 2020, p. 5). Given that participation is an important concept in the profession, occupational therapy interventions are oriented to support clients engaging in what matters to them (AOTA, 2020). This could range from catching a bus to go to work, going on holidays, or cooking a meal for the family on a given celebration. The OTPF-IV (AOTA, 2020) also indicates that participation happens in and through our daily occupations, which bring meaning and purpose to our lives. Participation does not occur in isolation or in a bubble, as it needs to be understood as the result or product of the ongoing interactions between people, what they want to do, and where they are engaging in them (AOTA, 2020).

Recently, the Canadian Association of Occupational Therapists invited the profession to revisit the idea of participation by reframing occupation as a relational construct. The Canadian Model of Occupational Participation (CanMOP) (Egan & Restall, 2022) brought attention to the notion that occupation very rarely occurs in isolation, and that through participation we relate to our surrounding circumstances (contexts/environments) (Egan & Restall, 2022). Based on this, as occupational therapists we must develop an understanding of how those circumstances can enable or severely restrict opportunities for participation (Egan & Restall, 2022).

In the context of the CanMOP, occupational participation is understood as "having access to, initiating, and sustaining valued occupations within meaningful relationships and contexts" (Egan & Restall, 2022, p. 76). The CanMOP asks us to consider how we can support our clients to access, initiate, and engage in occupations they want to participate in, as well as the considerations that will make their participation unique (Egan & Restall, 2022). For example, think about the occupation of having a meal. Would the client do it alone or with their family? At home, at a park, or at a restaurant? Frozen, or freshly made food? Are there any dietary considerations due to their health needs or cultural backgrounds? Are they eating with cutlery, chopsticks, or with their hands? Would the radio, television, or mobile/cell phones be allowed while eating?

Even though the notion of participation is widely acknowledged in occupational therapy theory (as discussed before) and in guiding our practice as it shapes the provision of client-centered practice, it is not equally or consistently researched in all areas of practice (O'Connor et al., 2021).

6.3 The Challenges of Defining Participation in Occupational Therapy

Cardoso da Silva and Correa Oliver (2021), as well as Magalhães (as cited by Castro de Jong et al., 2022), remind us that complex concepts and their definitions (many of which are used in our profession) must be situated and contextualized. Participation is no exemption, as seen in its use in recent reviews of emerging concepts such as occupational justice which can be understood as "[…] access to and participation in the full range of meaningful and enriching occupations afforded to others, including opportunities for social inclusion and the resources to participate in occupations to satisfy personal, health, and societal needs […]" (AOTA, 2020, p. 79). Access to a "full range of meaningful and enriching occupations" will vary from individual to individual, group to group, and community to community. What a "full range" of those occupations would be for us as the authors of this chapter will differ from your own expectations, lived experiences, or needs. This is further explained by Kjellberg et al. (2012) in their research on participation in the provision of client-centered services where participation is discussed in terms of independence, interdependence, and dependence. These appear to be shaped by contextual factors such as our location in the world and the actual possibilities to provide appropriate services (Kjellberg et al., 2012).

In the following section, examples of participation in Latin America from an occupational perspective will be provided. These fictional scenarios are based on the lived experiences of some of the co-authors and illuminate the rich and diverse nature of participation.

6.4 The South Is Not the North

Latin America corresponds to more than half of the surface of the American continent and is home to around 650,000,000 inhabitants in 30 nations (CEPALSTAT, 2018). The region is characterized by great cultural diversity, shaped by the co-existence of Indigenous communities and the legacy of colonization and subsequent waves of migration that arose from the exploitation and enslavement of our native, Indigenous, and black peoples who were kidnapped from the African continent (Ambrosio & Silva, 2022; Mailhe, 2019).

Historically, Latin American countries have had unstable political systems and economies riven by social inequality, a characteristic that has been exacerbated by the COVID-19 pandemic (CEPAL, 2022; Yasunaga, 2020).

The occupational therapy profession was initially established in Latin America in the late 1950s and early 1960s as a result of the polio epidemics (Monzeli et al., 2021). Over 60 years, the profession has navigated between the dominant theories from the Global North and local knowledge (Guajardo et al., 2015) and it is the latter than informs the authors' positionality. This position is based on the emergence of a movement within the profession called "occupational thera*pies* of the South" (Simó et al., 2016; Valderrama, 2019). This movement has emerged in those countries from what has been called the Global South, where life, health, and occupations are shaped in a particular way that differs from traditional views from within the discipline (Valderrama, 2019). The Global South, in the words of de Sousa Santos (2018), is a "metaphor that represents the global, systemic and unjust human suffering caused by capitalism, colonialism and patriarchy" (p. 275).

In contrast, the Global North represents the dominant views and values system in the world because "Eurocentric knowledge has legitimized the civilizing/normalizing mission based on the deficiencies and deviations from the normal civilized pattern of other societies" (Lander, 2000, p. 25). Understanding our history allows us to consider our identity and how it might differ from those of our clients or the lived experiences of occupational therapists in other regions. From this perspective, the occupational therapies of the South would be eminently critical and social, and the profession's work is to restructure the asymmetrical power relations between the different social actors. A restructuring that "brings us closer to occupations, human activities, and everyday life, considering varied contexts crossed by a series of sociohistorical and cultural processes and impacted by the crossroads of hegemonic systems of power" (Ambrosio & Silva, 2022, p. 9).

This is particularly relevant in terms of participation as the historical, political, economic, cultural, and social contexts in which occupational therapists live and work shape the way in which participation is experienced. The following sections include two case studies from Latin America that highlight individuals' experience of participation.

6.5 Youth Participation in Latin America

To provide some context, the adolescent and youth population of Latin America (i.e., those aged between 15 and 29 years old) is 133 million, of whom around 37 million live in poverty (Morales & Van Hemelryck, 2022). A large percentage (20.3%) is considered as "nor," i.e., they neither study nor work, while women in poverty aged 20–29 represent the most excluded (Camacho, 2014). Ethnic, racial, economic, and educational inequalities further perpetuate and accentuate difficulties and differences among this group (CEPAL, 2022; Morales & Van Hemelryck, 2022). In Nicaragua and Guatemala, illiteracy rates remain high in the youth population: 13.1% and 12.4% among Indigenous groups; and 7.4% and 9.5% in the mestizo and white populations, respectively (Lorente Rodríguez, 2019).

6.6 Meeting Cristina

Cristina is a 25-year-old woman from a small town in the north of Chile and the eldest of four siblings. Her mother is a nursing assistant and took care of her four children alone, after her husband left the family more than 15 years ago. The family lived in a vulnerable area of the city blighted by extreme poverty, i.e., people living on less than USD1.90/day and with high levels of criminal activity and drug dealing. Since a child, Cristina has been interested in reading every book that comes into her hands and she learnt from her mother that the only way to "escape" poverty was through formal education. Indeed, she is the first-generation university student to complete a law degree. Despite the scarcity of economic resources within the family, Cristina was able to finance her university course through scholarships and bank loans. Her excellent academic performance meant that she had no difficulties continuing her legal training post-graduation.

In Chile, located in the southwest corner of Latin America, this is not an isolated case as the country has experienced an exponential rate of expansion of participation in secondary education, particularly tertiary or higher education (INJUV, 2021). In less than 20 years, participation in tertiary education among the younger population increased from 10% to 50% in 2021 (CEPAL, 2022). For Cristina and other children and young people in Latin America, participation and active involvement in education represent the potential to completely transform lives and families, through improved well-being and a better quality of life.

In Cristina's case, she had to make some clear occupational choices from an early stage: to choose whether or not to consume substances, join a group of friends to commit crimes, drop out of school and work, etc. For Cristina, being actively involved in her education and achieving success gave meaning to her life. Positive outcomes in the occupational choice of student role are multidimensional: first, they reaffirm autonomy and independence; and second, they promote cognitive, cultural, emotional, social, and, over time, economic development.

In contrast, there are also children and young people for whom participation and involvement in education are unsuccessful and this happens for various reasons. Some abandon academic life for work in order to help out financially at home, while others leave education due to lack of motivation, school failure, or low expectations of better paid jobs (Morales & Van Hemelryck, 2022). In the case of women, adolescent pregnancy, marriage, early relationships, and care of older or younger family members are all factors that lead to the abandonment of formal education, the primary factor in social mobility

(CEPAL, 2022). Adolescent pregnancy is a known risk factor for maternal and infant mortality and contributes to the cycle of disease and poverty resulting from school dropout, less training, and, consequently, the acquisition of more precarious jobs (Binstock & Näslund-Hadley, 2013; World Health Organization, 2022). The same rationale explains the lack of attachment to education in teenage mothers who exhibit lower aspirations to work outside their home (Binstock & Näslund-Hadley, 2013) but for whom economic need (many must support their own home) forces them to access low-skilled jobs in precarious working conditions (Vaca Trigo, 2019). In a labor market where the informal sector is widespread, particularly in lower-skilled jobs, inadequate social and work safety protection is common (Binstock & Näslund-Hadley, 2013).

Compared to their peers who complete their education, adolescents who drop out of secondary or higher education are more likely to be financially and socially disadvantaged, highlighting the influence of participation in education on future health and well-being (Gómez et al., 2018). This is particularly relevant for occupational therapists as modifying environments and/or tasks that allow individuals and groups to access education is within the scope of the profession. As we have seen, participation in education in Latin America is influenced by various factors that include the personal, social, cultural, and economic.

6.7 Participation of Older People in Latin America

When we think of older people, we might have multiple and co-existent images. One of them is joy and satisfaction, the older years being a time to celebrate the effort made in those earlier vital stages (Hernández, 2009). At this stage of life, daily occupations will vary, from those centered on paid work and raising children (typical of adulthood), to those centered on the person, such as caring for one's own health or recreation (Aguilar-Parra et al., 2016). However, when it comes to being able to focus on these person-centered occupations, the social support networks of older people assume great importance (Pillemer et al., 2000). Where better social support networks exist, there are usually more opportunities to participate in meaningful occupations (Soriano et al., 2022). Societies with robust social security systems for older people also facilitate participation in and enjoyment of occupations (Leiva et al., 2020). However, being an older person in any part of the world represents a challenge, and in the context of Latin America a very particular one. While select countries in the region have some of the highest life expectancies, close to 80 years (Costa Rica, Chile, Uruguay), in others, life expectancy is closer to 70 years (Honduras, Belize), or as in the case of Haiti, one of the poorest countries in the world, barely over 60 years (Cardona et al., 2013). In this region, poverty is a determining factor in the older age group and influences all areas of occupational performance and participation (Paz & Arévalo, 2019). The average monthly pension of an older person in Latin America varies from around USD400 in Argentina, approximately USD200 in Chile, Bolivia, and Brazil, to around USD100 in Mexico and Paraguay (Arenas de Mesa, 2019). Aging in poverty adds specific challenges to the daily occupations of older people.

Therefore, for occupational therapists in these countries, the need to promote fairer and more inclusive contexts becomes ever more urgent, to ensure that older people can participate in meaningful occupations according to their potential, interests, and needs (del Barrio Truchado et al., 2020).

6.8 Meeting Luisa

Luisa is 70 years old and a former teacher who retired two years ago. She lives in the Magallanes region, located in southern Chile at the southernmost tip of the American continent. It is an area isolated from the rest of the country characterized by extreme climatic conditions, cold all year round and with winds so strong they often prevent people, especially older people, from venturing onto the streets due to the risk of falls. Luisa worked as a primary school teacher for 45 years, during which she got married and had two children. Today, her children are both professionals and they remember their mother as a hard-working person, who was at school from 8 o'clock in the morning until 6 o'clock in the afternoon, Monday through to Friday. Her salary was not high, but it allowed them to meet their basic needs and Luisa, despite her long working days, always tried to reconcile her work with her family occupations and obligations, for which her children are grateful. Her children have since moved to different areas of the country and her husband passed away three years ago. When she retired, Luisa began to receive a pension of close to USD400 per month (equivalent to the local currency), which is insufficient to cover her rent, private medical insurance, basic household services, and, for some years, the medicines she needs on a daily basis (for high blood pressure and Type II diabetes). Like many other people in the region, due to the lack of money, Luisa was forced to continue working. For the last six months, she has combined medical check-ups with her job as a cashier in a bakery near her home. She works 36 hours a week, from Monday to Saturday (10 am–4 pm). Luisa would prefer not to have to work, so she could spend more time with her friends and join groups with whom she can share her hobbies (reading and gardening). She is unable to, however, and as a result, she is not optimistic about her future and her long-term health. The little time she has free from paid work does not allow her to read or garden to the degree she would like. Luisa reads a couple of times a week when she is not too tired from working and she gardens on her only free day, Sunday. When asked about her dream, she says she would like to visit her children and grandchildren, but regards the prospect as utopian because she does not have the money to do it. She is also afraid that something could happen to her on a trip and she would be unable to afford the medical expenses.

Luisa has participated in significant occupations throughout her life, occupations that are now restricted due to the context in which she lives. This context is especially complex for the elderly in South America, mainly due to the economic situation most pensioners in this part of the world find themselves in, and that has a direct impact on their quality of life.

6.9 Conclusion

This chapter is intended as an open invitation to reflect on and carefully consider the notion of participation as used historically and currently in occupational therapy. While not exhaustive, the chapter highlighted some of the key considerations to address when thinking about the diverse nature of participation as used in the profession. This complexity is shaped by a growing body of knowledge that allows us to gain a rich understanding of how societal and global issues impact people's participation. Different bodies of knowledge emphasize, in unique ways, the key aspects of participation, from active engagement to social expectations and the relational/interactive notion of occupation to name just a few. The case scenarios illustrate how situated contexts and practices shape not only our clients' participation in occupation, but also allow us to critically consider how our own practices are shaped as a result. The co-authors' positionality and the scenarios from the Global South are another invitation to reflect on how the concept must be examined in a situated manner. As a reader, identify where are you standing – geographically, culturally, and politically, among other contextual characteristics – when looking at participation. Our only certainty in this is space to keep watching and learning as new developments in the understanding of participation continue to emerge. Embrace the challenges and enormous responsibilities that come with it!

6.10 Summary

- Occupational therapy conceptualizes participation as having close ties to the concepts occupation, health, and well-being.
- Wilcock (1998, 2006) formulated the occupational perspective in health through her vision on doing, being, becoming, and belonging; these four dimensions allow participation to embrace objective and subjective components.
- The World Federation of Occupational Therapists (2012) includes enabling participation in daily occupations as the profession's main goal.
- Participation occurs as a result or product of the ongoing interactions between people, what they want to do, and where they are engaging in them.
- The historical, political, economic, cultural, and social contexts in which occupational therapists live and work shape the way in which participation is experienced; an example of this is the impacts of the Global North and Global South.

6.11 Review Questions

1. What is participation according to the OTPF-IV and the CanMOP?
2. What are some commonalities and differences between the OTPF-IV and the CanMOP definitions of participation?
3. In the case scenarios presented, how do social and economic factors impact participation?
4. In the case scenarios presented, what are the valued occupations described by both individuals?
5. How are the concepts of agism, sexism, human rights, and occupational justice relevant to participation in the case studies given?

References

Aguilar-Parra, J. M., Padilla, D., & Manzano, A. (2016). Importancia de la ocupación en el desarrollo del mayor y su influencia en su salud. *International Journal of Developmental and Educational Psychology*, 1(1), 245–253. https://doi.org/10.17060/ijodaep.2016.n1.v1.232

Ambrosio, L., & Silva, C. R. (2022). Intersectionality: An American diasporic concept for occupational therapy. *Cadernos Brasileiros de Terapia Ocupacional*, 30, e3150. https://doi.org/10.1590/2526-8910.ctoen241431502

American Occupational Therapy Association. (2020). Occupational Therapy Practice Framework: Domain and Process (4th ed.). *American Journal of Occupational Therapy*, 74(S2), 7412410010p1–7412410010p87. https://doi.org/10.5014/ajot.2020.74S2001

Arenas de Mesa, A. (2019). *Los sistemas de pensiones en la encrucijada: Desafíos para la sostenibilidad en América Latina*. CEPAL.

Binstock, G., & Näslund-Hadley, E. (2013). Maternidad adolescente y su impacto sobre las trayectorias educativas y laborales de mujeres de sectores populares urbanos de Paraguay. *Papeles de Población, 19*(78), 15–40. https://www.scielo.org.mx/scielo.php?script=sci_arttext&pid=S1405-74252013000400003

Camacho, C. (2014). Desigualdad en el empleo y el trabajo. In H. de Zela, P. Esquenazi, A. Briones, & G. Ochoa (Eds.), *Desigualdad e inclusión social en las Américas: 14 ensayos* (pp. 255–275). Organización de los Estados Americanos.

Cambridge Dictionary (2022). *Definition of participation*. https://dictionary.cambridge.org/dictionary/english/participation

Cardona, D., Acosta, L. D., & Bertone, C. L. (2013). Inequidades en salud entre países de Latinoamérica y el Caribe (2005–2010). *Gaceta Sanitaria, 27*(4), 292–297. https://doi.org/10.1016/j.gaceta.2012.12.007

Cardoso da Silva, A. C., & Correa Oliver, F. (2021). Social participation in occupational therapy: Is it possible to establish a consensus? *Australian Occupational Therapy Journal, 68*(6), 535–545. https://doi.org/10.1111/1440-1630.12763

Castro de Jong, D., Sy, M. P., Twinley, R., Lim, K. H., & Borba, P. L. O. (2022). (Des)Connections between occupational justice and social justice: An interview with Gail Whiteford and Lilian Magalhães. *Cadernos Brasileiros de Terapia Ocupacional, 30*(spe), e30202202. https://doi.org/10.1590/2526-8910.ctoED302022022

CEPALSTAT. (2018). *Bases de datos y publicaciones estadísticas*. https://statistics.cepal.org/portal/cepalstat/dashboard.html?indicator_id=1&area_id=1&lang=es

Comisión Económica para América Latina y el Caribe. (2022). *Panorama social de América Latina 2021*. CEPAL.

del Barrio Truchado, E., Pinzón Pulido, S., Sancho, M., & Garrido Peña, F. (2020). Ciudadanía activa y personas mayores: Viejos conceptos, nuevos abordajes. Una revisión sistemática y metasíntesis cualitativa. *Revista Española de Geriatría y Gerontología, 55*(5), 289–299. https://doi.org/10.1016/j.regg.2020.01.001

de Sousa Santos, B. (2018). *Construindo as epistemologias do sul: Antologia esencial*. Volume I. CLACSO.

Egan, M., & Restall, G. (2022). The Canadian Model of Occupational Participation. In M. Egan & G. Restall (Eds.), *Promoting occupational participation: Collaborative relationship-focused occupational therapy* (pp. 73–95). Canadian Association of Occupational Therapists.

Gómez, M. I., Medina-Pacheco, B., & Hernández-Martínez, I. (2018). Autoconcepto y motivación en adolescentes que abandonan voluntariamente sus estudios de preparatoria. Una aproximación cualitativa. *Búsqueda, 5*(21), 135–145. https://doi.org/10.21892/01239813.400

Guajardo, A., Kronenberg, F., & Ramugondo, E. L. (2015). Southern occupational therapies: Emerging identities, epistemologies and practices. *South African Journal of Occupational Therapy, 45*(1), 3–10. https://doi.org/10.17159/2310-3833/2015/v45no1a2

Hernández, G. (2009). Cese de la actividad profesional y preparación para la jubilación. *Cuadernos de Relaciones Laborales, 27*(2), 63–81. https://revistas.ucm.es/index.php/CRLA/article/view/CRLA0909220063A/32229

Instituto Nacional de la Juventud. (2021). *Problemáticas y desafíos de las juventudes en Chile: Evidencias desde las Encuestas Nacionales de Juventud*. Departamento de Planificación y Estudios. INJUV.

Kjellberg, A., Kåhlin, I., Haglund, L., & Taylor, R. R. (2012). The myth of participation in occupational therapy: Reconceptualizing a client-centred approach. *Scandinavian Journal of Occupational Therapy, 19*(5), 421–427. https://doi.org/10.3109/11038128.2011.627378

Lander, E. (2000). *La colonialidad del saber. Eurocentrismo y Ciencias Sociales. Perspectivas Latinoamericanas*. CLACSO/UNESCO.

Larsson-Lund, M., & Nyman, A. (2017). Participation and occupation in occupational therapy models of practice: A discussion of possibilities and challenges. *Scandinavian Journal of Occupational Therapy, 24*(6), 393–397. https://doi.org/10.1080/11038128.2016.1267257

Leiva, A. M., Troncoso-Pantoja, C., Martínez-Sanguinetti, M. A., Nazar, G., Concha-Cisternas, Y., Martorell, M., Ramírez-Alarcón, K., Petermann-Rocha, F., Cigarroa, I., Díaz, X., & Celis-Morales, C. (2020). Personas mayores en Chile: El nuevo desafío social, económico y sanitario del Siglo XXI. *Revista Médica de Chile, 148*(6), 799–809. https://doi.org/10.4067/S0034-98872020000600799

Lorente Rodríguez, M. (2019). Problemas y limitaciones de la educación en América Latina. Un estudio comparado. *Foro de Educación, 17*(27), 229–251. http://doi.org/10.14516/fde.645

Mailhe, A. (2019). El mestizaje en América Latina durante la primera mitad del siglo XX. *Antíteses, 12*(24), 402–427. https://doi.org/10.5433/1984-3356.2019v12n24p402

Meyer, A. (1922). The philosophy of occupation therapy. Archives of Occupational Therapy. Reprinted in *American Journal of Occupational Therapy, 31*(10), 639–642.

Monzeli, G. A., Morrison, R., & Lopes, R. E. (2021). Historias de la terapia ocupacional en América Latina: La primera década de creación de los programas de formación profesional (C. Duarte Cuervo & G. A. Monzeli, Trad.). *Revista Ocupación Humana, 21*(2), 113–136. https://doi.org/10.25214/25907816.1134

Morales, B., & Van Hemelryck, T. (2022). *Inclusión laboral de las personas jóvenes en América Latina y el Caribe en tiempos de crisis: Desafíos de igualdad para las políticas públicas. Documentos de Proyectos (LC/TS.2022/34)*. CEPAL.

O'Connor, D., Lynch, H., & Boyle, B. (2021). A qualitative study of child participation in decision-making: Exploring rights-based approaches in pediatric occupational therapy. *PLoS ONE, 16*(12), e0260975. https://doi.org/10.1371/journal.pone.0260975

Paz, J., & Arévalo, C. (2019). Pobreza en las personas mayores. Un estudio multidimensional para Argentina. *Revista Latinoamericana de Población, 13*(25), 75–102. https://doi.org/10.31406/relap2019.v13.i2.n25.4

Pillemer, K., Moen, P., Wethington, E., & Glasgow, N. (2000). S*ocial integration in the second half of life*. Johns Hopkins.

Simó, S., Guajardo, A., Galheigo, S., & Garcia-Ruiz, S. (2016). *Terapias ocupacionales desde el sur. Derechos humanos, ciudadanía y participación*. USACH.

Soriano, A. A. L., Aliaga, A. C., & Vidal-Sánchez, M. I. (2022). La España despoblada y la vulneración de los derechos ocupacionales. *Journal of Occupational Science, 29*(2), XIII–XXII. https://doi.org/10.1080/14427591.2022.2044441

Vaca Trigo, I. (2019). *Oportunidades y desafíos para la autonomía de las mujeres en el futuro escenario del trabajo, serie Asuntos de Género*, No. 154 (LC/TS.2019/3). CEPAL.

Valderrama, C. (2019). Terapias ocupacionales del sur: Una propuesta para su comprensión. *Cadernos Brasileiros de Terapia Ocupacional, 27*(3), 671–680. https://doi.org/10.4322/2526-8910.ctoARF1859

Wilcock, A. (1998). Reflections on doing, being and becoming. *Canadian Journal of Occupational Therapy, 65*(5), 248–256. https://doi.org/10.1177/000841749806500501

Wilcock, A. (2006). *An occupational perspective of health* (2nd ed.). SLACK Incorporated.

World Federation of Occupational Therapists. (2012). *Definition of occupational therapy*. https://wfot.org/about/about-occupational-therapy

World Health Organization. (2019). *Participation as a driver of health equity*. WHO. https://apps.who.int/iris/bitstream/handle/10665/324909/9789289054126-eng.pdf?sequence=1&isAllowed=y

World Health Organization. (2022). *Adolescent pregnancy*. WHO. https://www.who.int/news-room/fact-sheets/detail/adolescent-pregnancy

Yasunaga, M. (2020). *La desigualdad y la inestabilidad política en América Latina: Las protestas en Ecuador, Chile y Colombia*. Boletín Instituto Español de Estudios Estratégicos. https://www.ieee.es/Galerias/fichero/docs_opinion/2020/DIEEEO22_2020MAYYAS_LatAm.pdf

CHAPTER 7

Practice Reasoning in Occupational Therapy

Introducing the Model of Occupational Therapy Reasoning

Craig Greber, Stephen Isbel, Justin Scanlan, and Jenniffer Garcia-Rojas

Abstract
This chapter introduces a new model of occupational therapy practice reasoning by reconstructing existing knowledge and scholarly work in the area. Through a case-based format, the chapter proposes a model that describes the practice reasoning process that occurs in occupational therapy, influenced by well-accepted conceptual models, practice process frameworks, and guiding factors. While the model draws upon existing literature in the area, it advances thinking about the practice reasoning process by reconceptualizing the way it is influenced by multiple guiding factors.

Authors' Positionality Statement
The authorship team recognizes that our positionality shapes the way we view the world and interpret the experiences of other people. We acknowledge that our positionality influences the way we create scholarly work and in the way I critique and understand the scholarly work of others. Our authorship teams comprise three male, Western, English-speaking, university-educated, professionally qualified, cisgendered, privileged scholars and one Latin American, Spanish-speaking, university-educated qualified and privileged female scholar.

The content of this chapter proposes a new way of organizing information we consider to make decisions in occupational therapy practice. We hope in doing so that any reader will feel included and respected in the way we have organized and presented the information. We acknowledge that the content is not completely free of bias but by stating our positionality, we hope to give readers confidence that we have made a concerted effort to acknowledge and address these biases in our writing.

> **Objectives**
> This chapter will allow the reader to:
>
> - Review the historical work done by occupational therapy scholars in coming to understand the reasoning process in occupational therapy.
> - Propose a new model of practice reasoning in occupational therapy: the Model of Occupational Therapy Reasoning.
> - Outline existing knowledge in the area of occupational therapy practice reasoning.
> - Demonstrate one way the Model of Occupational Therapy Reasoning could be applied in a client-based scenario.

> **Key terms**
> - practice reasoning
> - clinical reasoning
> - the Model of Occupational Therapy Reasoning

7.1 Introduction

Despite significant advances over the past three decades in understanding how occupational therapists engage in clinical and professional reasoning, studies on the topic have been diverse and there is no coherent understanding of the process in its entirety. Research has focused on many factors, including similarities and differences in reasoning between health disciplines, the unique characteristics of occupational therapist reasoning, differences between expert and novice practitioners, and the various aspects, or styles, of reasoning used by occupational therapists to understand situations. Some theorists have drawn on work from outside the occupational therapy profession such as cognitive science and decision-making theory. More recently, the place of context in occupational therapy reasoning has been discussed. Several scholars have presented models of occupational therapy reasoning that attempt to describe how occupational therapists engage in decisions about service delivery. While these have all proven useful in understanding the reasoning process, there is value in drawing together all the factors influencing a therapist's thinking into a comprehensive Model of Occupational Therapy Reasoning.

Unsworth (2012) encouraged deep exploration of ways that clinicians engage in reasoning in their everyday practice; therefore, this chapter brings together previous work on the topic, presents influential ideas generated from outside the profession, and reconstructs our understanding of these factors in a proposed model – the Model of Occupational Therapy Reasoning (see Figure 7.1) – that represents the way occupational therapists consider, make, and refine decisions in practice, along with the range of factors that guide them. The model synthesizes the content of previous models proposed by Unsworth (2004), Schell et al. (2018), Turpin and Iwama (2011), and Robertson (1996). It adds a representation of the complex thinking process that occurs

PRACTICE REASONING IN OCCUPATIONAL THERAPY

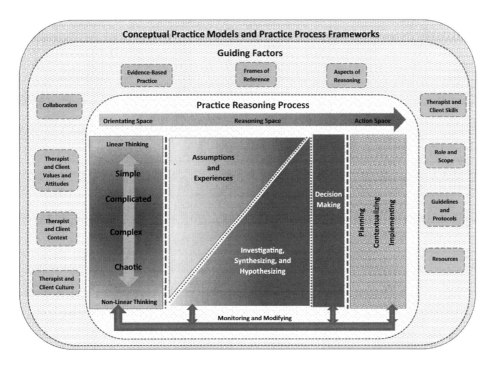

Figure 7.1 The Model of Occupational Therapy Reasoning.

when occupational therapists work with people to attain occupational goals, and provides a way of summarizing what is currently known about occupational therapy reasoning. The model should undergo further review and development as conversations about occupational therapy reasoning continue.

Throughout this chapter, the terms "clinical reasoning" and "professional reasoning" have been replaced by "practice reasoning". The authors have chosen this term to focus the discussion directly on the reasoning used during occupational therapy service delivery. The chapter aims to briefly describe the many factors that influence occupational therapy reasoning and proposes one way of synthesizing those factors into a representation of the reasoning process.

7.2 The Model of Occupational Therapy Reasoning

The model presented in Figure 7.1 illustrates the layered influences on occupational therapy practice reasoning, together with the cognitive processes that underpin service delivery. This chapter presents components of practice reasoning and reconstructs them in a unique way that demonstrates their contribution to the reasoning process. The discussion acknowledges previous research within and outside occupational therapy that informs the model's content and explains its application through two concurrent scenarios. While the scenario described suggests ways the model could inform one-to-one approaches to therapy, the authors contend that similar scenarios exist in indirect, coaching, or community service contexts that would be equally well served by the model.

The Model of Occupational Therapy Reasoning depicts the overarching influence of conceptual practice models and practice process frameworks, identifies the implicit and explicit factors that guide thinking, and describes the cognitive process of practice reasoning. These dimensions are represented as layers, each of which can be expounded on based on the excellent and exhaustive work engaged in previously by our colleagues.

7.3 Meet John and Max

The stories of John and Max will be used to highlight how the Model of Occupational Therapy Reasoning (Figure 7.1) can be applied to these two clients. You will meet John and Max and their respective occupational therapists as they go through a journey of rehabilitation over eight months. You will see that while the occupational needs and outcomes for John and Max are similar, the way in which practice reasoning occurs explains differences in the way occupational therapy services are delivered.

7.3.1 Background

John and Max have very similar backgrounds except that Max lives in Latin America and John lives in Australia. They both had car accidents at the age of 22 resulting in incomplete T8 spinal cord injuries. Prior to their injuries they were first-year students studying a Certificate of Tourism and Travel at local educational facilities, shared houses with friends, and worked in restaurants on weekends. At the start of their rehabilitation, both stated that they wanted to return to study and home. Tables 7.1 and 7.2 describe *some* of the critical events and decisions made with John and Max during their rehabilitation journeys.

7.3.2 John

Once medically stable, John was transferred to the acute rehabilitation ward where a multidisciplinary team guided his rehabilitation. The ward occupational therapist, Maureen, administered the Canadian Occupational Performance Measure (COPM) (Carswell et al., 2004). Occupation-focused goals were established for John to address his needs and once John was discharged from rehabilitation after four months he was referred to Mark (a driver-trained occupational therapist) with the goal of obtaining his driver's license. Finally, Jasmine (a private occupational therapist) was involved in a return-to-work program for John.

7.3.3 Max

Max was discharged from hospital when medically stable. The health system in his country does not have inpatient rehabilitation ward services, but Max was able to access public or private outpatient rehabilitation within the community while staying at home. He was admitted to a charity-based pediatric rehabilitation center that treats clients up to 24 years old, as it offered a more comprehensive service than the public rehabilitation unit at the local hospital. The occupational therapist from the spinal cord injury team, Andrea, performed an initial assessment that included an unstructured interview and administration of the Functional Independence Measure (FIM) (Ottenbacher et al., 1996) (a standardized assessment that must be applied to all clients in the center). Andrea first prescribed an appropriate wheelchair, given that Max was

Table 7.1 The Influence of Guiding Factors for John and Max

Guiding factor	John	Max
Therapist and client culture	John had three occupational therapists involved in his rehabilitation journey (Maureen, James, and Jasmine). All were born, raised, and trained in Australia. John has spent all of his life in Australia and has a very supportive family (two parents and two siblings).	Max had two occupational therapists involved in his rehabilitation process (Andrea and Maria). They were born, grew up, and studied occupational therapy in a Latin American country. Max, his parents, and two siblings are Latin American, and they have been very supportive, actively participating in Max's rehabilitation.
Therapist and client context	In Australia, the universal health care system (Medicare) covered the costs of John's hospital stay and employed occupational therapists to address his needs. He also had access to subsidized continence products and accessible public housing. He is a participant in the NDIS, which covers the cost of most of his equipment (wheelchair, commode, etc.).	The local health care system covered the costs of Max's hospital stay. He had access to specialized equipment and rehabilitation services through a charity-based non-government pediatric rehabilitation center. The National Disability Pension Scheme provides Max the equivalent of USD95 per month. He needs to afford the costs of continence products, adapted equipment, and home modifications.
Aspects of reasoning	All aspects of reasoning were used in John's journey, but primarily scientific and pragmatic reasoning. Scientific reasoning using published guidelines and protocols guided occupational therapy in the acute stages. Throughout the process of driver rehabilitation and the return-to-work phase, standardized assessments, legislation, and protocols were used. Pragmatically, John had access to public housing and the NDIS, but there were limits to the scope of modifications that were available for John, and the NDIS plan had limitations on the type of wheelchair and vehicle modifications that could be purchased.	Occupational therapists utilized all aspects of professional reasoning to work with Max, including scientific, narrative, and pragmatic reasoning. Research evidence was difficult to source so the therapist used practice evidence sources from her own experience and Max's personal experience. Pragmatically, the service scope and limited benefits offered by the local government determined the nature of services. Max received information and advice from his occupational therapist, but he had to afford home modifications, being supported by his family and friends. The therapists' consideration of these factors was informed by pragmatic reasoning.

(Continued)

Table 7.1 (Continued)

Frames of reference	The primary frame of reference used by all of the occupational therapists involved was the biomechanical frame of reference (Trombly, 1983). This is used when people like John experience occupational performance challenges due to changes in muscle strength, endurance, and range of motion.	The frames of reference used by all the therapists involved were the biomechanical (Trombly, 1983) and rehabilitative frames of reference (Gillen, 2014). The rehabilitative frame of reference is used with clients with permanent disabilities to maximize their independence, including concepts like adaptation, compensation, and environmental modifications.
Evidence-based practice	Throughout John's journey, his occupational therapists were guided in their decisions about assessment and intervention by the research evidence contained in publications from Icare (2017), Austroads (2016), and AOTA (2020b). John's therapists also drew on their own professional experience and John's own experiences as important forms of evidence.	Max's therapists faced some barriers accessing research evidence due to language barriers and limited availability of the research base. They used information from a manual that was developed by a local NGO *Accessible City*, which considered national norms and legislation on architectural barriers. Elements of the OTPF-4 (AOTA, 2020b) were considered. Max's therapists were forced to rely heavily on their own experience as an evidence base.
Collaboration	Decisions made throughout John's journey were always made in a multidisciplinary context. For example, a physiotherapist aided in the decision about wheelchair purchase in relation to John's upper limb strength and trunk stability. A social worker was important in securing appropriate accessible housing. John's family was also instrumental in collaborating in the occupational therapy process and influenced decisions about equipment, housing, and return to work.	Max's rehabilitation process was supported by a multidisciplinary team. While the wheelchair and pressure cushion were prescribed by the occupational therapist, the physiotherapist trained Max to increase upper limb strength and taught him how to maneuver the chair. The nurse taught Max how to manage continence products and safely perform self-catheterization. Max's family was actively involved in therapy sessions, taking turns to attend the center with Max, and helping him at home.
Therapist and client values and attitudes	From an early stage John was determined to get back to work and live independently as he highly valued these aspects of his life. He valued the role his family played in supporting him throughout his rehabilitation.	Max expected to return to work and get back to study. He wanted to stay in the shared house with his friends, but was open to moving back with his family where he received more support. (Most people around his age are still living in the family home.)

(Continued)

Table 7.1 (Continued)

Roles and scope	The roles and scope of each therapist were different. Maureen's role in the initial stages of rehabilitation focused on self-care occupations and mobility to enable discharge. James's primary role was to enable John to drive again using vehicle modifications under the appropriate Austroads (2016) guidelines. Jasmine's role was to enable John to re-enter the paid workforce.	The role of the occupational therapist in the Spinal Cord Injury team was to address all the needs that could arise during the process, with the exception of returning to work. As driving is not an area of practice in occupational therapy in Latin America, the therapist provided information so Max could solve the problem independently.
Therapist and client skills	While there are three occupational therapists involved in this case study, each had specific skills that aided decision making at specific points. Decisions about driving for example were beyond Maureen's skills, but James did not have the skills and knowledge to make decisions about a custom-made wheelchair.	The occupational therapist had developed knowledge and experience while working with clients with spinal cord injury. When facing challenges, Andrea received expert advice from senior colleagues. Although Max or his family and friends did not have the skills to make home modifications, following the advice of the therapist they used their abilities to adapt Max's home.
Resources	John and his occupational therapists went through their journey supported by a universal health care system and a social policy (NDIS) that gave considerable financial and material support. The decisions about equipment were made on the understanding that it would all be paid for through John's NDIS plan.	Given that Max is under 24 years old, he was able to access a pediatric rehabilitation center that provided him free-of-charge services and some equipment. Local government offered limited resources and funding, but that was restricted by long waiting lists. To solve the lack of resources, Max's family and friends organized a fundraising activity and assisted Max in completing his daily tasks and rehabilitation process.
Guidelines and protocols	Several guidelines and protocols were used throughout John's journey. For example, Icare (2017) and Spinal Cord Injury Australia (n.d.) provided guidance and tools to determine the needs and support for a person with all levels of spinal injury. This was used by all therapists but primarily by Maureen when she was working with John to decide on the equipment he would need for self-care occupations and mobility.	Some local guidelines have been developed by the rehabilitation team, which were built based on their clinical experience, local regulations, and some disciplinary information (AOTA, 2020b, 2020c). An accessibility manual published by a local NGO was used to inform Max about regulations for home modifications.

using a loan chair from the hospital that was too small and difficult to maneuver. Following a home visit, Andrea established that Max would have difficulty accessing all parts of his house with a wheelchair. Max's friends and family organized a fundraising activity (Bingo) to get the resources he needed and neighbors helped them to build a ramp, enlarge the door widths, and modify the bathroom while Max was in hospital to enable discharge.

Max owned an old car and intended to modify it so he could drive, but given the logistics and cost involved in modifying the car he did not proceed. He relied on family and friends for transportation. Finally, Max was referred to Maria, an occupational therapist from a return-to-work program in the same rehabilitation center. Maria conducted a job analysis and a formal return to work/study plan. As Max qualifies for the National Disability Pension Scheme (Chile), he received 300 Chilean Pesos (or about USD95) per month to cover the needs associated with his rehabilitation process.

John and Max shared the same occupational therapy goals, albeit in very different contexts and circumstances:

Acute phase (one to four months)

- To be independent in all self-care in four weeks.
- To be independent in self-catheterization in six weeks.
- To engage in all valued occupations using an appropriate wheelchair.
- To access all areas of an appropriate residence in four months.

Community phase (four to eight months)

- To drive an adapted vehicle to community-based occupations.
- To continue his study of a Certificate in Tourism and Travel at his local educational facility.
- To return to work with alternate duties.

The practice reasoning processes used by occupational therapists to address these goals for each client were informed, guided, and undertaken in unique ways that can be understood using the Model of Occupational Therapy Reasoning in Figure 7.1.

7.4 Conceptual Practice Models and Practice Process Frameworks

7.4.1 Occupational Therapy Conceptual Practice Models

Conceptual practice models in occupational therapy provide a structure or framework to guide thinking and decision making. Turpin and Garcia (2021) say that "models of practice provide guidance for combining knowledge and action" (p. 213), while Trede and Higgs (2008) state that models of practice are "mental maps that assist practitioners to understand their practice" (p. 32). As there are many factors influencing the practice reasoning process, coming to sound decisions can often be challenging. Using a conceptual model guides practitioners to make occupation-focused decisions while taking into account the complexities that can arise in varying contexts. Conceptual models also ground practitioners in the philosophy and values of occupational therapy, so the decisions made during the practice reasoning process reflect the unique contribution occupational therapy makes to individuals or communities.

Many conceptual practice models have been published in occupational therapy and a number of these are described in detail in Chapter 5. Models such as the Model of Human Occupation (Taylor, 2017), the Canadian Model of Occupational Participation (Egan & Restall, 2022), and the Person Environment Occupation Performance model (Baum et al., 2015) are informed by a biopsychosocial view of health that focuses primarily on the individual and how the broader socio-cultural environment affects health at an individual level. In contrast, the Kawa model (Iwama, 2006) has been developed from a collectivist perspective, meaning that the individual cannot be separated from the culture and society in which they live. Decisions about which model to use can be influenced by factors such as the occupational therapist's knowledge of the model, skill in applying the concepts, practice context, and preferences, and the background of the individual or community involved.

7.4.2 Occupational Therapy Practice Processes

Occupational therapy practice processes apply the ideas and thoughts that arise from conceptual practice models and provide a guide to implementing occupation-focused thinking arising from the models. Many of the practice models describe specific processes that can be used in conjunction with the associated model and have some common features, including evaluation, assessment, goal setting, intervention, measuring outcomes, and re-evaluation. Most processes recognize factors such as culture and the practice context as influences on the therapeutic relationship. Two examples of occupational therapy practice processes that are used to operationalize the concepts of practice models are the Occupational Therapy Practice Framework – 4th edition (OTPF-4) (AOTA, 2020a, 2020b, 2020c) and the Canadian Occupational Therapy Inter-relational Practice Process Framework (COTIPP) (Restall et al., 2022). The processes related to the OTPF-4 are described in Chapter 5, while the COTIPP processes are outlined in more detail in Chapter 5.

Conceptual practice models and practice process frameworks ensured that the therapists involved with John and Max maintained an occupation-focused perspective and worked with them in ways that align with occupational therapy theory and philosophy.

7.5 Guiding Factors

Doyle et al. (2013) highlighted the influence of many factors in the generation, synthesis, and interpretation of information used to inform the practice reasoning process. These included content and contextual factors, implicit and explicit knowledge and understandings, client and therapist perceptions, attitudes and values, and societal and organizational influences. These authors noted the importance of such factors in shaping the reasoning process and determining decisions made. In the Model of Occupational Therapy Reasoning, these factors are represented in an intermediate layer, guiding practice reasoning while also being influenced by conceptual understandings of occupational therapy practice.

7.5.1 Evidence-Based Practice

Evidence-Based Practice (EBP) is a process that uses multiple sources of evidence, including research evidence, clinical expertise, information from the practice setting, and the person's values and circumstances. The process that health professionals use to integrate all of this information has been called clinical reasoning by Hoffman and colleagues (Hoffman et al., 2017), and this chapter builds on this idea to include all practice areas (not just a clinical setting) in occupational therapy.

Reliance on research evidence alone is problematic in occupational therapy as it largely "ignores the individual narratives that characterise the very essence of occupational therapy" (Greber, 2021, p. 12). When research evidence is not clear or conclusive, occupational therapists have relied on information from the client, the practice setting, and their own experience to guide their reasoning. Clinicians, however, need to consider the efficacy of making decisions based upon practice evidence and should appraise the validity and reliability of those sources (Greber, 2021).

7.5.2 Therapist and Client Skills

Therapist and client skills are the capacities and capabilities that the therapist and the client bring into the professional encounter. For therapists, these skills can include experience in using particular interventions, certification in the use of specific procedures and techniques, and more general skills related to communication, reasoning, and planning. Clients also bring many skills into the professional encounter, including specific background knowledge and experience (they may be a builder or a physician) that could support interventions, but most frequently these skills relate to clients' (and families') expertise in managing their condition.

Integrating therapist and client skills into the reasoning process is essential, as overlooking the lived experience of clients may mean that inappropriate, unacceptable, or ineffective intervention options are prioritized, creating inefficiencies and reducing client adherence. It is important for the therapist to be appropriately skilled in specific intervention techniques (or engage services from others who do have those skills) to ensure safe service delivery. However, it is also important to ensure that preferred techniques are not chosen ahead of the most useful approach for the client's unique presentation.

7.5.3 Therapist and Client Values and Attitudes

Values are "a person's own set of principles which they consider of great importance", whereas attitude is "a way of thinking of feeling in regards to someone or something" (University of Reading, n.d.). People have different values and attitudes depending on factors that include their culture, past experiences, and current situation. This means a therapist will most likely have different values and attitudes than their client and this will affect the practice reasoning process. An example is when a client has values and attitudes that may be abhorrent to a therapist (for example, racist or homophobic views) making a therapeutic relationship impossible. In most cases, however, differences in values and attitudes between a therapist and client can be accommodated and in many cases embraced as part of the collaborative process that informs practice reasoning.

7.5.4 Therapist and Client Culture

The respective cultures of the occupational therapist and the client are an important guiding factor in practice reasoning. Culture goes beyond race and ethnicity and includes "any dimension of diversity, including class, gender, sexual orientation, and ability" (Hammell, 2013, p. 224). Cultural differences are often celebrated and embraced, but, unfortunately, they are often the source of conscious and unconscious biases that affect a multitude of human interactions, including in health care. Occupational therapy theorists have proposed that power imbalances exist due to cultural differences and these affect client–therapist relationships (Hammell, 2013). Seen from this perspective, practice reasoning informing decisions made with and for clients will be affected by the culture of both the client and the occupational therapist.

Therapists' reasoning is also influenced by social conceptions and attitudes toward illness or disability that prevail within the practice context (Shafaroodi et al., 2014), the social dynamics of interdisciplinary health care teams, and the local culture of particular settings (Kristensen et al., 2012). Additionally, professional culture has been identified as a key factor that frames practice reasoning, given the impact it has on the development of professional identity and "the acquisition of knowledge, affecting how and when knowledge is used, and to what end it may be used" (Peters et al., 2017, p. 874).

Occupational therapy has strived to develop a body of knowledge that supports practitioners' cultural competence when working with clients, which requires therapists to develop an understanding about, and be sensitive with, cultural differences (Taff et al., 2020). Contemporary debates within occupational therapy emphasize the need of moving from cultural competence to cultural humility, since cultural competence encompasses an understanding of culture as a limited concept that has to be comprehended and mastered (Agner, 2020). Conversely, cultural humility "acknowledges implicit and explicit bias and prejudices as a part of being human, and works toward identification of bias to promote positive change" (Agner, 2020, p. 2). It is important therefore to know that practice reasoning will be guided by therapist and client culture, and for the occupational therapist to reflect on their own cultural humility in this process.

7.5.5 Therapist and Client Context

When working with clients, occupational therapists need to consider information from the context in which they work, and factors from the client's context that might have an impact on the intervention and outcomes. Some elements that are often identified in the literature as shaping practice reasoning are related to the type of setting, physical and economic resources, time available, organizational regulations, managers' leadership styles, and support provided (Shafaroodi et al., 2014). The Model of Context-Specific Professional Reasoning proposed by Turpin and Iwama (2011) suggests that occupational therapists' practice reasoning is not only molded by the immediate context in which occupational therapists and clients work together, but also by the characteristics of a "multilayered" (p. 42) environment in which the setting works. It includes legislation and governmental processes and regulations, the existence of regulatory bodies (Turpin & Iwama, 2011), availability of support networks, social welfare, and safety within the community (Stark et al., 2015). Occupational therapists also need to consider information related to the client's context, such as housing and architectural conditions, family's economic resources, and level of caregiver's engagement (Shafaroodi et al., 2014, 2017; Stark et al., 2015).

In the case studies presented in this chapter, the contexts in which Max and John live and the practice context in which their occupational therapists work influence practice reasoning. See Table 7.1 for guiding factors specific to Max and John that influence practice reasoning.

7.5.6 Collaboration

Collaboration between the occupational therapist, client, caregivers, significant others, other members of the multidisciplinary team, and other service providers is essential to support reasoning processes. Effective interprofessional communication is associated with lower rates of adverse events in health care settings (Brandis et al., 2017) and better client outcomes (Foronda et al., 2016). Communication between service providers involved in supporting clients is also important in ensuring interventions or services are complementary, unnecessary duplication is avoided, and priority needs are addressed. This is true in all settings and requires focused attention to ensure effective liaison, especially where service providers are working in different settings or organizations.

While interprofessional communication and collaboration is essential, the most important stakeholders to involve in collaborative discussions are the client and their family/other chosen supports. As noted above, clients and families bring a wealth of knowledge from their lived experience and this knowledge informs the reasoning process. Collaboration with clients and families is essential for client-centered practice as without it interventions may not focus on the client's priorities or the intervention methods selected may not be considered useful to them. Lack of collaboration with clients and families can lead to poorer adherence with intervention recommendations and may slow or diminish progress. This collaboration also supports the client's knowledge of the intervention purpose, which can reduce adverse events and promote better congruence between service providers (as the client or their families can identify when different interventions may not be optimally aligned).

7.5.7 Guidelines and Protocols

Guidelines and protocols are developed to support best practice in service provision through "standardizing" approaches for similar clients in similar situations. Guidelines are generally developed by a panel of experts and include evidence-based recommendations to support decision making. Guidelines are often designed for integrated, multidisciplinary practice and are intended to be applicable across an entire country or region. However, protocols are often more localized and describe general expectations of roles and duties. Protocols can be multidisciplinary (e.g., a designated "care pathway" for a particular type of "patient" in a hospital setting) or focused on the processes undertaken by one professional group. Where guidelines and protocols are available, these can simplify practice reasoning by supporting the implementation of best practice and reducing what is referred to as "unwarranted clinical variation" (Harrison et al., 2019). However, guidelines and protocols should never replace the reasoning process. Blindly implementing recommendations or processes without considering other factors can lead to inappropriate interventions that increase the risk of adverse events or poor outcomes.

7.5.8 Resources

Resources available to the client and occupational therapist have a significant influence on the reasoning process. "Resources" include the availability and accessibility of services, funding, equipment, community support, and a range of other elements. Resource availability also includes clients' natural support systems and occupational therapists' access to professional support (e.g., supervision and guidance from more experienced clinicians). Such factors are often associated with pragmatic styles of reasoning that guide decisions in light of the resources available. Limited resources can be overcome by practice reasoning that leads to novel and creative ways of approaching a client's issues.

7.5.9 Frames of Reference

Hinojosa et al. (2019) described Frames of Reference (FoR) as a method of "organizing theoretical material and translating information into practice… The frame of reference is designed to first highlight traditionally used theories, then to relate that information to function, and finally to organize that information for the purpose of intervention" (p. 5). In the broadest of terms, an FoR is a standpoint from which to view and understand something. In practice reasoning, FoRs are used to consider a person's occupational performance from the perspective of specific theories about personal capacities – motor, sensory, cognitive, behavioral, and other standpoints that can explain causes of dysfunction and provide a means of improving performance. For example, jerky, uncontrolled hand movement when pouring tea could be viewed as the result of poor proprioception (sensory FoR), tremor (neurological FoR), upper limb instability (biomechanical FoR), or anxiety (psychological FoR). While the FoR a therapist uses influences practice reasoning, its selection should be based on other guiding factors.

7.5.10 Aspects of Reasoning

Various authors have explored and developed theories that describe the different styles of reasoning used by occupational therapists. "Aspects" of reasoning represent different reasoning strategies employed to think about situations and to consider potential solutions. Mattingly and Fleming (1994) have been among the most influential authors in this area, most notably in their description of the therapist with the "three track mind" (Fleming, 1994). These three "tracks" were labeled procedural, interactive, and conditional reasoning, and they proposed that therapists used different aspects of reasoning when faced with different types of situations.

Following Mattingly and Fleming's influential work, numerous authors, including Unsworth (2012) and Schell and Schell (2018), built on these concepts. Schell and Benfield (2018) summarized the state of knowledge and described five major aspects of reasoning: scientific, narrative, pragmatic, ethical, and interactive.

Scientific reasoning incorporates concepts from procedural, diagnostic, and hypothetico-deductive reasoning. These approaches use knowledge of the condition and its functional implications to guide intervention approaches, and this aspect of reasoning is most closely aligned with the "application of research evidence" from the evidence-based practice model (Hoffman et al., 2017).

Narrative reasoning involves understanding the "story" of clients – their perspectives about their situation and their occupational story prior to, concurrent with, and beyond their involvement with occupational therapy. This aspect of reasoning often involves "co-creation" of a desired future, especially for individuals who have lost hope or who cannot see a future beyond the consequences of their situation.

Pragmatic reasoning involves considering resource limitation or limitations associated with the practice context or role and scope of occupational therapy in the setting. Pragmatic reasoning encourages the therapist to determine the optimal approach given the limitations imposed on the reasoning process.

Ethical reasoning involves identifying and dealing with ethical dilemmas. This may involve managing different expectations between funders and clients, conflicting opinions among the multidisciplinary team, how much time can be spent with each client, and managing documentation processes to ensure the client receives optimal funding without including fabricated or misleading information.

Finally, interactive reasoning considers the relationships between the client, their family and supports, the occupational therapist, and the broader service system. This aspect of reasoning encourages the occupational therapist to focus on the importance of these relationships and how they can be used to optimize the reasoning process.

Depending on each situation, setting, and other influencing factors, particular aspects of reasoning will take priority. Schell and Benfield (2018) describe this as a "conditional" process that is informed by reflective processes over time.

7.5.11 Role and Scope

A number of professional bodies have attempted to describe the current and potential scope of practice for occupational therapy (American Occupational Therapy Association, 2021; Occupational Therapy Australia, 2017). Capturing the varied role and scope of occupational therapists has resulted in quite general descriptions. In some settings, the role is narrow and tightly specified, whereas in others, it is very broad and includes numerous activities that could be completed by other professionals. The role and scope of occupational therapists in each setting will be influenced by many factors, including funding, length of stay, team members and structure, traditional roles of professionals within that setting, and knowledge and awareness among the team about capabilities of professional groups. As noted above, interprofessional collaboration and communication can be effective in supporting efficient and effective service delivery by ensuring that unnecessary duplication is avoided and all priorities are addressed.

Role and scope limitations imposed on occupational therapists in select settings may mean that some priorities for clients may not be able to be addressed. If this is the case, then consideration should be given to advocating for flexibility in scope, or linking the client to other services that can support these priorities. The manner in which the various guiding factors influenced occupational therapy practice reasoning for John and Max is summarized in Table 7.1.

7.6 The Practice Reasoning Process

Mattingly (1991) described occupational therapy reasoning as "a largely tacit, highly imagistic, and deeply phenomenological mode of thinking" (p. 979). For this reason, it has been difficult to provide a definitive guide to the way occupational therapists integrate the many influences on their provision of services. Rather than providing a rigid depiction of the process, the inner parts of the model describe a structure for implementing those iterative modes to which Mattingly refers in flexible, individualized ways.

Occupational therapy practice reasoning occurs within the occupation-focused perspective imposed by conceptual practice models, and is organized by practice process frameworks that describe how the provision of services should proceed. The way the therapist engages in practice reasoning is guided by the factors identified above, making the process of practice reasoning unique for every therapist, client, and encounter. The practice reasoning process itself is depicted in the model as the innermost ring, influenced by, and, in turn, influencing, the outer layers of conceptual and guiding factors. The practice reasoning process requires the therapist and client to orient themselves to the person's needs, decide on strategies to address the person's needs, and implement effective actions. In the Model of Occupational Therapy Reasoning (see Figure 7.1), each of these processes occupies a separate space.

7.6.1 The Orienting Space

The practice reasoning process begins when the therapist identifies issues arising for a client, understands those within an occupation-focused perspective, and initiates the practice process.

Rogers (Rogers & Holm, 1991; Rogers, 2004) proposed framing a person's needs in an occupation-focused way that ensures practice reasoning is informed by overarching conceptual practice models. By using an occupational diagnosis, rather than a biomedical one, occupational therapists are able to organize their thinking in response to occupational needs. An occupational diagnosis inverts the biomedical diagnosis by recognizing occupation, rather than pathology, as the primary focus. An occupational diagnosis has four components:

1. Descriptive component: names the occupational performance issues that will be the focus of service delivery.
2. Explanatory component: describes what forms the barriers to occupational performance. These are often the tasks or activities that are currently problematic.
3. Cue component: includes the signs and symptoms the individual experiences that lead to difficulty performing the tasks and activities.
4. Pathological component: names the medical condition, situation, or circumstance that has led to occupational performance issues.

By framing the situation in this way, occupational therapists can focus primarily on their domain of concern (enhancing occupational performance) rather than being drawn into reducing symptoms or managing the person's condition. Cues and pathologies are only important to the extent that they influence occupational performance.

Consider the differences between a biomedically oriented diagnosis and an occupational diagnosis for John and Max (see Figure 7.2):

Developing an occupational diagnosis orients the therapist to the person's primary occupational needs and ensures practice reasoning proceeds in an occupation-focused manner. An understanding of the occupational diagnosis is influenced by considering

> **John**
>
> **Biomedical diagnosis:** John has a T8 spinal cord injury. He has impaired lower limb function, limited sensation, and impaired autonomic nervous system function. He cannot mobilize around the hospital ward and he is unable to attend to daily occupations such as self-care.
>
> **Occupational diagnosis:** John is unable to engage in daily occupations that require him to mobilize around the hospital ward, such as getting to the bathroom to attend to self-care. He is unable to walk or weight bear and he has impaired lower limb function, limited sensation, and autonomic responses as the result of a T8 spinal cord injury.

> **Max**
>
> **Biomedical diagnosis:** Max has a T8 spinal cord injury. He has impaired lower limb function, limited sensation, and impaired autonomic nervous system function. He is unable to self-catheterize and cannot use the bathroom for showering. Max is unable to complete self-care occupations such as dressing, showering, and bathing.
>
> **Occupational diagnosis:** Max is unable to engage in self-care occupations such as dressing, showering, and toileting. He is unable to self-catheterize and cannot access the bathroom for showering. Max cannot don underwear or pants when dressing. He has impaired lower limb function and limited sensation and autonomic responses as the result of a T8 spinal cord injury.

Figure 7.2 Biomedical versus occupational diagnosis.

the guiding factors. The therapist's and client's perception of the occupations is influenced by cultural and contextual factors. Orientation to the person's situation is informed by the various aspects of reasoning engaged in, each of which provides a different lens through which to understand the person, their occupations, and their limits in occupational performance. Similarly, identified barriers to occupation are understood through a synthesis of FoR, each of which provides a different explanation of the reasons for dysfunction. At a pragmatic level, the therapist's role and scope and the resources at hand influence the description of the person's occupational needs because they define the domain of concern that the therapist holds.

Orienting to the level of complexity of the person's situation is also important. Whiteford et al. (2005) noted that contemporary practice in occupational therapy occurs within a context of complexity. These authors argued that occupation cannot be understood within a reductionist paradigm, and proposed complexity theory as a way of understanding how occupational therapists negotiate their way through challenging practice scenarios where many factors interact within dynamic systems.

Orienting to the complexity of the person's situation is an important preliminary process. Smith et al. (2008) and Copley et al. (2010) identified the complexity and uncertainty often associated with occupational therapy reasoning. Several occupational therapy scholars have identified the differences between linear and non-linear perspectives (Champagne et al., 2007; Creek et al., 2005), agreeing that a non-linear orientation is most congruent with understandings of human occupation. Linear thinking applies to those situations that are highly repetitive and routine, and for which established guidelines or protocols are present. Novel decisions that require the development of new procedures have been described as non-linear. Linear thinking is reductionist in nature and is well served by reference to empirical evidence, while non-linear reasoning acknowledges the interaction of a range of factors and also requires synthesis of other forms of practice evidence. Linear thinking is best applied to simple problems, while non-linear thinking is required as problems become more complex (Champagne et al., 2007). The concept of linearity is an important but singular element in helping therapists orient to a situation and the reasoning processes required to address it.

Arising from the field of cognitive science, Snowden and Boone (2007) introduced the Cynefin Framework – a complexity model that makes sense of situations based on their level of disorder and unpredictability. The Cynefin Framework has been used to understand the effect of complexity on reasoning processes in medicine (Corazza & Lenti, 2021), health promotion (Van Beurden et al., 2013), mental health (Smit & Derksen, 2017; Stampfer, 2019) and general health care (Gray, 2017). It has not been embraced by occupational therapy scholars, yet it potentially brings much to the understanding of occupational therapy reasoning. The framework proposes four degrees of complexity that each require different reasoning approaches: simple, complicated, complex, and chaotic situations.

Simple situations are those that have an obvious relationship between cause and effect. The reasoning process is therefore straightforward and involves sensing the situation, categorizing the issue, and applying the appropriate response. Simple situations apply linear thinking.

Complicated situations also have a linear relationship between cause and effect, but the relationship is not obvious and requires analysis of the situation to identify which response is required from a range of known options. In those instances, the prospective actions lie within the lived experience of the therapist and the reasoning process involves a choice between the known alternatives.

Complex situations entail non-linear relationships between cause and effect, where activity in one part of the system can create large-scale effects on other parts, yet the relationship is an indirect one. Most issues addressed by occupational therapists are complex in nature because they occur within the context of a dynamic system. Managing complex situations requires the therapist to probe or investigate the system to identify the best way to respond. Gathering information is a key component of this type of reasoning and solutions to complex problems emerge as the result of creative thinking that synthesizes all the system's components.

Chaotic situations are those for which there is no apparent relationship between cause and effect. Order is created within chaotic systems by action that establishes resultant activity, which can then be observed and understood. When working in chaotic systems, therapists need to act and observe rather than probe and investigate. Acting and observing creates an opportunity to create relationships between cause and effect that don't pre-exist in a chaotic system.

The Cynefin Framework suggests that therapists should think differently about a situation depending on its complexity. Snowden and Boone (2007) advise against interpreting a situation based on a singular reasoning style. Appropriate reasoning can only occur when the complexity of the system is accurately assessed and the required reasoning processes are implemented. Snowden and Boone (2007) warned of the implications of misattributing complexity. Viewing a simple problem as complex would lead a therapist to engage in unnecessary analysis and use of resources. Conversely, viewing a complex problem as simple would lead the therapist to apply linear thinking to a non-linear system, making solutions narrow and insufficient.

In occupational therapy, it is important to recognize that complex medical histories do not necessarily imply complex occupational needs. As the Person-Environment-Occupation-Performance (PEOP) model assures us, where personal, environmental, occupational, and performance factors are congruent, occupational performance and participation can proceed without incident despite limits in personal capacities imposed by injury, illness, or circumstance. Using an occupational diagnosis rather than a biomedical one informs decisions about complexity because it centers the therapist on the degree of occupational dysfunction, rather than being focused on biomedical complexity.

As the complexity of a system increases, reasoning changes from linear thinking to non-linear thinking (Champagne et al., 2007). Simple problems are those that sit within the therapist's lived experience and have a ready solution at hand. Linear thinking allows rapid decisions to be made and actions implemented. As complexity increases, novel and customized solutions are required and these can only be developed through moving beyond linear thinking. The more complex the situation, the more novel the reasoning process and the less the therapist can rely on an understanding of linear relationships: non-linear thinking that generates new hypotheses becomes necessary. Orientating accurately to the complexity of the situation is therefore a pivotal step in the practice reasoning process.

The orientation space is a process by which a therapist understands the nature of occupational disruption and the complexity of factors impacting that disruption. By orienting appropriately to the situation, the therapist is able to:

- Conceptualize the reason for engagement with the person.
- Frame the person's needs in an occupation-focused way.
- Understand the complexity of the situation in readiness to engage in reasoning.

7.6.2 The Reasoning Space

Having oriented to the client's occupational needs, considered the guiding factors that influence the situation, and assessed the degree of complexity, the therapist is then able to make informed decisions about how best to respond. The reasoning space is therefore influenced by prior decisions about complexity.

When the nature of occupational dysfunction is perceived as simple, several theorists have noted that heuristics can be used to accelerate the reasoning process (Fleming, 1994; Mattingly, 1991; Robertson, 1996). Dale (2015) described heuristics as mental shortcuts that assist decision making by reducing the time spent researching and analyzing information. By linking the current situation to one in the therapist's previous experience, decisions can be made quickly and efficiently. It is important to note that the use of heuristics has been linked to superficial and inadequate decision making when the complexity of the problem is not sufficiently recognized (Dale, 2015). Heuristics speed up the decision-making process, but by relying more on assumptions and previous experience the quality of reasoning can be affected. Robertson (1996) suggested that the use of heuristics is more commonly a feature of experienced therapists' reasoning as they have memory of a wide range of similar situations and the actions used to address them.

As the level of complexity increases, and reasoning moves from linear to non-linear processes, therapists rely more on investigation, synthesis, and hypothesis generation to consider the best way to progress. As Snowden and Boone (2007) described, simple situations involve those occasions where previous experience or knowledge helps in understanding the most obvious cause of dysfunction and recognizing the most appropriate actions. Complicated situations have a less clear cause–effect relationship because the issue can be understood in multiple ways. The therapist's challenge is to consider which of a series of possible explanations might be correct in addressing the person's occupational needs. Assumptions and experiences can be used to guide that understanding and propose relevant actions. Simple and complicated reasoning use the pattern matching strategies described in Robertson's (1996) Model of Problem Solving in Occupational Therapy, but as situations become more complicated hypothesis generation requires a more substantial element of reasoning.

Complex situations require therapists to investigate barriers to occupation–capacities, environment, and occupational form – and then understand the dynamic nature of factors contributing to those barriers. The therapist faces the challenge of developing hypotheses that lead to the creation of novel therapeutic interventions through a synthesis of approaches and techniques. The result is an idiosyncratic, individualized action, developed through non-linear thinking. Robertson (1996) described a series of strategies used by occupational therapists to generate novel actions, including mental modeling and means-end analysis, which avoided the randomness associated with trial and error.

When situations are chaotic, a different approach is required. In a chaotic system, order can be created through action (Snowden & Boone, 2007). When a person's life is so disrupted that there is no clear order, the therapist acts first and observes the response to establish a better understanding of how the dynamic system functions. Those observations form the basis for developing hypothetical understandings of barriers to occupational performance, and then to deciding on actions to address them. The degree to which assumptions and experience are replaced by conscious cognitive processes is dependent on the level of complexity of the situation, and is influenced by a range of guiding factors.

Perceptions of complexity are influenced by the combined experience of client and therapist, As therapists build their lived experience, their conceptualization of complexity alters. Practice reasoning evolves through thoughtful reflection on therapeutic encounters, and increased professional experience reduces the number of occasions where high perceived complexity requires the generation of novel responses informed by synthesis and hypothesizing. The journey from novice to expert clinician therefore reflects an increasing reliance on experience and assumptions that can be generated from previous encounters as client needs become more familiar.

The second element of the reasoning space is the decision-making process. Smith et al. (2008) describe decision making as something that is the outcome of the reasoning process and leads to the development of action points. Decision making has historically been defined as the process of identifying and choosing between alternatives to fit the presenting goals and objectives (Edwards, 1954). As helpful as this might be, theories on decision making have sometimes been clouded by the inclusion of many other reasoning processes as part of decision making. In the context of this model, decision making is considered an essential but final element of the reasoning space because it involves choosing between a number of potential actions – a stance that is consistent with Smith et al.'s (2008) distinctions. This choice is informed by the preceding assumptions and experiences of the therapist and the cognitive processes involved in investigating, synthesizing, and hypothesizing. To a large extent, decision making remains similar regardless of the complexity of the situation, and although the number of potential options might vary from one encounter to another, the choices are reduced and prioritized by the reasoning process. This means the decision-making aspect of reasoning can be simplified by drawing effectively on existing assumptions and experience, and by effective investigation, synthesis, and hypothesizing. Decision making is therefore the relatively simple act of choosing, from a refined number of alternatives, the most appropriate actions to take.

The reasoning process in occupational therapy is a fluent and imprecise experience that is influenced by a number of factors that guide the therapist's thinking. When reasoning is simple and guided largely by assumptions and experiences, implicit factors such as culture, context, values, and attitudes, as well as explicit factors such as EBP and resources, flavor those assumptions. This can have both positive and negative effects. While it ensures reasoning remains culturally sensitive and contextually appropriate, it is also limited by the therapist's lived experiences and their personal values. As reasoning becomes less linear, the generation of hypotheses is informed by a host of procedural and pragmatic factors, unearthed through the use of multiple aspects of reasoning. The presence or absence of an evidence base, the role and scope of the therapist, the resources available, the frame of reference, and aspects of reasoning the therapist uses all limit and enable the hypotheses the therapist might generate. The more complex the situation and the more factors influencing reasoning, the more comprehensive but unpredictable the hypothesis generation process becomes.

7.6.3 The Action Space

Interventions in occupational therapy rarely proceed without the need for modification and amendment. Even when firm decisions have been made about how to proceed with intervention, those strategies still need to be planned, contextualized to the client, and then implemented.

Actions and interventions need to be delivered in an organized fashion that considers the need for grading, fading, or modifying those strategies over time. Often a series of strategies might be implemented to address components of an occupational performance issue. These might be implemented sequentially, simultaneously, or intermittently depending on the situation. For example, a therapist might implement environmental changes, or introduce assistive technology, while also building a client's capacity with a view to reducing or removing those changes in the long term. In many cases an occupational therapist might be called upon to address multiple issues for a client and these need to be prioritized and negotiated as part of the delivery of services. Guiding factors such as collaboration, client values, culture, and context might be influential in determining need and planning therapy.

Regardless of the evidence base available, or the presence of specific guidelines and protocols, actions to address occupational performance issues still need to be individualized to the person or community to which they will be provided. Compromises to intervention dosages or customization of equipment may be required to meet the unique needs of the individual.

Implementation of actions is often influenced by pragmatic factors, including resources, skills, and the role and scope of the therapist. A thorough practice reasoning process will identify and pre-empt barriers to implementation by thorough consideration of the many factors impacting service delivery.

7.6.4 Monitoring and Modifying

Implementation can be assumed to be the final stage in occupational therapy reasoning, but in reality the occupational therapy process is often a closed loop system whereby intervention gives rise to new information that provides feedback into the practice reasoning process. During implementation, unanticipated barriers or shortcomings might become obvious, new occupational performance issues might arise, and various parts of the reasoning process might require revision based on observed outcomes.

This formal feedback loop is identified in the model as the monitor and modify process, but several other minor feedback and revision processes also occur throughout the practice reasoning process. In the model, these minor feedback loops are identified by the broken lines that separate elements of the thinking space, and between processes occurring within those spaces. These signify the fluent back and forth process that often occurs between stages. For example, assessment information may cause the therapist to rethink the situation's complexity; guiding factors may modify the assumptions the therapist makes during the reasoning process; and intended actions may be reconsidered when contextualizing an intervention proves problematic.

More formal modifications to the reasoning process might follow the illustrated feedback loops. For example, attempts to generate hypotheses about the situation may illuminate hidden complications that require the therapist to reconsider perceptions of the situation's complexity. Alternatively, implementation of an action might reveal additional barriers to occupation that require formal consideration through a rekindling of the reasoning process. Formal and informal revisions ensure that practice reasoning is a dynamic process that is continually reshaped to address challenges to the client's occupations.

Table 7.2 presents the practice reasoning processes for John and Max during the acute stage of their recovery, in accordance with the Model of Occupational Therapy Reasoning. The table summarizes the ways in which the therapists, Maureen and Andrea, used the practice reasoning process component of the model to orient to the nature of their client's needs, consider and determine potential approaches, implement actions to address occupational goals, monitor the outcomes, and modify their reasoning. Rather than providing answers, the model guided the therapists in the practice reasoning process. Table 7.2 provides examples of how the process occurred in each scenario.

Table 7.2 The Practice Reasoning Process for John and Max

Thinking space	John	Max
Orienting space	Maureen framed John's occupational needs using an occupational diagnosis (see Figure 7.2). Due to Maureen's experience, she was able to make several assumptions about the nature of barriers to John's occupational performance, and this allowed her to view the situation as complicated, but not complex because the actions to be taken lay within her existing knowledge base.	In the acute setting, Andrea developed her occupational diagnosis for Max (see Figure 7.2). Andrea's moderate level of experience allowed her to make some assumptions about the best way to address Max's goals, but she considered some of his situation as complex because his unique needs required some novel actions that were not part of her existing experience.
Reasoning space	Maureen's reasoning was required when selecting a wheelchair. John had a T8 spinal cord injury and following physical assessments it was known that John had 4+/5 strength in all upper limb movements and good trunk stability. Having worked with many people with similar health conditions and similar movement capacities, Maureen was able to make several assumptions about John's ability to manually propel a wheelchair. This reduced the number of viable options and Maureen was able to choose between a small set of alternatives. Guiding factors such as resources and therapist role and scope influenced the decisions she and John made together.	Andrea had to reason appropriate approaches to enable Max to independently dress his lower limbs. Andrea's previous experience led her to assume Max could face difficulties completing dressing activities because of paraplegia. However, because Max's injury was an incomplete spinal cord transection she needed to investigate his physical capabilities. She discovered unique patterns of muscle activation and considered numerous adaptations to occupations before deciding on adapted techniques she believed would best meet Max's needs.
Action space	Maureen customized the wheelchair to John's unique needs. With the information above, along with other factors like John's preference of style and color, an appropriate titanium, rigid frame wheelchair and cushion was selected for John. As the wheelchair was going to be used every day for multiple occupations, Maureen knew from experience	Andrea trialed the techniques she believed would be most helpful for Max. Through collaboration, Max identified that dressing in bed was more efficient for him and he felt more competent, so dressing techniques were adapted.

(Continued)

Table 7.2 (Continued)

	that the NDIS would fund the cost of the wheelchair. John trialed some similar chairs with a local equipment supplier, obtained NDIS approval to purchase the chair, and it was ordered and delivered during his hospital rehabilitation phase.	
Monitoring and modifying	During initial use of the chair, minor modifications were made to enhance comfort and maneuverability.	Andrea observed that Max had more difficulty than she expected in undoing his trousers. Andrea reconsidered her interventions and adapted Max's pants, adding Velcro to overcome this issue.

7.7 Conclusion

The Model of Occupational Therapy Reasoning is a synthesis and reconstruction of the valuable work contributed by many authors within and outside of occupational therapy over many decades, and can be used to understand, critique, learn, and engage in occupational therapy practice reasoning. It is a general representation of a complicated process that underpins occupational therapy service delivery. It can be used to inform decisions, as well as to understand how those decisions were made, and while the scenarios described illustrate its application at a micro level, the authors contend that it can equally be used to depict the reasoning required for occupational therapists working at community and population levels. The model provides a representation of what we currently know about the tacit, imagistic, phenomenological process described by Mattingly (1991).

7.8 Summary

- The Model of Occupational Therapy Reasoning represents the way occupational therapists consider, make, and refine decisions in practice, along with the range of factors that guide them. It identifies the implicit and explicit factors that guide thinking and describes the cognitive process of practice reasoning.
- Conceptual models guide practitioners to make occupation-focused decisions while taking into account the complexities that can arise in varying contexts.
- Practice models have some common features, including evaluation, assessment, goal setting, intervention, measuring outcomes, and re-evaluation.
- Therapist and client skills are the capacities and capabilities that the therapist and the client bring into the professional encounter.
- The culture of the occupational therapist and the client is an important guiding factor in practice reasoning.
- When working with clients, occupational therapists need to consider information from the context in which they work and factors from the client's context that might have an impact on the intervention and outcomes.

- The Cynefin Framework is a complexity model that makes sense of situations based on their level of disorder and unpredictability.
- The concept of linearity is an important but singular element in helping therapists orient to a situation and the reasoning processes required to address it.
- The practice reasoning process involves several thinking spaces, including the orienting space, reasoning space, action space, and monitoring and modifying.

7.9 Review Questions
1. Why is practice reasoning important in occupational therapy?
2. Why are conceptual models of practice processes important in practice reasoning?
3. Give some examples of how the guiding factors in the Model of Occupational Therapy Reasoning influence the way the reasoning process occurs?
4. How are the orienting, reasoning, and action spaces different in the Model of Occupational Therapy Reasoning?

References

Agner, J. (2020). Moving from cultural competence to cultural humility in occupational therapy: A paradigm shift. *American Journal of Occupational Therapy, 74*(4), 7404347010p1–7404347010p7. https://doi.org/10.5014/ajot.2020.038067

American Occupational Therapy Association. (2020a). *Occupational Profile Template*. https://www.aota.org/~/media/Corporate/Files/Practice/Manage/Documentation/AOTA-Occupational-Profile-Template.pdf

American Occupational Therapy Association. (2020b). Occupational therapy practice framework: Domain and process (4th ed.). *American Journal of Occupational Therapy, 74*(Suppl. 2), 7412410010p1–7412410010p87. https://doi.org/10.5014/ajot.2020.74S2001

American Occupational Therapy Association. (2020c). *Domain and process: Contexts*. https://www.aota.org/practice/domain-and-process/contexts

American Occupational Therapy Association. (2021). Occupational therapy scope of practice. *American Journal of Occupational Therapy, 75*(Suppl. 3), 7513410020. https://doi.org/10.5014/ajot.2021.75S3005

Austroads. (2016). *Assessing fitness to drive for commercial and private vehicles*. Austroads Ltd.

Baum, C., Christiansen, C., & Bass, J. (2015). Person-Environment-Occupation-Performance (PEOP) Model. In C. Christiansen, C. Baum, & J. Bass (Eds.), *Occupational therapy: Performance, participation, well-being* (4th ed., pp. 49–56). Slack.

Brandis, S., Rice, J., & Schleimer, S. (2017). Dynamic workplace interactions for improving patient safety climate. *Journal of Health Organization and Management, 31*(1), 38–53. https://doi.org/10.1108/JHOM-09-2016-0185

Carswell, A., McColl, M. A., Baptiste, S., Law, M., Polatajko, H., & Pollock, N. (2004). The Canadian Occupational Performance Measure: A research and clinical literature review. *Canadian Journal of Occupational Therapy, 71*(4), 210–222. http://doi.org/10.1177/000841740407100406

Champagne, T. T., Ryan, J. K., Saccomando, H. M., & Lazzarini, I. (2007). A nonlinear dynamics approach to exploring the spiritual dimensions of occupation. *Emergence: Complexity and Organization, 9*(4), 29.

Copley, J. A., Turpin, M. J., & King, T. L. (2010). Information used by an expert paediatric occupational therapist when making clinical decisions. *Canadian Journal of Occupational Therapy, 77*(4), 249–256. https://doi.org/10.2182/cjot.2010.77.4.7

Corazza, G. R., & Lenti, M. V. (2021). Diagnostic reasoning in internal medicine: Cynefin framework makes sense of clinical complexity. *Frontiers in Medicine, 8*, 641093. https://doi.org/10.3389/fmed.2021.641093

Creek, J., Ilott, I., Cook, S., & Munday, C. (2005). Valuing occupational therapy as a complex intervention. *British Journal of Occupational Therapy, 68*(6), 281–284. https://doi.org/10.1177/030802260506800607

Dale, S. (2015). Heuristics and biases: The science of decision-making. *Business Information Review, 32*(2), 93–99. https://doi.org/10.1177/0266382115592536

Doyle, S., Bennett, S., & Gustafsson, L. (2013). Clinical decision making when addressing upper limb post-stroke sensory impairments. *British Journal of Occupational Therapy, 76*(6), 254–263. https://doi.org/10.4276/030802213X13706169932789

Edwards, W. (1954). The theory of decision making. *Psychological Bulletin, 51*(4), 380. https://doi.org/10.1037/h0053870

Egan, M., & Restall, G. (2022). The Canadian model of occupational participation. In M. Egan & G. Restall (Eds.), *Promoting occupational participation: Collaborative relationship-focused occupational therapy* (pp. 74–95). CAOT.

Fleming, M. H. (1994). The therapist with the three-track mind. In C. Mattingly & M. H. Fleming (Eds.), *Clinical reasoning: Forms of inquiry in a therapeutic practice* (pp. 119–136). F. A. Davis.

Foronda, C., MacWilliams, B., & McArthur, E. (2016). Interprofessional communication in healthcare: An integrative review. *Nurse Education in Practice, 19*, 36–40. https://doi.org/10.1016/j.nepr.2016.04.005

Gillen, G. (2014). Occupational therapy interventions for individuals. In B. A. B. Schell, G. Gillen, M. E. Scaffa, & E. S. Cohn (Eds.), *Willard and Spackman's occupational therapy* (12th ed., pp. 322–341). Lippincott Williams & Wilkins.

Gray, B. (2017). The Cynefin framework: Applying an understanding of complexity to medicine. *Journal of Primary Health Care, 9*(4), 258–261. https://doi.org/10.1071/hc17002

Greber, C. (2021). Critical appraisal of practice evidence: A professional imperative for occupational therapy. *New Zealand Journal of Occupational Therapy, 68*(1), 11–14.

Hammell, K. R. W. (2013). Occupation, well-being, and culture: Theory and cultural humility. *Canadian Journal of Occupational Therapy, 80*(4), 224–234. https://doi.org/10.1177/0008417413500465

Harrison, R., Manias, E., Mears, S., Heslop, D., Hinchcliff, R., & Hay, L. (2019). Addressing unwarranted clinical variation: A rapid review of current evidence. *Journal of Evaluation in Clinical Practice, 25*(1), 53–65. https://doi.org/10.1111/jep.12930

Hinojosa, J., Kramer, P., & Howe, T. (2019). Structure of the frame of reference: Moving from theory to practice. In P. Kramer, J. Hinojosa, & T. Howe (Eds.), *Pediatric frames of reference in occupational therapy* (4th ed., pp. 3–19). Wolters Kluwer.

Hoffmann, T., Bennett, S., & Del Mar, C. (2017). Introduction to evidence-based practice. In T. Hoffmann, S. Bennett, & C. Del Mar (Eds.), *Evidence-based practice across the health professions* (3rd ed., pp. 1–15). Elsevier.

Icare (Insurance and Care NSW). (2017). *Guidance on the support needs for adults with spinal cord injury* (3rd ed.). www.icare.nsw.gov.au/treatment-and-care/what-we-do/guidelines-and-policies

Iwama, M. K. (2006). *The Kawa Model: Culturally relevant occupational therapy*. Churchill Livingstone Elsevier.

Kristensen, H. K., Borg, T., & Hounsgaard, L. (2012). Aspects affecting occupational therapists' reasoning when implementing research-based evidence in stroke rehabilitation. *Scandinavian Journal of Occupational Therapy, 19*(2), 118–131. https://doi.org/10.3109/11038128.2011.556197

Mattingly, C. (1991). What is clinical reasoning? *American Journal of Occupational Therapy, 45*(11), 979–986. https://doi.org/10.5014/ajot.45.11.979

Mattingly, C., & Fleming, M. H. (1994). *Clinical reasoning: Forms of inquiry in a therapeutic practice*. F. A. Davis.

Occupational Therapy Australia. (2017). *Position paper: Occupational therapy scope of practice framework*. Occupational Therapy Australia. https://otaus.com.au/publicassets/725

829df-2503-e911-a2c2-b75c2fd918c5/Occupational%20Therapy%20Scope%20of%20 Practice%20Framework%20(June%202017).pdf

Ottenbacher, K. J., Hsu, Y., Granger, C. V., & Fiedler, R. C. (1996). The reliability of the functional independence measure: A quantitative review. *Archives of Physical Medicine and Rehabilitation, 77*(12), 1226–1232. https://doi.org/10.1016/S0003-9993(96)90184-7

Peters, A., Vanstone, M., Monteiro, S., Norman, G., Sherbino, J., & Sibbald, M. (2017). Examining the influence of context and professional culture on clinical reasoning through rhetorical-narrative analysis. *Qualitative Health Research, 27*(6), 866–876. https://doi.org/10.1177/1049732316650418

Restall, G., Egan, N., Valavaara, K., Phenix, A., & Sack, C. (2022). The Canadian occupational therapy inter-relational practice process framework. In M. Egan & G. Restall (Eds.), *Promoting occupational participation: Collaborative relationship-focused occupational therapy* (pp. 120–150). CAOT.

Robertson, L. J. (1996). Clinical reasoning, part 1: The nature of problem solving, a literature review. *British Journal of Occupational Therapy, 59*(4), 178–182. https://doi.org/10.1177/030802269605900407

Rogers, J. C. (2004). Occupational diagnosis. In M. Molineux (Ed.), *Occupation for occupational therapists* (pp. 17–31). Wiley.

Rogers, J. C., & Holm, M. B. (1991). Occupational therapy diagnostic reasoning: A component of clinical reasoning. *American Journal of Occupational Therapy, 45*(11), 1045–1053. https://doi.org/10.5014/ajot.45.11.1045

Schell, B. A. B., & Benfield, A. (2018). Aspects of professional reasoning. In B. A. B. Schell & J. W. Schell (Eds.), *Clinical and professional reasoning in occupational therapy* (2nd ed., pp. 127–144). Wolters Kluwer.

Schell, B. A. B., & Schell, J. W. (2018). Professional reasoning as the basis of practice. In B. A. B. Schell & J. W. Schell (Eds.), *Clinical and professional reasoning in occupational therapy* (2nd ed., pp. 3–22). Wolters Kluwer.

Schell, B. A. B., Unsworth, C., & Schell, J. (2018). An ecological model of professional reasoning. In B. A. B. Schell & J. W. Schell (Eds.), *Clinical and professional reasoning in occupational therapy* (2nd ed., pp. 23–50). Wolters Kluwer.

Shafaroodi, N., Kamali, M., Parvizy, S., Mehraban, A. H., & O'Toole, G. (2014). Factors affecting clinical reasoning of occupational therapists: A qualitative study. *Medical Journal of the Islamic Republic of Iran, 28*, 8.

Smit, E. D., & Derksen, J. J. (2017). Vignette research on messy and confusing problems in primary mental healthcare. *Europe's Journal of Psychology, 13*(2), 300. https://doi.org/10.5964/ejop.v13i2.1212

Smith, M., Higgs, J., & Ellis, E. (2008). Factors influencing clinical decision making. In J. Higgs, M. A. Jones, S. Loftus, & N. Christensen (Eds.), *Clinical reasoning in the health professions* (3rd ed., pp. 89–100). Butterworth Heinemann Elsevier.

Snowden, D. J., & Boone, M. E. (2007). A leader's framework for decision making. *Harvard Business Review, 85*(11), 68.

Spinal Cord Injury Australia (n.d.). *Supporting people with SCI and other neurological conditions.* Spinal Cord Injury Australia. https://scia.org.au/

Stampfer, H. (2019). Advocating for mental health doublespeak. *Australian & New Zealand Journal of Psychiatry, 53*(5), 479–480. https://doi.org/10.1177/0004867418818750

Stark, S. L., Somerville, E., Keglovits, M., Smason, A., & Bigham, K. (2015). Clinical reasoning guideline for home modification interventions. *American Journal of Occupational Therapy, 69*(2), 6902290030p1–6902290030p8. https://doi.org/10.5014/ajot.2015.014266

Taff, S. D., Grajo, L. C., Kniepmann, K., Carson, N., Jackson, D., Deforge, M., Chakraborty, S., Gray, J. M., & Amin-Arsala, T. (2020). Educator's guide for addressing cultural awareness, humility and dexterity in occupational therapy curricula. *American Journal of Occupational Therapy, 74*(S3), 7413420003–7413420003p19. https://doi.org/10.5014/ajot.2020.74S3005

Taylor, R. (2017). *Keilhofner's model of human occupation.* Wolters Kluwer.

Trede, F., & Higgs, J. (2008). Clinical reasoning and models of practice. In J. Higgs, M. Jones, S. Loftus, & N. Christensen (Eds.), *Clinical reasoning in the health professions* (3rd ed., pp. 31–41). Elsevier.

Trombly, C. (1983). *Occupational therapy for physical dysfunction*. Williams & Wilkins.

Turpin, M., & Garcia, J. (2021). Occupational therapy models of practice. In T. Brown, H. Bourke-Taylor, S. Isbel, R. Cordier, & L. Gustaffson (Eds.), *Occupational therapy in Australia: Professional and practice issues* (2nd ed., pp. 213–225). Routledge.

Turpin, M. J., & Iwama, M. K. (2011). *Using occupational therapy models in practice: A field-guide*. Elsevier Health Sciences.

University of Reading (n.d.). *Definitions of values, belief and attitude*. https://overcorp.com.au/?page_id=488

Unsworth, C. A. (2004). Clinical reasoning: How do pragmatic reasoning, worldview and client-centredness fit? *British Journal of Occupational Therapy, 67*(1), 10–19. https://doi.org/10.1177/030802260406700103

Unsworth, C. A. (2012). Research and scholarship in clinical and professional reasoning. In B. A. B. Schell & J. W. Schell (Eds.), *Clinical and professional reasoning in occupational therapy* (2nd ed., pp. 477–491). Wolters Kluwer.

Van Beurden, E. K., Kia, A. M., Zask, A., Dietrich, U., & Rose, L. (2013). Making sense in a complex landscape: How the Cynefin Framework from complex adaptive systems theory can inform health promotion practice. *Health Promotion International, 28*(1), 73–83. https://doi.org/10.1093/heapro/dar089

Whiteford, G., Klomp, N., & Wright-St Clair, V. (2005). Complexity theory: Understanding occupation, practice and context. In G. Whiteford & V. Wright-St Clair (Eds.), *Occupation and practice in context* (pp. 3–15). Elsevier.

SECTION TWO

Contemporary Perspectives on Human Occupation

CHAPTER 8

Bringing Critical Perspectives into Occupation-based Practices

Lisette Farias, Gail Teachman, Rebecca M. Aldrich, Roshan Galvaan, and Debbie Laliberte Rudman

Abstract
Critical perspectives provide concepts and a lens that can be used to problematize and reformulate occupational issues, practices, and assumptions that maintain an individualist focus and neglect socially inequitable conditions that differentially affect groups in society. Critical perspectives provide a broader understanding of the socioeconomic and political conditions that shape occupation. Numerous examples have emerged in the literature to support the value added by integrating these perspectives into *occupation-based practices*.[1] Applying critical perspectives can contribute to social transformation by shifting ways of thinking and doing, such that the socioeconomic and political roots of occupational inequities are addressed. This chapter interweaves critical reflexive vignettes and examples of the authors' work to exemplify how critical perspectives have helped reframe issues and solutions in ways that expand beyond a primary focus on individual doing. This chapter builds on previous work that calls for continuous reflexivity and problematization of socially dominant norms as strategies to resist individualistic tendencies and contribute to enacting social transformation and promoting equity-oriented practices.

Authors' Positionality Statement
We (the chapter authors) have employed a range of critical perspectives to challenge dominant ways of doing occupation-based practices in and across different contexts. Given the diversity and depth of critical perspectives, this chapter does not aim to provide an exhaustive overview but rather draws on selected critical perspectives to explore their features and value for occupation-based practices. Geographically, our experiences are grounded in diverse places such as Chile/Sweden, the United States of America, Canada, and South Africa. While we share some positionalities (university-educated, professionally qualified, cisgendered, socioeconomically privileged), we also bring varied individual positionalities (non-Western, Western, Amerindian/Latinx, White, Black, Spanish-speaker, English-speaker, able-bodied). We recognize that the ideas shared in this chapter are influenced by a range of social, political, and

DOI: 10.4324/9781003504610-10

cultural views of human occupation, social equity, and social transformation, including Westernized understandings that have become predominant within occupational therapy through historical processes of colonization. Consistent with the intent of critical theoretical perspectives to question the "status quo" and promote more equitable ways of living together, we offer this material in the hope of promoting critical, inclusive, culturally sensitive, anti-racist, gender-affirming, and respectful dialogue.

> **Objectives**
> This chapter will support readers to:
>
> - Identify key features of critical theoretical perspectives that distinguish them from other approaches guiding occupation-based practices.
> - Explain the value that critical theoretical perspectives add to conceptualizing and addressing socioeconomic and political conditions that shape occupation.
> - Highlight the relations between the uptake of critical perspectives and socially transformative occupation-based practices.

> **Key terms**
> - **socially transformative practices**
> - **occupation-based practices**
> - **critical reflexivity**
> - **problematization**
> - **epistemology**

8.1 Introduction

The ways occupational therapists *frame* or conceptualize inequities shape possibilities and boundaries for what they propose as appropriate and relevant ways to practice (Laliberte Rudman et al., 2022). This means that when inequities are framed as individual rather than social problems, practices to address those inequities will tend to be focused on individual doing (Gerlach et al., 2018). This chapter describes how critical theoretical perspectives *frame* inequities in ways that illuminate the socioeconomic and political conditions that shape occupation. Our focus on the value of critical perspectives reflects growing interest in enacting socially responsive occupation-based practices and optimizing the potential of occupation to contribute to *social transformation* (see also Chapter 14). The fundamental assumption underlying this chapter is that critical theoretical perspectives support analyses of occupations that reveal inequitable conditions across social groups and prompt (new) insights, awareness, and possible actions to address those inequities.

We start by clarifying key terms, including "critical theoretical perspectives", "social transformation", and "socially transformative practices". *Critical theoretical perspectives*, also referred to as critical social theory, denote an evolving group of theoretical approaches (e.g., Marxism, postmodernism, feminism, and critical race theory). Common to these theories is a focus on revealing inter-group power relationships that result from historical, socioeconomic, political, and cultural processes and systems (e.g., colonialism, capitalism, and patriarchy). By drawing attention to patterns of social privilege, disadvantage, and oppression produced through those dynamic relations, critical approaches aim to provide a basis for social transformation (Farias & Aldrich, 2021).

Social transformation refers to a process of engaging with critical perspectives to consider power as complex, dynamic, and multiple. As such, social transformation not only questions "why things are not right as they are", but seeks to identify hidden structures, assumptions, and practices that need to be altered to promote equity. *Socially transformative practices* seek to promote equity by developing partnerships and enacting *social or collective practices* and counterhegemonic forms of knowledge, together with those experiencing disparities, to build on their efforts of resistance (see more about social or collective practices in Chapter 14). This implies that social transformation does not always involve a reversal of power relations but a strengthening of the negotiating power of people/communities within these relations (Farias et al., 2016).

This chapter is organized into four main sections. In the first section, we set out the main tenets of critical theoretical perspectives, bringing examples of problematization of "positive" aging, and the idealized notion of children's "normal" development in occupational therapy. In the second section, we describe ways of problematizing an individualistic perspective through a focus on the notions of inclusion, independence, and individual "behavior". In the third section, we discuss the potential of creating new framings that move beyond individualized solutions, using examples addressing long-term unemployment and individual "choices". The fourth section presents an application of critical perspectives to educational practices to reframe assumptions about what contributed to successful participation in education as a foundation for future transformative practices. The chapter concludes with summary arguments reinforcing the importance of ongoing critical reflexivity and critical awareness of the implications of individualistic frames for the occupational possibilities of particular social groups.

8.2 Critical Epistemology
8.2.1 A View from Somewhere

I (the first author) come from a region that continues to suffer the consequences of historical colonialism – a process that denies Indigenous communities their knowledge and tries to reform them to European standards of thought and practice. This personal background has made me aware of the power relations that privilege some voices over others. Because of my background, I find critical perspectives helpful to disrupt dominant understandings of occupation and practice resulting from European/colonial processes. Yet, I am increasingly concerned with the ways the profession continues to internalize dominant views that value European standards of knowledge. This type of epistemology disregards collectivist values, lived experiences, and traditional wisdom, promoting a decontextualized view of knowledge that limits the ways knowledge can be questioned or critiqued.

Epistemology refers to the assumptions about knowledge and processes of knowing that, for example, are embraced in the development of a profession and disciplinary knowledge, setting the agenda for who is deemed a knower/expert and what knowledge is considered legitimate or worthy of pursuing (Kinsella & Whiteford, 2009). Understanding the underlying epistemological assumptions of critical perspectives is key to engaging with collective and counterhegemonic forms of knowledge that are often located outside the dominant status quo (Santos, 2014). For instance, positivist epistemology, which is dominant within the Western model of "science", positions ideal occupational therapy practitioners as unbiased observers administering assessment protocols that accurately measure components of "true" performance. Critical epistemology, in contrast, suggests that there is a need to unlearn the notion that reality or performance can be studied and captured as "it is" without influencing or being influenced by it. Applying this to assessment practices, critical epistemology questions the possibility of "unbiased" assessors/assessments and highlights the need for critical reflexivity regarding whose knowledge and ways of understanding occupation are privileged and marginalized within an assessment (Laliberte Rudman et al., 2022).

Critical epistemologies are historically grounded in the work of Karl Marx (Marx, 1996). Marx argued that ideology, or common sense, is not objective but, instead, is subjective and shaped by one's situated sociopolitical and cultural circumstances. As such, knowledge is inherently always situated and comes from "somewhere". Dominant forms of knowledge, for Marx, are partial and cannot represent a full picture of reality; rather, they reflect and serve the interests of privileged groups in society. Based on this understanding, the critical inquirer's role is to look "behind the appearances of reality as it is taken to be, to reveal the hidden mechanisms of social inequality, thereby contributing to the liberation of oppressed groups" (Farias & Laliberte Rudman, 2016, p. 35).

To reveal these mechanisms, critical perspectives use problematization as a tool to examine why things are as they are, and who is silenced, privileged, or marginalized by the status quo. *Problematization* is an analytic strategy that questions how some ways of knowing come to be accepted as "natural", "right", and "logical", thus making alternative understandings invisible and "unthinkable". Critical approaches are premised on the assumption that problematization of "why things are as they are" is a necessary step toward contesting and unlearning dominant beliefs, norms, or practices, creating space to visualize how things could or should be. For example, Laliberte Rudman (2017) has drawn upon critical theory (specifically Foucault's theorization of governmentality[2]) to question the occupations held out as ideal and responsible within contemporary discourses of so-called "positive" aging. This theoretical framework illuminates how certain "retirees"' behaviors, needs, and desires are idealized and related to body monitoring, self-improvement, risk management, and lifestyle maximization. Simultaneously, such a framing of "retirees" obscures other possibilities for "aging well".

By adopting a critical perspective, Laliberte Rudman's work advances an understanding of the ways that "positive" aging can be harmful to adults who lack the bodily, financial, social, and other resources required to take up the expected "duty to age well".

Beliefs, norms, and ways of doing related to "aging well" can be internalized and, if left unquestioned, inadvertently contribute to inequities by shaping occupation-based practices in inaccessible or exclusionary ways.

Based on a conceptualization of power as complex, dynamic, and multiple, socially transformative practices seek to (re)formulate/transform social beliefs, social relations, and practices within structures that support injustices. *Critical reflexivity* is therefore another tool for problematizing and reflecting on how certain knowledge and practices are socially embraced and constructed. For instance, drawing upon critical disability perspectives, Phelan (2011) noted that for occupational therapists working with children, practices oriented around a progression through "normal" developmental stages discount the unique trajectories associated with neurological differences and fail to account for the child's unique context. Phelan proposed a shift away from overreliance on idealized notions of normal development and increased acknowledgment of the sociopolitical mechanisms that produce disability. Enacting this shift challenges occupational therapists to move beyond dualisms of disability/ability or dependence/independence to attend to the broader social relations and structures that construct disability. This type of critical reflexivity allows practitioners to interrogate the frameworks and models that are embraced as part of occupation-based professional knowledge, as well as the underlying assumptions regarding the essence of human doing that shape occupation-based practices.

8.3 Problematizing Individual Solutions

8.3.1 Inclusion Framed as an Individual Journey toward "Normality"

> At age 22, Jack had completed high school and had a part-time job. He had been diagnosed at a young age with cerebral palsy and used a speech-generating device along with gestures, facial expressions, and some limited vocalizations to communicate. His communication device was mounted on his power wheelchair; he controlled both using a head switch. Jack had participated in an independent-living training program organized by a children's rehabilitation center. As part of the program, he stayed for a week, with attendant support, in a college residence. He described this as an important experience: "I 'found myself' finally…and I stayed on budget". He said he hoped to live on his own in the future and noted: "My parents are not going to be around forever!" Jack had attended his local high school and graduated with a diploma at age 21. It took him a full year to complete courses that were typically scheduled for one term. Jack described his time in high school as emotionally and physically painful, but he said he was also immensely proud of this accomplishment. In his final year of school, he was elected by his peers as "Prom King". Building on experience he gained through a high school co-op course, Jack had secured a part-time job as a disability advocate for a local school board and proudly shared: "I'm a working man now!"

This vignette, drawn from research about how disabled youth in Canada experience and understand "inclusion" (Teachman et al., 2020), provides an opportunity for readers to problematize the normative assumptions influencing Jack's understanding of inclusion. His narrative shows how he has internalized ideas about being as "normal" and independent as possible in order to be included. Such assumptions reinforce the notion that disability is an individual deficit to be "overcome" at all costs. Jack's sense of being successful is linked with broader social expectations about productive occupations for young adults (e.g., independent living, graduating from high school, and working). His pride around securing a paid job can be interpreted as an achievement that, for Jack, serves as evidence of the ways he has successfully persevered to maintain precarious social positions in mainstream educational spaces, even though this positioning was emotionally and physically painful.

For Jack, dominant views of inclusion are set as an "individual journey" that people with disabilities need to navigate on their own. The journey required that he and his family invest heavily and continually in various rehabilitation and educational endeavors. This view of inclusion as "individually" driven comes at a high cost, a cost that often remains invisible within health care, education, and other systems. The price of "inclusion" when seen as an individual journey toward "normal" ways of being, and in particular, "normal" occupational expectations, involves arduous and ongoing struggles to meet the standards expected of non-disabled persons, regardless of the personal costs. In this individualized framing of "inclusion", persons labeled "disabled" are continually required to "overcome" impairments to avoid being categorized as tragic, unfortunate, and "in need of inclusion". Because Jack, like all persons, is immersed in broader social messages, he internalizes the sense that engaging in the occupational roles expected throughout the life span is the "ideal" way of achieving inclusion, but this framing places the work of being included on people with disabilities and fails to value other ways of being and doing as an adult.

Part of our role as health-related professionals should involve problematizing individualistic views that place the responsibility for inclusion on those being marginalized. Through biomedically focused training and socialization, occupational therapists, like other professionals, tend to uncritically internalize ways of thinking about the individual/body and disease/problems (Farias, 2020). Biomedicine is primarily focused on biological, neurological, and physiological processes as if these were disconnected from the sociopolitical and cultural constructions of health and illness. This view is problematic since a focus on body parts as fully representative of health assumes that disease, and its consequences for occupation, are the result of viruses, toxins, and a person's genetics, behavior, or lifestyle, disregarding the role played by social conditions (i.e., poverty, social exclusion, inadequate public policies, and health services). This view is also problematic since the healthy body becomes a sign "of good decision-making" by those with the capacity to follow the "right" advice and consume the "right" products.

In a further example, consider how biomedical portrayals of alcoholism as the result of "unhealthy" behavior and an individual disease state contribute to practices that pathologize and blame the person for their lifestyle or "poor choice". As such, uncritically framing alcoholism as a problem that resides within the individual can result in blaming the individual for not "solving" his/her problem, or for being "part of the problem and not the solution". Problematizing such portrayals through reframing alcohol use as an occupation has generated insights regarding how this occupation is situated within broader forces, such as consumerism, sociocultural expectations, colonialism, inequitable alternative occupational opportunities, and geographic isolation (Cloete & Ramugondo, 2015).

The examples shared in this section highlight the need for practices to shift beyond approaches that locate causes and solutions solely at an individual level toward those that account for contextual forces that promote and constrain occupational possibilities.

8.4 Creating New Framings
8.4.1 Who "Counts" as Worthy of Employment Services and Support?

Within many nations, including Canada and the United States, long-term unemployment has been defined to include only those without formal paid employment who demonstrate motivation for work, particularly through "active" job-seeking. Being counted as "long-term unemployed" often determines eligibility for income support and employment support services. This narrow definition masks the employment experiences of many citizens within socioeconomic contexts where precarious forms of labor marked by underemployment, cyclical engagement in insecure employment, and restricted workers' rights, are escalating, particularly for collectives who face pervasive forms of discrimination tied to race, age, ability status, citizenship status, and other markers of difference. It also masks the diverse occupational inequities faced by individuals and collectives who are most "at risk" in the precarious labor market, for example, concerning secure housing, food security, and social belonging. Fully understanding the complexity of precarity in work, that is, insecure, unstable, or absent work opportunities, and addressing associated occupational inequities, requires a reframing that acknowledges and addresses diverse struggles to participate in work in ways that generate security, hope, and diverse forms of occupational engagement.

Creating new frames is essential to finding new ways of thinking that can guide equity-oriented and socially transformative practices. Yet, it can be challenging to reformulate certain frames that have been naturalized as "true" within most Western societies. The vignette in this section reflects the critical intent of a program of research led by Laliberte Rudman and Aldrich which challenges who is addressed and what occupations are attended to within government policies regarding income support and employment support services (Aldrich et al., 2020). Through collaborative engagement with persons who self-identified as long-term unemployed, employment support service providers, and organizational and governmental stakeholders, this work seeks to challenge the narrow framing of "who counts" as struggling with sustainable employment. It also proposes reframing this social issue by resisting jumping to specific solutions from an "expert" perspective instead of first questioning how policymakers have defined long-term unemployment as a problem of individual motivation and skill deficiencies, and how this framing perpetuates solutions that fail to address the complex conditions that sustain employment precarity.

As another example, a common frame within occupational therapy portrays individuals as having "choices" to act in ways that promote their health (Murthi & Hammell, 2021). These individual "choices" are usually grounded in occupational possibilities, i.e., "ways and types of doing that come to be viewed as ideal and possible within a socio-historical context, and that come to be promoted and made available within environments" (Laliberte Rudman, 2006, p. 188). For example, normative guidelines on what people can and should do to maintain their health and productivity, such as healthy eating or physical activity guidelines, target individuals and communities in efforts to shape "ideal" choices for a range of everyday occupations, resulting in both social pressures and neglect of the conditions and resources required to take up ideals. This messaging tends to be directed at some people more than others, e.g., those who are viewed as "incapable" of choosing "good" occupations, i.e., children, the poor, women, the unemployed, and Indigenous peoples (Power & Polzer, 2016). This notion of choice as an individual endeavor, inherent to some occupational therapy models, narrowly focuses on an individual's occupational choices with little or no consideration of the contextual forces that shape those choices (Galvaan, 2015).

Based on this frame, a "client's" lack of collaboration or "non-compliance with a self-management program" could be interpreted by occupational therapists as a "problem" linked to individual choice. This framing neglects factors outside the individual that work against their choices, or that render the choices offered inappropriate. Rushing to "solve" this problem risks (a) perpetuating dominant views that portray individuals as inherently capable of self-managing; (b) blaming individuals for "choosing" not to follow the "right" programs; (c) overlooking health insurers', researchers', and policymakers' responsibility for framing the problem in this way; (d) framing "unhealthy" people as "bad citizens" who are burdens to society; and (e) diminishing individuals' voices and credibility without taking into consideration the factors that shape or create health-related "decisions" about occupations (e.g., collective wisdom, lack of time, and availability of resources).

However, occupational therapists can also work to create new frames that challenge individualistic understandings of occupational choice, foregrounding the influences of social, political, and cultural factors that shape everyday life (Galvaan, 2015). The following vignette illustrates the power of reframing assumptions about what contributes to successful participation in education (Galvaan, 2016):

> The legacy of racially segregated access to education during apartheid in South Africa is still apparent and has been referred to as the persistence of a dual economy of schooling (Shalem & Hoadley, 2009). In this dual economy of schooling, most of the black population in South Africa continues to access low-income schools with inadequate infrastructure, large teacher:student ratios, and a curriculum that does not respond well to students' needs. School completion and pursuing a post-school qualification are often accepted as a route out of poverty, emphasizing individuals lifting themselves out of negative social conditions rather than questioning and changing these social conditions. For occupational therapists working in schools, the traditional approaches to treating learners would perhaps focus on individual sessions that improve learners' fine motor, gross motor, or visual perception skills. Adopting a critical theoretical perspective shifts this individual focus to questioning how the framing of education limits learning. It also implies challenging the narrative that occupational choice is merely a matter of individual agency. This leads to re-thinking what may need to be included in the school curriculum or what changes may be made to the delivery of the curriculum to create a less constraining context for learning. The rhetoric that "through hard work, access and opportunity are equitably available", is thus reframed.

In occupational therapy literature, Indigenous scholars such as Emery-Whittington (2021) have argued for (re)framing practices to respond to the socio-historical stigmatization and oppression of Indigenous people, as a way of decolonizing the profession of occupational therapy and its prioritization of White, settler values, norms, knowledges, and ways of being and doing in the world. For instance, occupational therapy scholars note "how everything from assessment norms to orthosis materials assumes Whiteness, and how values such as occupational balance and categories of occupational domains are steeped in White Western culture" (Beagan et al., 2022, p. 53). By creating a new framing of individuals' doing, especially of people belonging to communities that have been historically marginalized/colonized, it is possible to draw attention to the socio-political, historical, and cultural conditions that oppress and marginalize individuals and communities. For example, reframing recovery from substance abuse as an occupational transition for men in Zimbabwe (Nhunzvi et al., 2019) amid prevailing cultures of substance abuse brought to awareness how this transition is entangled with the profound effects of a drawn-out economic crisis and lack of paid work on everyday life and well-being.

In this way, critical perspectives can provide a new frame or rationale that shifts the ways individuals are framed/judged to be responsible and, instead, considers and addresses broader socioeconomic, political, or historical conditions. As examples, using participatory approaches, Trentham and Neysmith's (2018) work with senior citizens raised awareness of how agism frames occupational possibilities in ways that limit their participation in health systems and other social arenas, while Benjamin-Thomas et al.'s (2022) work with children in India pointed to historical, social, and political framings of disability that constrain community responses to issues of environmental degradation and occupational marginalization.

8.5 Applying a Critical Approach to Educational Practice
8.5.1 Creating Critically Oriented Learning Environments

> Creating dedicated, facilitated spaces for dialogue about Equity and Diversity within the University of Cape Town occupational therapy curriculum allows students and academic facilitators to reflect on situations as a collective. One example of these spaces is quarterly sessions with each occupational therapy class. Students have used these spaces to question the way that clinical or practice learning placements are allocated and to question curriculum decisions. Although identifying actions towards resolving the problems raised is one important part of these spaces, unpacking the taken-for-granted assumptions that underpin the problems is foregrounded. This opportunity to build our capacities to be critically reflexive as part of a class, that is, as a collective, provides a foundation for embracing this process as part of our professional identities.

To support future practitioners' development of critical skills to analyze occupation in relation to socioeconomic and political conditions, integration of critical perspectives into occupational therapy education is essential. The vignette in this section is based on the work of Galvaan and colleagues at the University of Cape Town (Galvaan, 2012; Ngcobo et al., 2018). It exemplifies how critical perspectives can be applied to occupational therapy education through concrete activities within the curriculum to support students' reflection and questioning of clinical practice and curriculum decisions (Galvaan, 2012). It illustrates how integration of critical perspectives can occur in many ways, including using critical pedagogical theories to shape learning environments; facilitating learning activities that help students develop critical reflexivity and awareness; and utilizing content that demonstrates the application of critical perspectives to topics related to clinical practice.

As a foundation for teaching and learning activities, educators can draw on pedagogical theories to support students' comfort with critical questioning. Freire,[3] whose pedagogical theory emphasizes the importance of reforming the "banking"/receiving method of learning, argued that when students "receive" knowledge through passive listening and acceptance of facts, the process reinforces a lack of critical thinking and ownership in students. He argued that teachers can support students' development of critical awareness or "conscientization" through active participation in reflection and interpretation of their experiences (Farias & Aldrich, 2021). The above example from the University of Cape Town demonstrates how educators can build students' abilities to question how certain ideas are "taken-for-granted" in their clinical practice. This educational approach builds on students' consciousness of how broader issues of power shape their everyday life, extending this understanding to question their learning and construction of professional identities.

Mezirow's[4] transformative learning theory (1991) provides another tool for creating critically oriented learning environments. Mezirow advocates using "disorienting dilemmas" to help students challenge assumptions and beliefs, explore alternative perspectives, and transform the way they understand the world. A disorienting dilemma can be based on an ethical issue experienced by students in their clinical practice, or infused in the classroom through cases. The point is to embrace "discomfort" with learned ways of practicing that do not fit students' experiences. In contrast to traditional or banking methods of learning, which focus on adding to "what we already know", transformational learning seeks to transform "what we know", a process that can occur gradually across several cumulative experiences, or from a sudden powerful experience. The questioning and reformation of students' frames are essential to support processes of personal and social transformation.

Learning activities that include exploration and transformation of students' values and assumptions have the potential to develop students' abilities to rethink their decision making, attitudes, and understandings of power as future occupational therapists. For example, occupational therapy practitioners need to develop and manage their relations with others by using professional reasoning, empathy, and a client-centered, collaborative approach (AOTA, 2020). To enact empathy and collaboration, practitioners need to consciously attend to issues of power, striving to create relationships within which individuals and communities can take control over the decision-making process (AOTA, 2020). This means critical theoretical perspectives can raise awareness of a therapist's values concerning collaboration before enacting collaborative practice approaches.

8.5.2 Developing Alternative Ways of Practicing by Applying Critical Perspectives
Learning activities that help students problematize taken-for-granted ways of thinking and doing in occupational therapy can provide a foundation for considering alternate ways of practicing. Professional models and theories that are presented in occupational

therapy curricula help students and practitioners "make sense" of people's situations and attribute significance to their experiences. However, these same models also play a key role in shaping perceptions, beliefs, expectations, and purposes about professional roles, scope of practice, and groups of clients. They provide students with a "line of action" that, once programed, risks being unreflexively and automatically applied from one client to another, thereby reinforcing framings that reject/judge ways of living or doing that do not fit with preconceptions of what is "healthy" or "good" (Kiepek et al., 2019).

This risk can be ameliorated by changing how professional models, frameworks, and theories are introduced: rather than presenting them as fixed, final, and universal, educators can open spaces for students to identify and question the underlying assumptions and influences that shape these guiding texts. Through discussion and reimagining of assumptions underlying professional models, theories, and frameworks, students can develop a critical consciousness concerning the advancement of practices that avoid reproducing inequities arising from stereotypes and unquestioned ideas. This, in turn, may help create a critical mass of occupational therapists who practice in this way.

Since educational institutions play a significant role in perpetuating marginalization of knowledge from outside the dominant Western sphere, educators can work to dismantle this dominance and contribute to the decolonization of occupational therapy education. Educators can use critically informed tools to examine how educational content and curriculum may perpetuate the dominance of particular voices, worldviews, and values. Specifically, educators can intentionally infuse content from non-Western or colonized writers to promote knowledge that has been historically oppressed or excluded from occupational therapy education (Simaan, 2020). Drawing on critical perspectives, educators can also design learning activities that challenge students' (dominant) understandings of occupation by incorporating local and global encounters (Aldrich, 2015) and creating learning activities that allow students to co-learn across global regions (Aldrich & Peters, 2019). Integrating multiple opportunities for co-learning across contexts can help students develop critical consciousness and reflexivity (Aldrich & Grajo, 2017). As occupational therapy is increasingly paying attention to questions of power, rights, and equity, educators can adopt a critical stance to question the underlying assumptions of theories and models, incorporate international dialogue, and acknowledge multiple ways of understanding occupation.

8.6 Conclusion

This chapter has demonstrated how critical theoretical perspectives can be integrated into occupation-based practices to support socially transformative and equity-oriented work in occupational therapy and occupational science. Understanding the epistemological assumptions and values underpinning these perspectives is essential to the development and enactment of practices that can respond to problematic socioeconomic and political conditions that inequitably shape occupation. Other examples of how specific critical perspectives are expressed in practice are presented in Chapters 14 and 15.

8.7 Summary

- Utilizing critical theoretical perspectives can support socially responsive and equity-oriented practices across the spectrum of professional practice, education, and research.

- Understanding the epistemological assumptions and values underpinning critical perspectives is essential to the development and enactment of practices that align with socially transformative goals.
- Critical theoretical perspectives support the analysis and problematization of occupational issues to reveal inequitable conditions among groups in society and prompt (new) insights and awareness that are needed to address inequities.
- Increasing awareness of the root causes of occupational issues can facilitate enacting practices that avoid blaming individuals for social conditions outside their control or choice, and address root causes located in social, economic, and political conditions.

8.8 Review Questions
1. What are the main features of critical theoretical perspectives?
2. What is the end goal of practices aligned with these perspectives?
3. How can critical reflexivity support the goal of practices commensurate with critical perspectives?
4. Why is it important to include critical reflexivity within professional practices?
5. How can critical theoretical perspectives be integrated into occupational therapy education?

Notes
1 Throughout the chapter, the term occupation-based "practices" will be used to refer to the spectrum of professional education, practice, and research endeavors in occupational therapy and occupational science.
2 Michel Foucault's work on governmentality, as part of his broader work addressing the relations of power through which "truths" are constructed, examined the diverse social actors, inclusive of and beyond the State, implicated in the governance of everyday life. This work, extended by other governmentality scholars, attends to the discourses, technologies, and practices that shape how particular types of subjects come to understand their social positions and their possibilities for being and doing (Power & Polzer, 2016).
3 Paulo Freire was an educationalist who launched literacy programs among peasant people in Brazil in the 1960s. Freire believed that the marginalization of a certain group in society is produced by those in power with the aim of oppression and is perpetuated by the absence of reflective participation or "culture of silence" by those who are disempowered (Freire, 1970). To break this culture, he argued that people need to be empowered through "conscientization", i.e., encouraging individuals to transform their reality through dialogue, reflection, and action.
4 Jack Mezirow was an adult educator engaged in fostering democratic social action through community development. Mezirow's theory was introduced in 1978 and arose from a "disorienting dilemma" in his life. Personally, Mezirow was intrigued by witnessing his wife return to higher education in the context of the women's movement of the 1970s. His subsequent studies of women re-entering community colleges revealed that change in these women occurred, not only in gaining skills but a transformation in how they were thinking and the focus of their thinking.

References
Aldrich, R. M. (2015). Course redesign to promote local and global experiential learning about human occupation: Description and evaluation of a pilot effort. *South African Journal of Occupational Therapy, 45*(1), 56–62. http://doi.org/10.17159/2310-3833/2015/v45no1a10

Aldrich, R. M., & Grajo, L. C. (2017). International educational interactions and students' critical consciousness: A pilot study. *American Journal of Occupational Therapy, 71*(5), 7105230020p1–7105230020p10. https://doi.org/10.5014/ajot.2017.026724

Aldrich, R. M., & Peters, L. (2019). Using occupational justice as a "linchpin" of international educational collaborations. *American Journal of Occupational Therapy*, 73(3), 7303205100p1–7303205100p10. https://doi.org/10.5014/ajot.2019.029744

Aldrich, R. M., Rudman, D. L., Park, N. E., & Huot, S. (2020). Centering the complexity of long-term unemployment: Lessons learned from a critical occupational science inquiry. *Societies*, 10(3), 65. https://www.mdpi.com/2075-4698/10/3/65

American Occupational Therapy Association. (2020). Occupational therapy practice framework: Domain and process – 4th edition. *American Journal of Occupational Therapy*, 74(Supplement 2), 7412410010p7412410011–7412410010p7412410087. https://doi.org/10.5014/ajot.2020.74S2001

Beagan, B. L., Sibbald, K. R., Bizzeth, S. R., & Pride, T. M. (2022). Systemic racism in Canadian occupational therapy: A qualitative study with therapists. *Canadian Journal of Occupational Therapy*, 89(1), 51–61. https://doi.org/10.1177/00084174211066676

Benjamin-Thomas, T. E., Rudman, D. L., McGrath, C., Cameron, D., Abraham, V. J., Gunaseelan, J., & Vinothkumar, S. P. (2022). Situating occupational injustices experienced by children with disabilities in rural India within sociocultural, economic, and systemic conditions. *Journal of Occupational Science*, 29(1), 97–114. https://doi.org/10.1080/14427591.2021.1899038

Cloete, L. G., & Ramugondo, E. L. (2015). "I drink": Mothers' alcohol consumption as both individualised and imposed occupation. *South African Journal of Occupational Therapy*, 45(1), 34–40. http://www.scielo.org.za/scielo.php?script=sci_arttext&pid=S2310-38332015000100006&nrm=iso

Emery-Whittington, I. G. (2021). Occupational justice – colonial business as usual? Indigenous observations from Aotearoa New Zealand. *Canadian Journal of Occupational Therapy*, 88(2), 153–162. https://doi.org/10.1177/00084174211005891

Farias, L. (2020). The (mis)shaping of health: Problematizing neoliberal discourses of individualism and responsibility. In H. Hosseini, J. Goodman, S. C. Motta, & B. K. Gills (Eds.), *The Routledge handbook of transformative global studies* (pp. 268–281). Routledge.

Farias, L., & Aldrich, R. (2021). Critical theory: Resources for questioning and transforming everyday life. In S. Taff (Ed.), *Philosophy and occupational therapy: Informing education, research, and practice* (pp. 155–162). Slack.

Farias, L., & Laliberte Rudman, D. (2016). A critical interpretive synthesis of the uptake of critical perspectives in occupational science. *Journal of Occupational Science*, 23(1), 33–50. https://doi.org/10.1080/14427591.2014.989893

Farias, L., Laliberte Rudman, D., & Magalhães, L. (2016). Illustrating the importance of critical epistemology to realize the promise of occupational justice. *OTJR: Occupation, Participation and Health*, 36(4), 234–243. https://doi.org/10.1177%2F1539449216665561

Freire, P. (1970). *Pedagogy of the oppressed* (M. Bergman Ramos, Trans.). Continuum International Publishing Group.

Galvaan, R. (2012). *Critical teaching and learning methods*. Essay submitted for module in Teaching and Learning in Higher Education, University of Cape Town.

Galvaan, R. (2015). The contextually situated nature of occupational choice: Marginalized young adolescents' experiences in South Africa. *Journal of Occupational Science*, 22(1), 39–53. https://doi.org/10.1080/14427591.2014.912124

Galvaan, R. (2016). Embracing an occupational perspective to promoting learning in context. *South African Journal of Higher Education*, 29(3), 281–293. https://doi.org/10.20853/29-3-498

Gerlach, A., Teachman, G., Rudman, D., Huot, S., & Aldrich, R. (2018). Moving beyond individualism: Critical perspectives in occupation-focused research and practice. *Scandinavian Journal of Occupational Therapy*, 25(1), 35–43. https://doi.org/10.1080/11038128.2017.1327616

Kiepek, N. C., Beagan, B., Rudman, D. L., & Phelan, S. (2019). Silences around occupations framed as unhealthy, illegal, and deviant. *Journal of Occupational Science*, 26(3), 341–353. https://doi.org/10.1080/14427591.2018.1499123

Kinsella, E. A., & Whiteford, G. E. (2009). Knowledge generation and utilisation in occupational therapy: Towards epistemic reflexivity. *Australian Occupational Therapy Journal, 56*(4), 249–258. https://doi.org/10.1111/j.1440-1630.2007.00726.x

Laliberte Rudman, D. (2006). Positive aging and its implications for occupational possibilities in later life. *Canadian Journal of Occupational Therapy, 73*(3), 188–192. https://doi.org/10.1177/000841740607300305

Laliberte Rudman, D. (2017). The duty to age well: Critical reflections on occupational possibilities shaped through discursive and policy responses to population aging. In N. Pollard & D. Sakellariou (Eds.), *Occupational therapy without borders: Integrating justice with practice* (2nd ed., pp. 319–327). Elsevier.

Laliberte Rudman, D., Aldrich, R. M., & Kiepek, N. (2022). Evolving understandings of occupation. In M. Egan & G. Restall (Eds.), *Promoting occupational participation: Collaborative relationship-focused occupational therapy* (pp. 13–30). Canadian Association of Occupational Therapists.

Marx, K. (1996). *Das Kapital* (F. Engels, Ed.). Regnery Publishing.

Mezirow, J. (1991). *Transformative dimensions of adult learning*. Jossey-Bass.

Murthi, K., & Hammell, K. W. (2021). 'Choice' in occupational therapy theory: A critique from the situation of patriarchy in India. *Scandinavian Journal of Occupational Therapy, 28*(1), 1–12. https://doi.org/10.1080/11038128.2020.1769182

Ngcobo, S., Bourn, E., & Galvaan, R. (2018, May 21–25). Becoming an occupational therapist: *Critically thinking about who we are and what we bring in contexts of diversity* [Paper presentation]. World Federation of Occupational Therapists Congress, Cape Town, South Africa.

Nhunzvi, C., Galvaan, R., & Peters, L. (2019). Recovery from substance abuse among Zimbabwean men: An occupational transition. *OTJR: Occupation, Participation, and Health, 39*(1), 14–22. https://doi.org/10.1177/1539449217718503

Phelan, S. K. (2011). Constructions of disability: A call for critical reflexivity in occupational therapy. *Canadian Journal of Occupational Therapy, 78*(3), 164–172. https://doi.org/10.2182/cjot.2011.78.3.4

Power, E. M., & Polzer, J. (2016). *Neoliberal governance and health: Duties, risks, and vulnerabilities*. McGill-Queen's University Press.

Santos, B. d. S. (2014). *Epistemologies of the south: Justice against epistemicide*. Paradigm Publishers.

Shalem, Y., & Hoadley, U. (2009). The dual economy of schooling and teacher morale in South Africa. *International Studies in Sociology of Education, 19*(2), 119–134. https://doi.org/10.1080/09620210903257224

Simaan, J. (2020). Decolonising occupational science education through learning activities based on a study from the Global South. *Journal of Occupational Science, 27*(3), 432–442. https://doi.org/10.1080/14427591.2020.1780937

Teachman, G., McDonough, P., Macarthur, C., & Gibson, B. E. (2020). Interrogating inclusion with youths who use augmentative and alternative communication. *Sociology of Health & Illness, 42*(5), 1108–1122. https://doi.org/10.1111/1467-9566.13087

Trentham, B. L., & Neysmith, S. M. (2018). Exercising senior citizenship in an ageist society through participatory action research: A critical occupational perspective. *Journal of Occupational Science, 25*(2), 174–190. https://doi.org/10.1080/14427591.2017.1402809

CHAPTER 9

The Situated Nature of Human Occupation

Rebecca M. Aldrich, Lisette Farias, Roshan Galvaan, Debbie Laliberte Rudman, and Gail Teachman

Abstract
Arguments about human occupation have always acknowledged that context influences various dimensions of what people can do, are expected to do, and cannot do. Occupational science and occupational therapy literature published through the early 2000s particularly emphasized how immediate physical, social, and temporal environments shaped people's occupational engagements. In recent years, scholars have shown how consideration of broader conditions, such as social power relations, yields more fulsome explanations of how occupation is both shaped by *and* helps to (re)shape life contexts. These "situated" approaches have generated increasingly rich and complex knowledge about occupation's political, social, cultural, and historical embeddedness and significance. Through selected examples about cooking and food provisioning occupations, this chapter provokes critical reflexivity regarding evolving understandings about the situated nature of human occupation and how they can inform occupation-based practices from individual to systemic levels.

Authors' Positionality Statement
The information included within this chapter provides a non-exhaustive overview of ideas about the situated nature of human occupation. As authors of this chapter, our writing about the situated nature of occupation is informed by our research and positionalities. We have worked and lived in different global locations and contexts, including Canada, Chile/Sweden, South Africa, and the United States of America. We share collective (university-educated, professionally qualified, cisgendered, socioeconomically privileged) and individual (non-Western, Western, Amerindian/Latinx, White, Black, Spanish-speaker, English-speaker, able-bodied) positionalities as a group of authors. We recognize that a range of social, political, and cultural views of human occupation, including Westernized understandings that have become predominant through historical processes of colonization, influence our thinking and writing. In drafting this chapter, we have made a concerted effort to include material that embraces a diverse

range of perspectives; however, we acknowledge that this chapter's contents cannot be completely bias free or representative of every cultural, racial, gender, economic, political, or social reality. Still, we hope that this material will promote critical, inclusive, and respectful learning and dialogue among readers.

> **Objectives**
> This chapter will allow the reader to:
>
> - Describe how "the situated nature of human occupation" extends knowledge about relationships among people, occupations, and contexts.
> - Explain how particular epistemological movements and values, such as pluralism, postmodernism, and decoloniality, inform understandings about the situated nature of human occupation.
> - Apply understandings about the situated nature of human occupation to an example.
> - Discuss how embracing the situated nature of occupation opens new opportunities for occupation-based practices.

> **Key terms**
> - context
> - situation
> - occupational possibilities
> - occupational consciousness
> - occupational choice
> - dialectical
> - postmodern
> - decolonial

9.1 Introduction

Occupational therapists and occupational scientists have long considered how immediate physical and social environments afford or constrain individual engagement in occupation. For example, when addressing the occupation of cooking, scholars and practitioners have acknowledged that people choose and prepare meals based on what food and tools are available, as well as what cuisines are familiar within people's families, communities, or cultures. These ideas primarily evidence a unidirectional focus regarding contextual influences on occupation, i.e., they highlight how material conditions or connections with others shape what people do and how they do it. Although this focus has helped present occupation as a complex phenomenon, it does not fully explain the relationships among occupation and context. Since the early 2000s, scholarly inquiries about power relations and social structures have enriched accounts of occupation, showing how context shapes occupation *and* occupation shapes context. Returning to the example of cooking, more nuanced understandings of this occupation might explore the root causes of why some people have a wider array of cooking options and supports as compared to others; how social expectations dictate who can or should cook; and how cooking not only facilitates survival and identity expression but can also reinforce historical trauma or change people's positions and statuses in society. By adopting ideas that emphasize the multifaceted "situated" nature of occupation, occupational scientists and occupational therapists can explain occupation's role in creating and perpetuating situations of oppression and also explore its potential to help foster more equitable conditions for all people.

The chapter begins with an overview of selected terminology and ideas about relationships among people, occupations, and life contexts. The discussion then highlights how various approaches to knowledge and related value propositions have informed understandings about the situated nature of occupation. The chapter ends by inviting readers to explore how embracing the situated nature of human occupation can (re)shape occupation-based practices.

9.2 Setting the Stage
9.2.1 Defining and Representing the Interrelations of Person, Occupation, and Context

As a foundation for understanding the situated nature of human occupation, it is important to review how the terms "person", "environment", and "context" have been defined, conceptualized, and related to each other in occupational therapy frameworks and models. As one example, the fourth edition of the American Occupational Therapy Association's (AOTA, 2020) *Occupational Therapy Practice Framework: Domain and Process* (OTPF-4) uses "context" as an umbrella term to refer to "the complete makeup of a person's life as well as the common and divergent factors that characterize groups and populations" (p. 76). In the OTPF-4, "context" is inclusive of "environmental" and "personal" factors, with "environmental" factors encompassing "physical, social, and attitudinal surroundings" (p. 35) and "personal" factors encompassing "unique features of the person that are not part of a health condition or health state" (p. 39). The OTPF-4 separates "context" from "performance patterns" (i.e., clients' habits, roles, routines, and rituals) and "client factors" (i.e., clients' values and beliefs as well as body structures and functions), thus setting many client-level phenomena apart from contextual factors.

The segmentation of human and contextual factors permeates many models that guide occupational therapy practice, including the *Canadian Model of Occupational Performance and Engagement* and the *Model of Human Occupation* (Hammell, 2020a). Separating the components of conceptual models and frameworks has a practical function: it can help identify and draw attention to the range of factors that warrant consideration and analysis. However, representing components as distinct in frameworks and models also risks implying that those components exist apart from each other in reality. Frameworks and models that represent components may discretely, in turn, foster practices that address components sequentially or in isolation. Such a practice approach can be problematic because phenomena in everyday life are not so neatly separable (Dickie et al., 2006). For example, attempting to modify a client's cooking-related habits, roles, routines, rituals, values, or beliefs in isolation of familial, cultural, or societal expectations or economic conditions can lead to occupation-based practices that are not adopted, unsustainable, irrelevant, oppressive, or prevent the use of cooking as a means to negotiate cultural values, express identities, or create relationships with others.

Apart from navigating representational challenges, occupational therapy conceptual frameworks and models must contend with the constraints of written language. English-language occupational therapy and occupational science literature often presents the terms "context" and "environment" as interchangeable (Johnson & Dickie, 2019), reflecting colloquial use of the terms as synonyms. However, these terms have different definitions, with "context" primarily referring to broader situational elements or conditions (Cambridge Dictionary, n.d.a) and "environment" primarily referring to concrete aspects of the natural world (Cambridge Dictionary, n.d.b). As with artificially separating human and contextual factors in conceptual frameworks and models, using terminology interchangeably carries implications: conflating "context" with "environment" can gloss over important sociopolitical and historical influences and narrow attention to the physical, immediate micro-level of interaction(s). The terms "contextualized" and "situated" are likewise interchanged in scholarship on occupation, with similar vagueness resulting from using these terms as synonyms.

In an effort to make clear arguments in this chapter, and recognizing the complexities of representation and limitations of semantics, we use "context" to encompass the physical, spatial, geographic, temporal, historical, social, cultural, relational, institutional, and political conditions through which people live their lives. Consistent with interpretations of John Dewey's transactional perspective in both occupational science and grounded theory writings (Aldrich & Laliberte Rudman, 2016), we use the term "situation" to reference particular instances of dynamic relationships among human and contextual elements in the world, with the term "situated" acknowledging that occupation is always implicated in those dynamic relationships.

9.3 Evolving Ideas about "Occupation in Context" and "Occupation as Situated"

9.3.1 Occupation "in" Context: Reinforcing Distinctions between People and Environment

Conceiving of occupation as a "situated" phenomenon requires seeing occupation within the complex, multi-layered whole of relations that make up daily life. How is this different from understanding occupation as occurring "in context"? Historically, understandings about occupation and context were based on ideas that foregrounded human agency and emphasized humans' drive for control and mastery over the environment (Hocking, 2021). Such ideas about occupation and context reflect a stance of individualism, which sees each person as enacting occupations in unique ways and bearing personal responsibility for successes and challenges separate from contextual influences (Gerlach et al., 2018; Hammell, 2020a). Individualistic understandings prioritize the influence of a person's motivation, roles, or (ill)health condition on occupational performance or experiences. For example, when encountering clients whose circumstances necessitate changes to cooking approaches, occupational therapists who draw on an individualistic perspective may try to ascertain how clients' different physical, social, cultural, and geographic contexts allow or restrict the clients' participation and engagement in cooking. Occupational therapy professionals may look at clients' histories to understand how events over time led clients to value cooking; what contextual elements need to be adapted to facilitate clients' re-engagement in cooking; or what alternative occupations may have similar functions and value to clients if re-engagement in cooking is deemed not possible. This approach reflects a view of occupation occurring *in* context, facilitating separate, if parallel, analyses of client and contextual factors that prioritize clients' control in reshaping their engagement in cooking.

However, occupational therapists and occupational scientists have begun to recognize limitations associated with this approach. As noted in the previous section of this chapter, the reality (ontology) of the world is messy, and that "messiness" must be accounted for in the foundations of occupation-based practices. As a starting point, scholars have suggested rebalancing the relative level of influence attributed to individual and contextual factors when considering how occupation is shaped. For instance, Galvaan (2015) drew on Pierre Bourdieu's sociological theory to explain how occupational choice is influenced by contextual conditions related to social position and status. This conceptualization of occupational choice illuminated how the value attributed to different social positions within societies sets conditions that facilitate or limit which occupational choices people can and do make.

Galvaan's (2015) approach departed from earlier individualistic constructions of choice as primarily a product of self-interest, volition, motivation, roles, or personal skills, instead showing how occupational choice is situated relative to economic, social, historical, and political contextual conditions. Galvaan's research also illustrated how occupations contribute to contexts, showing how engagement in occupation can either resist or reinforce existing conditions in people's lives. Applied to the example of a client whose engagement in cooking is altered, perspectives like Galvaan's (2015) opens up possibilities for occupational therapists to consider how changes in a client's cooking necessarily influence that client's contexts, given the situatedness of occupations. For example, changes in a client's cooking can reshape familial expectations about who is responsible for cooking and how cooking should occur.

9.3.2 Another Approach: Emphasizing Relations among People, Occupations, and Contexts

Rather than viewing occupation as something that happens *in* a context that is fundamentally distinct from human beings (Cutchin, 2004), contemporary scholarship has moved toward illustrating the multiple influences that link people, occupations, and life contexts. Scholars have begun to embrace theoretical perspectives that frame people, occupation, and context as mutually constitutive – that is, as being what they are only because of their relationships with each other (Aldrich, 2008; Hermosilla & Valderrama, 2022). Drawing on such perspectives has helped redirect focus beyond separate personal and environmental influences on occupation, instead emphasizing relations among situational elements wherein each element is inextricably linked to and shapes other elements. This relational focus has helped occupational therapists and occupational scientists generate new frameworks and models that foreground relations among humans, contexts, and occupations, such as Fisher and Marterella's (2019) *Transactional Model of Occupation*. This relational focus has also provided new entry points for occupational therapists and occupational scientists to explore why many people do not have the power to change problematic elements of their contexts; why adapting to problematic contextual elements might not be a feasible goal;

and how contextual conditions shape differential possibilities for occupation (Gerlach et al., 2018; Hocking, 2021).

Embracing a more relational perspective allows occupation to be understood as "occur[ring] at the level of the situation" (Johnson & Dickie, 2019, p. 305) and as always involving relations between human and non-human elements (Aldrich & Laliberte Rudman, 2016). As such, seeing occupation as a "situated" phenomenon shifts away from oversimplified understandings of the relation among people, occupations, and contexts, instead viewing them as a dialectical, i.e., as intimately interconnected and interdependent within an ongoing dynamic transaction (Hammell, 2020a; Laliberte Rudman & Huot, 2013). Understanding occupation as a situated phenomenon brings attention to *how* situational relationships unfold through people's engagement in occupations (Madsen & Josephsson, 2017).

9.3.3 Adding Depth to Relational Understandings through a Focus on Systems of Power

To deepen understandings about the interconnectedness and interdependence of people, occupations, and contexts, scholars have drawn on critical social perspectives to explain the active, negotiated relationships that "situate" occupation within broader conditions and power relations (Farias & Laliberte Rudman, 2019; Galvaan, 2021; Laliberte Rudman & Huot, 2013). Such work has led to the generation of new concepts such as occupational possibilities (Laliberte Rudman, 2010) and occupational consciousness (Ramugondo, 2015), which have raised awareness of the dialectical transactions of individual and collective doing, historical context, and power relations. For example, occupational possibilities (Laliberte Rudman, 2010; Laliberte Rudman & Huot, 2013) describe how social systems and structures promote certain types of doing as ideal and possible for particular people and groups, while simultaneously framing other occupations as non-ideal or not possible. In a similar vein, occupational consciousness (Ramugondo, 2015) describes how ways of engaging in occupation can mirror and sustain societal norms and practices, including dominant practices of coloniality that sustain oppression. By highlighting how dominant practices become dominant, the concept of occupational consciousness draws attention to the doing of all persons involved in oppressive power relations, showing the ways people internalize and normalize situated preferences, as well as how individual and collective "doings" can resist or challenge dominant practices of coloniality that sustain oppression.

Based on these deeper understandings about how social positions, resources, power relations, and occupations reciprocally shape each other, scholars have emphasized the importance of politicizing occupation (Laliberte Rudman, 2018). Politicizing occupation raises awareness of how human doing is relational and affects other people's possibilities for doing, being, becoming, and belonging. Taking a political approach to occupation has helped occupational scientists and occupational therapists extend beyond viewing occupation as an objective, neutral action that is largely self-determined; instead, scholars and practitioners have attended to the ways in which people's occupations can hinder, force, or marginalize others' ways of being or doing, identifying occupation as a potential mechanism of deprivation, alienation, marginalisation, social control, and imbalance (Nilsson & Townsend, 2010).

By paying attention to the role of occupation in producing injustices, scholars and practitioners have opened paths for addressing and transforming the mechanisms through which power stigmatizes and/or marginalizes individual and community doing. This politicization of occupation can inform "situated" practices aimed at transforming sociopolitical systems and structures to create more occupationally just conditions. As one example, colonization practices have long sought to erase Indigenous food practices and relations to land in many nations, with enduring effects on emotional, spiritual, and physical health and wellbeing (Cote, 2016). A recognition of how food practices, including cooking, are sites for the reproduction of oppressive power relations can be the foundation for enacting occupational therapy in ways that support access to traditional foods and work with communities to revitalize Indigenous food practices (Fijal & Beagan, 2019).

9.4 Expanding Understandings of Occupation as Situated
9.4.1 Ontological and Epistemological Underpinnings

Shifting toward understanding occupation as "situated" requires more than adding consideration of broader contextual elements (Galvaan, 2021; Laliberte Rudman, 2018). At a fundamental level, it involves re-examining the assumptions that have underpinned how occupation has been conceptualized, studied, and used in practices (Farias & Laliberte Rudman, 2019; Gerlach et al., 2018). Ontological and epistemological assumptions – i.e., assumptions about the reality of a phenomenon, what can be known about a phenomenon, and what forms of knowledge about a phenomenon are valuable – set boundaries on how occupation comes to be understood (Aldrich et al., 2021; Farias & Aldrich, 2021). Put another way, the beliefs that people hold about what is "real", what "counts" as knowledge, and how knowledge is best generated, shape what can be learned about occupation.

For much of their existence, occupational therapy and occupational science have been shaped by positivist and post-positivist epistemological approaches. These approaches assert that truths exist in the world as universal facts and can be identified and understood through linear processes of observation and experimentation. Combined with the dominance of Eurocentric perspectives, which give priority to the experiences and ideas of cultures originating in Western European countries, the historical emphasis on positivism and post-positivism in occupational therapy and occupational science led to a search for universal, objectively measurable, and static features of occupation, often resulting in understandings that were de-contextualized, dualistic, reductionistic, and ethnocentric (Gerlach et al., 2018; Laliberte Rudman, 2018). As articulated by Farias and Aldrich (2021), understandings that frame "occupation as solely the product of human action, giving primacy to individuals' abilities to engage in occupations, and neglecting contextual factors that shape occupational experiences" (p. 158) align with, privilege, and impose Western, Anglophonic perspectives. Although such framings can be useful and relevant to particular circumstances, they do not fully represent the nuance and complexity of occupation as it is manifested and experienced around the world.

Several non-positivistic approaches have been drawn on to enhance understandings of occupation as "situated". For example, postmodern theory, which is grounded in ideas that knowledge is always situated, partial, and dynamic, has opened the door to pluralism in scholarship on occupation, rejecting the search for universal truths and embracing different ways of doing, being, becoming, and knowing. Informed by theorists such as Foucault and Deleuze, postmodern perspectives can inform ongoing critical reflexivity regarding what is taken-for-granted and spoken or written as "truths" about occupation, helping to unpack the situatedness of occupation and celebrate diverse understandings of how occupation is experienced, negotiated, and enacted through contexts (Aldrich et al., 2021).

Similar to postmodern approaches, critical perspectives (also known as critical social theory or a critical paradigm) have been drawn on to highlight how what is taken-for-granted as the reality of occupation is itself shaped through power relations over time. As described more fully in Chapter 8, critical perspectives illuminate how dominant knowledge privileges the experiences, views, and needs of particular groups in society while marginalizing others. Critical scholars such as Habermas, Freire, and Tuhiwai Smith have asserted that knowledge is inherently contextual and therefore always tied to values and power relations. As such, the theories created by these scholars have provided a basis to question and transform contextually situated power relations that privilege certain ways of understanding occupation, ultimately advancing knowledge about occupation's diverse expressions (Farias & Aldrich, 2021; Laliberte Rudman, 2018).

Embracing additional epistemologies (knowledges) and ontologies (realities) to situate human occupation can also facilitate transformative action. Mobilizing change in people's capabilities to access and engage in occupations requires shifting societal systems and structures. Decolonial perspectives, which provide an alternate approach to dominant Eurocentric perspectives, offer one avenue for initiating such shifts. Decolonial perspectives recognize that coloniality of power came to exist through "racial social classification of the world population under Eurocentered world power" (Quijano, 2007, p. 171). This coloniality persists through the invisible but exclusionary systemic forms of knowing, doing, and being that remain evident in occupations. In this ongoing coloniality, White supremacist racial and capitalist hierarchies persist in setting standards for what is valued. These standards divide humans, exploiting differences, and creating competition for the purposes of control over protecting capitalist and colonial ideals.

Colonial standards embedded in education, information, and economic systems capture the minds of colonized persons (Asante, 2006), thus maintaining coloniality. In turn, this contributes to the silencing and exclusion of Indigenous, anti-racist, and transformative discourses and practices in disciplines such as occupational science and the profession of occupational therapy (Emery-Whittington, 2021). Perspectives rooted in coloniality advance false binaries between knowledge and practice, govern what counts as knowledge, often reinforcing hierarchies about what is studied, who contributes to knowledge generation, and how this occurs. To decolonize means to break with such patterns, or as Mignolo (2007) put it, to delink. Delinking from and disrupting patterns of coloniality occurs by dismantling power relations and knowledges that reproduce race, gender, and geopolitical hierarchies in the modern, colonial world (Maldonado-Torres, 2017). Delinking further involves conceptual and practice shifts to ways of knowing, doing, and being that have been framed as struggles toward generative disruption (Galvaan, 2021). Through authentic dialogic engagements that foreground the voices and experiences of oppressed people, generative disruption contributes to beginnings from which diverse possibilities can emerge.

9.5 Putting Understandings into Practice

9.5.1 Exemplifying the Situated Nature of Human Occupation

Thus far, this chapter has addressed what it means to see occupation as a situated phenomenon and how situated understandings arose through broader movements away from Eurocentric individualism and positivism toward epistemic pluralism, postmodernism, and decolonization. To culminate this discussion, we offer an example to help readers envision possibilities that stem from seeing occupation as a situated phenomenon. The example focuses on one type of occupational engagement – food provisioning – during the COVID-19 pandemic that began in 2020 and was ongoing as much of this chapter was being drafted. As a background to the example, the next paragraph provides a brief overview of how the COVID-19 pandemic intersected with broader inequities and calls for change in occupational science and occupational therapy.

Long before the COVID-19 pandemic emerged, the inequitable impacts of pandemics on marginalized social groups were recognized as a public health concern (Blumenshine et al., 2008). As the COVID-19 pandemic unfolded and its inequitable impacts became increasingly severe, there was also increased conscientization of the need to eradicate systemic racism, led by the Black Lives Matters movement in response to the deaths of multiple Black people at the hands of United States police officers. Early calls to focus occupation-based practices on the COVID-19 pandemic recognized the need to attend to issues of inequity and marginalization (Hammell, 2020b). Bolstered by the increased attention to systemic racism, many international occupational therapy and occupational science associations pledged their commitment to working toward a more equitable status quo.

Scholars probed the Eurocentric knowledge foundations of occupational science and occupational therapy, recognizing how assumptions associated with White supremacy undermined diverse understandings and limited possibilities for change. Resonating with decolonial perspectives, these contestations and calls to eradicate systemic forms of racial discrimination placed accountability on individuals, collectives, and institutions to change discriminatory policies and dismantle racist power structures (Galvaan & van der Merwe, 2021).

9.5.2 Example

Food provisioning is a complex and often invisible occupation that requires strategic planning and expert use of skills, especially for people who have limited financial resources (Beagan et al., 2018). At the outset of the COVID-19 pandemic, when many governments instituted stay-at-home orders to manage the evolving public health crisis, people had to change how they secured food for themselves, their families, and their communities. Persons with limited income who already experienced food insecurity could not access commonly used cheap local food markets and street vendors. Children who would have had access to school meals were also left in need. Many people had to rely on charity or scarce government or non-profit organization-issued food parcels for survival, while people with some finances had to purchase food from more expensive supermarkets. Rather than go to grocery stores, markets, and restaurants, some people were able to utilize grocery and restaurant delivery applications on their mobile phones or computers.

However, such "choices" and options were not equitably distributed; for example, people without financial resources, with limited digital literacy, with homes in remote locations, or without reliable access to home internet or mobile data plans could not easily adapt their food provisioning occupations in this way. In some contexts, grocery delivery options were simply non-existent or too expensive. This meant that people risked breaking the stay-at-home orders to access food. People who relied on community resources such as food pantries were further disadvantaged by stay-at-home orders that limited their abilities to access such resources in person.

In recognition of these inequitable impacts of COVID-19 stay-at-home orders, communities, institutions, and governments developed several solutions to support access to food resources. At the neighborhood level, community members created grassroots food pantries and collection points at local stores and organizations, and social media networks were used to spread the word about available resources to non-internet-connected people. At the institutional level, non-profit organizations coordinated volunteers to pack and deliver meal kits or prepared meals to unhoused persons, people in need, and people residing in remote or under-resourced communities.

At the governmental level, municipal and federal governments authorized emergency funds to bolster food subsidies for people with limited financial resources, although such subsidies were inadequate in some countries and did not always reach the intended beneficiaries. At first glance, these solutions all appeared to address the food provisioning problems brought on and intensified by the COVID-19 pandemic; however, they did not reflect a situated understanding of the occupation of food provisioning. Food provisioning does not simply involve accessing food in particular contexts: it entails working through situational affordances and constraints that shape people's abilities to gather foods that meet nutritional and cultural needs, and can be prepared using existing tools and capacities.

The grassroots food pantries and delivered meal kits described above offered solutions to the problem of food access, but the types of food donated or delivered might not have met individual or collective needs, or aligned with the tools and knowledge that recipients used to prepare food. Expanded governmental food subsidies may have provided some relief or increased individual and family resources for acquiring food, but they did not address larger infrastructural issues that limited some people and communities from ordering groceries through websites or mobile phone applications and did not increase overall food security. Moreover, these kinds of solutions for food provisioning challenges in the early months of the COVID-19 pandemic did not address the broader power relations that have long fueled inequitable impacts on this occupation for different groups in society.

Understanding food provisioning as a situated occupation provides opportunities to reimagine solutions that address the dynamic, interrelated elements that differentially shaped everyday life for various communities prior to and at the onset of the COVID-19 pandemic. Such reimagining can be guided by the following questions:

1. What relationships among people, their occupations, and everyday life contexts are salient when considering how to support food provisioning?
2. How might interpretations of food provisioning as a situated occupation influence the actions occupational therapists and occupational scientists take at individual, community, and societal levels to address current and future food insecurity needs?

Preliminary answers to these questions highlight a broader array of factors that can be considered. For example, a situated approach to food provisioning might recognize that people need transportation resources to access the variety of foods, food vendors, and community organizations that provide nutritional and culturally relevant ingredients for meals that people can prepare given their circumstances. A decolonizing approach to food provisioning would further aid occupational therapists in supporting ongoing critical reflexivity about what types of foods and food practices they assume to be "healthy", "appropriate", and "culturally necessary", opening up space to engage with and support diverse ways of food provisioning. Respecting Indigenous knowledge and local expertize in how best to provide food might involve, for example, paying attention to the energy requirements for preparing different meals or working with communities to inform organizations about meals that are preferred or could assist with meeting family, cultural, and community commitments. Likewise, considering religious beliefs that shape which ingredients are permissible to use and how to prepare meals would help inform both direct food provision and broader plans and policies to support food provision.

Thus, taking a situated approach to food provisioning opens possibilities for moving beyond a focus on an individual's food preparation abilities and completion of kitchen assessments to considering how diverse contextual elements, such as neighborhood characteristics, family situations, loss of significant others, and various types of accessibility issues shape meanings and opportunities for this occupation. Occupational therapists addressing food provisioning in the context of a public health crisis could work with communities to mobilize people to collectively use limited available resources and strategize about increasing food access. This could involve forming alliances and networks within communities and among organizations and institutions, e.g., negotiating for local community members to use local school facilities to cook for their communities.

Occupational therapists could also contribute to social movements and organizations that agitate for policy shifts to advance food security; for example, by promoting access to sustainable food production beyond the end of a pandemic. Recognizing supply chain disruptions, rising fuel prices, and changes to public transportation schedules as important contextual influences on the occupation of food provisioning facilitates more considered solutions, such as pairing food subsidies with transportation supports or working with community groups to organize shared "grocery runs" for local neighborhood communities. Building on situated understandings in this way creates opportunities to not only respond to emergent needs but create solutions that redress inequitable contextual conditions and pave the way for social transformation.

9.6 Conclusion

This chapter has addressed how situated understandings of occupation extend beyond ideas about occupation occurring in context, bolstered by pluralistic, postmodern, and decolonizing approaches. Through an explanation of evolving terminology and epistemologies, this chapter has described various approaches to situating occupation in the dynamic relations of the world. Drawing on an example exploring needs for food provisioning during the COVID-19 pandemic, this chapter illustrated how embracing the situated nature of human occupation facilitated more opportunities for practicing in ways that pursued equity and social transformation.

9.7 Summary

- Occupational engagement is a negotiated process shaped by reciprocal relations of human, non-human, and contextual situational elements.
- Seeing occupation as a situated phenomenon requires questioning dominant assumptions that separate individual influences from contextual influences.
- Epistemological movements that disrupt positivism, such as pluralism, postmodernism, and decoloniality, can help enhance situated understandings of occupation.
- Seeing occupation as a situated phenomenon provides grounding for occupation-based practices that aim to promote equity and transformation.

9.8 Review Questions

1. What does it mean to say that human occupation is "situated", and how does this differ from saying that occupation occurs "in context"?
2. Why is it important to understand occupation as a situated phenomenon?
3. How do epistemological movements, like positivism or postmodernism, shape how and what we know about occupation as a situated phenomenon?
4. How might understanding occupation as "situated" influence considerations and approaches taken in occupational therapy practices?
5. What is the connection between seeing occupation as "situated" and engaging in practices that support equity and transformation?

References

Aldrich, R. M. (2008). From complexity theory to transactionalism: Moving occupational science forward in theorizing the complexities of behavior. *Journal of Occupational Science, 15*(3), 147–156. https://doi.org/10.1080/14427591.2008.9686624

Aldrich, R. M., & Laliberte Rudman, D. (2016). Situational analysis: A visual analytic approach that unpacks the complexity of occupation. *Journal of Occupational Science, 23*(1), 51–66. https://doi.org/10.1080/14427591.2015.1045014

Aldrich, R. M., Laliberte Rudman, D., & Bonsall, A. (2021). Postmodernism: Foundations for problematizing and reimagining conditions of possibility. In S. D. Taff (Ed.), *Philosophy and occupational therapy: Informing education, research, and practice* (pp. 201–207). Slack.

American Occupational Therapy Association (AOTA). (2020). Occupational therapy practice framework: Domain and process – 4th edition. *American Journal of Occupational Therapy, 74*(Supplement 2), 7412410010p7412410011–7412410010p7412410087. https://doi.org/10.5014/ajot.2020.74S2001

Asante, M. (2006). Foreword. In G. J. Sefa Dei & A. Kempf (Eds.), *Anti-colonialism and education: The politics of resistance* (pp. ix–x). Sense Publishers.

Beagan, B. L., Chapman, G. E., & Power, E. (2018). The visible and invisible occupations of food provisioning in low income families. *Journal of Occupational Science, 25*(1), 100–111. https://doi.org/10.1080/14427591.2017.1338192

Blumenshine, P., Reingold, A., Egerter, S., Mockenhaupt, R., Braveman, P., & Marks, J. (2008). Pandemic influenza planning in the United States from a health disparities perspective. *Emerging Infectious Diseases, 14*(5), 709–715. https://doi.org/10.3201/eid1405.071301

Cambridge Dictionary. (n.d.a). Context. https://dictionary.cambridge.org/dictionary/english/context

Cambridge Dictionary. (n.d.b). Environment. https://dictionary.cambridge.org/dictionary/english/environment

Cote, C. (2016). 'Indigenizing' food sovereignty. Revitalizing Indigenous food practices and ecological knowledges in Canada and the United States. *Humanities, 5*(3), 57–71. https://doi.org/10.3390/h5030057

Cutchin, M. P. (2004). A Deweyan case for the study of uncertainty in health geography. *Health & Place*, 10(3), 203–213. https://doi.org/10.1016/j.healthplace.2003.06.001

Dickie, V., Cutchin, M. P., & Humphry, R. (2006). Occupation as transactional experience: A critique of individualism in occupational science. *Journal of Occupational Science*, 13(1), 83–93. https://doi.org/10.1080/14427591.2006.9686573

Emery-Whittington, I. G. (2021). Occupational justice—Colonial business as usual? Indigenous observations from Aotearoa New Zealand. *Canadian Journal of Occupational Therapy*, 88(2), 153–162. https://doi.org/10.1177/00084174211005891

Farias, L., & Aldrich, R. M. (2021). Critical theory: Resources for questioning and transforming everyday life. In S. D. Taff (Ed.), *Philosophy and occupational therapy: Informing education, research, and practice* (pp. 155–162). Slack.

Farias, L., & Laliberte Rudman, D. (2019). Practice analysis: Critical reflexivity on discourses constraining socially transformative occupational therapy practices. *British Journal of Occupational Therapy*, 82(11), 693–697. https://doi.org/10.1177/0308022619862111

Fijal, D., & Beagan, B. L. (2019). Indigenous perspectives on health: Integration with a Canadian model of practice. *Canadian Journal of Occupational Therapy*, 86(3), 220–231. https://doi.org/10.1177/0008417419832284

Fisher, A. G., & Marterella, A. (2019). *Powerful practice: A model for authentic occupational therapy*. Center for Innovative OT Solutions.

Galvaan, R. (2015). The contextually situated nature of occupational choice: Marginalised young adolescents' experiences in South Africa. *Journal of Occupational Science*, 22(1), 39–53. https://doi.org/10.1080/14427591.2014.912124

Galvaan, R. (2021). Generative disruption through occupational science: Enacting possibilities for deep human connection. *Journal of Occupational Science*, 28(1), 6–18. https://doi.org/10.1080/14427591.2020.1818276

Galvaan, R., & van der Merwe, T. R. (2021). Re-orienting occupational therapy: Embracing generative disruption and revisiting a posture that acknowledges human dignity. *South African Journal of Occupational Therapy*, 51(2), 99–103. https://scielo.org.za/scielo.php?script=sci_abstract&pid=S2310-38332021000200013

Gerlach, A., Teachman, G., Laliberte Rudman, D., Aldrich, R. M., & Huot, S. (2018). Expanding beyond individualism: Engaging critical perspectives on occupation. *Scandinavian Journal of Occupational Therapy*, 25(1), 35–43. https://doi.org/10.1080/11038128.2017.1327616

Hammell, K. W. (2020a). *Engagement in living: Critical perspectives on occupation, rights and well-being*. Canadian Association of Occupational Therapists.

Hammell, K. W. (2020b). Engagement in living during the COVID-19 pandemic and ensuing occupational disruption. *OT Now*, 22(4), 7–8. https://www.wfot.org/assets/resources/Hammell-ENGAGEMENT-IN-LIVING-DURING-THE-COVID-19-PANDEMIC-AND-ENSUING-OCCUPATIONAL-DISRUPTION1.pdf

Hermosilla, A., & Valderrama, C. (2022). Collective occupations and nature: Impacts of the coloniality of nature on rural and fishing communities in Chile. *Journal of Occupational Science*, 29(2), 252–262. https://doi.org/10.1080/14427591.2021.1880264

Hocking, C. (2021). Occupation in context: A reflection on environmental influences on human doing. *Journal of Occupational Science*, 28(2), 221–234. https://doi.org/10.1080/14427591.2019.1708434

Johnson, K. R., & Dickie, V. (2019). What is occupation? In B. A. B. Schell & G. Gillen (Eds.), *Willard and Spackman's occupational therapy* (13th ed., pp. 320–330). Wolters Kluwer.

Laliberte Rudman, D. (2010). Occupational terminology. *Journal of Occupational Science*, 17(1), 55–59. https://doi.org/10.1080/14427591.2010.9686673

Laliberte Rudman, D. (2018). Occupational therapy and occupational science: Building critical and transformative alliances. *Cadernos Brasileiros de Terapia Ocupacional*, 26(1), 241–249. http://dx.doi.org/10.4322/2526-8910.ctoEN1246

Laliberte Rudman, D., & Huot, S. (2013). Conceptual insights for expanding thinking regarding the situated nature of occupation. In M. P. Cutchin & V. A. Dickie

(Eds.), *Transactional perspectives on occupation* (pp. 51–63). Springer. https://doi.org/10.1007/978-94-007-4429-5_5

Madsen, J., & Josephsson, S. (2017). Engagement in occupation as an inquiring process: Exploring the situatedness of occupation. *Journal of Occupational Science, 24*(4), 412–424. https://doi.org/10.1080/14427591.2017.1308266

Maldonado-Torres, N. (2017). On the coloniality of human rights. *Revista Crítica de Ciências Sociais, 114*, 117–136. https://doi.org/10.4000/rccs.6793

Mignolo, W. (2007). Delinking: The rhetoric of modernity, the logic of coloniality and the grammar of de-coloniality. *Cultural Studies, 21*(2–3), 449–514. https://doi.org/10.1080/09502380601162647

Nilsson, I., & Townsend, E. (2010). Occupational justice-bridging theory and practice. *Scandinavian Journal of Occupational Therapy, 17*(1), 57–63. https://doi.org/10.3109/11038120903287182

Quijano, A. (2007). Coloniality and modernity/rationality. *Cultural Studies, 21*(2–3), 168–178. https://doi.org/10.1080/09502380601164353

Ramugondo, E. L. (2015). Occupational consciousness. *Journal of Occupational Science, 22*(4), 488–501. https://doi.org/10.1080/14427591.2015.1042516

CHAPTER 10

Equity, Disadvantage, Justice, and Human Occupation

Sharon Gutman

Abstract
This chapter examines the ways in which societal inequity, disadvantage, poverty, and minority intersect to prevent people from full and desired occupational participation. The chapter explores how societal structures that preserve racial, ethnic, and gender injustices impact occupational participation throughout all developmental stages from childhood to late adulthood. Health care professionals, including occupational therapists, must understand the ways in which disadvantage and poverty have adversely impacted the lives of patients and clients to facilitate their desired function and community participation.

Authors' Positionality Statement: See Chapter 1, Section 1.9

Objectives
This chapter will allow the reader to:

- Understand the terms inequity, disadvantage, social injustice, and occupational injustice as they relate to occupation and occupational participation.
- Understand how systemic racism has been embedded into the culture of Western society and has barriered the equal occupational participation of minority groups over centuries.
- Understand how inequity and poverty adversely impact the occupational participation of people throughout the lifespan – childhood, adolescence, adulthood, and late adulthood.
- Understand the meaning of intersectionality and how those affected by it experience heightened forms of discrimination that obstruct desired occupational participation.

> **Key terms**
> - inequity
> - social injustice
> - occupational injustice
> - critical race theory
> - intersectionality

10.1 Introduction

Inequity, disadvantage, and social and occupational injustices adversely impact people's ability to participate in desired, meaningful daily life activities, or occupations. Equity means that all people in a society are fairly included and have equal access to the same opportunities and environmental conditions that facilitate personal growth, educational attainment, health care, safe housing, and employment opportunities. In an equitable society, all people – regardless of race, ethnicity, gender orientation, sex, religion, age, socioeconomic status, and disability – are ensured equal conditions under which to reach their full potential and participate in society in meaningful and desired ways.

Inequity is the unfair and unequal treatment of certain societal groups with the intent to marginalize or exclude them from societal participation and prevent the attainment of resources (e.g., education, health care, safe housing, and livable wage employment) needed to prosper and secure higher socioeconomic status. Social injustice is the act of denying the same rights, civil liberties, and societal opportunities ensured for certain people, to groups that have been marginalized by the larger society. Social injustices are commonly committed by groups in power to maintain their status (and the privileges associated with status) while preventing others in lower, less influential societal positions from attaining resources to prosper. Governments, political groups, religious organizations, large and wealthy corporations, and socioeconomically privileged groups often knowingly and unwittingly commit acts of social injustice to maintain their power and prevent marginalized groups from reaching higher socioeconomic status. Examples of historical and present social injustices include slavery; removing Native/Indigenous peoples from their land and excluding them from societal participation; underfunding educational systems in low socioeconomic areas; incarcerating higher percentages of minority groups; denying voting rights for people of color or creating obstacles that make voting inaccessible; preventing access to or creating barriers to the attainment of livable wage employment; and preventing same-sex couples from having the same legal rights as heterosexual partners (Lavalley & Johnson, 2022).

Occupational injustice is the prevention of marginalized groups from participating in societal roles and activities that are needed or desired to enhance quality and meaningfulness of life (Durocher et al., 2014). Historical and present examples of occupational injustices include restricting career options for women and people of color; preventing Native/Indigenous peoples from engaging in their cultural occupations by forcibly displacing them from their First Nation lands and segregating them in impoverished areas (e.g., relegated to reservations); and discriminating against gender diverse and sexually diverse people by denying or terminating employment and housing, and illegalizing the ability to participate in the roles of married spouse and health care proxy. Occupational injustices also occur commonly in the penal system in which prisoners are denied the participation in appropriate and sufficient daily activities needed to manage stress and conflict, and attain skills needed to return to civilian life.

10.2 Western Society's Creation of Systems of Social and Occupational Injustice

Critical race theory suggests that Western society has created a social system in which people of color have historically been oppressed through systemic racism. Systemic racism is the embedding of subjugation and discrimination in a society's social structures with the intent to oppress people of color to prevent them from rising in socioeconomic status. Overtime, the policies, prevailing attitudes, beliefs, and laws of a society designed to oppress marginalized races, become so thoroughly embedded into a society's cultural norms that they are no longer recognized or questioned as discriminatory. Examples of systemic racism include underfunded schools in low socioeconomic areas; laws that maintain the minimum wage at a level below poverty; police policies that profile people of color; higher percentages of arrests, incarceration, and police violence against Black and Brown people (e.g., African American, West Indian, Jamaican, Haitian, Hispanic, Lantinx, Mexican, Arab, and other Middle Eastern Americans); and banking systems that discriminate against people of color by denying mortgages and loans, and charging higher interest rates (Delgado & Stefancic, 2017).

Systemic racism in Western society has its roots in British colonization and slavery which also became embedded as cultural norms in United States' history. Systemic racism, however, extends beyond the subjugation of Black races and includes the Native peoples of the Americas and Australia. In the United States and Canada, Native peoples were persecuted, expulsed from their ancestral lands, and forced to live in restricted areas, or reservations, often in unlivable conditions. The Native/Indigenous peoples of the Americas continue to be a marginalized and socioeconomically impoverished group to this day. A similar history of colonization and subjugation was perpetrated by British colonists against Aboriginal Australians, who were dispossessed from their original First Nation lands and forced to live in conditions of economic disadvantage (Feagin, 2013).

The systemic oppression and discrimination of groups, however, has not been limited to race alone. Women have also been a historically oppressed group, being denied voting rights in many Western countries until the early 20th century, and having restricted access to post-secondary higher education and most career opportunities until the 1970s. Even in the present day, women earn only 80% of men's salaries for the same job (Barroso & Brown, 2022). One of the most marginalized and discriminated groups in Western society has historically been people identifying as gender and sexually diverse (or people identifying as lesbian, gay, bisexual, transgender, queer or questioning, intersex, and asexual). Gender and sexually diverse people, until approximately only a decade ago, have been denied the ability to legally marry, adopt children, serve as health care proxies for long-term unmarried spouses, and were subject to blatant housing and employment discrimination. Sexism and homophobic and transphobic discrimination have been so thoroughly embedded into a patriarchal and heteronormative society, that it has been invisible and unquestioned until the women's movement of the 1970s and the gay rights movement, beginning in the 1960s, challenged prevailing systemic inequity and social injustice (Strauss et al., 2020).

10.3 How Intersectionality Impacts Inequity, Disadvantage, and Injustice

Intersectionality is the overlap or combining of marginalized groups, and commonly heightens the severity of an individual's or group's experience of disadvantage and discrimination. For example, transgender Black women report the highest levels of discrimination and disadvantage in studies examining the experience of gender diversity in heteronormative societies (Biello & Hughto, 2021). Black and Brown women report the lowest levels of earnings among all employees for the same work (United States Census Bureau, 2021). Similarly, studies have shown that Black men are the most racially profiled by police and are three times more likely to be a victim of police violence (Kaiser Family Foundation, 2022). Intersectionality commonly intensifies the experience of inequity and injustice for disempowered groups in which members self-identify with more than one stigmatized category. Such individuals report that societal discrimination is amplified and difficult to attribute to a specific stigmatized characteristic.

10.4 How Inequity, Disadvantage, and Injustice Impact Occupational Participation

In many Western, capitalistic societies in which members are expected to be independent wage earners who can self-sufficiently secure all economic and material needs, a strong belief system has been embedded into the culture that suggests that any person who works hard enough can be successful. This belief has become so ingrained into cultural narratives that its plausibility is rarely questioned. Instead, the belief that anyone can achieve success if they work sufficiently hard has been fueled by rare accounts of people who pulled themselves out of poverty to become powerful and wealthy – multimillionaire industrialists, celebrity athletes, and superstar entertainers.

The reality, however, is that for those born into poverty and who are forced to grow up in neighborhoods rife with crime, violence, and drug use; where public school systems are grossly inadequate and the high school completion rate is low; and where Black adolescent males have a higher likelihood of being the victim of violence than entering college, then the rags to riches tale is more myth than reality. Poverty is often intergenerational, as infrastructure systems in low socioeconomic areas tend to maintain conditions of disadvantage over time – unsafe neighborhoods, lack of affordable housing, food insecurity, poor public education systems, inadequate and inaccessible health care, and under- and unemployment. Children growing up in such conditions are at a heightened risk for school dropout, juvenile delinquency and criminal involvement, teen pregnancy, single adolescent parenting, homelessness, and substance use.

If the barriers to the attainment of higher socioeconomic status are already exigent, they become almost insurmountable for those with prison records. This is a critical recognition, as Black and Brown people are overrepresented in the penal systems of many Western countries, particularly the United States. In the United States, Black Americans are five times as likely to be incarcerated as their White counterparts, while Latinx Americans are 1.3 times as likely (Nellis, 2021). Several reasons have been put forth by scholars to account for this overrepresentation: a history of White subjugation over Black people stemming from slavery; policing policies in which minority groups have

EQUITY, DISADVANTAGE, JUSTICE, AND HUMAN OCCUPATION

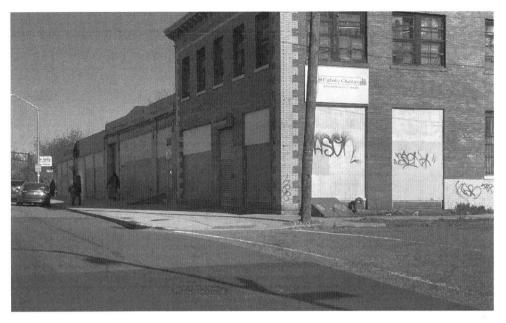

Figure 10.1 Impoverished communities are commonly characterized by lack of livable wage employment opportunities, crime, drug use, and proximity to environmental pollutants.

Source: Photo by Sharon Gutman, chapter author, and used with her permission.

historically been profiled and arrested for misdemeanor crimes; and the mass incarceration of Black people beginning in the 1970s which both lengthened prison sentences and increased the use of imprisonment for a variety of felonies. Having a prison record severely reduces the likelihood of obtaining employment and securing affordable housing once former felons return to the community. The presence of a prison record also significantly reduces lifetime earnings and adversely affects the life opportunities of the children of formerly incarcerated parents. Prior imprisonment additionally increases the likelihood of future arrests and incarceration.

Proponents of critical race theory have argued that Western society's infrastructure was designed to oppress people of color and maintain their state of disadvantage over time. Impoverishment becomes a cyclic, intergenerational phenomenon that is embedded in a dominant White, heteronormative culture. The obstacles and barriers set in place to preserve such oppression – ineffective school systems, housing and food insecurity, crime and drug ridden neighborhoods, lack of livable wage employment opportunities –become nearly insurmountable for people with few resources and even less societal influence and strength (Delgado & Stefancic, 2017) (see Figure 10.1).

10.5 How Inequity, Disadvantage, and Injustice Impact the Occupations of Childhood

The United States leads the Western world's child poverty rates with one in seven children living in poverty (an estimated 11 million) (Haider, 2021). Canada (1.3 million children living in poverty), Australia (731,000 children), and the United Kingdom (4.3 million children) have lower percentages of child poverty, with approximately

12–14% of children falling below their respective country's poverty line (Davidson et al., 2020; Francis-Devine, 2021; Hillel & Sarangi, 2021; OECD, 2022). Children of color were the most likely to experience poverty with Black, Hispanic, and First Nation children experiencing the highest poverty levels.

10.5.1 Occupations of Play

Growing up in poverty affects all aspects of a child's daily life, including the availability of food and nutrients, a home in which to live, schools in which to learn basic educational skills, neighborhoods and playgrounds in which to be safe, and communities in which their parents can obtain livable wage employment. Play is one of the central occupations of childhood; however, if children grow up in neighborhoods pervaded by violence, they may feel scared to play outside, walk to school, or enter stores. Neighborhood playgrounds and parks may be unsafe and children may be restricted to play in their homes. Play allows children to explore their environments and facilitates learning about the world. When children do not feel safe to play in their own neighborhoods, however, they may grow up learning that the world is an unsafe and frightening place. A child growing up in a disadvantaged area may also experience their home as unsafe for a variety of reasons, including the threat of home invasion; street violence spilling into the home; lack of temperature control and clean water; and rodent and insect infestation. Housing in low socioeconomic areas is also more likely to possess health risks such as lead paint and pipes, and proximity to environmental waste sites and highways yielding toxic air pollution (Feagin, 2013).

The home life may be chaotic without established routines. Children may be left to fend for themselves or neglected if parents are burdened by low-wage work, cannot afford childcare, do not have parenting skills, or may experience a mental illness that is untreated. When both the neighborhood and home environments are unsafe, children may become anxious, fearful, and angry. Children may fear losing or may have lost family members to violence. If they have been victims of violence or abuse, they may experience post-traumatic stress disorder (PTSD) and play may then mirror the violence that they have experienced or become an outlet for anger. Anger that is compounded day after day and left untreated can turn into conduct disorders in the school system. If the school system feels punitive to the child and exacerbates the child's anger rather than allaying it, anger may eventually provoke the child into acts that later involve them in the criminal justice system. In such cases, the larger societal system seems to breed the resentment, wrath, and socially inappropriate behaviors in children that it seeks to punish when they reach adolescence and adulthood.

10.5.2 Occupations of Learning, Education, and School

Education and learning are also primary and critically important occupations of childhood. Families living in poverty, however, commonly experience food insecurity and children may go to school and spend the school day hungry. Without sufficient nutrition to support cognitive functions, children who are hungry frequently have difficulty with attention, concentration, and learning. Such children may rapidly fall behind grade-level competencies, prompting labels of learning disorders. Children who are chronically hungry may also develop disruptive classroom behaviors for which they are labeled with conduct disorders. Conversely, learning disorders and attention deficit hyperactivity disorder (ADHD) that have an authentic neurologic basis may go undetected or unaddressed in under-resourced schools and may exacerbate a child's ability to maintain pace with grade-level academic competencies. Schools in low socioeconomic regions are commonly underfunded, short-staffed, and ill-equipped to address the myriad childhood issues stemming from poverty (Feagin, 2013).

One of the most significant problems in low socioeconomic school systems is low literacy. The National Assessment of Education Progress (2015) suggests that approximately 64% of fourth-grade students in the United States read below grade level, and Black and Hispanic children living in low socioeconomic areas are overrepresented in this estimate (Nitardy et al., 2015). These percentages are critical, as reading and school performance are directly associated with adult economic and quality of life markers. For example, 85% of minors in the criminal justice system report reading difficulties (Formby & Paynter, 2020), and 75% of incarcerated adults could not read or write sufficiently to earn a high school diploma (Bureau of Justice Statistics, 2003; Lockwood et al., 2015).

Low-level literacy, poor academic performance, and school dropout are often embedded in intergenerational cycles of poverty and housing insecurity (Bennett et al., 2013). The parents of impoverished children, who likely have been failed by the same underfunded and low-resourced schools as their children, commonly possess low-level literacy skills and basic academic competencies. Consequently, they may be at a loss to help their own children learn academic skills such as reading, writing, math, and science. They may be similarly unable to role model skills needed to succeed in school (such as time management, study skills, and organization) and may not understand how to help their children create daily routines to complete homework and school assignments. If the home environment is chaotic because of noise, too much activity, clutter, and insufficient space, it may not support the child's participation in homework and study activities (see Figure 10.2).

For children whose families have become homeless and are residing in shelters, family life is completely disrupted, and any semblance of routine has likely been lost. The ability to complete homework when displaced from the home environment to a crowded, noisy, and possibly unsafe shelter is an unrealistic expectation, particularly if children are left to their own devices to create routines that support school participation without assistance from caregivers. Chronic family homelessness and successive foster care placements present children with multiple disruptions to their educational attainment that almost ensure school dropout, school failure, or high school graduation without basic writing and reading skills. The consequences of childhood homelessness and multiple foster care placements on adult life trajectories cannot be underestimated. High school dropouts are three times more likely to be unemployed than their peers who received college degrees (United States Bureau of Labor Statistics, 2019), and adults who attained only a General Educational Development certificate (i.e., GED) or high school diploma have lifetime earnings of approximately one half the salaries of those with college educations (United States Bureau of Labor Statistics, 2021).

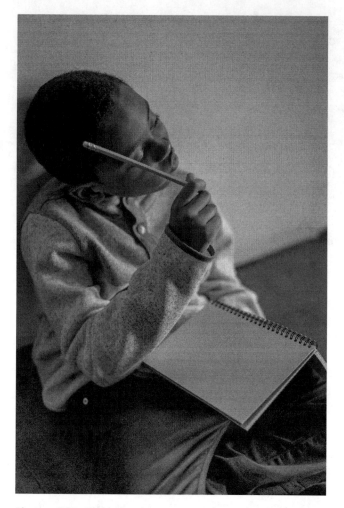

Figure 10.2 Children who are a product of disadvantaged homes, communities, and school systems may not have the support needed to create daily routines to participate in educational activities such as homework and school assignments.

Source: Photo by Katerina Holme and image used under license from pexels.com.

10.6 How Inequity, Disadvantage, and Injustice Impact the Occupations of Adolescence

10.6.1 Occupations of Learning, Education, and School

As children enter adolescence, a central occupation continues to be learning and school participation. If children transition to adolescence with significant gaps in foundational educational skills (e.g., reading, writing, and math), the demands of high school-level coursework commonly become more onerous as adolescents fall further behind grade-level competencies. In the immediacy of daily life, this situation may prompt adolescents to psychologically or physically withdraw from school engagement, be unable to attend to and focus on class activities, or demonstrate inappropriate or disruptive behaviors in the classroom. Such adolescents may become irate with a school system that has failed them; and many are labeled with anger management problems and fail to receive the emotional and psychological support they need to better deal with the hardships encountered since childhood. If parents, educators, and school administrators – who are likely overworked and lacking needed resources – adopt punitive responses as assistance, they may inadvertently heighten the adolescent's resentment and resistance. It is important to understand that although adolescents may be able to identify their feelings of animosity and distrust, they commonly do not have the analytical skills and insight to understand how years of systemic disadvantage have contributed to those feelings. Similarly, the adults in the adolescent's life (parents, educators, and school officials) – who likely experienced comparable hardships while growing up – may have their own emotions of anger that have not been consciously analyzed.

The persistent presence of ADHD and learning disabilities (e.g., dyslexia, dysgraphia, auditory and language processing disorders, and visual-perceptual problems) in adolescence, particularly if unaddressed or ineffectively addressed, will continue to exacerbate the attainment of basic reading and writing skills needed for adult daily living. By the time a child with undiagnosed learning difficulties or ADHD reaches adolescence, that adolescent has likely received and internalized messages that they are unintelligent and incapable of constructing a successful adult life. Although most Western countries have legislation that mandates special services for children with learning disabilities in public school systems, schools in low socioeconomic areas may be unable to attract or retain service providers. Adolescents with ADHD and learning disabilities may therefore not receive the educational assistance to which they are entitled. Such adolescents may never learn that they are in fact intelligent and capable of learning using alternative educational strategies. Adolescents who have been told since childhood that they are powerless to succeed in the school system and adult life, report feelings of internalized self-defeat and possess higher school dropout rates (Haider, 2021).

The compounded effects of years of destitution, food and housing insecurity, and school difficulties can commonly fuel depression, anxiety, and hopelessness. The occurrence of victimization, chronic abuse, and the loss of family members to violence – all prevalent experiences of adolescents growing up in poverty – can trigger PTSD and severe mental health problems that can further heighten the risk of school failure. As noted above, underfunded and low-resourced schools may be unable to address such mental health problems with their adolescent students, prompting such students to withdraw further from the school system. A disproportionate amount of Black and Brown adolescents in Western society, compared to their White counterparts, turn to substance use, likely to manage the stresses of disadvantage. Substance use will worsen an adolescent student's school performance and may facilitate behaviors that increase the risk of involvement in the juvenile justice system (United States Department of Housing and Urban Development, 2021).

10.6.2 Occupations of Leisure, Recreation, and Socialization with Peer Groups

In adolescence, the occupations of leisure, recreation, and socialization shift from the family of origin to the peer group, and more activities are carried out in the community. Impoverished areas, however, may be crime ridden and dangerous, lack safe parks and playgrounds, and lack community centers with adult-supervised recreational activities (see Figure 10.3). It is not uncommon for existing community centers in impoverished neighborhoods to be closed due to lack of funding and staff shortages.

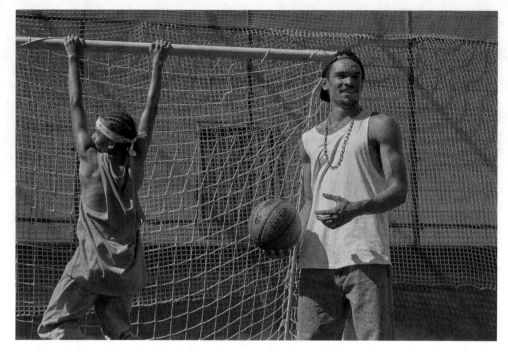

Figure 10.3 Community and school systems in disadvantaged areas may not be able to provide safe spaces and activities in which adolescents can socialize with each other and engage in enjoyable occupations. If deprived of these occupational environments, adolescents may turn to non-sanctioned, adverse occupations such as substance use, crime, and violence.

Source: Photo by Cottonbro and image used under license from pexels.com.

Similarly, underfunded schools are often unable to offer an array of adult-supervised clubs and sports programs that could provide safe, skill-building activities.

When the community and school systems in disadvantaged areas cannot furnish safe spaces and activities in which adolescents can socialize with each other in enjoyable occupations that can promote self-esteem, interpersonal skills, and teamwork, adolescents may turn to the adverse occupations prevailing in a community – such as substance use, crime, and violence. Some adolescents in low socioeconomic areas report feeling compelled to join gangs to protect themselves and their families. In such situations, gang membership – and the inherent violence and criminal activity demanded by participation – is traded to secure protection in a perilous environment (Haider, 2021).

Risk factors for adolescent substance use in disadvantaged communities include having a family member who uses drugs or alcohol; lacking parental or family member monitoring of activities and friends; associating with friends who use substances; ongoing and persistent feelings of anxiety and depression; and identification as gender and sexually diverse in an unsupportive, heteronormative community. Engagement in substance use is also associated with higher percentages of adolescent sex, unprotected sex, victimization, and teenage pregnancy. Teenage females who have children are more likely to drop out of school and become homeless. Children born to adolescent parents who cannot adequately care for them are commonly placed on a path of successive foster care placement, victimization, school incompletion, and juvenile and adult incarceration – thus, maintaining the cycle of disadvantage that appears embedded in the larger dominant, social structure (Haider, 2021).

These adverse occurrences can be attenuated with positive adult mentorship, involvement in team sports programs, assistance with academics, and school participation. Adult mentorship and guidance, particularly with mentors of similar racial and ethnic backgrounds, can help minority adolescents to develop positive identities, self-esteem, and confidence. Mentorship programs can assist minority youth to better understand their experience of oppression and construct paths to overcome societally embedded barriers. The opportunity for adolescents of color to participate in team sports and related leisure activities can be instrumental in helping to shape positive identities (particularly if the school system has failed in this regard); build skills such as perseverance, responsibility, dedication, and commitment; enhance an adolescent's ability to work collaboratively with team members and develop interpersonal skills; and serve as a positive stress management strategy. Adolescents of color also benefit from small group or individualized assistance with schoolwork in which comprehension is enhanced through visual, auditory, and kinesthetic strategies that target an adolescent's learning needs (Haider, 2021).

10.6.3 Intersectionality and the Impact of Gender Diversity on Occupational Participation

Adolescents who both live in poverty and identify as gender and sexually diverse are overrepresented among the homeless youth population in Western countries. Approximately 20%–40% of adolescents experiencing homelessness in North America self-identify as gender and sexually diverse, with the highest percentages of this range reported in disadvantaged urban areas. Gender and sexually diverse youth are 120% more likely to experience homelessness compared to their same age, heterosexual, cisgender peers. When youth self-identify as both gender and sexually diverse and Black or Brown, the risk for homelessness nearly doubles (National Conference of State Legislators, 2021).

A primary reason for this disproportionately high rate of homelessness among gender and sexually diverse adolescents of color include discrimination and rejection by family members and caregivers in response to gender identity disclosure. Many gender and sexually diverse adolescents of color report abuse in response to gender-nonconforming behaviors perpetrated by foster home guardians and peers in the school system (Robinson, 2021). Years of cumulative abuse and bullying by homophobic and transphobic caregivers and peers commonly result in mental health concerns, including depression, substance use, and suicidality. Gender and sexually diverse minority youth report the highest rates of mental health concerns in comparison to their same-age, cisgender peers, with transgender minority youth reporting the highest rates (National Alliance on Mental Illness, 2021).

While the home, neighborhood, and school environments may hold inherent dangers from crime, violence, and drugs for all minority youth, gender and sexually diverse adolescents of color report a heightened experience of daily threat because of their gender identity. They may feel ostracized from their school system and peer group, and the typical adolescent occupations of dating and sexual exploration commonly occur clandestinely. When bullying becomes sufficiently severe to force gender and sexually diverse minority youth to leave the home of parents or guardians, they not only lose shelter, food, and protection from the elements, but also participation in occupational roles such as high school student and the ability to learn the essential life skills needed to transition to adulthood.

Homelessness for gender and sexually diverse minority youth may take the form of street sleeping (or rough sleeping), couch surfing (or sleeping in a series of impermanent conditions), and transitioning through temporary shelters. During periods of homelessness, gender and sexually diverse youth of color are at a heightened risk of victimization and unsafe behaviors, including survival sex (trading sex for shelter and food), unprotected sex, sex with intravenous drug using partners, and sex with strangers. These types of survival behaviors can increase the risk for HIV and sexually transmitted diseases, sexual exploitation, and physical assault (Keuroghlian et al., 2014).

Many of the same discriminatory and abusive behaviors that occurred in the family or foster care home, reoccur in juvenile shelter systems where violence is often perpetrated by homophobic and transphobic peers, and where sex-segregated shelters commonly implement policies and practices that are insensitive and potentially dangerous to gender and sexually diverse youth (e.g., assigning shelter bed placements based on birth sex rather than self-identified gender, and failing to provide private showering facilities and gender-neutral bathrooms).

Years of cumulative trauma and discrimination, severed family relationships and lack of support safety nets, and intermittent periods of homelessness or shelter residence often result in depression and anxiety disorders, substance use problems, and significant educational and life skill deficiencies. Researchers have found that gender and sexually diverse adolescents of color who are homeless benefit most from shelter programs that are sensitive to gender diversity; offer private or gender-neutral bath- and bedrooms; and provide educational and employment assistance, financial education, life skill development, substance use harm reduction strategies, and education about safe sex practices (Abramovich, 2016). Even with such assistance, however, gender and sexually diverse adolescents of color continue to face inequity and societal barriers as they transition into adulthood in the form of housing and employment discrimination, and reduced access to or bias in health care services and education.

10.7 How Inequity, Disadvantage, and Injustice Impact the Occupations of Adulthood
The primary occupational roles of adulthood include family member (e.g., parent, spouse, offspring, and sibling) and employed worker.

10.7.1 Occupational Participation in Families
Adults of color living in poverty commonly have histories of family relationships that have been torn apart by crime, mass incarceration of Black and Brown people, drug use, and unemployment. Some scholars have suggested that the fractionation of family relationships that is characteristic of many impoverished Black homes today has its historical roots in slavery, when the families of slaves were severed by slave owners who sold and separated them. While it was common for slave owners to maintain the unity of Black children with their mothers to ensure caregiving responsibilities, Black men were divided from the family through the slave trade, and their roles as fathers and spouses were ruptured. Black women of the same and extended families unified

to provide each other with the emotional and physical support needed to raise children amidst the horrors of bondage and extreme abuse. The single-mother household in which a racial minority mother raises children with the assistance of extended family (e.g., grandmothers and siblings) continues to this day. In the United States and the United Kingdom, approximately 64% of Black children live in single-mother homes in low socioeconomic regions (Annie E. Casey Foundation, Kids Count Data Center, 2022; Office for National Statistics, 2021). This percentage drops to 46% in Canada (Statistics Canada, 2004) – just four percentage points below half of all Black Canadian children.

Reasons for the continued severance of Black families in Western countries today point toward systemic racism and embedded social structures that serve to derail the economic stability of Black men and women. For example, in many urban areas, lack of livable wage opportunities exists for Black men in particular; Black women tend to have higher employment rates, although earnings are the lowest among all races and genders. Mass incarceration rates of Black men also likely account for both the unavailability of men as marriage partners and their perceived economic instability by their female counterparts. Moreover, the existence of a prior prison record, as previously noted, further reduces employment and housing opportunities. It appears that the social and legal structures of Western countries may undermine Black men's ability to remain within the family unit as spouses and fathers (Lloyd et al., 2021).

10.7.2 Historical and Current Societal Barriers to Building Wealth: Occupational Participation in Employment, Home Ownership, and Transferring Wealth Intergenerationally

Although the abolition of slavery in the United States was meant to ensure equality, generations of Black people faced newly constructed obstacles in the form of Jim Crow segregation laws, sharecropping (in which landlords rented portions of land to impoverished Black men and demanded a percentage of profits from land use), prison labor camps, housing discrimination, voting barriers, and banking discrimination (in the form of mortgage and business loan denials or exorbitant interest rates). These institutions were designed largely by southern sympathizers with the intent to prevent Black men and women from attaining economic stability and mobility.

The historical disparity in wealth persists to the present day in which Black Americans own approximately one-tenth the wealth owned by White Americans. Having access to accumulated assets is a form of critical security, as it allows people to overcome difficult life situations such as transitioning between jobs, moving to a new location for school or work, paying for post-secondary higher education, surviving loss of work due to a protracted illness, and saving to ensure economic stability for retirement. Present-day societal barriers that impede Black adults from building wealth include employment and housing discrimination, unethical mortgage lending practices that obstruct home ownership, lack of livable wage employment opportunities, mass incarceration policies, and inadequate public school systems that reduce pathways to college. As a result of societal barriers that impede the ability to build personal savings, Black adults are more likely to fall behind on bills and become indebted during times of emergency. A lack of accumulated assets not only adversely impacts adults living in poverty, but it also detrimentally affects future generations, as parents of color are not able to transfer assets to children to help them become economically stabile and attain higher education and home ownership.

It should be noted that while the experience of many impoverished Black Americans has been discussed as an example of the ways in which inequity and disadvantage affect occupational participation in Western society, both Latinx and First Nation peoples have also been excluded from opportunities to build wealth and become economically stable. Similar disparities in wealth accumulation, ownership, and intergenerational transference also exists in Canada, the United Kingdom, and Australia, where people of color – compared to White peers – report reduced employment opportunities and lower income for comparable work (Zucman, 2019).

10.7.3 The Intersection of Low Literacy, Race, and Poverty

Low literacy, being a member of a racial minority group in Western society, and poverty are all connected. It is estimated that approximately 8.7 million disadvantaged elementary and high school students read below grade level. Children who cannot read at grade level in their second year of elementary school are unlikely to ever become grade-level readers, and adolescents who cannot read proficiently by eighth grade are at high risk for school failure. As adults, low-level readers are more likely to be unemployed, homeless, and have higher incarceration rates (National Assessment of Educational Progress, 2015).

Low-level literacy and poverty affect all forms of daily occupation: employment seeking; interpreting and paying bills; health care access and usage; deciphering transportation signage and maps; purchasing foods; and using package directions to prepare meals, launder clothing, take medication appropriately, and use cleaning products safely. The inability to read proficiently is one of the highest predictors of chronic disadvantage and is an occupational injustice maintained through institutional racism. One of the most blatant forms of institutional racism in Western society is the failing public school system that cannot adequately prepare children in the most basic educational skills because of underfunding, lack of resources, and staff shortages. The cumulative effects of low literacy; lack of livable wage employment opportunities; housing discrimination; mortgage lending practices that deter home ownership; police violence; and mass incarceration policies result in a recipe for chronic, intergenerational poverty and homelessness (United States Department of Housing and Urban Development, 2021).

10.7.4 The Societal and Occupational Injustice of Homelessness

In the United States, on any given night, it is estimated that approximately 580,500 people are homeless (United States Department of Housing and Urban Development, 2021). In Canada the number of homeless people is estimated at 235,000 (Strobel et al., 2021), 274,000 in the United Kingdom (Shelter, the National Campaign for Homeless People, 2022), and 116,000 in Australia (Australian Institute of Health and Welfare, 2022). Most people who are homeless in Western countries are people of color, including First Nation peoples, and the connection between systemic racism and homelessness is unarguable. Homelessness is perhaps the most severe form of societal exclusion in which people are denied the basic necessity of shelter, consistent and nutritious meals, sanitary toileting and bathing, and the ability to sleep without fear of harm. Although shelter systems

EQUITY DISADVANTAGE, JUSTICE, AND HUMAN OCCUPATION

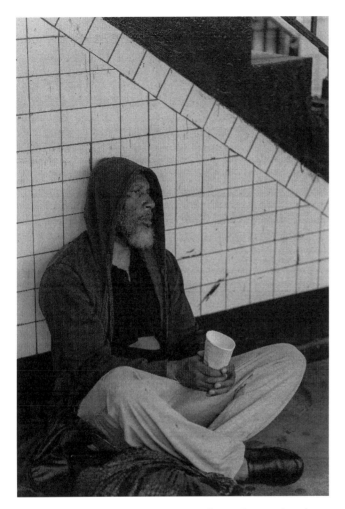

Figure 10.4 Homelessness is a severe form of societal exclusion where people are often denied the basic necessities of shelter, consistent and nutritious meals, sanitary toileting and bathing, as well as the opportunity to sleep without fear of harm.

Source: Photo by Timur Weber and image used under license from pexels.com.

attempt to provide these basic necessities, many homeless people avoid temporary shelter residences due to the high rate of potential violence, theft, drug use, and chaos. Chronic homelessness prematurely ages people causing severe systemic organ disease, mental health disorders, and musculoskeletal conditions (see Figure 10.4). Homeless adults have a mortality rate 3–4 times greater than their average White counterparts and a life expectancy of about 50 years (Salhi & Doran, 2021).

10.8 How Inequity, Disadvantage, and Injustice Impact the Occupations of Late Adulthood

It is not surprising, given a lifetime of systemic racism and the health inequities and occupational justices associated with it, that the average life expectancy of Black men and women is approximately four years less than their same-age White peers, with

Black men having the lowest life expectancy at 72 years (Bond & Herman, 2016). For people of color who survive into late adulthood, a lifetime of food insecurity, poor nutrition, and chronic stress has likely contributed to diseases such as diabetes, cardiovascular conditions, high blood pressure, asthma, and chronic pain syndromes. Elders may have encountered and continue to experience bias and inaccessible health care systems in which health care professionals of non-minority races may be less likely to listen to and take their concerns seriously, be willing to prescribe pain medication, and provide treatment congruent with patient desires. Elders living in impoverished areas may feel unsafe to go outside their homes and may have lost family support due to violence and illness. Food shopping, obtaining needed medical care and medicine, and socializing with others may be hindered by unsafe communities.

Minority elders' homes may also be unsafe and they may live in conditions posing high risk for falls and other safety hazards. For example, the home may have outside or indoor steps that have become too difficult for elders to negotiate, indoor lighting may be poor and aggravate elders' visual conditions, the bathtub and toilet may be too difficult to sit on or rise from, and cluttered floors or steps may pose fall risks. Other home safety concerns may include cluttered kitchen stoves which pose a fire hazard, too many electrical cords in single outlets, and windows that are too difficult to open in case of fire. Elders may be unable to afford air conditioning in the extreme heat of summer, or live in tenements with poor heating in winter.

Many elders may become isolated because of a fear of venturing outside their homes into unsafe communities, while loss of family and friends to violence, incarceration, and illness may leave elders without a safety support net. Other elders may be required to become guardians or caregivers of grandchildren when parents cannot afford or provide childcare because of single parenting. The most disadvantaged minority elders have likely been unable to save for an economically stable retirement and are dependent on social security and government subsidies that are often too little to ensure access to even basic resources.

For those elders who identify as gender or sexually diverse, particularly transgender, housing, employment, and health care discrimination have likely occurred as common experiences throughout adolescence and adulthood, and continued to occur well into late adulthood. Gender and sexually diverse minority elders report that a lifetime of employment discrimination has frequently left them without the security of retirement funds. Many also report that they continue to experience housing discrimination, even in assisted living facilities. Gender and sexually diverse elders, particularly those identifying as transgender, additionally express fear of traversing an already unsafe community because of homophobic and transphobic violence. Many describe that late adulthood is often a time of heightened isolation, as family relationships have long been severed, friends within the gender and sexually diverse community have passed away, and the larger heteronormative community continues to be a place of rejection and the threat of violence (Boggs et al., 2017).

10.9 Conclusion

Inequity, disadvantage, and injustice are embedded in the fabric of Western society's laws, institutional policies and practices, and prevailing attitudes – whether explicit or implicit. Inequity, disadvantage, and injustice uphold a culture of systemic racism, in which the most impoverished community members – who are primarily Black, Brown, and First Nation peoples – have historically been denied the same opportunities for socioeconomic mobility and occupational participation as that of the larger, dominant White group. Although the forms of oppression have changed over time, socioeconomic subjugation continues to the present day and adversely impacts all daily occupational participation from childhood to late adulthood. The same occupational participation in society that is taken for granted by a privileged, dominant White group is often unattainable or tenuous for people of color living in poverty – being able to go to a public school to attain basic reading and writing skills, living in a community free from the threat of daily violence, having access to livable wage employment opportunities and affordable housing in safe neighborhoods, and being able to attain economic security that could serve to help one's children and provide security in retirement.

As occupational therapists, we must acknowledge the impact of systemic racism in our patients' and clients' lives and explore our own implicit biases as health care professionals. We must help youth in the school system who may be academically compromised, lacking a home environment that supports educational attainment, struggle with food insecurity and psychosocial trauma, and have little understanding of how to bridge the gap between high school and college or vocational training. We must also help youth who are struggling with their gender diversity in a heteronormative school environment, as well as students whose families are homeless and residing in temporary shelter. We must make sure that our disadvantaged elders are safe within their homes and have secure methods to obtain needed resources within the community such as food and health care. We must also ensure that our adult and senior clients possess functional literacy and can participate in all desired occupations that require reading print. Additionally, we must increase our work with homeless adults, children, and families to help them attain the skills needed to transition from homelessness to supported housing.

Our roots as a profession were immersed within the community working with marginalized groups, including disabled veterans needing to reintegrate into society, adults with chronic mental illness living lifespans in sanitariums, and impoverished immigrant populations desiring assistance to adapt to Western society and attain community skills. As occupational therapists, we have the competencies needed to help the most disadvantaged among us to attain daily life skills to participate in desired occupations that have historically been denied or barriered. We need to use our professional skills to mitigate the occupational injustices that have been committed against the most powerless and disadvantaged of our society.

10.10 Summary
- Inequity, disadvantage, and social and occupational injustices adversely impact people's ability to participate in desired, meaningful daily life activities, or occupations.
- Critical race theory suggests that Western society has created a social system in which people of color have historically been oppressed through systemic racism.
- Other historically marginalized groups, such as women and people identifying as gender and sexually diverse, have also experienced blatant discrimination and oppression that have limited their full occupational participation in Western society.
- Examples of systemic racism include underfunded schools in low socioeconomic areas; laws that maintain minimum wage at a level below poverty; police policies that profile people of color; higher percentages of arrests, incarceration, and

- police violence against Black and Brown people; and banking systems that racially discriminate against people of color by denying mortgages and loans and charging higher interest rates.
- Intersectionality is the overlap or combining of marginalized groups, and commonly heightens the severity of an individual's or group's experience of disadvantage and discrimination.
- Living in poverty affects all aspects of children's, adolescents', and adults' daily lives, including the availability of food and nutrients, a home in which to live, schools in which to learn basic educational skills, neighborhoods and communities in which to be safe, opportunities to attain livable wage employment, and the ability to save for an economically stable and secure retirement.
- As occupational therapists, we must acknowledge the impact of systemic racism in our patients' and clients' lives and explore our own implicit biases as health care professionals. We must use our own professional competencies to assist the most disadvantaged among us to participate in desired occupations that have historically been denied or barriered.

10.11 Review Questions

1. What are historical and present-day examples of social and occupational injustice experienced by minority groups (including people of color, women, and gender and sexually diverse people)?
2. What is intersectionality and how has it impacted the occupational participation of people who self-identify as members of two or more marginalized groups?
3. How does inequity, disadvantage, and injustice impact the occupations of childhood, adolescence, adulthood, and late adulthood?
4. What is the intersection of low literacy, race, and poverty, and how do these three combined factors impact occupational participation in society throughout a lifetime?
5. What are examples of ways in which occupational therapists can assist marginalized groups to attain the skills and resources needed to overcome barriers embedded in the larger society?

References

Abramovich, A. (2016). Preventing, reducing and ending LGBTQ2S youth homelessness: The need for targeted strategies. *Social Inclusion*, 4(4), 86–96. https://doi.org/10.17645/si.v4i4.669

Annie E. Casey Foundation, Kids Count Data Center. (2022). *Children in single-parent families by race in the United States.* https://datacenter.kidscount.org/data/tables/107-children-in-single-parent-families-by-race#detailed/1/any/false/1729,37,871,870,573,869,36,868,867,133/10,11,9,12,1,185,13/432,431

Australian Institute of Health and Welfare. (2022). *Homelessness and homelessness services.* https://www.aihw.gov.au/reports/australias-welfare/homelessness-and-homelessness-services

Barroso, A., & Brown, A. (2022). *Gender pay gap in US held steady in 2020.* Pew Research Center. https://www.pewresearch.org/fact-tank/2021/05/25/gender-pay-gap-facts/

Bennett, I. M., Frasso, R., Bellamy, S., Wortham, S., & Gross, K. (2013). Pre-teen literacy and subsequent teenage childbearing in a US population. *Contraception*, 87(4), 459–464. https://doi.org/10.1016/j.contraception.2012.08.020

Biello, K. B., & Hughto, J. M. (2021). Measuring intersectional stigma among racially and ethnically diverse transgender women: Challenges and opportunities. *American Journal of Public Health*, 111(3), 344–346. https://doi.org/10.2105/AJPH.2020.306141

Boggs, J. M., Dickman Portz, J., King, D. K., Wright, L. A., Helander, K., Retrum, J. H., & Gozansky, W. S. (2017). Perspectives of LGBTQ older adults on aging in place: A qualitative investigation. *Journal of Homosexuality*, 64(11), 1539–1560. https://doi.org/10.1080/00918369.2016.1247539

Bond, M. J., & Herman, A. A. (2016). Lagging life expectancy for black men: A Public Health imperative. *American Journal of Public Health*, 106(7), 1167–1169. https://doi.org/10.2105/AJPH.2016.303251

Bureau of Justice Statistics, US Department of Justice. (2003). *Educational and correctional populations*. https://bjs.ojp.gov/content/pub/pdf/ecp.pdf

Davidson, P., Saunders, P., Bradbury, B., & Wong, M. (2020). *Poverty in Australia 2020: Part 1, Overview*. ACOSS/UNSW Poverty and Inequality Partnership Report. https://povertyandinequality.acoss.org.au/wp-content/uploads/2020/02/Poverty-in-Australia-2020_Part-1_Overview.pdf

Delgado, R., & Stefancic, J. (2017). *Critical race theory* (3rd ed.). New York University Press.

Durocher, E., Rappolt, S., & Gibson, B. E. (2014). Occupational justice: Future directions. *Journal of Occupational Science*, 21(4), 431–442. https://doi.org/10.1080/14427591.2017.1294016

Feagin, J. (2013). *Systemic racism: A theory of oppression*. Routledge.

Formby, A. E., & Paynter, K. (2020). The potential of a library media program on reducing recidivism rates among juvenile offenders. *National Youth-At-Risk Journal*, 4(1), 14–21, Article 3. https://files.eric.ed.gov/fulltext/EJ1269471.pdf

Francis-Devine, B. (2021). *Poverty in the UK: Statistics*. House of Commons Library. https://researchbriefings.files.parliament.uk/documents/SN07096/SN07096.pdf

Haider, A. (2021). *The basic facts about children in poverty*. Center for American Progress. https://www.americanprogress.org/article/basic-facts-children-poverty/

Hillel, I., & Sarangi, L. (2021). 2021: *Report card on child and family poverty in Canada. No one left behind: Strategies for an inclusive recovery*. Campaign 2000. https://campaign2000.ca/wp-content/uploads/2021/11/C2000-2021-National-Report-Card-No-One-Left-Behind-Strategies-for-an-Inclusive-Recovery-AMENDED.pdf

Kaiser Family Foundation. (2022). *Poll: 7 in 10 Black Americans say they have experienced incidents of discrimination or police mistreatment in their lifetime, including nearly half who felt their lives were in danger*. https://www.kff.org/racial-equity-and-health-policy/press-release/poll-7-in-10-black-americans-say-they-have-experienced-incidents-of-discrimination-or-police-mistreatment-in-lifetime-including-nearly-half-who-felt-lives-were-in-danger/

Keuroghlian, A. S., Shtasel, D., & Bassuk, E. L. (2014). Out on the street: A public health and policy agenda for lesbian, gay, bisexual, and transgender youth who are homeless. *American Journal of Orthopsychiatry*, 84(1), 66–72. https://doi.org/10.1037/h0098852

Lavalley, R., & Johnson, K. R. (2022). Occupation, injustice, and anti-Black racism in the United States of America. *Journal of Occupational Science*, 29(4), 487–499. https://doi.org/10.1080/14427591.2020.1810111

Lloyd, C. M., Alvira-Hammond, M., Carlson, J., & Logan, D. (2021). *Family, economic, and geographic characteristics of Black families with children*. https://www.childtrends.org/publications/family-economic-and-geographic-characteristics-of-black-families-with-children

Lockwood, S. K., Nally, J. M., Ho, T., & Knutson, K. (2015). Racial disparities and similarities in post-release recidivism and employment among ex-prisoners with a different level of education. *Journal of Prison Education and Reentry*, 2(1), 16–31. http://doi.org/10.15845/jper.v2i1.703

National Alliance on Mental Illness. (2021). *LGBTQI*. https://www.nami.org/Your-Journey/Identity-and-Cultural-Dimensions/LGBTQI

National Assessment of Educational Progress. (2015). *2015 mathematics and reading assessments.* http://www.nationsreportcard.gov/reading_math_2015/#reading?grade=4

National Conference of State Legislators. (2021). *Youth homelessness overview.* https://www.ncsl.org/research/human-services/homeless-and-runaway-youth.aspx

Nellis, A. (2021). *The color of justice: Racial and ethnic disparity in state prisons.* The Sentencing Project. https://www.sentencingproject.org/publications/color-of-justice-racial-and-ethnic-disparity-in-state-prisons/

Nitardy, C. M., Duke, N. N., Pettingell, S. L., & Borowsky, I. W. (2015). Racial and ethnic disparities in educational achievement and aspirations: Findings from a statewide survey from 1998 to 2010. *Maternal and Child Health Journal, 19*(1), 58–66. https://link.springer.com/content/pdf/10.1007/s10995-014-1495-y.pdf

Office for National Statistics. (2021). *Proportion of children in lone parent families by ethnic group, England and Wales, 2019.* https://www.ons.gov.uk/peoplepopulationandcommunity/birthsdeathsandmarriages/families/adhocs/12947proportionofchildreninloneparentfamiliesbyethnicgroupenglandandwales2019

Organization for Economic Cooperation and Development. (2022). *OECD 6C data. Poverty rate.* https://data.oecd.org/inequality/poverty-rate.htm#indicator-chart

Robinson, B. A. (2021). "They peed on my shoes": Foregrounding intersectional minority stress in understanding LGBTQ youth homelessness. *Journal of LGBT Youth*, 1–17. https://doi.org/10.1080/19361653.2021.1925196

Salhi, B. A., & Doran, K. M. (2021). Homelessness. In H. J. Alter, P. Dalawari, K. M. Doran, & M. C. Raven (Eds.), *Social emergency medicine* (pp. 235–253). Springer. https://doi.org/10.1007/978-3-030-65672-0_14

Shelter, the National Campaign for Homeless People. (2022). *274,000 people in England are homeless, with thousands more likely to lose their homes.* https://england.shelter.org.uk/media/press_release/274000_people_in_england_are_homeless_with_thousands_more_likely_to_lose_their_homes#:~:text=More%20than%20274%2C000%20people%20are,are%20currently%20without%20a%20home

Statistics Canada. (2004). *Spotlight: Black population.* https://www150.statcan.gc.ca/n1/pub/11-002-x/2004/03/07604/4072460-eng.htm

Strauss, P., Cook, A., Winter, S., Watson, V., Toussaint, D. W., & Lin, A. (2020). Associations between negative life experiences and the mental health of trans and gender diverse young people in Australia: Findings from Trans Pathways. *Psychological Medicine, 50*(5), 808–817. https://doi.org/10.1017/S0033291719000643

Strobel, S., Burcul, I., Dai, J. H., Ma, Z., Jamani, S., & Hossain, R. Statistics Canada. (2021). *Health Reports. Characterizing people experiencing homelessness and trends in homelessness using population-level emergency department visit data in Ontario, Canada.* https://www150.statcan.gc.ca/n1/en/pub/82-003-x/2021001/article/00002-eng.pdf?st=7iFycVBl

United States Bureau of Labor Statistics, Department of Labor. (2019). *TED: The Economics Daily.* https://www.bls.gov/opub/ted/2019/44-6-percent-of-high-school-dropouts-and-72-3-percent-of-college-graduates-employed-in-august-2019.htm?view_full

United States Bureau of Labor Statistics, Department of Labor. (2021). *Career Outlook. Data on display. Education pays, 2020.* https://www.bls.gov/careeroutlook/2021/data-on-display/education-pays.htm

United States Census Bureau. (2021). *Work experience: People 15 years old and over, by total money earnings, age, race, Hispanic origin, sex, and disability status.* https://www.census.gov/data/tables/time-series/demo/income-poverty/cps-pinc/pinc-05.html

United States Department of Housing and Urban Development. (2021). *The 2020 annual homeless assessment report (AHAR) to Congress.* https://www.huduser.gov/portal/sites/default/files/pdf/2020-AHAR-Part-1.pdf

Zucman, G. (2019). Global wealth inequality. *Annual Review of Economics, 11*, 109–138. https://doi.org/10.1146/annurev-economics-080218-025852

CHAPTER 11

Undoing Coloniality

An Indigenous Occupation-based Perspective

Isla G. Emery-Whittington

Abstract
Decoloniality is a commitment to disengage in unethical colonial and oppressive harms while dismantling the everyday structures that reproduce such harms. As the profession's status quo, coloniality has limited the potential of occupation to heal and liberate. Disrupting colonial ways of being, as expressed occupationally, requires manifestly different relationships, language, infrastructure, goals, and values. This chapter examines links between occupation and colonialism, exploring the praxis of being colonially occupied as well as the under-theorization of colonialism. Doing colonialism is explicated alongside barriers to making fair space for global knowledges; a preparation step in safely and humanely appreciating global knowledges. Despite coloniality's capture of the profession's theories and systems, decolonial praxis flourishes where critical consciousness and anti-oppressive collaborations grow. Decolonized occupation is a platform for connection and reconnection to each other and life purpose.

Author's Positionality Statement
I am a Māori cis woman from Aotearoa New Zealand, and I am decolonizing. In the 30 years that I have studied, researched, practiced, theorized, and taught as an occupational therapist, I am regularly racially targeted and too often have occupational opportunities withheld by systems and colleagues. Despite this, along with a growing number of Indigenous practitioners and educators, I work to decolonize occupation in theory and practice within and beyond the profession. My teachings are invitations to colleagues and their communities to radically reconsider decolonized occupation as abundant accessible sites of healing.

ISLA G. EMERY-WHITTINGTON

> **Objectives**
> This chapter uses process and content to:
>
> - Platform decolonial methods of studying and writing, by inviting the reader to examine their relationship with coloniality.
> - Examine the relationship between coloniality and everyday occupations.
> - Examine the status quo of coloniality in the profession.
> - Highlight decolonial praxis in the profession.

> **Key terms**
>
> - decoloniality
> - coloniality
> - oppression
> - antiracism
> - occupation

11.1 Introduction

This chapter is about toil, joy, risk, and growth inherent in a process of de-centering "coloniality as the status quo". Decoloniality is a path less traveled and is littered with challenges that test the spirit, body, and relationships. However, unspoken and unexamined, coloniality has been a formidable and unshakable foundation to occupation for generations. Coloniality shapes what humans do because it requires human bodies, minds, and families to guard, limit, and seed its everyday occupational expression. Thus, decoloniality necessarily calls for different ways of doing as well as refusal to participate in colonial doings. The reader is invited to take time sitting with, and dwelling in, ideas that have been chosen and placed in the format of this text. The title, abstract, objectives, and positioning signal the intention of this chapter: to examine how occupational therapy and occupational science uphold coloniality and to spotlight the decolonial praxis that occurs despite coloniality.

This chapter is structured so that the reader is supported to seriously examine their personal investment and relationship to colonialism. The first section explores colonial approaches to knowledge, values, and beliefs, and the importance of a shared language of decoloniality. The chapter continues with a theoretical discussion and examination about occupation and colonialism, and how the profession upholds coloniality. This is followed with a brief examination of the profession's early steps in decolonization and contemporary efforts to making space for global knowledges. The chapter concludes with an exploration of decolonial approaches being utilized in the profession.

11.2 Being in Relationship with Coloniality and Decoloniality Is Praxis

It is a diabolical phenomenon that coloniality is so widely practiced through everyday occupation and yet for many of the global north parts of the profession, it is not well understood. Consequently, language and processes to develop the profession's understanding appear limited, experimental, and "best guesses". This is partly because the profession is using colonial worldviews, imagination, and processes to decolonize; an impossible task. As a mostly regulated health profession of highly trained practitioners, we need to expect more of ourselves than a stumble, trip, and fall into a fantasized decoloniality.

Decoloniality requires thoughtful, purposeful planning, and an understanding of how we learn and do decoloniality. An important starting point is recognizing that the global minority/north is en masse practicing coloniality via everyday occupations. Recent approaches to understanding coloniality in the profession have not shied away from acknowledging colonial history and acknowledge the impact on Indigenous lives (e.g., Egan & Restall, 2022; Hammell, 2020). Certainly, from a colonized perspective, occupations founded in coloniality are obvious, recognizable, certain, habitual, well-practiced, and frequently harmful.

However, settler colonial societies continue to deny coloniality which makes the work of examining one's personal and professional engagement with it all the more tricky. Honest scrutiny and understanding of how colonialism operates in one's life is an exact antidote to coloniality because at its fundamental core, coloniality prefers opacity and severance of relationships to self, purpose, lands, histories, and each other. Thus, examination of one's relationship with coloniality needs to be simultaneously deeply personal, intentionally collaborative, and expansively collective. This section supports the reader to explore their own engagement to coloniality and decoloniality through a series of questions, and explication of decolonial approaches to knowledge. The reader is encouraged to consider values, ethics, and social positioning in relation to decolonial occupational therapy praxis and to invite trusted peers into those considerations.

11.3 Settler Colonialism, Coloniality, and Decoloniality

This text is interested in settler colonialism because it is a driver of the dominant global north arrangements in occupational therapy. Tuck and Gaztambide-Fernández (2013) described settler colonialism as "the specific formation of colonialism in which the colonizer comes to stay, making himself the sovereign, and the arbiter of citizenship, civility, and knowing" (p. 73). As a "warmup" exercise for antiracism workshops, Dr Heather Came, activist scholar, invites attendees to consider and discuss the question, "What is your relationship to settler colonialism?". The question directly engages the work of examining one's relationship, benefits, oppression, inheritance, and forced associations with colonialism, however much denied.

> **11.1 Textbox: What Is Your Relationship to Coloniality?**
>
> Consider the lands, territories, and, where applicable, the Indigenous communities where you study or practice. When and how are Indigenous communities noticed, acknowledged, and responded to? What are the words, language, and processes used? What is your family's inheritance and/or relationship to settler colonialism? How do you feel about this and coloniality? What does that mean for your practice?

Ramugondo (2018) provided a deft analysis of coloniality in relation to occupation and posed the following: "If full humanness refers to a thinking and knowledgeable being, then occupational therapy must have a problem with the framing of certain beings as incapable of thinking, or less knowledgeable" (Ramugondo, 2018, p. 87). Coloniality relies on such ideological framing, resources, systems, minds, and bodies. Ramugondo's (2015, 2018) theoretical examinations and explorations rightly assume that occupation is problematic, or rather, that colonial theories and expressions of occupation are. Hence, as occupational therapists and occupational scientists, it is necessary to establish one's personal and professional engagement in coloniality.

Importantly, decolonial academics show that coloniality does not wish to be known, have its sites examined, nor its boundaries mapped. Instead, it wants to be served and reproduced often, from the background and without examination, which makes everyday occupation the perfect vehicle. Everyday occupations are where colonialism is transmitted generation to generation, by way of conversation and gesture, approval, and disapproval, "hidden in plain sight" (Emery-Whittington, in press). Hence, if one is not decolonizing everyday occupations, then it is doubtful that one is decolonizing curriculum, research, or practice. Decoloniality requires different epistemologies and pedagogies, learning infrastructures, audit tools, and membership from those that are created by, and for, coloniality.

There is a direct link between decoloniality and values. Values are the place one "goes home to" and where we lean into when change or challenge occurs. As decolonial praxis becomes more usual, values act like guardrails to ensure a perspective beyond the window of coloniality and into wide vistas of global contexts. Knowing one's values requires a habit of thoughtfulness about how one is in relation to opportunities, choices, dilemmas, and difficulties, but especially when one encounters folk who hold relatively less power and privilege to us.

Occupational therapy programs tend to lean into Western ethics when facilitating discussions about ethics and values. This means that students may not be aware of alternative sets of ethics that guide colleagues and communities outside the global north. Making sense of values and ethics in settler colonial societies is tricky especially where settler colonialism is denied or minimized. Certainly, ignoring settler colonialism in the design and facilitation of health programs is a characteristic of colonially led curricula. However, in the recent trend for decoloniality in curricula, it is expected that global ethics and values are designed into the program across content and processes.

11.2 Textbox: What Is Your Relationship to Decoloniality?

What are the values that guided you to pursue occupational therapy as a possible career? How have you become aware of the shared and personal values that guide you? How do your values align or become re-prioritized over time? In relation to oppression and privilege, how do you make sense of your guiding values? Who supports you to unpack this?

The process of knowing oneself, of identifying one's values and ethics, and learning to be fully cognizant of one's impact on the world, must be intentionally taught and role-modeled. Further, praxis that is based on values must be observed and mentored in our peers, community, lecturers/educators, and professional body every day. For instance, when learners observe educators taking direct action in the face of expressions of social injustice on campus, racism during a lecture, and ableism over lunch, it fosters a sense of "how to" and gives the expectation of decoloniality. This then leads to further direct actions, whereas observing educators only "talking about" injustice sans direct action creates a sense that "talking about injustice" is a sufficient response to, or worse is, injustice.

Decoloniality is a praxis of unlearning and undoing coloniality across everyday occupations, and spans entire ways of being, thinking, appreciating, doing, and belonging. Yet, there is no singular universal way of doing, being, and becoming decolonial because oppression is slightly different everywhere and bespoke responses are necessary. However, a consistent theme of decoloniality is daily refusal to support any expression of oppression and its harms, especially coloniality. A natural slope where decolonial praxis aligns and flows toward is the agreement that coloniality causes people to be treated inequitably (Reid, 2021). Thus, a decolonial inquiry is not "is colonialism present here?" but instead, "can we locate, map, and name the sites of colonialism in our practice spaces?" and following that "by what means?" and "what values and knowledge might scaffold a decolonial inquiry?".

11.4 A Decolonial Approach to Knowledge and Learning

Where is knowledge from? From where does knowledge arise and what does it take to perceive knowledge? Every tradition and society have taught and learned, held, treasured, and guarded knowledge over many centuries. A decolonial approach to knowledge and learning requires serious considerations of questions around knowledge because colonialism has contended that the only kind of knowledge that is of value is that which has arisen among its own core sites. Conversely, some traditions ascribe to the importance of trusting that knowledge evolves for good reason within local, bespoke situations and are expressed through occupations in the manner that makes sense, even if that sense is unknown to outside observations. This is a very different approach to knowledge in Western spaces where knowledge is considered "generalizable" and at times applied universally.

Therefore, a decolonial approach to knowledge and learning is first and foremost local and appreciative of the spaces – physical, ancestral, historical, spiritual, collective – that grow and hold knowledge. Just like coloniality is different in different contexts, so too must decoloniality be. Thus, efforts to create a generalized approach to "the" decolonial curricula, "the" decolonial chapter, etc., deserve a level of skepticism and critique.

Decoloniality is about considered action, reflection, and further action and is not about filling a "knowledge gap". The notion of a "knowledge gap" has limited the profession's growth to new and emerging engagement and development regarding decoloniality. Rather, limited growth exists because the profession is still arriving at decolonial work with colonially fashioned skills, processes, and attitudes to global south knowledge. Instead, this chapter is about arriving at decoloniality because there is a collective sense of indignation at the unexamined maintenance of coloniality in the profession and the harm that this causes every day.

The "knowledge gap trap" is one that assumes an ability and capacity to receive all kinds of knowledge that relate to any culture, anywhere, anytime and their many and varied ways of knowing beyond our own. Importantly, not all knowledge is or should be available to all (Tuck & Gaztambide-Fernández, 2013). From an Indigenous vantage, some knowledge is only able to be sought after and held by certain people and at certain times. In addition, only after long periods of observation of the person's character, enacted values, and way of relating to their community and knowledge will knowledge be shared.

Indigenous perspectives of knowledge differ to that which seeds and maintains Western-oriented occupational therapy programs. In Western systems, identified knowledge bearers are those that can rely on social, cultural, and financial capital which may or may not consider their character and values. Decolonial praxis however requires the occupational therapist to understand what historical trauma and historical privilege continue to afford and deny (Borell et al., 2018). As comforting as checklists and identified knowledge gaps may be, decoloniality requires relationships to be built or restored while being cognizant of the mechanisms that perpetuate and crave coloniality.

With regard to the profession's early and developing engagement with decoloniality, many publications introduce the reader to decolonial thinking, writings, and ways of being from beyond the profession. Indigenous academics and colleagues such as Elelwani Ramugondo, Chontel Gibson, Angie Phenix, Kaarina Valavaara, and Juman Simaan, among others, are also examining occupational theory and decoloniality. Notably, much of what is written by non-Indigenous writers regarding decoloniality – as scientists and connoisseurs of everyday occupation – excludes how one is decolonizing one's own everyday lives, homes, and communities. Instead, there is a narrowed focus on decolonizing occupational therapy curricula and education programs rather than how decolonization is occurring in personal lives beyond the classroom, project, or research.

Many occupational therapy publications regarding professional knowledge and practice aim to capture and share new contemporary insights. However, not all cultures believe that poiēsis, or the act of bringing something new into creation, is what is occurring. Rather, knowledge is always occurring in relation to what already is, and some knowledge is considered to be accessible only through humility and toil. Further, revelations of learning arise from and already exist in other-worldly realms waiting for the learner to perceive it. Manifested learning then has wisdom added over time via many hands, hearts, and minds, which ensures that it is refined, improved, and makes sense for the community.

Everyday occupation is the profession's scope and focus, but it occurs in the context of coloniality and racism. This means that coloniality is also the backdrop to our understandings and language of occupation, occupational therapy, and the foundational sciences that inform it. Somewhat predictably, language regarding decoloniality and occupation remains somewhat unexplored and underdeveloped. However, the development of decolonial praxis, including language, will be greatly enhanced by sharing personal and professional experiences of decoloniality. The following section invites the reader to examine social positioning based upon an exploration of values.

11.5 Social Positioning
Examination of who we are in relation to colonialism is essentially an exercise in deeply understanding who we are in relation to each other and the world around us. This work

is antiracist, intersectional, and collectivist because it is the opposite of colonialism where the multiple and varied differences in human appearance and character have been used as a categorization of human value. Social positioning is a critical practice that values relationships and connections to topics and issues of the day. Hammell (2020) implored critical occupational therapists to recognize that what is said, and how we view what is said and known, comes from somewhere.

When an author or speaker states their social position in relation to the topic at hand, colleagues can get a sense of the authority, relationships, and connections that are in play. Social positioning can be conveyed as a statement before a written text or spoken word and functions to build trust. As well, trustworthiness is enhanced by the author or speaker who has taken the time to curate words that honestly and clearly convey connection to the topic at hand. For Indigenous decolonial scholars this includes reciprocal relationships with local folk who are connected to and knowledgeable of the territories where they practice. Non-Indigenous practitioners would do well to bring thoughtful consideration of Indigenous and/or local folk upon whose lands the institution is situated (Stewart-Ambo & Yang, 2021).

> **11.3 Textbox: Social Positioning and Background**
>
> Social positioning and background impact how one views and relates to terms such as "family", "power", "relationship", "privilege", and "landback". Meditating on such terms may bring to mind certain images and perhaps trigger feelings. What are the images and feelings that arise when you consider each of these terms? What meaning do you make from these and how does your understanding of your social positioning impact this?

11.6 Understanding Race and Racism

Despite a quarter century since the American Anthropological Association's (AAA) 1998 Statement on Race clarifying that "race as a biological concept" is disproven, it continues to scaffold and structure social power. Indeed, as much as race is contemporarily considered a "folk belief" that "led to countless errors" (AAA, 1998), the idea of race and therefore racial superiority is still very much in play. Racism is a socially constructed set of ideologies that lives occupationally and needs "race" to lend a plausible morality and justification of violent exploitation practices against human folk and their territories. Such violence and its justifications extend to the environment and Indigenous territories for the benefit of Western cultures and societies (Te Kāhui Tika Tangata Human Rights Commission, 2022). Racism halts, changes, and denies connection between groups and communities of people, between people and their territories, and between people and their stories, identities, and histories.

Racism is expressed occupationally and at times enforced violently but is still a fledgling concern in occupational therapy. Hence poor engagement across theories, models, and practices signals that the profession agrees with, supports, or is at least not outraged by its own reproduction of racism. As a social determinant of health (Commission on Social Determinants of Health, 2007) racism has attracted a huge and growing base of research and evidence across health and justice sectors. Racism can now be measured for physiological impacts and psychological distress (e.g., Marsh et al., 2010) and overall well-being (Williams & Mohammed, 2013). Racism is an entirely avoidable social harm (Borell et al., 2009) and as the profession has no plan to end racism and oppression, it will continue to violate and inhibit the profession's growth and harm our communities.

A consequence of unaddressed and denied racism means that occupational therapy clinics and classrooms continue to be sites of racism. Upon entry to training programs, some learners are already well started on their work toward social justice, while some are newly exposed to the need for it. Occupational therapy needs a plan to ensure that students who know a great deal about oppression and inequities are not expected to "teach"/"share" among peers who can be still learning how to listen deeply and respectfully. A culturally safe classroom would not leverage colonial power to make labor requests on students and would instead be prepared to address racism every time in real time as a usual function of the pedagogy. The decolonial educator would anticipate situations where oppression might occur and work to end its expression by putting into place pedagogical structures, role-modeling, and conversations that address expressions of coloniality anytime it appears (Blaise, 2010).

What then might the goal of understanding and explicating one's engagement with coloniality (oppression and racism) and decoloniality look like? As previously mentioned, decoloniality is not about broadening the mind. The goal is to create a post-colonial community – that is well-versed and practiced in sharing power – who protects and cares for our shared home: Planet Earth. Therefore, decolonial praxis requires that space is made for all historically excluded communities, whose place is not to fill a knowledge gap, yet demonstrate how to be in relationship. Making space means becoming well-versed in invisible yet everyday expressions and reproductions of colonialism which successfully sever relationships and connections. The following section highlights decolonial thinking by colleagues who have explicated links between occupation and coloniality from ancient, Indigenous, and critical perspectives.

11.7 Links between Occupation and Coloniality

Decolonial scholars and practitioners across the globe have contributed theoretical examinations to the profession regarding the links between occupation and coloniality. Ramugondo (2015) made the case for occupational consciousness and alongside mentors and colleagues expanded the analysis to coloniality and decoloniality in 2018. Gibson (2020) brought clarity to racism and antiracism as expressed occupationally within the profession and Simaan (2020) shared Indigenous knowledge as decoloniality despite terrors of denied military occupation. These contributions highlight how analysis of coloniality as expressed occupationally are themselves simultaneously anti-oppressive and deeply connecting.

Colonization also can be understood as occupational stages (Emery-Whittington, 2021). That is, colonization begins with occupations of market research where researchers scout and record the homes and territories of "encountered" communities. The second occupational stage of colonization is often led by militaries which occupy, seize, steal, and illegally claim the homes and territories of the communities. The third occupational stage of colonization is often aimed at children of the communities who are forced to spend days, weeks, months, and years learning the colonizer's language and everyday occupations. Their parents are pre-occupied with colonial tools such as land loss, alcohol, religion, low/no waged employment, bureaucracy, and imposed justice, education, and health systems. The final occupational stage of colonization is where the colonizer's language, traditions, histories, and ideologies of supremacy take up residence in the mind, often replacing those of the community and creating irreconcilable tensions. These tensions are a result of fresh daily colonial harms and expressions and, over time, can themselves become a source of transmitted colonial harm onto one's own communities.

11.8 How the Profession Upholds Coloniality

The following section is drawn from a collection of observations over three decades of how coloniality is upheld in occupational therapy and occupational science. The collection is roughly ordered into four parts; a map of sorts, if coloniality is the destination. The four parts are a colonial worldview's system of *beliefs*, a colonial worldview's *characteristics*, a colonial worldview's *goals*, and a colonial worldview's *protections*.

11.8.1 Beliefs

Privilege and supremacy are essential foundational values of a colonial worldview. They are fixed beliefs that despite irony and harm caused are foundational to colonial practices which are enacted and reproduced daily. As enduring beliefs, privilege and white supremacy occur and recur for centuries in settler colonial spaces. Borell and colleagues (2018) have included the temporal reach of privilege in their working definition of historical privilege:

> The complex and collective structural advantages experienced over time and across generations by a group of people who share an identity, affiliation, or circumstance. These structured advantages may include financial and economic rewards, as well as legal, social and cultural freedoms that were denied to others. (p. 26)

Examples of privilege and white supremacy in the profession include curriculum (Grenier, 2020), "calls to action" sans structural change (Kronenberg, 2021), regular development of theories and tools that ignore and deny colonialism (Emery-Whittington, 2021; Hammell, 2011), and apologies for racist deeds during public gatherings that include no plans for further action. In addition, colonial beliefs, underlying values, and outward expressions of these can appear to be open for examination and critique, especially where and when harm is both public and undeniable. But those examinations are often short-lived and quickly moved on from despite being incommensurate with espoused ethics and published codes of conduct.

Like many health professions founded on Western traditions and values, occupational therapy, and latterly occupational science, struggle to respond systematically to white supremacy and privilege. Part of the struggle is attributable to the pervasive sense of sufficiency; that what needs to be known, theorized, taught, and practiced are for the most part already within the profession's grasp. If there is more to learn, that can be later added as improvements to the "core" (values, curricula) or "foundations" (theories and scope) that already exist. There is an over-confidence in what is and an under-estimation of what could be. This type of an approach presumes that the status quo is not racist, oppressive, exclusionary, stigmatizing, discriminatory, limiting, unjust, or harmful. This means that even small and ineffective areas of "learning and growth" attract attention, funding, and celebration despite unproven impact. The danger in early celebrations without evidence of positive change is that vulnerable and historically excluded communities might reduce protections from racialized targeting and, in so doing, experience more harm than is usual.

Hammell's 2020 book titled *Engagement in living: Critical perspectives on occupation, rights, and wellbeing* and the Canadian Association of Occupational Therapists' book *Promoting occupational participation: Collaborative relationship-focused occupational therapy* (Egan & Restall, 2022) both outline and promote a critical approach to occupational therapy. An important aspect of a critical approach to practice is the recognition that up to now, global north parts of the profession have not needed to consider colonialism. This is a direct result of privilege and supremacy, and despite being new considerations for some they are nonetheless contexts of occupation. The shape and expressions of coloniality can differ depending on the contexts, but supremacy and privilege underlie most.

11.8.2 Characteristics

Power – especially colonial power – is easier to fathom when one does not have it. Coloniality is immediately recognizable in how welcome one is made to feel over time – or not – and how one's identities and cultures are acknowledged and celebrated – or not. Language chosen, atmosphere, and patterns of communication that build community all paint a picture of how power is shared or wielded. Inclusiveness, exclusiveness, relatedness, and distance as usual and expected ways of being are readily perceived and understood. How a professional space acknowledges or ignores colonialism also signals colonial power.

From my experience, coloniality is characteristically contradictory such as requesting "cultural advice" and then rejecting said advice, creating spaces to "hear, understand and learn" and then becoming defensive and at times aggressive during such discussions. Harts (2021) referred to the all-encompassing and often traumatic backdrop that is working as a Black woman in the United States, in workplaces that support racist and oppressive policies and practices. Racialized targeting and trauma can and does occur – and perhaps especially so – when a workplace hires a single "diverse" voice. The single voice typically becomes isolated from the community they represent, overburdened with an increasing workload, on limited hours with sometimes reasonable – but often late – support from colleagues when racialized targeting occurs.

Another characteristic of coloniality is a particular focus on cultural competency (Grenier et al., 2020). New Zealand institutions have pursued the goal of finding and employing "cultural experts" to support growth of non-Indigenous colleagues' cultural competency and readiness to work with Indigenous peoples. One of the presumptions of this approach to learning is that knowing something "about" Indigenous language, culture, and Indigenous health models is what the Indigenous communities most desire and need from these institutions. It also presumes that coloniality has been understood, mapped, learning processes and plans strategized, and then collaboratively actioned. Grenier (2020) argued that cultural competency has little evidence of significant positive impact for those it is purported to benefit, rather it embeds coloniality. These peculiar approaches to understanding coloniality make more sense when the goals of coloniality are clarified.

11.8.3 Goals

The main goals of coloniality are to gain and grow resources and power, which are believed to be finite and therefore must also be guarded and hoarded. These types of goals are unable to exist in harmony alongside nature. Gaining, guarding, and hoarding resources and power are inherently genocidal and ethnocidal, and require discrimination and supremacy to endure. What this means in the context of a health profession such as occupational therapy is a question still to be wrangled with.

Certainly, power sharing with historically excluded communities is not well demonstrated nor practiced, as evidenced by the lack of people of color in executive roles and decision-making spaces across the profession in governance, education, research, and clinical spaces. Lack of power and resource sharing is obvious in settler colonial spaces and global communities that are set up and controlled by settler colonials. Moreover, when disparities are highlighted, it can result in aggression and harm. Perhaps this explains a lack of a major revolt or movement against such colonial harms in the profession. To be sure, coloniality finds several ways to protect itself.

11.8.4 Protections

The profession has deployed a number of protections for coloniality, including appearing neutral, fair, and respectable, employing a singular "Diversity, Equity and Inclusion (DEI) hire" and controlling how coloniality and racism is allowed to be discussed. For instance, Beagan (2021) noted that as a new scholar to the discipline, upon submitting papers to occupational therapy journals, editors required that the word "perceived" was placed in front of the word "racism". Guiding language is an expected editorial task. However, when unacknowledged settler colonialism is the context of the writing, particular norms around how coloniality is allowed to be discussed means that coloniality is likely being protected.

Another protection of colonial harm is to create the appearance of civility and fairness such as promoting the idea of "a neutral position on racism". Although unsupported by neuroscience (Blaise, 2010), there is a presumption of innocence for the perpetrator and ascribed "misunderstanding" for the person of color who raises concerns about racism. Blaise (2010) argued that "being color blind" is an impossibility from a neuroscience perspective and can instead increase racial tensions. As a white educator, they noted that there is a difference between trying to avoid racism with taking actions to end racism in the classroom. Blaise (2010) noted that by trying to "see everyone as the same" and designing the curriculum to only include the "universal traditional canon", they had inadvertently made those who were not like them invisible.

When denial of oppression is no longer plausible, protections for coloniality turn to distractions and derailments. Distractions include hyper-focus on the messenger, who is typically a person from a historically excluded community, rather than what they are saying. In addition, deferring to policy/procedure/budget restrictions or creation of new steps/processes/guidelines also serve to delay right action and justice. Another protection is to appear to want to do decoloniality with promises of preparing to learn, planning to have a plan, and "having" a diversity/antiracism policy/champion. All function to appear as if positive change is, or soon will, occur while keeping power exactly where it is.

The employment of colleagues of color as cherry-picked "diversity hires" supports the colonial appearance of "learning". Unsurprisingly, few organizations have evaluated nor disseminated the impact of such employment situations. "Having" folk employed as the "diversity expert" is a cynical but predictable colonial characteristic because of the demands placed on the (often) sole practitioner and the historically excluded communities they represent. A too common characteristic is that such folk have limited experience and/or inclination to challenge the status quo and over time the person becomes overburdened and/or increasingly loyal to the mainstream organization, especially where salary and/or career opportunities are dependent on their continued loyalty.

In addition, job interviews for such positions tend to focus on how the person can support the cultural competency of the department/section/team. Organizations who are serious about their decolonial journey would ensure the interview process centers around the community, not a singular position. Instead, collaborative relationships with communities building trust over time would pre-empt creation of such positions. The organization itself might be interviewed for fit and expertize as much as the "community hire".

Where decoloniality is a stated goal, it is important to examine carefully who is in power in national, regional, and world institutions, and who are the speakers/chapter authors/representatives of "global voices". Coloniality is protected by people enacting roles that uphold coloniality. Is the way your country, its people, circumstances, and issues represented portrayed accurately and collaboratively?

Protections are not only about saving face or appearances of respectability. Protections can also include not-doing, delay, or withholding of opportunities and resources such as slow moves to look after colleagues who are racially targeted. This form of colonial harm goes beyond the racially targeted and vicariously impacts bystanders and allies. Such events also reveal how prepared allies are to stand with the racially targeted and, for some, they are found wanting. All is not lost however if the racially targeted are supported with honest discussions, healing actions, and meaningful changes to infrastructure in a timely fashion.

11.4 Textbox: Decolonial Approaches to Practice and Decoloniality at Home

In what ways does your home reflect connection? When tired or under pressure, where do you seek and find connection? Who supports you to reconnect with your purpose and unique contribution? How do you support others to seek and maintain supportive connections?

Decoloniality is deeply contextual and relies on a steady honest examination of our social positioning and privilege. It requires leaning in to unlearning (Zafran, 2021) and being mindful of early messaging and messages conveyed over one's lifetime. Recalling what teachings occur at home, work, and community spaces can be as simple as considering closely what we hear ourselves say, especially among family. How do we teach children to perceive and respond when they encounter folk who are weaker, stronger, slower, faster, poorer, richer than them? What meanings do we support them to make with regard to coloniality and decoloniality?

As much as coloniality is expressed occupationally, it is also true that decoloniality is practiced every day, in small habitual, yet disruptive ways. For example, before writing and study sessions, meetings, lectures, clinic appointments, and large speaking events, I take a moment to call to mind and connect with the main purpose and goal of the next action. I pray, consider wise words of an ancestor or trusted guide and these often bring clarity and peace that help me get a sense of my contribution to a shared purpose. Intentional, regular, and routine connection is a core tenet of decoloniality; connecting to one's own purpose for that purpose to connect to greater goals for the collective. Reverent reconnection to a greater purpose and deep considerations of relationship with purpose, society, and the planet, ensures that one can move beyond the pretenses and shallowness of individualism.

As mentioned above, sharing about decolonial praxis from the perspective of the non-Indigenous professional is still emerging. As an Indigenous woman and antiracism trainer, I have observed non-Indigenous folk posing honest questions about antiracist praxis to me. However, their listening is radically deeper when one of my non-Indigenous team members shares about how they are decolonizing their lives – personally and professionally. From my perspective, the minutiae, joys, challenges, failures, and eventual return to meaning and purpose of antiracist praxis are cherished by learners. It is a profound experience to witness this kind of sharing because it is humble, vulnerable, and powerful.

11.9 From "Talking about Culture" to Cultural Safety

Prior to calls for critical occupational therapy, the profession regarded and disseminated literature concerning Indigenous peoples from the perspective of non-Indigenous practitioners (e.g., Nelson, 2007; Thibeault, 2002). The topic of concern was often identified by the non-Indigenous researcher and community voices were interpreted and shared without Indigenous authorship. As well, a common conclusion included the importance of critical reflection upon cultural worldviews. The benefit of such research design for marginalized folk is unclear due to a lack of research showing how critical reflexivity led to structural change.

Following early descriptions of the "other", discussions about historically excluded or marginalized communities began to be reported through a lens of occupational injustice (e.g., Whiteford, 2005). The practice of researching, writing, and learning about historically excluded communities aligns with cultural competency – a practice that centers the individual practitioner's skills and knowledge. However, if learning about the colonized and marginalized communities was sufficient, then tourism alone would have solved inequity and racism by now. As previously discussed, cultural competence is a predictable characteristic of a colonial worldview; instead of making space for and appreciating global knowledges, a cultural competence lens diminishes them to how understandable, packageable, and colonially useful their service could be.

Around the same time that occupational justice was beginning to take root, the Social Occupational Therapy movement in South America, particularly in Brazil, was gaining strength. The collective and collaborative focus was built on long traditions of critique of social injustices (Lopes & Malfitano, 2020). Iwama (2003, 2006) and Hammell (2009, 2011, 2020) engaged and examined taken-for-granted assumptions of occupational therapy practice in the Western world, and collections of writings such as *Occupational therapies without borders* (Kronenberg et al., 2011) furthered such examinations. Indeed, the number of contributions to critical occupational therapy increased markedly following the murder of Mr George Floyd in 2020 (Wijekoon & Peter, 2023). Critical examination of colonial structures, theories, models, and tools that uphold colonialism is now well underway (e.g., Grenier et al., 2020; Hendricks et al., 2023; Turcotte & Holmes, 2023).

It is argued that cultural competence provides a plausible distraction from two central aspects of cultural safety: sharing power and centering the experience of people who receive health services rather than staff skills and knowledge. In programs and clinics that seek to create cultural safety, one would experience and witness power sharing with the most vulnerable. The *experience* of equity in practice – of power shared in the moment – is an entirely different experience that draws in and heals all who are witness and central to the moment.

Cultural safety was explored and shared in 1992 by Kaja Jungersen, an Indigenous woman of Aotearoa New Zealand and an occupational therapist. With power being so central to cultural safety, structural analysis and decision making are also key aspects of cultural safety. Cultural safety gets behind distractions of cultural competence to the colossal but unanswered question of settler colonial legitimacy in Indigenous lands and territories. Certainly, the profession, like many, has yet to grapple meaningfully with the "unresolved business of Indigenous sovereignty…" (Bond et al., 2021, p. 86) and what that means for everyday occupation.

At the core of critical occupational therapy is the reasonable assumption that unless an institution has purposefully and specifically designed in decoloniality, then it is likely reproducing the colonial status quo. The performance of equity in boardroom presentations, conferences, and publications without meaningful examination and analysis is an odd strategy in the face of need. There is a direct correlation between the profession's performative calls for decolonial praxis with ongoing racialized and oppressive harms to Black and Indigenous People of Color (BIPOC) colleagues and communities. It turns out that the performance of decoloniality is in effect coloniality.

Coloniality gets to reproduce without mitigations because of the lack of power sharing, leadership, and strategy to do so. Certainly, decoloniality is relational and a team sport that requires many working together toward an agreed goal. It is possible that local, national, and now international collectives and affinity groups to support, provide leadership, and healing for the profession is the pathway forward. Knowledge shared and generated within such collectives are anti-colonial and growing, as seen in the rise of Māori OT Network, DisruptOT, BAMEOTUK, ABLEOTUK, and more (Emery-Whittington et al., 2023).

Knowing one's sphere of influence and using this strategically alongside peers who are actively decolonizing is a powerful way to engage in decolonial praxis. Attending to particular literature, citing conscientiously (Mott & Cockayne, 2017), developing language of decolonial praxis, and healing from harms are all aspects of decolonial collectives. Examination of social positioning and privilege prior to building relationships with global colleagues and knowledges builds trust and trustworthiness among collectives. These kinds of collegial spaces can make and safely hold space for global knowledges where coloniality is displaced and potentially undone.

11.10 A Brief Note to BIPOC Colleagues

If healing in this day and age is like water, then decoloniality is the cup that carries it. However, as Western occupational therapy institutions turn to global south ways of understanding and practicing, it is essential that global south communities do not pour our epistemologies, pedagogies, and praxis into half-rendered cups. The need to "appear to be doing equity" is strong and can often pull BIPOC students and colleagues away from vital work with our own communities. Centering the question "*In what ways does this work benefit my community?*" ensures that the voices and desires for our decoloniality stay at the core of our focus. Indeed, if occupational balance can exist in capitalist societies, global south efforts of creating a decolonial profession must be balanced with uplifting our own communities. Whether or not those with colonial power ready themselves to engage in vastly different ways of being, doing, and belonging, those that remember and identify with knowledge and collectivist practices of caring for and protecting Earth Mother must continue to do so.

Addressing coloniality means being mindful of the relationship we have with it, finding and mapping it, acknowledging its harms and barriers to equity, and collaborating across institutions to end it. Sometimes it involves going within and finding any stereotypes and colonial stories that have become – through no fault of our own – internalized (Emery-Whittington & Davis, 2023). Maintaining regular contact with community elders, territories, and nature heals and brings clarity in difficult times. Collegial healing circles can be pivotal in supporting racially targeted BIPOC colleagues to negotiate pathways back to our healed selves. Finally, while occupational therapy is beginning its journey into antiracist decolonial praxis, it is not without cost to BIPOC colleagues. Unthinking public commentary, fully engaged defamation, refusal to reflect on advice, and rage at the boardroom table mean that the work of undoing coloniality and inequity falls to every occupational therapist and occupational scientist.

11.11 Conclusion

"It is significant that racism is part of colonialism throughout the world; and it is no coincidence" (Memmi, 1965, pp. 69–70). Whenever coloniality's presence is denied and minimized it greatly impacts the ability to critically examine its manifestations, mechanisms, and patterns. Occupational therapy and occupational science have a unique contribution to understanding the links between coloniality, decoloniality, and occupation. However, a major barrier to unlocking the potential and healing of everyday occupation is the profession's deep and rarely acknowledged investment in, and practice of, coloniality.

Despite this, a growing number of global south theorists, practitioners, and global north colleagues are forming and joining anti-oppressive decolonial collectives. Manifestly different relationships, power-sharing arrangements, infrastructure, and goals are guiding the movement away from the reproduction of colonial harm such as performative calls for change. These collectives show how fair space for global knowledges can be made, appreciated, and looked after through practices of connectedness and relationship. They are themselves holding space and a vision for the whole profession whether global leaders and their resources believe, join, or value decoloniality or not. Recolonization of spaces is always possible but less likely when decolonized occupation is used as a platform for connection and reconnection to each other and life purpose.

11.12 Summary

- Understanding one's relationship and investment in coloniality is crucial to decolonial praxis.
- Coloniality prefers disconnection and ignorance, while decoloniality requires relationship and new ways of knowing.
- Knowledge is culturally framed and for occupational therapy, colonially constructed.
- Occupation is the means by which coloniality is transmitted.
- The profession upholds coloniality through core beliefs, characteristics, goals, and protective measures.
- Decoloniality begins at home and resides in the language and processes we utilize every day.
- Decolonial collectives can promote growth, facilitate healing, and be the relationships we are both held to and actively support.

11.13 Review Questions

1. Write a brief social positioning statement and share with a trusted friend. What do you notice about that process?
2. How would you describe the difference between cultural competence and cultural safety to a classmate? Please share.
3. In the past month, how have you consciously shared power? What happened and how was equity enhanced?
4. How have your educators, supervisors, or managers role-modeled inclusive antiracist praxis?
5. Who are five authors that critique settler colonialism that you could follow or cite? Do any of them write or publish in languages other than English?

References

American Anthropological Association. (1998). *Statement on race*. https://tinyurl.com/53kadh3v

Beagan, B. L. (2021). Commentary on racism in occupational science. *Journal of Occupational Science, 28*(3), 410–413. https://doi.org/10.1080/14427591.2020.1833682

Blaise, D. (2010). The perils of colour blindness. In J. Marsh, R. Mendoza-Denton, & J. A. Smith (Eds.), *Are we born racist? New insights from neuroscience and positive psychology* (pp. 71–74). Beacon Press.

Bond, C. J., Singh, D., & Tyson, S. (2021). Black bodies and bioethics: Debunking mythologies of benevolence and beneficence in contemporary Indigenous health research in colonial Australia. *Journal of Bioethical Inquiry, 18*(1), 83–92. https://doi.org/10.1007/s11673-020-10079-8

Borell, B., Moewaka Barnes, H., & McCreanor, T. (2018). Conceptualising historical privilege: The flip side of historical trauma, a brief examination. *AlterNative: An International Journal of Indigenous Peoples, 14*(1), 25–34. https://doi.org/10.1177/1177180117742202

Borell, B. A. E., Gregory, A. S., McCreanor, T. N., Jensen, V. G. L., & Moewaka Barnes, H. (2009). It's hard at the top but it's a whole lot easier than being at the bottom: The role of privilege in understanding disparities in Aotearoa/New Zealand. *Race/Ethnicity: Multidisciplinary Global Contexts, 3*(1), 29–50. https://www.jstor.org/stable/25595023

Commission on Social Determinants of Health. (2007). Achieving health equity: From root causes to fair outcomes. *The Lancet, 370*(9593), 1153–1163. https://doi.org/10.1016/S0140-6736(07)61385-3

Egan, M., & Restall, G. (Eds.). (2022). *Promoting occupational participation: Collaborative relationship-focused occupational therapy*. Canadian Association of Occupational Therapists.

Emery-Whittington, I. G. (2021). Occupational justice: Colonial business as usual? Indigenous observations from Aotearoa New Zealand. *Canadian Journal of Occupational Therapy, 88*(2), 153–162. https://doi.org/10.1177%2F00084174211005891

Emery-Whittington, I. (in press). Decoloniality in action: A Kaupapa Māori occupational analysis of colonization. In S. Baptiste & S. Shann (Eds.), *International handbook of occupational therapy*. Taylor & Francis.

Emery-Whittington, I., & Davis, G. (2023). Rapua te kurahuna: An occupational perspective of internalised oppression. *AlterNative: An International Journal of Indigenous Peoples, 19*(4), 762–770. https://doi.org/10.1177/11771801231206209

Emery-Whittington, I., Leite Junior, J., & Ivlev, S. (2023). Antiracism as means and ends. In M. Ahmed-Landeryou (Ed.), *Antiracist occupational therapy: Unsettling the status quo* (pp. 119–136). Jessica Kingsley Publishers.

Gibson, C. (2020). When the river runs dry: Leadership, decolonisation and healing in occupational therapy. *New Zealand Journal of Occupational Therapy, 67*(1), 11–20. https://search.informit.org/doi/10.3316/informit.162982618221927

Grenier, M.-L. (2020). Cultural competency and the reproduction of white supremacy in occupational therapy education. *Health Education Journal, 79*(6), 633–644. https://doi.org/10.1177/0017896920902515

Grenier, M.-L., Zafran, H., & Roy, L. (2020). Current landscape of teaching diversity in occupational therapy education: A scoping review. *American Journal of Occupational Therapy, 74*(6), 7406205100p1–7406205100p15. https://doi.org/10.5014/ajot.2020.044214

Hammell, K. W. (2009). Sacred texts: A sceptical exploration of the assumptions underpinning theories of occupation. *Canadian Journal of Occupational Therapy, 76*(1), 6–13. https://doi.org/10.1177%2F000841740907600105

Hammell, K. W. (2011). Resisting theoretical imperialism in the disciplines of occupational science and occupational therapy. *British Journal of Occupational Therapy, 74*(1), 27–33. https://doi.org/10.4276/030802211X12947686093602

Hammell, K. W. (2020). *Engagement in living: Critical perspectives on occupation, rights, and wellbeing*. Canadian Association of Occupational Therapists.

Harts, M. (2021). *Right within: How to heal from racial trauma in the workplace*. Seal Press.

Hendricks, F., Singleton, M., Clark, A., Mishin, M., & Epps, M. (2023). A narrative review of student evaluations of teaching in decolonial praxis: Implications for occupational therapy higher education. *The Open Journal of Occupational Therapy, 11*(1), 1–16. https://doi.org/10.15453/2168-6408.1969

Iwama, M. (2003). Toward culturally relevant epistemologies in occupational therapy. *American Journal of Occupational Therapy, 57*(5), 582–588. https://doi.org/10.5014/ajot.57.5.582

Iwama, M. K. (2006). *The Kawa Model: Culturally relevant occupational therapy*. Elsevier.

Jungersen, K. (1992). Culture, theory, and the practice of occupational therapy in New Zealand/Aotearoa. *American Journal of Occupational Therapy, 46*(8), 745–750. https://doi.org/10.5014/ajot.46.8.745

Kronenberg, F. (2021). Commentary on JOS Editorial Board's anti-racism pledge. *Journal of Occupational Science, 28*(3), 398–403. https://doi.org/10.1080/14427591.2020.1827483

Kronenberg, F., Pollard, N., & Sakellariou, D. (Eds.). (2011). *Occupational therapies without borders: Volume 2 – Towards an ecology of occupational-based practices*. Elsevier.

Lopes, R. E., & Malfitano, A. P. S. (2020). *Social occupational therapy: Theoretical and practical designs*. Elsevier Health Sciences.

Marsh, J., Mendoza-Denton, R., & Smith, J. A. (Eds.). (2010). *Are we born racist?: New insights from neuroscience and positive psychology*. Beacon Press.

Memmi, A. (1965). *The colonizer and the colonized*. Beacon Press.

Mott, C., & Cockayne, D. (2017). Citation matters: Mobilizing the politics of citation toward a practice of 'conscientious engagement'. *Gender, Place and Culture, 24*(7), 954–973. https://doi.org/10.1080/0966369X.2017.1339022

Nelson, A. (2007). Seeing white: A critical exploration of occupational therapy with indigenous Australian people. *Occupational Therapy International, 14*(4), 237–255. https://doi.org/10.1002/oti.236

Ramugondo, E. L. (2015). Occupational consciousness. *Journal of Occupational Science, 22*(4), 488–501. https://doi.org/10.1080/14427591.2015.1042516

Ramugondo, E. L. (2018). Healing work: Intersections for decoloniality. *World Federation of Occupational Therapists Bulletin, 74*(2), 83–91. https://tinyurl.com/2hs9ss4b

Reid, P. (2021). Structural reform or a cultural reform? Moving the health and disability sector to be pro-equity, culturally safe, Tiriti compliant and anti-racist. *The New Zealand Medical Journal (Online), 134*(1535), 7–10.

Simaan, J. (2020). Decolonising occupational science education through learning activities based on a study from the global south. *Journal of Occupational Science, 27*(3), 432–442. https://doi.org/10.1080/14427591.2020.1780937

Stewart-Ambo, T., & Yang, K. W. (2021). Beyond land acknowledgment in settler institutions. *Social Text 146, 39*(1), 21–46. https://doi.org/10.1215/01642472-8750076

Te Kāhui Tika Tangata Human Rights Commission. (2022). *Maranga mai! The dynamics and impacts of white supremacy, racism, and colonisation upon tangata whenua in Aotearoa New Zealand*. https://tikatangata.org.nz/our-work/maranga-mai

Thibeault, R. (2002). Fostering healing through occupation: The case of the Canadian Inuit. *Journal of Occupational Science, 9*(3), 153–158. http://doi.org/10.1080/14427591.2002.9686503

Tuck, E., & Gaztambide-Fernández, R. A. (2013). Curriculum, replacement, and settler futurity. *Journal of Curriculum Theorizing, 29*(1), 71–89. https://journal.jctonline.org/index.php/jct/issue/view/20

Turcotte, P.-L., & Holmes, D. (2023). The shadow side of occupational therapy: Necropower, state racism and colonialism. *Scandinavian Journal of Occupational Therapy*, 1–14. https://doi.org/10.1080/11038128.2023.2264330

Whiteford, G. E. (2005). Understanding the occupational deprivation of refugees: A case study from Kosovo. *Canadian Journal of Occupational Therapy, 72*(2), 78–88. https://doi.org/10.1177/000841740507200202

Wijekoon, S., & Peter, N. (2023). Examining racial, ethnic, and cultural diversity in occupational science research: Perspectives of persons of color. *Journal of Occupational Science, 30*(3), 322–341. https://doi.org/10.1080/14427591.2022.2119269

Williams, D. R., & Mohammed, S. A. (2013). Racism and health 1: Pathways and scientific evidence. *American Behavioral Scientist, 57*(8), 1200–1226. https://tinyurl.com/bddyj64p

Zafran, H. (2021). Lost in translation: The languages of a critical occupational therapy. *Occupational Therapy Now, 23*(6), 23–25.

CHAPTER 12

Critical Disability Studies Perspectives on Human Occupation

Marjorie Désormeaux-Moreau, Bethan Collins, Laura Yvonne Bulk, Susan Mahipaul, Stephanie LeBlanc-Omstead, and Tal Jarus

Abstract
This chapter introduces concepts central to disability studies and related areas that historically have not been included within mainstream occupational therapy and occupational science literature. Core to the understanding of how critical disability discourse relates to occupational therapy is recognizing the privileging of certain types of knowledge that have occurred within our profession which have, in effect, silenced critical disability perspectives (epistemic injustices). The chapter highlights concepts, including ableism and disablism, and, using independence as an example, it highlights how occupational therapy and occupational science knowledge could include concepts from within critical disability and related discourses.

Authors' Positionality Statement
We are a collective/group of disabled, chronically ill, mad, and neurodivergent-identifying occupational therapists and occupational scientists who have found community through and with each other in recent years. While it is true that we, as authors, each have *lived experiences* of the phenomena of disability, chronic illness, madness, and neurodivergence between us, the perspectives shared in this chapter are rooted in our collective *experiential knowledges* – or a critical (often politicized) evaluation of these experiences. The kinds of phenomena and experiences of which we write have been theorized extensively in the fields of critical disability studies (CDS), critical autism studies (CAS), and mad and neurodiversity studies, as well as disability/mad justice. We draw on these theories to interpret and create meaning from our collective experiences, not just our individual experiences. We are white women, from different parts of the Global North, who have had the privilege of occupational therapy education and have undertaken higher-level study and research.

Authors' note: In this chapter, "we" always refers to the authors. Also, for various reasons – which are similar to those mentioned by researchers in the field of Deaf studies – many authors dissociate CAS from CDS.

> **Objectives**
> This chapter will:
>
> - Introduce the concepts of critical disability studies and related fields.
> - Explore the impact of epistemic injustice as it relates to knowledge within critical disability studies and their consideration within occupational therapy and occupational science.
> - Define ableism, disablism, and related concepts.
> - Examine the concept of independence as discussed within occupational therapy and critical disability discourses.

> **Key terms**
>
> - critical disability studies
> - critical autism studies
> - mad studies
> - epistemic injustice
> - ableism
> - disablism
> - independence
> - interdependence

12.1 Introduction

> It should not be surprising that critical disability theorists perceive occupational therapists' neoliberal-inspired and ableist ideologies of self-reliance and independence to be both disempowering and out of step with disabled people's values, priorities and needs.
>
> *(Hammell, 2023, p. 750)*

Historically, knowledges from fields associated with disability studies have existed in parallel with those of occupational science and occupational therapy, intersecting only with difficulty (Grenier, 2021; Hammell, 2023). This chapter aims to introduce knowledges associated with critical disability studies (CDS) and proposes that these knowledges can be used to influence occupational therapy and occupational science theory and practice. We recognize that readers will be diverse, some with extensive knowledge of critical disability-related discourses, some with experiential knowledge and for others, concepts in this chapter may be less familiar or new. To support the reader, we have included Table 12.1 with definitions of terms and sources of further reading. Terms defined in Table 12.1 are marked with an asterisk (*) as they appear in the text.

Table 12.1 Definitions and Resources

Term	Definition	Further resources
Ableism	A system of assigning value to people's bodies and minds based on societally constructed ideas of normalcy, productivity, desirability, intelligence, excellence, and fitness. These constructed ideas are deeply rooted in eugenics, anti-Blackness, misogyny, colonialism, imperialism, and capitalism. This systemic oppression that leads to people and society determining people's value based on their culture, age, language, appearance, religion, birth or living place, "health/wellness", and/or their ability to satisfactorily re/produce, "excel" and "behave". You do not have to be disabled to experience ableism.	Working definition by @TalilaLewis Updated January 2022, developed in community with disabled Black/negatively racialized folk, especially @NotThreeFifths. Read more: bit.ly/ableism2022
Crip	A fluid and ever-expanding term used in disability communities and activism. Individuals with physical and sensory impairments, neurodivergence, and mental distress and diversity may claim crip to resist systemic able-bodied oppression within a society that refuses to, or does not want to, accommodate disabled (non-normative) bodyminds.	Kafer, A. (2013). *Feminist, queer, crip.* Indiana University Press. McRuer, R. (2006). *Crip theory: Cultural signs of queerness and disability.* New York University Press.
Crip wisdom	The knowledge and "lifegiving ways disabled, Deaf, sick, chronically ill and neurodivergent folk mentor each other, giving each other lifesaving wisdom that no doctor's office will". It is about the wisdom to slow down, creating movements, and staying at the pace of our slowest members, including disabled, parents, older folks, poor folks, caregivers, etc.	Tovah. (October 13, 2016). *Sins Invalid's "Birthing, Dying Becoming Crip Wisdom" Features Crip Art, Activism, Love & Liberation.* https://www.autostraddle.com/sins-invalids-birthing-dying-becoming-crip-wisdom-features-crip-art-activism-love-and-liberation-354749/
Critical autism studies (CAS)	A field that aims at "investigating power dynamics that operate in Discourses around autism, questioning deficit-based definitions of autism, and being willing to consider the ways in which biology and culture intersect to produce 'disability'" (p. 1337).	Waltz, M. (2014). Worlds of autism: Across the spectrum of neurological difference. *Disability & Society, 29*(8), 1337–1338. https://orcid.org/10.1080/09687599.2014.934064

(*Continued*)

Table 12.1 (Continued)

Critical disability studies (CDS)	CDS centers on academics and activists spanning multiple interdisciplinary fields (including cultural studies and humanities, feminist, postcolonial and queer thinkers, etc.). Disability is viewed as socially constructed, embodied, and impacted by societal and political power relations. Disability is interpreted through the lived experiences of disabled, chronically ill, and neurodivergent people.	Goodley, D. (2013). Dis/entangling critical disability studies. *Disability & Society, 28*(5), 631–644. https://doi.org/10.1080/09687599.2012.717884 Meekosha, H., & Shuttleworth, R. (2009). What's so "critical" about critical disability studies? *Australian Journal of Human Rights, 15*(1), 47–75. https://doi.org/10.1080/1323238X.2009.11910861
Disability	As in Disability Studies: The social disadvantages and exclusions that people with impairment face in all areas of life: employment, housing, education, civil rights, transportation, negotiation of the built environment, and so forth (p. 10).	Thomas, C. (2014). Disability and impairment. In J. Swain, C. Thomas, C. Barnes, & S. French (Eds.), *Disabling barriers, enabling environments* (3rd ed., pp. 9–16). Sage.
Disability justice	A disability justice framework understands that: ■ All bodies are unique and essential. ■ All bodies have strengths and needs that must be met. ■ We are powerful, not despite the complexities of our bodies, but because of them. ■ All bodies are confined by ability, race, gender, sexuality, class, nation state, religion, and more, and we cannot separate them. What has been consistent across disability justice – and must remain so – is the leadership of disabled people of color and of queer and gender non-conforming disabled people.	Invalid, S. (2019). *Skin, tooth, and bone: The basis of movement is our people – a disability justice primer* (2nd ed.). Sins Invalid.
Disabled occupations	The occupations unique to disabled people that reflect the disability-related work and care that is invisible and hidden from society. Coupled with normative violence, disabled occupations include expecting individuals to overcome adversity, undergo unnecessary treatments, and interventions to be normal (p. 8).	Mahipaul, S. (2022). Accounting for our history: Ableism & White supremacy in occupational therapy. *Occupational Therapy Now, March/April 25*(2), 7–10. https://caot.ca/document/7758/OT%20Now_Mar_22.pdf

(Continued)

Table 12.1 (Continued)

Disablism	Refers to the *social* imposition of *avoidable restrictions* on the life activities, aspirations, and psycho-emotional well-being of people categorized as "impaired" by those deemed "normal". Disablism is *social-relational* in character and constitutes a form of *social oppression* in contemporary society – alongside sexism, racism, ageism, and homophobia. As well as enacted in person-to-person interactions, disablism may manifest itself in institutionalized and other socio-structural forms (p. 11).	Thomas, C. (2014). Disability and impairment. In J. Swain, C. Thomas, C. Barnes, & S. French (Eds.), *Disabling barriers, enabling environments* (3rd ed., pp. 9–16). Sage.
Epistemic injustice	Epistemic injustice refers to the distinct wrong done to someone in their capacity as a knower; restricting their ability to engage in the basic everyday practices of knowing, conveying knowledge to others, and making sense of personal and social experiences. Due to unequal epistemic power relations, certain groups have greater power to determine what constitutes valid knowledge, and whose knowledge should count.	Fricker, M. (2007). *Epistemic injustice: Power and the ethics of knowing.* Oxford University Press. Kidd, I. J., Medina, J., & Pohlhaus, G. (2017). Introduction. In I. J. Kidd, J. Medina, & G. Pohlhaus, Jr. (Eds.), *Routledge handbook of epistemic injustice.* Routledge.
Experiential knowledge	Involves more than just lived experience, but more importantly, a critical/political understanding of that lived experience (p. 24). Note, experiential knowledge is not synonymous with practical knowledge. Developed from lived experience, through analysis which may sometimes take the form of rigorous, systematized reflection over time. Involves a constructed as well as critical/political understanding of situations. Not to be confused either with lived experience, narrative, or testimony, nor practical knowledge.	LeBlanc-Omstead, S., & Mahipaul, S. (2022). Toward more socially accountable service user involvement education: Embracing critical disability studies. *Occupational Therapy Now, March/April 25*(2), 24–26. https://caot.ca/document/7758/OT%20Now_Mar_22.pdf Gardien, È. (2017). Qu'apportent les savoirs expérientiels à la recherche en sciences humaines et sociales? *Vie Sociale, 4*(20), 31–44. https://doi.org/10,391 7/vsoc.174.0031

(*Continued*)

Table 12.1 (Continued)

Independence	Informed by neoliberal individualism, a mainstream Western definition of independence is doing or engaging alone, without human or non-human companions. The disabled living movement and CDS scholars promote an alternative perspective of independence being about choice and autonomy to make decisions about what to do and how to do it. For the disabled living movement, independence is therefore not related to whether or not there is human or other assistance. In occupational therapy, there have been different explanations of independence that attempt to bridge concepts of choice and competence or doing alone.	Collins, B. (2017). Independence: Proposing an initial framework for occupational therapy. *Scandinavian Journal of Occupational Therapy*, 24(6), 398–409. https://doi.org/10.1080/11038128.2016.1271011 Reindal, S. M. (1999). Independence, dependence, interdependence: Some reflections on the subject and personal autonomy. *Disability and Society*, 14(3), 353–367. https://doi.org/10.1080/09687599926190 Goble, C. (2004). Dependence, independence & normality. In C. Barnes (Ed.), *Disabling barriers, enabling environments* (pp. 41–46). Sage.
Interdependence	Interdependence "is not just me 'dependent on you'. It is not you, the benevolent oppressor, deciding to 'help' me" (para. 8). Interdependence is relational and involves giving and receiving in material and beyond material ways. As an alternate to doing alone, Interdependence has been proposed as a means to understand choice and autonomous doing, regardless of whether there is co-occupation, human assistance, or "help".	Collins, B. (2017). Independence: Proposing an initial framework for occupational therapy. *Scandinavian Journal of Occupational Therapy*, 24(6), 398–409. https://doi.org/10.1080/11038128.2016.1271011
Mad	A reclaimed, politicized term to describe broader social, cultural, and liberatory approaches to thinking about and responding to medicalized experiences of mental distress and diversity (widely known as "mental illness" within psy-systems).	LeFrançois, B. A., Menzies, R., & Reaume, G. (Eds.). (2013). *Mad matters: A critical reader in Canadian mad studies*. Canadian Scholars' Press.
Mad studies	A field of scholarship, theory, and activism about the lived experiences, history, cultures, and politics of people who may identify as Mad,	Beresford, P. (2020). 'Mad', mad studies and advancing inclusive resistance. *Disability & Society*, 35(8),

(*Continued*)

Table 12.1 (Continued)

	mentally ill, psychiatric survivors, consumers, service users, patients, neurodiverse, and disabled. Mad studies refer to a body of knowledge that has emerged from psychiatric survivors, Mad-identified people, antipsychiatry academics and activists, critical psy- professionals, and radical therapists. This body of knowledge is wide ranging and includes scholarship that is critical of the mental health system and biomedical approaches to the domain widely known as "mental illness" or "mental health", and substitutes instead a framework of "madness".	1337–1342. https://doi.org/10.1080/09687599.2019.1692168 LeFrançois, B. A., Menzies, R., & Reaume, G. (Eds.). (2013). *Mad matters: A critical reader in Canadian mad studies*. Canadian Scholars' Press.
Neurodivergence	Sometimes used as a descriptive term to refer to forms of cognitive difference (divergence); sometimes used as a social identity. Refers to a cognitive, affectual, and sensory functioning that differs (diverges) from that of the majority which represents the predominant neurotype (often described as "neurotypical"). It is an alternative to the "neurodevelopmental disorders" idea that is encompassed by standard medical models. The adjective "neurodivergent" is not to be confused with the adjective "neurodiverse", which refers to neurodiversity among a group, and therefore describes a group, a community, or a society that includes individuals presenting with various neurotypes.	Bertilsdotter Rosqvist, H., Stenning, A., & Chown, N. (2020). Introduction. In H. Bertilsdotter Rosqvist, N. Chown, & A. Stenning (Eds.), *Neurodiversity studies: A New critical paradigm* (1st ed., pp. 218–220). Routledge. Diamond, E. (2023). *Neurodiverse vs neurodivergent: Understanding the differences and celebrating the spectrum*. https://www.psychreg.org/neurodiverse-neurodivergent-understanding-differences-celebrating-spectrum/
Neurodiversity	A polysemic term that is used to refer to: (i) neurological diversity (in other words, to a genetic manifestation of diversity); (ii) a paradigm aiming to depathologize and politicize neurodivergence; as well as (iii) a new way of conceiving function and dysfunction. "Neurodiversity orien- tations tacitly assume neurodivergence as a potentially valuable form of human existence" (Bertilsdotter Rosqvist et al., 2020, p. 7).	Chapman, R. (2020). Defining neurodiversity for research and practice. In H. Bertilsdotter Rosqvist, N. Chown, & A. Stenning (Eds.), *Neurodiversity studies: A new critical paradigm* (1st ed., pp. 218–220). Routledge.

(Continued)

Table 12.1 (Continued)

		Bertilsdotter Rosqvist, H., Stenning, A., & Chown, N. (2020). Introduction. In H. Bertilsdotter Rosqvist, N. Chown, & A. Stenning (Eds.), *Neurodiversity studies: A New critical paradigm* (1st ed., pp. 218–220). Routledge.
Neurodiversity studies	A new interdisciplinary field that aims to address the epistemic and ideological rules that determine and produce "normal" and "others" according to scientific, cultural, and social practices. Neurodiversity studies are interested in both "centralizing cognitive marginality and marginalizing the cognitive center" (Bertilsdotter Rosqvist et al., 2020, p. 228).	Bertilsdotter Rosqvist, H., Stenning, A., & Chown, N. (2020). Neurodiversity studies. Proposing a new field of inquiry. In H. Bertilsdotter Rosqvist, N. Chown, & A. Stenning (Eds.), *Neurodiversity studies: A new critical paradigm* (1st ed., pp. 226–229). Routledge.
Normalcy / normality	An oppressive concept within society that is built on the taken-for-granted concept of society's norms (i.e., skin color, able-bodied for ability, and heterosexual relations for sexual expressions) and what society believes constitutes a *normal life*. Marginalized people will always be on the margins of what we call normalcy/normality, which is built on beliefs – physical and attitudinal – that exclude disabled people and render them unable to achieve, or try hard to achieve, a "good life".	McDonald, J. E. (2016). Intersectionality and disability. In J. Robertson & G. Larson (Eds.), *Disability and social change: A progressive Canadian approach.* Fernwood Publishing. Titchkosky, T. (2007). *Reading and writing disability differently: The textured life of embodiment.* University of Toronto Press.
Normative violence / the violence of normativity	The belief that disability is a problem within the individual (and within society) that ought to be overcome. This need to overcome can take the form of treatments, surgeries, therapies, medications (often invasive), or feeling forced to hide and pass for *normal*.	Titchkosky, T. (2007). *Reading and writing disability differently: The textured life of embodiment.* University of Toronto Press.
Oppression	The unjust treatment and/or control of marginalized people that create barriers and unjust experiences in disabled people's lives based on stereotypes of ability, class, gender, and race.	McDonald, J. E. (2016). Intersectionality and disability. In J. Robertson & G. Larson (Eds.), *Disability and social change: A progressive Canadian approach.* Fernwood Publishing.

(*Continued*)

Table 12.1 (Continued)

Sanism	Describes the systematic subjugation of people who have received mental health diagnoses or treatment. Sanism may result in various forms of stigma, blatant discrimination, and a host of microaggressions. Individuals with mental health issues experience low expectations and professional judgment that they are incompetent, unable to care for themselves, that they need to be supervised and assisted, and can be unpredictable, violent, and irrational.	LeFrançois, B. A., Menzies, R., & Reaume, G. (Eds.). (2013). *Mad matters: A critical reader in Canadian mad studies.* Canadian Scholars' Press. Beresford, P. (2020). 'Mad', mad studies and advancing inclusive resistance. *Disability & Society, 35*(8),1337–1342. https://doi.org/10.1080/09687599.2019.1692168

We hope that the removal of definitions from the body of the chapter not only provides a complete, easy-to-use index, but will also support the flow and usability of the chapter.

As noted in our author positionality statement, we identify as a collective of disabled*, chronically ill*, mad*, and neurodivergent*-identifying occupational therapists/scientists. We are among those who recognize the dearth of critical disability* and critical autism*, and mad* and neurodivergent-informed* perspectives for understanding human occupation; and that the implications of such knowledges are "urgent, vital, and immense" (Harrison et al., 2021, p. 5). The lack of engagement with these vast and rich bodies of critical knowledge is perhaps most apparent to us as clinicians, educators, and researchers.

Alongside recognizing the lack of integration of critical disability and related discourses, we are simultaneously keenly aware of our precarious positionality within disabilities studies and occupational therapy/science spaces (Mahipaul & Kimpson, 2021). We have experienced – both individually and collectively – othering, suppression, and denial of our perspectives, voices, identities, and body/minds in both occupational therapy and science. Throughout this chapter, we use identity-first language (i.e., d/Disabled, m/Mad, n/Neurodivergent, d/Deaf, and b/Blind) to locate ourselves within our respective critical fields, to situate our experiences within socially and politically constructed norms, and to demand our personhoods within ableist* environments (Aubrecht, 2012; Linton, 1998; Oliver, 1990). The combined use of lower and upper cases (e.g., d/Disabled) as a common noun is inspired by a long-term convention observed in d/Deaf communities (Ladau, 2021).

For those not yet acquainted with CDS*, neurodiversity studies*, or mad studies* (and related fields), these create foundational knowledge that forms the basis for the way disability, madness, and neurodivergence are understood. This foundational knowledge challenges the uncritical perspective that it is non-disabled professionals or "experts" who are best suited to theorize and educate about disability. The absence of CDS-informed knowledge around human occupation has historically resulted in those whose experiences align more closely with the critical knowledges found in CDS or in mad studies, having little choice but to smother their testimony, or altogether disengage from their experiential knowledges for the sake of professional acceptance.

This disengagement results in a denial of our belonging within occupational science and occupational therapy as valid *knowers*, constituting an epistemic injustice* that harms us as individuals, and arguably threatens the foundations of occupational science and occupational therapy knowledge(s).

In the process of our working together, we recognize our very different lived experiences; we have come to understand and value our shared experiential knowledge*. Our individual scholarship within critical disability, critical autism, and mad studies has enabled us to shift from perspectives that situate problems within the person and an individualized understanding of our lived experience, to an understanding and experiential knowledge* that actively draws on the scholarship of others to recognize the societal (and professional) barriers to occupational engagement. We have transitioned from knowing through experience alone to knowing through integration and sharing of scholarship and experience. We argue that integration of critical disability, critical autism, and mad studies scholarship could support our profession to similarly move from an individual perspective, informed (to a greater or lesser extent) by snapshots of lived experience, to perspectives of human occupation that genuinely integrate and recognize the theory and knowledges of d/Disabled people and critical disability scholarship.

12.2 Epistemic Injustice: Troubling Valid Knowledge(s)

Epistemic injustice* is suggested as a useful theoretical lens to understand and illustrate the challenges experienced by disabled, mad, and neurodivergent people to develop and communicate experiential knowledges* within health professions education, research, and practice (Carel & Kidd, 2014; Fletcher & Clarke, 2020; Kidd & Carel, 2017; LeBlanc & Kinsella, 2016; Liegghio, 2013; Miller Tate, 2019; Molas, 2016; Newbigging & Ridley, 2018; Scrutton, 2017; Scully, 2018). Epistemic injustice refers to the distinct "wrong done to someone specifically in their capacity as a knower" (Fricker, 2007, p. 155); restricting their ability to engage in the basic everyday practices of knowing, conveying knowledge to others, and/or actively participating in the production of a collective knowledge base (Dotson, 2011; Fricker, 2007; Pohlhaus, 2017). The last of these – the inability to actively participate in the production of a collective or accepted knowledge base – can be understood as *contributory injustice*.

Contributory injustice is not simply a matter of people (who are considered marginalized or equity-seeking, e.g., those who possess experiential knowledge of disability or occupy disabled identities) lacking adequate conceptualizations and language, or "having no contribution to make" (Miller Tate, 2019, p. 97). Rather, among themselves, marginalized people are often able to make sense of and articulate aspects of their experience relatively effortlessly, yet remain unable to communicate these with the same ease or effectiveness in mainstream discourse (Pohlhaus, 2012, p. 722). For example, we are able to discuss our (shared and divergent) experiences and knowledges of being people who are disabled, mad, neurodivergent, and chronically ill within our collective. We can theorize and explain the experiences. However, the ability to articulate this to and within our profession is challenging. Contributory injustice is often perpetuated by what Pohlhaus (2012) called *willful hermeneutical ignorance*, which occurs when dominantly situated knowers (e.g., health professionals within health care contexts) refuse to make the efforts necessary to understand parts of the world which can only be known from positions other than their own.

Health professionals play an important role in fostering epistemic justice and bringing knowledge of marginalized people into the mainstream (Katzman & LeBlanc-Omstead, 2019; Kurs & Grinshpoon, 2018; LeBlanc & Kinsella, 2016; Miller Tate, 2019; Scrutton, 2017). Promoting epistemic justice requires conscious effort: there needs to be recognition that the status quo privileges some knowledges, the "majority knowledge". In health and social care settings, the majority knowledge tends to be generated by non-disabled professionals. Promoting epistemic justice, where the knowledges of marginalized people are fully acknowledged, requires redress at a systemic level (Scully, 2018, p. 16). Disabled, chronically ill, mad, and neurodivergent knowers, for whom mainstream epistemic resources are too often ill-fitting, are well positioned to "notice inadequacies in our epistemic resources" and draw attention to "whole parts of the world for which dominantly held resources are not very suitable" (Pohlhaus, 2012, pp. 719–720).

Thus, the very existence of this chapter – one written from the perspectives of disabled, chronically ill, mad, and/or neurodivergent authors – within a textbook on human occupation, where we rarely, if ever, encounter such perspectives, represents a shift toward epistemic justice. Our recognition that this chapter is, to our knowledge, the first of its kind within occupational science and occupational therapy comes with an acceptance that what we can reasonably accomplish within these pages is an introduction or starting point for those who wish to rethink human occupation from a CDS-informed perspective. Thus, for the purposes of this chapter, we have opted to conflate – to an extent – the knowledges stemming from CDS, mad studies, critical autism studies (CAS), as well as disability and mad justice, positioning these as an experientially informed body of knowledge, alternative to the professional, "objective", expert knowledge that continues to be privileged in our understandings of occupational science and therapy. Drawing from these collective knowledges, we introduce and define the important concepts of ableism*, disablism*, (neuro)ableism*, and sanism*, calling attention to their presence in occupational therapy and science, as well as their broader impact on marginalized people and communities, as intersecting and inseparable from other forms of oppression.

12.3 Engaging with, Firmly Situated, and Belonging within CDS

Throughout the 1960s and 1970s, activists in the Disability Rights Movement highlighted that biomedical perspectives and approaches are pervasive. Biomedical perspectives situate the "cause" of disability (and any disadvantage that arises from disability) as due to individual impairment or difference. These biomedical perspectives underpin the understanding of disability evident in governmental and social policies, health care, education, and legislation. Unlike acute illness where fixing the impairment is an appropriate treatment approach, disability rights activists highlight that disability is not inherently an individual "problem", neither is it an "abnormality" to be cured, fixed, or eradicated within the person. Instead, disability (and any resulting disadvantage) is caused by societal structures that do not take account of difference (e.g., Union of the Physically Impaired Against Segregation and The Disability Alliance, 1975). As such, theorists have situated disability as a social construct, initially explained through the social model of disability* (Oliver, 1990; Thomas, 2014).

Biomedical perspectives underpin disabling and deeply rooted social practices that harm disabled people. Biomedical perspectives tend to arise from assumptions about what is "normal", good, and accepted/acceptable. Disabled people are expected to behave, achieve, and engage in manners considered "normal" and this normal is often undefined. Messages to aspire to some form of "normal" – pervasive within the *individual/medical model of disability** – include the expectation that disabled people wish to be "cured", that they (*we*) should undergo (and should want to undergo) invasive and extensive treatment and rehabilitation to be "normal". This includes expectations to meet social norms and representations, to perform certain occupations considered typical, and to perform those occupations in specified ways (e.g., independently*). There is an expectation that disabled people consent to medications, painful surgeries, and therapies that can reduce behaviors perceived as disruptive because they are not understood and/or increase function, or the ability to perform occupations valued by normative society. These messages are experienced and enacted as power through authority and specialist knowledge (including medical, rehabilitation, social work, educational, and legislative professionals) and are exceptionally difficult to resist (Shildrick, 2012; Thomas, 2014). Disabled, mad, and neurodivergent people are taught that they are broken, devalued, deficient, incapable, unintelligent, unproductive, weak, unstable, dependent, and burdensome on society and its systems.

Critical perspectives of disability, madness, and neurodivergence question society's concepts of "normal" and "acceptable". Concepts of what is normal and acceptable are continually shaped by ableism. Ableism is insidious, with "firm historical roots resulting in systems of oppression designed by people in power that still underpin society and beliefs in current times" (Mahipaul, 2022, p. 8). Ableist principles are underpinned by the same ideologies as those of white supremacy, colonialism, heteronormativity, patriarchy, and capitalism. Within these deeply rooted oppressive frameworks, society has come to view disability, madness, and neurodivergence on biomedical terms, as something to be cured, fixed, or eradicated and if these fail for disability to be overcome, hidden, and erased. Therefore, the very question *"whose body/minds are worthy and belong?"* is reinforced by policies, social networks, government supports, social services, and physical environments (Shildrick, 2012; Thomas, 2014).

Value-laden and ableist* belief systems fuel efforts to control disabled people. These belief systems most harshly impact Indigenous, racialized, immigrant, and refugee communities (Sins Invalid, 2019; Withers et al., 2019) because of cumulative discrimination due to intersectionality and membership of minority social groups. For example, racialized disabled people are taught to hide their disability experience as they are already perceived as "other", when white disabled people may use their disability experience to access services. Neoliberal systems – underpinned by values of self-sufficiency and capitalist priorities – have tended to funnel people into either isolated living (wherein care is downloaded onto family) or occupation-limiting institutions. Ableist ideologies justify the creation of institutions to "house" disabled people in hospitals, rehabilitation centers, group homes, and prisons, which further entrench systemic oppression and invasive control experienced by disabled people, often exclusively determined and controlled by professionals (Grenier, 2021; Hammell, 2023).

From the perspective of occupation, neoliberal ideologies can limit occupational possibilities and opportunities, rendering occupations valued by an individual as impossible. This leads to multiple occupational injustices. Rooted in (neuro)ableist* and sanist* harmful biases, neoliberal systems modulate occupational choices. This means that occupational choices available may not be in line with the potential and aspirations of disabled individuals and communities. This results in disabled people's exclusion from meaningful occupations, their forced participation in purposeless activities, and limited participation in low-status or low-valued occupations. These constitute occupational marginalization, occupational alienation, and occupational apartheid (see Durocher et al., 2014).

Society teaches disabled people to construct themselves as "useless", unvalued, to be pitied, and dependent and incapable of caring for themselves. Ableism not only teaches us that disabled people experience disability because they have not tried or refuse to try harder, following the same rhetoric according to which "poor individuals are lazy, incompetent, and irresponsible; that people experience racism because they are dangerous, threatening or choose to be victimized; [and] that women experience inequality because they exaggerate gender gaps, are weak, and are too emotional/hysterical" (Mahipaul, 2022, p. 7). Ableism acts as the very foundation to the perspectives that disable and harm disabled people within society.

Disabled people experience disablism* as social restrictions and exclusions imposed on them directly by those in society who can and choose to conform to a "normal" status, not only in the way their bodies and brains are but also in the way they engage and achieve their occupations. Carol Thomas (2012) defines disablism as follows:

> *Social-relational* in character and constitutes a form of *social oppression* in contemporary society – alongside sexism, racism, ageism, and homophobia. As well as enacted in person-to-person interactions, disablism may manifest in institutionalised and other socio-structural forms.
>
> *(p. 211)*

These institutionalized and socio-structural practices emerge particularly within neoliberalist approaches where ableism and neoliberal discourses combine to valorize independence as a social standing and social identity. A person is attributed merit, social approval, and value (i.e., human status) based on their whiteness, wealth, cisgender (preferably masculine) and heteronormative orientation, productivity, potential to sell labor-power, ability, sanity, and capacity to conform to *societally constructed* norms (Mahipaul, 2022). These socially constructed norms reinforce the cyclical nature of how ableism, disablism, and the biomedical approach all fuel each other, and are particularly rooted within medical and rehabilitation knowledge foundations (Hammell, 2006; Oliver, 1996).

Work in occupational therapy and occupational science has started to move in directions that reflect on and bump up against hidden assumptions and biases that are often created in normative environments (e.g., colonial, Western, Eurocentric, gendered, and governmentality). These are discussed in Chapters 8–11. Overall, many scholars within the field have voiced a commitment to recognize the profession's role and complicity in shaping and maintaining practices, policies, and institutions that led to oppression and control of all people who could not fit the dominant paradigm of what was imagined/accepted as humanness and personhood (Hammell, 2023). However, as part of this work, disability often remains in the background, or can be missing/erased entirely (Pooley & Beagan, 2021), which is all the more ironic given that occupational therapists, in particular, work primarily with people who, for the most part, were born with or have acquired a condition on the basis of which they experience disability.

Our embodied and experiential knowledges, and the knowing we have garnered from our respective critical studies of disability, madness, and neurodivergence inform our understandings of concepts such as normality, independence, engagement, doing, participating, and belonging. These often sit in significant tension with the ways these concepts/theories are understood and taught within occupational science and occupational therapy. What follows is an exploration of this tension, using the concept of independence – in relation to concepts of interdependence and community – as an exemplar for illustrating the implications of approaching human occupation through a CDS-informed lens.

12.4 Independence, Dependence, Interdependence

Many occupational scientists and occupational therapists foster conformism* through their work, which is informed by ableist* expectations regarding normality – ways of engaging in occupations and who engages in what occupations. Overall, disabled, neurodivergent, and mad people are expected to engage in sanctioned occupations that will help them approximate the (neuro)ableist sanist norm, and are expected to do their upmost to fake normality and engage in occupations independently (alone). While it is assumed that they all desire to approximate the norm or *pass* as normal, and it is also considered that disability is only acceptable when it approaches societally constructed norms. For example, assessments are often predicated on ableist and sanist expectations of what are acceptable occupations, such as typical self-care occupations, work, and certain leisure occupations.

Disabled, neurodivergent, and mad people often experience limitations to their occupational possibilities because there are assumptions regarding, and limits on, what disabled, neurodivergent, and mad people are expected to do. What occupations are sanctioned for people with particular disabilities varies from those that are sanctioned for non-disabled people (see Chapter 13). For example, although it is shifting slowly, disabled, neurodivergent, and mad people are not expected in health professional roles, and as previously mentioned their experiential expertise is therefore missing from those professions (Battalova et al., 2020; Jarus et al., 2023). People with particular disability experiences are typically additionally expected by those around them to engage in specific occupations, often those aimed at achieving an ableist norm, and specific productive roles are assumed to be more or less appropriate for people with particular disability experiences.

Independence has long been assumed to be a goal of occupational therapy intervention (Collins, 2017) but it is not at all clear where this assumption comes from or upon what knowledges it is based. As the discussion of epistemic injustice in this chapter highlights, much information about human occupation is based on knowledge from Western cultures and privileges professional biomedical perspectives, rather than experiential knowledge of disabled people (Hammell, 2023). Independence is one aspect of taken-for-granted knowledge in occupational therapy that can be questioned and critiqued using CDS as well as mad and neurodivergent studies.

Independence in terms of performing human occupation can be interpreted differently, depending on the knowledge base used. Reindal (1999), for example, highlights the difference between a "professional view" and the "independent living view" of independence when performing human occupations. In the professional view, which is situated within a medical model of disability, independence is characterized as doing *alone*, without interaction with other human or non-human actors. There is even debate in occupational therapy about whether independent performance includes that which is done using adaptive equipment. This professional view of independent occupational performance thus draws on a medical and rehabilitation professional knowledge base, and inherently assumes this form of independence as a vital aspect of normality. The independent living perspective, however, describes independence as choice and autonomy in *the way* occupations are performed and perhaps what occupations are performed (Collins, 2017; Reindal, 1999). This perspective draws on experiential knowledge of disabled people and, as being independent is choosing what to do and how to perform chosen occupations, there is no assumed normal.

The professional view of independence can be highly problematic when considered through CDS, mad, or neurodivergent-informed perspectives. There are assumptions about which occupations are considered "normal" to be performed alone, typically as characterized in Western cultures. In occupational therapy and occupational science, there are assumptions that many or most personal self-care occupations are typically performed alone, and further that it is desirable to perform these occupations alone. Bathing and grooming are examples of occupations that are expected to be performed alone, yet historical perspectives and those outside of a mainstream Western culture highlight many examples of where bathing and grooming can be communal acts and ritualized acts (see Chapter 25).

Critical disability-, mad-, and neurodivergence-informed perspectives might encourage occupational scientists and occupational therapists to critique the concept of independence and the use of this concept by questioning which occupations are considered *normal* to perform or engage in interdependently, and for whom it is acceptable to receive supports and in which occupations. For example, many leisure occupations are expected to be done with others. Sex is an example of an occupation normatively expected to be done with another and sexual acts which are engaged in alone are often not sanctioned. Non-disabled people are permitted supports for their occupational engagement (e.g., glasses, a calculator, or a bicycle), whereas supports required by disabled people are stigmatized (e.g., a sighted guide or wheelchair). According to a critical disability and specifically a disability justice perspective, and from Indigenous perspectives, humans are *interdependent* occupational beings. Assumptions of capacity are made based on individuals' abilities to perform normalized versions of occupations in normalized assumed ways which can have implications for individuals.

As an example, in many Western countries, a role of occupational therapists is to make judgments on the appropriateness of living accommodation, often based on whether or not a person can perform a pre-designated list of activities of daily living "independently" as measured using tools such as the Barthel Index or the Functional Independence Measure. These measures are of *doing alone* rather than choices regarding modes of doing. A CDS perspective might further suggest that these assessments are lacking in that they do not measure the societal and institutional factors impacting the person or community's *doing,* nor do they address their belonging (see Chapter 25). Classifying interdependent performance of some occupations (such as self-care) as deviant is based in ableist, ageist, and white supremacist assumptions. Older adults who move from engaging in self-care alone to engaging in these occupations with another person's assistance are perceived as more *child-like*, and, similarly, disabled people who engage in self-care occupations with another person's assistance are infantilized. Disabled mothers are stigmatized and questioned regarding their fitness for motherhood – questions that are interweaved with assumptions regarding parenting that do not involve interdependence* with other community members (see Box 12.1).

> **Box 12.1 Example**
>
> One of my participants in my doctorate, which admittedly is a few years ago now, was being asked by the occupational therapist to learn how to put her bra on. She said: 'It's a bit of a riddle really, but I suppose I have to do it myself'. She already had access to personal assistance but somehow the occupational therapist made the decision that it is the 'norm' to be able to put a bra on independently. And, therefore, she had spent time in occupational therapy approximating some kind of 'normality' rather than doing the things that were meaningful to her.
>
> It's normal to play tennis with somebody else, it's normal to do lots of other activities with people, but for some reason it is not normal to do activities of daily living with someone else.

12.5 Conclusion

This chapter attempts to bridge fields built on differing, often opposing, knowledge paradigms. Occupational therapy has roots within (the still dominant) biomedical modes of thought where the individual is viewed as a problem in need of rehabilitation/remediations in pursuit of approximating an ableist norm. The pre-eminent focus on individual-first/person-first orientations and the individualization of occupation (Rudman, 2013) in occupational science and therapy is in opposition to a CDS perspective. Occupational therapy has been complicit in upholding and shaping the normative standards that create the image of what a social "normal" ought to be (Hammell et al., 2021; Mahipaul, 2022; Shildrick, 2012). CDS and mad or neurodivergent perspectives are rooted in recognizing the heterogeneity and embodied nature of disability; how social practices can exclude and erase individuals; and questioning what mobilizes these normative exclusions.

The complexity of this work is deeply rooted within cultures and communities that are rich in their diversities. A discussion of the rich complexity of postmodern/structural theories on disability and disablement are beyond the scope of this chapter. We would, however, encourage the reader to recognize how these knowledges (knowledge communities) create foundations/road maps to dismantling disablement, ableism, and sanism inherent in the policies, biomedical discourses, and individualizing approaches within the field of occupational therapy. We are still viewed as *exceptional*, not fitting within certain molds that make up how society is and who invariably *should* belong within the multiple possibilities of what it is and means to be human. CDS and mad or neurodivergent-informed perspectives highlight this social practice not because we are *different* but because it opens the door to highlight how our embodied selves challenge/unpack what a modern society defines as, or imagines, a proper human to be (Shildrick, 2012).

We, as a group, are keenly interested in and aware of how each one of us embodies our disability and theorizes this embodiment as central to occupational science and occupational therapy education, research, and practice. We understand deeply what it feels like to live (belong) within societies that are "so unsettled by non-normative forms of embodiment" (Shildrick, 2012, p. 31). CDS and mad or neurodivergent-informed perspectives not only challenge mainstream normative society, but also disability politics that solely focus on disability as exclusively socially constructed. We do not wish to say with this chapter that only those of us who are disabled, mad, and neurodivergent occupational scientists and occupational therapists should speak authoritatively on occupational engagement and disability, madness, and neurodivergence. We need, however, to trouble whose voices are heard, which knowledges matter, and for those in dominant positions (oppressors) to interrogate how they have benefited from power to shape knowledge foundations that do not include discourses from those who have been viewed as lesser than and historically subjugated; people such as the very authors of this chapter. Thus, we attempt to break with an epistemic injustice that exists in our disciplines to instead promote disabled, chronically ill, mad, and neurodivergent-identifying occupational therapists and occupational scientists' epistemic agentivity.

12.6 Summary

- Certain types of knowledge are privileged in occupational therapy/science and this has silenced critical disability perspectives. The injustice caused by excluding certain knowledges is known as epistemic injustice. Occupational therapists and scientists need to recognize where knowledge comes from and critique this.
- Occupational therapy has its roots in a biomedical perspective, which describes disability as being a result of impairment or difference within the person. A biomedical perspective states that the way to fix disability is to manage the impairment. Disability activists state that disability is a social construct and the way to fix the restrictions caused by disability is by creating an environment that includes disabled people.
- Ableism is a system of assigning value to people's bodies and minds based on assumptions about what is normal, desirable, acceptable, and productive. Ableism is rooted in neoliberal, colonial, white, middle-class values, and is closely linked to racism and misogyny. Ableism results in systemic oppression as experienced by disabled people (and non-disabled people) whose bodies, minds, or ways of doing things are not considered good enough. Occupational therapists need to be aware of their value systems to reduce the impact of ableism on those with whom they interact.
- Disablism is the social disadvantages that people with impairments experience due to inaccessible environments and social structures, such as in work, housing, access to transportation, access to buildings, and engagement in community occupations. Occupational therapists and scientists should recognize the impact disablism can have on occupation and work with disabled people to dismantle barriers.

- Many aspects of occupational therapy could be critiqued from a perspective of CDS. One example is the concept of independence. When defined as doing alone and when the value of independence is assumed, occupational therapists' focus on enabling independent performance risks being oppressive and ableist.

12.7 Review Questions

1. What is epistemic injustice and why is this relevant for occupational therapists and occupational scientists?
2. How do approaches to "fixing" disability differ between biomedical and disability rights perspectives?
3. What is ableism? Give some examples of what may be ableist assumptions.
4. What are the different ways that independence can be defined and why is it important to understand the client's way of defining and valuing independence?

References

Aubrecht, K. (2012). Disability studies and the language of mental illness. *Review of Disability Studies: An International Journal*, 8(2), 31–44. https://www.rdsjournal.org/index.php/journal/article/view/98

Battalova, A., Bulk, L. Y., Nimmon, L., Hole, R., Krupa, T., Lee, M., Mayer, Y., & Jarus, T. (2020). "I can understand where they're coming from": How clinicians' disability experiences shape their interaction with clients. *Qualitative Health Research*, 30(13), 2064–2076. https://doi.org/10.1177/1049732320922193

Carel, H., & Kidd, I. J. (2014). Epistemic injustice in healthcare: A philosophical analysis. *Medicine, Health Care and Philosophy*, 17(4), 529–540. https://doi.org/10.1007/s11019-014-9560-2

Collins, B. (2017). Independence: Proposing an initial framework for occupational therapy. *Scandinavian Journal of Occupational Therapy*, 24(6), 398–409. https://doi.org/10.1080/11038128.2016.1271011

Dotson, K. (2011). Tracking epistemic violence, tracking practices of silencing. *Hypatia*, 26(2), 236–257. https://doi.org/10.1111/j.1527-2001.2011.01177.x

Durocher, E., Gibson, B. E., & Rappolt, S. (2014). Occupational justice: A conceptual review. *Journal of Occupational Science*, 21(4), 418–430. https://doi.org/10.1080/14427591.2013.775692

Fletcher, A., & Clarke, J. (2020). Integrated care systems as an arena for the emergence of new forms of epistemic injustice. *Ethical Theory and Moral Practice*, 23(5), 723–737. https://doi.org/10.1007/s10677-020-10111-1

Fricker, M. (2007). *Epistemic injustice: Power and the ethics of knowing*. Oxford University Press.

Grenier, M.-L. (2021). Patient case formulations and oppressive disability discourses in occupational therapy education. *Canadian Journal of Occupational Therapy*, 88(3), 266–272. https://doi.org/10.1177/00084174211005882

Hammell, K. W. (2006). *Perspectives on disability and rehabilitation: Contesting assumptions; challenging practice*. Elsevier.

Hammell, K. W. (2023). A call to resist occupational therapy's promotion of ableism. *Scandinavian Journal of Occupational Therapy*, 30(6), 745–757. https://doi.org/10.1080/11038128.2022.2130821

Hammell, K. W., Jarus, T., Bulk, L. Y., Collins, B., Grenier, M.-L., & Mahipaul, S. (2021). Letter to the editor. *Canadian Journal of Occupational Therapy*, 88(4), 279–282.

Harrison, E. A., Sheth, A. J., Kish, J., VanPuymbrouck, L. H., Heffron, J. L., Lee, D., Mahaffey, L., & Occupational Therapy and Disability Studies Network. (2021). Disability studies and occupational therapy: Renewing the call for change. *American Journal of Occupational*

Therapy, 75(4), 7504170010. ttps://research.aota.org/ajot/article/75/4/7504170010/12524/Disability-Studies-and-Occupational-Therapy

Jarus, T., Krupa, T., Mayer, Y., Battalova, A., Bulk, L., Lee, M., Nimmon, L., & Roberts, E. (2023). Negotiating legitimacy and belonging: Disabled students' and practitioners' experience. *Medical Education, 57*(6), 535–547. https://doi.org/10.1111/medu.15002

Katzman, E., & LeBlanc-Omstead, S. (2019). Considering epistemic justice in the quest for client-centered practice. *Occupational Therapy Now, 21*(2), 9–10.

Kidd, I. J., & Carel, H. (2017). Epistemic injustice and illness. *Journal of Applied Philosophy, 34*(2), 172–190. https://doi.org/10.1111/japp.12172

Kurs, R., & Grinshpoon, A. (2018). Vulnerability of individuals with mental disorders to epistemic injustice in both clinical and social domains. *Ethics & Behavior, 28*(4), 336–346. https://doi.org/10.1080/10508422.2017.1365302

Ladau, E. (2021). *Demystifying disability: What to know, what to say, and how to be an ally*. Ten Speed Press.

LeBlanc, S., & Kinsella, E. A. (2016). Toward epistemic justice: A critically reflexive examination of 'sanism' and implications for knowledge generation. *Studies in Social Justice, 10*(1), 59–78. https://doi.org/10.26522/ssj.v10i1.1324

Liegghio, M. (2013). A denial of being: Psychiatrization as epistemic violence. In B. A. LeFrancois, R. Menzies, & G. Reaume (Eds.), *Mad matters: A critical reader in Canadian mad studies* (pp. 122–129). Canadian Scholars' Press.

Linton, S. (1998). *Claiming disability: Knowledge and identity*. New York University Press.

Mahipaul, S. (2022). Accounting for our history: Ableism & White supremacy in occupational therapy. *Occupational Therapy Now, 25*(2), 7–10. https://caot.ca/document/7758/OT%20Now_Mar_22.pdf

Mahipaul, S., & Kimpson, S. (2021). Inhabiting borderlands: Living/exploring tensions in being both disabled women and health professionals. In D. Driedger (Ed.), *Still living the edges: A disabled women's reader* (pp. 172–186). Inanna.

Miller Tate, A. J. (2019). Contributory injustice in psychiatry. *Journal of Medical Ethics, 45*(2), 97–100. https://doi.org/10.1136/medethics-2018-104761

Molas, A. (2016). Silent voices, hidden knowledge: Ecological thinking and the role of mental health advocacy. *Dialogue: Canadian Philosophical Review, 55*(1), 87–105. https://doi.org/10.1017/S0012217316000160

Newbigging, K., & Ridley, J. (2018). Epistemic struggles: The role of advocacy in promoting epistemic justice and rights in mental health. *Social Science & Medicine, 219*, 36–44. https://doi.org/10.1016/j.socscimed.2018.10.003

Oliver, M. (1990). *The politics of disablement*. Macmillan.

Oliver, M. (1996). *Understanding disability: From theory to practice*. Palgrave.

Pohlhaus, Jr., G. (2012). Relational knowing and epistemic injustice: Toward a theory of willful hermeneutical ignorance. *Hypatia, 27*(4), 715–735. https://doi.org/10.1111/j.1527-2001.2011.01222.x

Pohlhaus, G. (2017). Varieties of epistemic injustice 1. In I. J. Kidd, J. Medina, & G. Pohlhaus, Jr. (Eds.), *Routledge handbook of epistemic injustice* (pp. 13–26). Routledge.

Pooley, E. A., & Beagan, B. L. (2021). The concept of oppression and occupational therapy: A critical interpretive synthesis. *Canadian Journal of Occupational Therapy, 88*(4), 407–417. https://doi.org/10.1177/00084174211051168

Reindal, S. M. (1999). Independence, dependence, interdependence: Some reflections on the subject and personal autonomy. *Disability and Society, 14*(3), 353–367. https://doi.org/10.1080/09687599926190

Rudman, D. L. (2013). Enacting the critical potential of occupational science: Problematizing the 'individualizing of occupation'. *Journal of Occupational Science, 20*(4), 298–313. https://doi.org/10.1080/14427591.2013.803434

Scrutton, A. P. (2017). Epistemic injustice and mental illness. In I. J. Kidd, J. Medina, & G. Pohlhaus, Jr. (Eds.), *Routledge handbook of epistemic injustice* (pp. 347–355). Routledge.

Scully, J. L. (2018). From "She would say that, wouldn't she?" to "Does she take sugar?" Epistemic injustice and disability. *IJFAB: International Journal of Feminist Approaches to Bioethics, 11*(1), 106–124. https://doi.org/10.3138/ijfab.11.1.106Shildrick, M. (2012). Critical disability studies: Rethinking the conventions for the age of postmodernity. In N. Watson, A. Roulstone, & C. Thomas (Eds.), *Routledge handbook of disability studies* (pp. 30–41). Routledge.

Sins Invalid. (2019). *Skin, tooth, and bone: The basis of movement is our people* (2nd ed.). Sins Invalid.

Thomas, C. (2012). Theorising disability and chronic illness: Where next for perspectives in medical sociology? *Social Theory & Health, 10*(3), 209–228. https://doi.org/10.1057/sth.2012.7

Thomas, C. (2014). Disability and impairment. In J. Swain, C. Thomas, C. Barnes, & S. French (Eds.), *Disabling barriers, enabling environments* (3rd ed., pp. 9–16). Sage.

Union of the Physically Impaired Against Segregation and The Disability Alliance. (1975). *Fundamental principles of disability*. Authors. https://disabledpeoplesarchive.com/wp-content/uploads/sites/39/2021/01/001-FundamentalPrinciplesOfDisability-UPIAS-DA-22Nov1975.pdf

Withers, A. J., Ben-Moshe, L., Brown, L. X., Erickson, L., da Silva Gorman, R., Lewis, T. A., & Mingus, M. (2019). Radical disability politics. In R. Kinna & U. Gordon (Eds.), *Routledge handbook of radical politics* (1st ed., pp. 178–193). Routledge. https://doi.org/10.4324/9781315619880-15

CHAPTER 13

Occupation and Social Sanctioning

Niki Kiepek, Cristian Mauricio Valderrama Núñez, Tanya Elizabeth Benjamin-Thomas, Michael Palapal Sy, and Marcel Nazabal Amores

Abstract

This chapter explores discussions around non-sanctioned occupations, alongside the dark side of occupation, and the figured world of occupation. These terms emerged at a time when occupational therapists were increasingly voicing skepticism about exclusively positive framings of occupation that claimed occupations *inherently* contributed to *improved* health and well-being. Contemporaneously, occupational therapy scholars in Latin America were also confronting assumptions around occupations as beneficial to the health and well-being of individuals and communities, as well as its individualist ideology and the perception that occupations are mediators between people and their social and natural environment. In this chapter, notions of ocupaciones colectivas and ocupaciones transgresoras are discussed as promoting understandings around the transformational potential of occupations to promote equity and inclusion among marginalized or oppressed social groups. Developing reflexive awareness to the situated nature of these concepts can mitigate potential harms and risks around oppression to individuals and societies.

As the scope of occupational therapy broadens to increasingly diverse settings with diverse populations, it is imperative to develop complex and nuanced understanding of occupations, experiences, and meanings that are not constrained by attending only to positive framings on human doing. Genuine attempts to understand occupations from the perspectives of individuals and collectives will contribute to improved partnerships and increase the relevance of occupational therapy approaches. Through such expanded understandings on occupation, occupational therapists may be better situated to work toward addressing complex circumstances in relation to occupation beyond the individual.

Authors' Positionality Statement

The authors are from diverse backgrounds with each author bringing a unique perspective. Niki Kiepek is a university-educated occupational therapist and identifies as a White, female, able-bodied, economically secure, second generation Canadian from a working-class background. Cristian Mauricio Valderrama Núñez is a university-educated occupational therapist and the son of non-professional trade workers who raised him in the context of a dictatorship in Chile. Tanya Elizabeth Benjamin-Thomas is an occupational therapist who grew up in India with educational opportunities in English-speaking, private institutions, as well as graduate education at Canadian and American universities. Michael Palapal Sy is an internationally educated Filipino occupational therapist and having lived in a developing country for 30 years, he currently lives and works in Switzerland. Marcel Nazabal Amores was raised by his professional parents in the hardships of the Cuban regime; years after receiving his university education in Havana, he emigrated to Canada where he is a novice scholar and musician in the minority Latino community. We came together as a group to share diverse and situated perspectives, recognizing the richness of multiple world views when seeking to understand occupation. We largely sought consensus through a collaborative writing process; however, the content may not reflect the full perspectives of all authors. The process of writing this chapter involved virtual meetings with simultaneous interpretation between scholars who speak Spanish and English. All sections of the chapter were translated into both English and Spanish to facilitate the full participation of all authors in the writing and revision processes. In this chapter, we have only represented English and Spanish language literature, but we imagine related ideas have emerged independently in other literature as well.

Objectives

This chapter will aim to:

- Guide readers to critically reflect on ideas around non-sanctioned occupations and the dark side of occupation as interlinked with historical, culturally, and socially situated norms, values, and assumptions.
- Introduce readers to Latin American scholarship around ocupaciones colectivas and ocupaciones transgresoras.
- Foster curiosity and commitment to develop more comprehensive and complex understandings around experiences and meanings of human occupation, extending beyond positive connotations of occupation for individuals and collectives.
- Recognize occupations as situated in complex contexts that can shape and produce social inequities, injustice, oppression, and harm. Such awareness promotes occupational therapy approaches that aim to achieve meaningful and lasting improvements.

Key terms

- **non-sanctioned occupations**
- **dark side of occupation**
- **figured world of occupation**
- **ocupaciones colectivas**
- **ocupaciones transgresoras**

13.1 Introduction

In this chapter, we present an overview of the notions "figured world of occupation", "dark side of occupation", and "non-sanctioned occupations", and briefly explore how these ideas have been taken up in peer-reviewed publications. These specific terms emerged in Canada and the United Kingdom and are largely circulated within English language publications. We thus introduce how similar ideas contemporaneously emerged in Latin American and Spanish language occupation-related scholarship, drawing on the concepts of ocupaciones colectivas and ocupaciones transgresoras, and attending to areas of conceptual convergence and divergence. We conclude with a discussion of potential implications for occupational therapy.

Understandings around "figured world of occupation", "dark side of occupation", "non-sanctioned occupations", ocupaciones colectivas, and ocupaciones transgresoras will shift over time, as will our own personal beliefs and interpretations. We recognize that readers bring their own lived experiences and unique perspectives to this topic. By the nature of the topics discussed in this chapter – particularly "social sanctioning" – we acknowledge that some occupations may elicit discomfort or be unsettling for some readers. In naming certain occupations, we aim to legitimize the study of these activities as relevant to occupation-related scholarship and practice; however, this should not be interpreted as indiscriminate legitimization of the occupation itself. The word "sanction" is intended to be understood as a social process, not an adjective that classifies occupations into fixed categories.

13.2 Conceptualizations of "Occupation"

"Occupation" is a historically and socially situated concept. Despite efforts to establish concrete, fixed definitions, concepts are fluid and definitions change over time and hold varied meanings across contexts. In 1993, Wilcock, a scholar in the Global North, defined occupation as purposeful activity that served to

> provide for immediate bodily needs of sustenance, self-care and shelter; to develop skills, social structures and technology aimed at safety and superiority over predators and the environment; and to exercise personal capacities to enable maintenance and development of the organism.
>
> *(Wilcock, 1993)*

More recently, occupation was defined by Laliberte Rudman and colleagues (2022) as "a wide-ranging expanse of everyday and extraordinary doings of individuals and groups, which have implications for individuals, societies, and the earth" (p. 15). This broad framing envisions expanding conceptualizations of occupation beyond Western values and ideologies that privilege individualism and objective scientific rationality, and neglect ethical obligations of reciprocity in human relationships with nature (Laliberte Rudman et al., 2022).

Goals of occupational therapy have been wide ranging, and participation in occupations has predominantly been framed as having positive impacts on health, well-being, and social justice (Stewart et al., 2016). As such, occupational therapy has centered on improving individual and collective performance and participation in occupations. In contexts of competition for research funding and professional prestige, it is not surprising that the health-promoting potential of occupation has been a relative focus of occupation-related scholarship. The emergence of occupational science in the late 1980s afforded opportunities for scholars to seek expanded understandings of occupation, which may have created a landscape to uncouple occupation from "positive" health and well-being.

In the early 2000s, scholarship emerged that explicitly contested occupations as inherently positive. Hocking (2009) stated that the meaning of occupation may be "mainstream or contested, highbrow or commonplace, sacred or profane, as a site of celebration, emancipation, oppression, weary drudgery, struggle, or degradation of the environment" (p. 145). Ramugondo (2015) argued that "human occupation may very well be central to oppression and coloniality, in that *doing* is the most visible enactment of unequal intersubjective relations" (p. 494). By acknowledging diverse experiences, occupation became increasingly understood as complex and multifaceted.

In 2008, Russell's study about tagging framed it as a "familiar" and "ordinary" occupation engaged in by youth, though typically viewed as a "maladaptive behaviour" by "authorities" (p. 87). This is, arguably, one of the first articles published in occupational science that explicitly featured an occupation dominantly constructed as "deviant" and "not socially acceptable", contesting such interpretations in relation to factors such as censorship, colonization, and physical deprivation (p. 95). This was followed by Kiepek and Magalhães' (2011) publication that defined addictions and impulse control disorders as occupations. It is worth noting the authors largely conformed to dominant conceptualization regarding criteria defining occupation; however, in future publications about substance use by Kiepek and colleagues, several of these constructs, such as the "meaning" of occupation, are challenged (Kiepek, Beagan, Patten et al., 2022).

A review of occupational therapy and occupational science scholarship reveals skepticism around portraying occupations as exclusively positive and as inherently contributing to improved health and well-being. In 2013, Twinley introduced the concept of the "dark side of occupation" as "the things some people do that may not always promote good health, may not always be productive", including occupations that are considered "anti-social; criminal; deviant; violent; disruptive; harmful; unproductive; non-health-giving; non-health-promoting; addictive and politically, socially, religiously or culturally extreme" (p. 302). Kiepek and colleagues (2014) conducted a critical discourse analysis that examined the *figured world* of occupation. They observed tendencies among scholars of occupation to identify occupations as "positive" and to emphasize relationships with enhanced health and well-being; however, the authors conclude "occupations are complexly related to health, well-being and social justice and the implications of those relationships are subjective, contextually situated, and defy efforts to categorize occupations as 'good' or 'bad,' 'healthy' or 'unhealthy'" (p. 412).

Kiepek and colleagues (2019) later introduced the term *non-sanctioned occupations* to "encompass occupations that, within historically and culturally bound contexts, tend to be viewed as unhealthy, illegal, immoral, abnormal, undesired, unacceptable, and/or inappropriate" (p. 2). The authors acknowledged that the term non-sanctioned implies a dualism "that likely fails to reflect the complexity of processes that shape social ideals, and that such a categorization is dynamic across time, social groups, and contexts" (Kiepek et al., 2019, p. 2). Yet, the term offers a language from which to confront the "silencing" of occupations discussed within occupation-based scholarship

OCCUPATION AND SOCIAL SANCTIONING

that do not conform to dominant social values, ideology, and hegemony, and calls for expanded understandings on such occupations and their situated nature.

Despite coining the term "non-sanctioned", Kiepek (2021) later cautioned that

> when an occupation or aspect of occupation is labelled 'non-sanctioned' or 'dark,' we have cast the occupation as being somehow unhealthy, immoral, illegal, to have an undesirable outcome, or on the fringe of dominant social norms – in other words, something that does not conform with values underlying the concept of a general 'occupation'.
>
> *(p. 4)*

As such, it is considered prudent to avoid rhetorical use of the terms "non-sanctioned" or "dark"; instead, occupational therapists are encouraged to describe contextual forces that inform occupational participation, which might include sociocultural norms and values and other historic, economic, and political forces that contribute to engagement in particular occupations. These types of factors inform how occupations are understood, experienced, classified, and responded to. It is important to examine how assumptions and determinations about the social sanctioning of occupations, and individual and social impacts of occupational participation, are influenced by one's positionality. "Positionality" refers to relative differences in social positions and power that shape personal identities, worldviews, access, and privilege.

13.3 Influence of "Dark Side", "Figured World", and "Non-sanctioned" Conceptualizations

To explore the influence of "dark side", "figured world", and "non-sanctioned" on future scholarship, we undertook a brief search of peer-reviewed articles that cited each of the three articles introducing these notions. As of February 2022, *Wiley Online Library* reported 46 citations of Twinley (2013) and *Taylor and Francis Online* reported 26 citations of Kiepek et al. (2014) and 31 citations of Kiepek et al. (2019). There was overlap in citations, with 17 articles citing two, or even all three, articles; in total, we reviewed 79 articles. It is not our intent to provide a systematic review in this chapter, but we are able to describe our general observations.

For some authors, citing one of the three papers served to position various ways of being and doing as "occupations". This effectively legitimized particular areas of study not otherwise addressed within existing occupational therapy or occupational science literature. Topics included restricted and repetitive behaviors among children with autism; ritualistic and obsessive behaviors associated with eating disorders; occupations emerging from boredom; substance abuse; sex work; fighting or aggression. The notion that occupations may not invariably contribute to improved health was a topic that arose a number of times. We observed that the terms "dark side" and "non-sanctioned" tended to be used synonymously, despite differences in theoretical and philosophical underpinnings. The concept of the "dark side" lends to an analysis of the nature of occupations, whereas the concept of "non-sanctioned" focuses on societal factors and social processes that shape occupations and perspectives about occupations (see Box 13.1).

> **Box 13.1 Critical Reflection – Kiepek**
>
> To resist conferring underlying assumptions of deviance or wrongness, one may refrain from using the terms "dark side" and "non-sanctioned", and simply (and perhaps more accurately) use the term "occupation". In blinded manuscript reviews about my research on substance use and criminalized occupations, it is not uncommon that well-intended, supportive reviewers recommend I cite literature around the "dark side" or "non-sanctioned occupations". Yet, when the intent of my research is to suspend positioning of the occupation as inherently problematic, endorsing these concepts would discretely and implicitly introduce and reinforce unwanted assumptions and biases.

The term "dark occupations" was sometimes used in the articles we reviewed, with citations attributed to Twinley. While the term "dark occupation" had already entered colloquial and academic literature (Matt Finch/Mechanical Dolphin, 2018), Twinley (2020) has since clarified, "[Dark occupation] is not my concept, nor what I chose to name it… I would never suggest we should label other people's occupations as 'dark'" (p. 1), expressing her concern that this term could convey a value judgment about a subjective experience.

It is notable that almost all articles that cited this scholarship were published in English, with the exception of one German source and two in French. To some extent, this reflects the predominance of English in international occupation-based journals. However, it is important to not lose sight of the fact that the ideas of "dark-side", "figured world", and "non-sanctioned" emerged in Anglophone cultures and may not reflect diverse worldviews. Increasingly, critical occupation-based scholarship points to the dominance of privileged perspectives about occupation as shaped and informed by factors such as educational status, literacy levels, language use, gender, race, class, ability status, and geographical locations of scholars, among others, that acknowledge certain types of doing as more or less relevant to occupational therapy, which risks diverse worldviews being delegitimized, "silenced, obscured, and negated" (Laliberte Rudman et al., 2022, p. 15).

For the purpose of this chapter, it was not feasible to explore all the ways in which "figured world", "dark side", and "non-sanctioned", or similar ideas may be emerging in non-English scholarship. However, we share contemporary developments in Latin America and in the following section we discuss how Latin American scholarship has approached and addressed the study of occupations which fall outside dominant norms.

13.4 Conceptualizations in Latin American Scholarship

Notions of "non-sanctioned occupations" and "the dark side of occupation" are not greatly used or discussed in the Latin American context. Contemporaneous with the introduction of the "figured world" and "dark side" scholarship, some scholars in Latin America explicitly confront assumptions around occupations as being beneficial to the health and well-being of individuals and communities, its underlying individualist ideology, and the perception that occupations are mediators between people and their social and natural environment. We introduce the select work of Latin American scholars, whose work is largely published in Spanish, but acknowledge that this does not represent the full scope of theoretical development in this region (e.g., see Nascimento (1990) for earlier work from Brazil).

In 2013, Valderrama Nuñez and Riquelme contested occupation as a means to achieve optimal health and well-being. Instead, occupations are viewed as a subjective social phenomenon situated within specific relationships. Occupations are the result of dynamic, historically situated intersubjective experiences that occur across the lifespan and are partially determined by existing social, economic, and political conditions. Comprehensive understandings of occupation require critical analysis of contextual conditions and the impact on individuals and collectives. For instance, when analyzing occupations of paid employment, it is important to examine diverse factors such as daily schedule, opportunity for benefits and unionization, contract details, level of responsibility, salary, and training opportunities. Variation among these types of conditions impacts the extent to which paid employment is experienced as health inducing or as producing discomfort, illness, or harm. A fundamental consideration of perceptions of positive "meaning" relates to dominant ideology and social norms, where ideology is defined as "a system of ideas, beliefs and assumptions that operates below one's level of conscious awareness and, by being taken for granted, appears to constitute normal common sense" (Hammell, 2006, p. 205).

Being employed in a job with poor working conditions can have positive meaning, particularly in capitalist societies where income is needed to meet the daily needs of families and employment options are scarce. At the same time, it is associated with meanings related to the perpetuation and reinforcement of social inequities and oppression. When interpreting perceptions of subjective well-being, it is important to take into consideration social discourses and values around being and doing. Social discourses include practices (e.g., language, dance, music, and custom) through which "individuals imbue reality with meaning" (Ruiz, 2009, p. 2).

Guajardo (2014) offers three important critical reflections that challenge dominant perspectives about occupation. First, it is argued that portraying occupations as natural promoters of health and well-being suggests a romantic and naive view that would only be justified in the practice of occupational therapy. Rather than perceiving occupations as inherently good and healthy, they are better understood as historical and situated products that arise within certain material conditions. Dominant contemporary contexts are largely embedded in capitalist social systems, alongside colonialism and patriarchy, and these social systems are thought to generate inequalities, exclusion, and alienation, Guajardo argues that occupations are shaped by and embed these characteristics, and that occupations do not exist outside or separate from social systems. Second, occupation does not occur in isolation; it is a cultural product that emerges through social relationships in the context of people's lives. The term "singularity of occupation" relates to individual expression of social relationships. Third, Guajardo proposes that occupations are "actors", not "objects" of study. From this perspective, occupations are not a "thing" or a mediator between people and the environment. People perform occupations; therefore, occupations exist when we, the people, express ourselves in our being and doing in the world. Occupation exists as long as there are people who occupy themselves – in other words, occupation is the place where human experience and existence is produced and/or reproduced.

The concept of ocupaciones colectivas was discussed by Tolvett (2017) based on their experiences engaging in community work during the Chilean dictatorship. Ocupaciones colectivas are social practices – those actions in everyday doing – in spaces that are shared and cohabitated with others. Ocupaciones colectivas can contribute to a sense of belonging, identity, socio-emotional support, and psychosocial well-being when performed with a purpose toward liberation from oppressive conditions. At the same time, ocupaciones colectivas may contribute to experiences of psychosocial harm, exclusion, and marginalization when enacted in ways that oppress and dominate. As such, ocupaciones colectivas are situated within a dynamic continuum that may or may not produce benefits according to historical contexts and meanings that people and communities attribute to the occupations. Illicit activity engaged in by youth, for example, can contribute to a positive sense of identity and belonging associated with shared values which emerge through engaging together in particular activities. At the same time, participating in illegal situations can risk personal integrity, generate violence, and result in formal and informal social punishment.

In Chile, occupation is understood from different perspectives. Some scholars choose to use the word ocupaciones, with the collective nature implied, while others use the term ocupaciones colectivas explicitly. In this chapter, we have chosen not to translate the term to "collective occupations" to retain the unique cultural connotations of ocupaciones colectivas as conceptualized and examined in Latin America. The concept aligns with Ramugondo and Kronenberg's (2015) definition of collective occupations as "Occupations that are engaged in by individuals, groups, communities and/or societies in everyday contexts; these may reflect an intention towards social cohesion or dysfunction, and/or advancement of or aversion to a common good" (p. 10). These authors assert that "Repressive social orders are thus perpetuated by collective human occupations and vice versa" (p. 10). Guajardo et al. (2015) share perspectives on collective occupation from a Global South, summarizing "There is nothing in me that is not in us" (p. 7). These authors conceptualize occupation beyond the individual, explaining

> if the subject is a product of a particular occupational field ('we are human occupation'), then all action in the professional realm must assume that there is no individual human occupation that is not social, and that any intervention requires assuming collective occupational perspectives for understanding human occupation as a personal, individual fact (p. 7).

Ocupaciones colectivas responds to the naive portrayal of occupations as naturally promoting health and well-being. Instead, occupations are understood as historically situated products that arise from within certain material conditions. Resisting romanticized notions of occupation creates opportunities to explore varied aspects of occupation from individual and societal perspectives. Tolvett (2017) describes ocupaciones colectivas as dynamic and flowing through different junctures, such as benefit/harm, functionality/dysfunctionality, inclusion/exclusion, and support/alienation. Reflecting on the notions of "the dark side", "figured world", "non-sanctioned occupations", and ocupaciones colectivas these ideas invite discovery, analysis, and reflection on the ways in which human occupations emerge and are shaped by conditions and social relationships established between people and the physical, material, symbolic, and natural environment. Deep analysis uncovers contradictions in experiences of occupations which are embedded in social systems and are frequently unequal, unjust, and exclusionary toward historically vulnerable social groups.

A distinctive meaning of ocupaciones colectivas within Latin American scholarship arises from collective action as a form of resistance and means of survival. Lines are drawn between obedience and submission or rebellion and fight. Resistance can be a driver toward achieving desire for betterment, access to rights, freedom, justice, and living with dignity. The notion of ocupaciones colectivas can inform understandings of various global occurrences, such as the planting of olive trees by Palestinians as an act of resistance in the context of war, uprisings, military occupation, segregation, and displacement (Simaan, 2017). Other examples are evident in Chile with regard to parents' efforts to access medicinal cannabis for their children (Valderrama Núñez, 2019) and participation in ancestral artisanal practices within dominant social practices that promote capitalist, economically motivated environmental extractivism (Valderrama Núñez et al., 2021). These ocupaciones colectivas, or non-sanctioned occupations, can promote the rediscovery or re-establishment of a sense of community within systems and society that tend to promote individuality and hedonism (Fredes & Palacios, 2019; Valderrama Núñez, 2019).

Another related concept within Latin American scholarship relates to ocupaciones transgresoras which are defined as occupations that transgress social and moral norms, but that provide meaning, shared values, and give voice and motivation for resistance among particular social groups that are often marginalized or excluded within society (De La Fuente, 2019; Tolvett & Dreyer, 2014). It is relevant to note that notions of ocupaciones transgresoras and non-sanctioned occupations are embedded within, not separate from, dominant perspectives. Accordingly, judgments, whether implicit or explicit, underpin understanding about the degree of acceptability of participation in occupation. There is inherent controversy in defining what is transgressed, sanctioned, or non-sanctioned.

These concepts should be used with caution, as they can further categorize as problematic social groups who perform such non-sanctioned occupations, or ocupaciones transgresoras, that disrupt the established social order. Thus, we are not only discussing intangible social constructs; people who live and engage in such occupations may suffer exclusion or discrimination for being associated with occupations labeled as non-sanctioned or transgresoras. By reproducing these constructs, we could contribute to the perpetuation of discrimination or exclusion for people who participate in such occupations. At the same time, oppression, injustice, harm, and violation of human rights can arise and be perpetuated through ocupaciones colectivas, ocupaciones transgresoras, and non-sanctioned occupations. It is not our intention to convey a presumption that occupations aligned with these constructs inherently lead to positive social transformation.

If we argue that occupaciones transgresoras, ocupaciones colectivas, or non-sanctioned occupations are solely transformative or harmful, we may then question who defines what is beneficial and harmful, and what values inform those definitions. Such decisions and perceptions can be controlled by those in power – often absent of involvement of people in more marginalized social positions – serving to protect elite privileges, peace, assets, and interests.

It can be understood that processes of social sanctioning are governed and shaped through dominant worldviews that can promote and work to produce a monoculture (Santos, 2010), where lifestyles and occupation that do not conform to dominant perspectives on what is right and good can be denied and regulated. Individual and collective values can be undermined by dominant legal and/or social positionings and/ or worldviews that either assume or impose "wrongness". In society, there can exist counter-hegemonic and resistive forces produced by social movements, collectives, communities, and people in their daily lives to resist conditions created by dominant forces that shed light on diverse ways of doing and ways of being. Thus, attending to the less examined (or "dark side", so to speak) aspects of ocupaciones colectivas and ocupaciones transgresoras may encourage diverse and complex meanings.

Complex approaches to understanding human occupation can lead toward social transformation, one form of which involves acknowledging, recognizing, and facilitating contextual understandings of multiple ways of doing and meaning. In seeking to understand occupations, it is important to honor the voice and perspectives of those who are oppressed and avoid representations that "other" or frame the occupation as somehow subjected or "different" from a particular "norm". Arising from transformed understanding of diverse ways of being and doing is the potential for social transformation, such as a sense of hope for improved social conditions and equity among people who are oppressed, marginalized, and vulnerable, a change in law or policy, access to resources, and so on. Ocupaciones colectivas and ocupaciones transgresoras share potential transformational means toward achieving equity and inclusion among marginalized or oppressed social groups, and may act as forms of resistance.

This is not to claim that all occupations are beneficial or without harm. Rather, it is important to engage in critical reflexivity and examine *how* the use of such constructs, social framings of, and participation in, certain occupations are shaped by social, political, and economic contexts. Also, to consider *who* might benefit and *who* might be harmed from defining and participating in particular occupations in particular ways. Failure to do so can perpetuate harm and oppression at individual to societal levels through discrimination and violation of human rights.

13.5 Governance of Individuals and Collectives through Occupation

In this section, we introduce societal power structures that influence the ways in which certain occupations may become understood as non-sanctioned and subject to resistance. Briefly, we explore the means through which occupations are produced, how occupations end up being more or less accepted, and the social processes that govern and rule how people act and how they are judged (and even punished) for performing these actions. For instance, what is defined as a "crime" typically affects marginalized and impoverished groups negatively and disproportionally (Crocker & Johnston, 2010). We discuss social normalization through the lens of cultures and then briefly explore the influence of patriarchy, capitalism, and colonialism on what is considered acceptable and not acceptable.

13.5.1 Deliberations around Social Sanctioning

We ask you to imagine a spectrum that ranges from "not at all socially sanctioned" to "completely socially sanctioned". Consider where you would place the following occupations on this spectrum:

- Refugee rescue efforts.
- Political protest.

- Drug use.
- Child begging.
- International tourism.
- Biking to commute to work.
- Street busking.

The social sanctioning of each of these occupations varies depending on social, cultural, historical, and political contexts.

We present refugee rescue efforts, drug use, and child begging as three examples. First, at the time of writing, millions of Ukrainians have been forced to flee their homes and seek refuge in neighboring countries and abroad, in a context of relatively high international support. At the same time, in some European countries, it is a crime to undertake rescue efforts to save refugees and help them across international borders, with humanitarian volunteers facing up to 15 years in prison (Gordon & Larsen, 2022). Most, if not all countries, have strict regulations about who can and cannot access refuge within their borders.

Second, drug use is subject to different controls across countries and cultures, and throughout history, drug use has been embedded in many traditional, religious, and ceremonial rituals. In many countries, certain "drugs" are classified as illegal, some are produced, distributed, and taxed by the government, and others are prescribed for therapeutic (or medicinal) use. Alcohol is one of the highest risk "drugs" for personal and social harm, yet is viewed in certain contexts and cultures as more socially sanctioned than substances like amphetamines and LSD, which pose relatively less potential for harm (Nutt et al., 2010).

Third, in several countries, particularly in the Global South, it is not uncommon for children to participate in public begging, or mendicancy. This occurs despite national and international efforts to institute policies and laws to mitigate child labor and child trafficking and to improve conditions for children, such as access to education. While some children are forced into begging as a result of violence or coercion by adults, others beg to meet personal survival needs, and in some cultures child begging is viewed as a means to teach humility or religious values (Delap & Anti-Slavery International, 2009).

We remind readers that naming and exploring a full range of human doing as occupation does not mean that we are expected to accept or condone all occupations. Each person is guided by a set of moral values and specific non-negotiable beliefs about what is right or wrong, shaped by the world around us. Through these examples, we aim to convey that the relative social sanctioning of a discrete occupation is not fixed, but varies over time and across cultures, influenced by diverse moral and societal perspectives. Occupations that are considered non-sanctioned under one set of conditions may be sanctioned under another set of conditions.

We suggest it is important to critically reflect on the diverse ways in which occupations are viewed as more or less sanctioned, and to interrogate *why* they are viewed that way. For instance:

- Do these occupations pose unacceptable (or perceived) risk of harm to self or others?
- Whose interests are served when this occupation is deemed disruptive or harmful?

- Who is punished or suffers when this occupation is deemed disruptive or harmful?
- Are these occupations unjust or oppressive?
- Do these occupations arise from or produce inequities?
- As an occupational therapist, can I condone this occupation?
- Is it my personal or professional role to promote a change in others' participation in this occupation? Why do I believe this?
- Is it my personal or professional role to address implications arising from participation in this occupation?

As noted, a disadvantage of a term like "non-sanctioned" is that it conveys and creates a dualism that can be problematic. It positions certain occupations as less desirable and others as more desirable; however, such distinctions are rarely reflective of lived experiences. The degree to which an occupation is formally and informally promoted or condemned relates to various forces, including historical, cultural, sociopolitical, and power. For instance, effective from January 2023, British Columbia, a Canadian province, will decriminalize possession of small amounts of illicit drugs for personal use (Paterson, 2022). Arguments for decriminalization generally promote cessation of criminal charges and/or imprisonment for possession of illicit substances, alongside improved access to social and health resources. Substance use disproportionately impacts people who experience poverty and are homeless, diagnosed with a mental health disorder, racialized, have a history of being removed from their families through child custody services, and/or have a developmental delay; thus, criminalization of drugs effectively criminalizes "poverty" (St. Denis, 2020). Despite drug use being associated with potential harms to health and well-being, individual and societal harms that arise from it being *defined* as a crime exacerbate, and sometimes cause, negative consequences. Unfortunately, decriminalization is unlikely to eliminate the social stigmatization and marginalization experienced by people who use illicit substances and the associated inequities.

Interrogation about why occupations are more or less sanctioned extend to those predominantly viewed as appropriate or acceptable. Many contemporary industrial and capitalistic occupations have direct and indirect impacts on environmental sustainability, pollution, and extinction (Atapattu et al., 2021). International tourism is an example of a privileged and classist occupation not available to many, and it is generally viewed as an inherent right of people who have the financial resources and legal permission to cross international borders. While this can be an economic advantage to the receiving country and foster increases in cross-cultural understanding, air travel and tourism are associated with carbon emissions, negative ecological impacts on land, waters, and local species, restrictions on local residents accessing desirable land and resources, and the devaluing and denigrating of cultural and spiritual sites. Even local modes of transportation, such as personal vehicles and trains, present risk of personal and environmental harm. Roads and railways have an extensive worldwide footprint that results in high rates of collision and mortality among wildlife, including birds, reptiles, and mammals (Popp & Boyle, 2017). Degrees of social sanctioning are therefore related to a number of factors associated with social values, health, well-being, justice, power, control, and anthropocentrism.

13.5.2 Social Inequities

Social groups that have historically experienced relative marginalization, social exclusion, and oppression include, among others, children, the elderly, women, Indigenous people, racialized people, disabled persons, people who have immigrated, people who live in rural regions, people who identify as LGBTQIA2S+ (lesbian, gay, bisexual, transgender, queer and/or questioning, intersex, asexual, two-spirit, and the countless affirmative ways in which people choose to self-identify), and people who live in impoverished conditions. Some theorists point to three primary modes of "modern domination", which are "capitalism (exploitation of labor power), colonialism (racism, slave labor, accumulation by dispossession), and patriarchy" (Atapattu et al., 2021, p. xvii). From a Global South perspective, capitalism, patriarchy, and colonialism are violently imposed in territories (Santos, 2018). Although European expansion and the practices of conquering civilizations across the American, African, and Asian continents occurred historically, modern domination continues through adapted, transformed, and reinvented social processes.

Oppressive forces materialized in day-to-day lives become normalized through doing and knowing. Examples include adult-centrism, gender inequities, ableism, and racism.

- Adult-centrism limits children's right to voice their opinion and participation in family matters. In some contexts, children are considered the property of the parents, transforming them into objects and actualizing their existence. Children's rights to occupational participation are unjustly regulated by their parents and other dominant social institutions, leading to occupational injustices through forced participation or marginalization in occupations.
- Sex and gender inequities influence the types of occupations people engage in and which occupations are more or less socially acceptable. Globally, women are more likely than men to be responsible for housework and caregiving and earn a lower wage than men in paid employment (Lexartza Artza et al., 2019).
- Ableist, capitalistic ideologies discriminate based on people's ability status and impede and exclude participation in socially valued occupations, such as work, education, sports, and community participation (Van Aswegen & Shevlin, 2019).
- Racism is one of the most complex forms of discrimination that affects populations. White supremacy dominates capitalist production and has historically functioned to subordinate knowledges, customs, and worldviews of racialized groups. Slavery and servitude were the main (sanctioned) occupations of ethno-racial groups for many years. Racialized people continue to experience inequities in employment opportunities (Sanchez-Rivera, 2020), such as being relegated to low-skilled occupations, prevented from accessing education, and forced to adopt the customs and culture of the dominant group (i.e., Western languages, beliefs, and values) (Ambrosio et al., 2021).

Although invisible, power underlies occupational possibility and occupational choice. Critical reflexivity is a means to identify the influence of power on subjectivities, lifestyles, interactions with others and the earth, social values, and the social sanctioning of occupation.

13.6 Implications for Occupational Therapy

Farias and colleagues, in Chapter 8, argue that critical scholarship can contribute to social transformation by problematizing dominant norms to resist individualistic tendencies and, thereby, shift ways of thinking and doing. This involves critical reflection aimed at avoiding the (re)production of ethnocentrism in practice, not just in theory (Farias & Laliberte Rudman, 2016). Developing critical and complex understandings of the various dimensions of occupation can inform, shape, and transform how occupational therapists approach their work with clients from diverse backgrounds and experiences. At minimum, interrogating our own ideas of what is or is not socially sanctioned, by reflecting on our own values and attempting to genuinely understand others' perspectives, will help us to approach our work with compassion and empathy.

When working with diverse populations, occupational therapists may consider therapeutic approaches to elicit and listen to experiences around various and complex occupations. It is important to create spaces for people to genuinely disclose the types of occupations they engage in and to share complex meanings, situatedness, and implications that may conform to and/or counter dominant understandings (see Box 13.2).

Box 13.2 Critical Reflection – Marcel Nazabal Amores

In the context of a dictatorship, state power is sustained through repressive forces, demagogic manipulation of politics, persecution, and unlawful prosecution to control and oppress their citizens. This is particularly harmful to those who oppose and claim their universal rights of freedom before such unjust ideologies. Long-term exposure to such regimes forces people to implement adaptative strategies that show content with the system at a superficial level but true beliefs are hidden to socially survive under these conditions. Civilians under totalitarian governments often distrust and fear the police, military, and civil espionage, and experience these feelings in their daily doings to fulfill their basic needs (e.g., obtaining food and household goods) which are often bought in the underground ("illegal") economy. In this environment individuals and families may develop trauma that carries forward even after emigrating or escaping from hostile countries. For example, some immigrants or refugees that have fled dictatorships may react with fear toward authorities in new countries as a result of prior traumatic experiences. Therefore, instead of seeking protection or help in certain circumstances, they may attempt to troubleshoot in a similar way that warranted "safety" in their home country, but which may not fit the sociopolitical context of the receiving nation. Understandings of diverse contexts and experiences could bring a critical perspective to bear for occupational therapists working alongside clients from similar hostile backgrounds.

Occupational therapists may be in positions of relative social privilege that can be harnessed to influence social and political change. Beyond their work with individual clients, occupational therapists may engage in advocacy to inform and alter service delivery models, policies, and laws. We need to work toward the transformation of social structures that directly and indirectly contribute to injustices, violence, trauma, and environmental degradation. Throughout time, there have been oppressive forces that provide certain groups with advantages while oppressing others; for example, slavery, indentured labor, human trafficking, constraints around women's rights, violence toward people who identify as non-binary, residential schools, and war (see Box 13.3).

> **Box 13.3 Bridging Research and Practice**
>
> Three of the chapter authors have undertaken research about substance use that can serve as examples for impacts on occupational therapy practices.
>
> Sy et al. (2020) undertook research on substance use in the context of the Philippine War on Drugs that resulted in the extrajudicial deaths of over 9,000 people. The research found that drug use could enhance a person's productivity and economic participation, particularly for those working in jobs requiring stamina, long hours, and arduous labor. From the perspective of social transformation, occupational therapists might promote emancipatory and interprofessional approaches using strategies such as multi-voicedness, codesigning, open discussion, and goal setting/care planning through interprofessional teams to encourage, support and sustain the (re)integration into society of citizens who use drugs.
>
> Benjamin-Thomas et al. (2022) carried out participatory action research with children with disabilities in rural India as co-researchers to investigate how substance abuse within their community contributed to household and community violence and environmental degradation. This "non-sanctioned" occupation was positioned as predictable occupational choices and taken-for-granted ways of being shaped by socioeconomic inequities. Additionally, inter-related occupational issues of garbage disposal and accumulation within villages contributed to substance use among young children. Occupational therapists could work in schools to discuss the situated nature and implications of drug abuse at individual to community levels, as well as develop occupation-based environmental programs. From a social transformation perspective, occupational therapists could join advocacy efforts to address systemic issues informing cycles of socioeconomic inequities.
>
> Kiepek, Beagan, Ausman et al. (2022) uncovered gendered differences in how Canadian women with professional careers reported advantages of substance use. Women reported greater responsibility for household maintenance and childcare, with substances acting as a "reward for surviving the day". From an individual perspective, an occupational therapist might assess the person's routine, consider introducing alternative relaxation strategies, and explore options to re-distribute some responsibilities to others. From the perspective of social transformation, occupational therapists might reflect on how they perpetuate gendered roles in teaching, research, and practice, such as the implicit exclusion of fathering (White, 2020).

13.7 Conclusion

The contemporaneous emergence of scholarship around ocupaciones transgresoras, ocupaciones colectivas, non-sanctioned occupations, the dark side of occupation, and the figured world of occupation reflects an underlying shift in understandings of occupation. Broadening definitions and understandings of occupation opens up possibilities for deeper and more complex understanding of people, the things they do, and the contexts in which occupations occur.

Occupational therapy and occupational science researchers are encouraged to consider how these ideas might inform the design of research projects and the types of questions asked. Understandings of diverse occupations should ideally come from the perspective of those who participate in these occupations, and it is important to consider how divergent and non-dominant perspectives might be silenced when not explicitly addressed as part of the data-collection process or analysis. It may be advantageous to engage in practice-based inquiry among communities of practitioners and scholars (Whiteford, 2020).

These types of insights may also align with approaches to social occupational therapy, which is described in Chapter 15. By incorporating these ideas into entry-level occupational therapy education, graduates may be better equipped to practice in role-emergent areas such as shelters for people who are unhoused or precariously housed, child protection services, court diversion programs, and more. Through engaging in critical reflexivity, we imagine novel and innovative occupation-based programs that promote dignity of life and well-being for individuals and collectives.

13.8 Summary

- The emergence of notions such as "the dark side of occupation", "figured world of occupation", "non-sanctioned occupations", ocupaciones transgresoras, and ocupaciones colectivas indicate a shift away from viewing occupations as having exclusively positive connotations for individuals and collectives.
- Notions of non-sanctioned occupations, ocupaciones transgresoras, and ocupaciones colectivas share similarities in attending to the social positioning of certain occupations that arise from context and conditions. However, while literature around non-sanctioned occupations tends to view sanctioning as arising from situated contexts, the literature around ocupaciones transgresoras and ocupaciones colectivas explicitly confronts oppressive forces, with participation in occupations viewed as deliberate acts of power and resistance.
- Deep understandings of ocupaciones colectivas, ocupaciones transgresoras, and non-sanctioned occupations require not only inquiry about the meanings and experiences of those participating in the occupations, but also critical inquiry about the context, social and political ideology, laws, social norms, cultural apparatus, and other factors that influence and shape individual and collective meanings, as well as understandings about implications from such participation.
- By analyzing occupations as situated in complex contexts that can produce social inequities, injustice, oppression, and harm, occupational therapists will be better positioned to respond to individual and collective needs and support meaningful and lasting improvements.

13.9 Review Questions

1. In what ways might ideas around the dark side of occupation, figured world of occupation, non-sanctioned occupations, ocupaciones transgresoras, and ocupaciones colectivas impact and shape current understandings of occupation?

2. What is the importance of critically interrogating why an occupation may (or may not) be viewed as socially sanctioned, when engaged in by certain individuals or collectives in particular contexts?
3. What personal and social values, assumptions, and beliefs influence your own judgment around the social sanctioning of occupations?
4. If an occupation is assessed to produce social inequities, injustice, oppression, and harm, how might this influence occupational therapy approaches?
5. In what ways are non-sanctioned occupations, ocupaciones colectivas, and ocupaciones transgresoras envisioned and positioned as forms of resistance that hold transformative potential to achieve equity among marginalized or oppressed social groups?
6. Describe the limitations of rhetorically naming an occupation as non-sanctioned or dark. What factors should be examined when describing the socially situated nature of occupations as more or less condoned, sanctioned, or accepted?

References

Ambrosio, L., Riquelme, V., Morrison, R., Gonçalves, A., & Silva, C. (2021). La urgencia de una Terapia Ocupacional Antirracista. *Revista de Estudiantes de Terapia Ocupacional, 8*(1), 1–17. http://www.reto.ubo.cl/index.php/reto/article/view/116/103

Atapattu, S. A., Gonzalez, C. G., & Seck, S. L. (2021). Intersections of environmental justice and sustainable development: Framing the issues. In S. A. Atapattu, C. G. Gonzalez, & S. L. Seck (Eds.), *The Cambridge handbook of environmental justice and sustainable development* (pp. 1–22). Cambridge University Press.

Benjamin-Thomas, T. E., Rudman, D. L., McGrath, C., Cameron, D., Abraham, V. J., Gunaseelan, J., & Vinothkumar, S. P. (2022). Situating occupational injustices experienced by children with disabilities in rural India within sociocultural, economic, and systemic conditions. *Journal of Occupational Science, 29*(1), 97–114. https://doi.org/10.1080/14427591.2021.1899038

Crocker, D., & Johnston, V. M. (2010). *Poverty, regulation and social justice: Readings on the criminalization of poverty*. Fernwood Publishing.

De La Fuente, P. P. (2019). Mujeres jóvenes y construcción de ocupaciones transgresoras: Una mirada de las trayectorias de vida desde Terapia Ocupacional. *Revista Chilena De Terapia Ocupacional, 19*(2), 112–113. https://doi.org/10.5354/0719-5346.2019.56980

Delap, E., & Anti-Slavery International. (2009). *Begging for change*. https://www.antislavery.org/wp-content/uploads/2017/01/beggingforchange09.pdf

Farias, L., & Laliberte Rudman, D. (2016). A critical interpretive synthesis of the uptake of critical perspectives in occupational science. *Journal of Occupational Science, 23*(1), 33–50. https://doi.org/10.1080/14427591.2014.989893

Fredes, F., & Palacios, M. (2019). Fútbol de barrio como okupación colectiva: Sentido de comunidad, territorio e identidades juveniles. In W. S. Acosta & L. D. S. Ocampo (Eds.), *Discriminaciones socioculturales globales: Entre el fútbol y la política* (pp. 195–210). CLACSO.

Gordon, E., & Larsen, H. K. (2022). 'Sea of blood': The intended and unintended effects of criminalising humanitarian volunteers assisting migrants in distress at sea. *Disasters, 46*(1), 3–26. https://doi.org/10.1111/disa.12472

Guajardo, A. (2014). Una terapia ocupacional crítica como posibilidad. In V. Santos & A. Donatti (Eds.), *Cuestiones contemporáneas de terapia ocupacional en América del Sur* (pp. 159–165). Editorial CRV.

Guajardo, A., Kronenberg, F., & Ramugondo, L. E. (2015). Southern occupational therapies: Emerging identities, epistemologies and practices. *South African Journal of Occupational Therapy, 45*(1), 1–9. http://doi.org/10.17159/2310-3833/2015/v45no1a2

Hammell, K. W. (2006). *Perspectives on disability & rehabilitation: Contesting assumptions, challenging practice*. Churchill Livingstone/Elsevier.

Hocking, C. (2009). The challenge of occupation: Describing the things people do. *Journal of Occupational Science, 16*(3), 140–150. https://doi.org/10.1080/14427591.2009.9686655

Kiepek, N., Beagan, B., Ausman, C., & Patten, S. (2022). "A reward for surviving the day": Women professionals' substance use to enhance performance. *Performance Enhancement & Health, 10*(2), 100220. https://doi.org/10.1016/j.peh.2022.100220

Kiepek, N., Beagan, B., Patten, S., & Ausman, C. (2022). Reflecting on conceptualisations of 'meaning' in occupational therapy. *Cadernos Brasileiros de Terapia Ocupacional, 30*, e3156. https://doi.org/10.1590/2526-8910.ctoARF24193156

Kiepek, N., & Magalhães, L. (2011). Addictions and impulse-control disorders as occupation: A selected literature review and synthesis. *Journal of Occupational Science, 18*(3), 254–276. https://doi.org/10.1080/14427591.2011.581628

Kiepek, N., Phelan, S., & Magalhães, L. (2014). Introducing a critical analysis of the figured world of occupation. *Journal of Occupational Science, 21*(4), 403–417. https://doi.org/10.1080/14427591.2013.816998

Kiepek, N. C. (2021). Innocent observers? Discursive choices and the construction of "occupation". *Journal of Occupational Science, 28*(2), 235–248. https://doi.org/10.1080/14427591.2020.1799847

Kiepek, N. C., Beagan, B., Rudman, D. L., & Phelan, S. (2019). Silences around occupations framed as unhealthy, illegal, and deviant. *Journal of Occupational Science, 26*(3), 341–353. https://doi.org/10.1080/14427591.2018.1499123

Laliberte Rudman, D., Aldrich, R. M., & Kiepek, N. (2022). Evolving understandings of occupation. In M. Egan & G. Restall (Eds.), *Promoting occupational participation: Collaborative relationship-focused occupational therapy* (pp. 11–30). Canadian Association of Occupational Therapists.

Lexartza Artza, L., Chaves Groh, M. J., Carcedo Cabañas, A., y Sánchez, A. (2019). La brecha salarial entre hombres y mujeres en América Latina. En el camino hacia la igualdad salarial. Organización Internacional del Trabajo.

Matt Finch/Mechanical Dolphin. (2018). *Bex Twinley: The dark side of occupation*. https://mechanicaldolphin.com/2018/08/03/bex-twinley-the-dark-side-of-occupation/

Nascimento, B. A. N. (1990). O mito da atividade terapêutica. *Revista de Terapia Ocupacional da USP, 1*(1), 17–21.

Nutt, D. J., King, L. A., & Phillips, L. D. (2010). Drug harms in the UK: A multicriteria decision analysis. *The Lancet, 376*(9752), 1558–1565. https://doi.org/10.1016/S0140-6736(10)61462-6

Paterson, S. (2022, May 31). *"Health care over handcuffs": B.C. first to decriminalize simple drug possession*. https://bc.ctvnews.ca/possession-of-small-amounts-of-illicit-drugs-will-be-decriminalized-in-b-c-1.5925897

Popp, J. N., & Boyle, S. P. (2017). Railway ecology: Underrepresented in science? *Basic and Applied Ecology, 19*, 84–93. https://doi.org/10.1016/j.baae.2016.11.006

Ramugondo, E. (2015). Occupational consciousness. *Journal of Occupational Science, 22*(4), 488–501. https://doi.org/10.1080/14427591.2015.1042516

Ramugondo, E. L., & Kronenberg, F. (2015). Explaining collective occupations from a human relations perspective: Bridging the individual-collective dichotomy. *Journal of Occupational Science, 22*(1), 3–16. https://doi.org/10.1080/14427591.2013.781920

Ruiz, J. (2009). Sociological discourse analysis: Methods and logic. *Forum: Qualitative Social Research, 10*(2), 1–31. http://nbn-resolving.de/urn:nbn:de:0114-fqs0902263

Russell, E. (2008). Writing on the wall: The form, function and meaning of tagging. *Journal of Occupational Science, 15*(2), 87–97. https://doi.org/10.1080/14427591.2008.9686614

Sanchez-Rivera, R. (2020). The legacies of 'race' science, anti-Chinese racism, and COVID-19 in Mexico. *Bulletin of Latin American Research, 39*(S1), 35–38. https://doi.org/10.1111/blar.13173

Santos, B. d. S. (2010). *Descolonizar el saber, reinventar el poder*. Ediciones Trilce. http://www.boaventuradesousasantos.pt/media/Descolonizar%20el%20saber_final%20-%20C%C3%B3pia.pdf

Santos, B. d. S. (2018). Introducción a las epistemologías del sur. In M. P. Meneses & K. Bidaseca (Eds.), *Epistemologías del Sur* (pp. 25–62): Ciudad Autónoma de Buenos Aires: CLACSO. http://biblioteca.clacso.edu.ar/clacso/se/20181124092336/Epistemologias_del_sur_2018.pdf

Simaan, J. (2017). Olive growing in Palestine: A decolonial ethnographic study of collective daily-forms-of-resistance. *Journal of Occupational Science*, 24(4), 510–523. https://doi.org/10.1080/14427591.2017.1378119

St. Denis, J. (2020, July 29). Vancouver votes to 'decriminalize poverty.' Over to you, police and province. *The Tyee*. https://thetyee.ca/News/2020/07/29/Vancouver-Votes-Decriminalizing-Poverty/

Stewart, K. E., Fischer, T. M., Hirji, R., & Davis, J. A. (2016). Toward the reconceptualization of the relationship between occupation and health and well-being. *Canadian Journal of Occupational Therapy*, 83(4), 249–259. https://doi.org/10.1177/0008417415625425

Sy, M. P., Bontje, P., Ohshima, N., & Kiepek, N. (2020). Articulating the form, function, and meaning of drug using in the Philippines from the lens of morality and work ethics. *Journal of Occupational Science*, 27(1), 12–21. https://doi.org/10.1080/14427591.2019.1644662

Tolvett, M. P. (2017). *Acerca de sentido de comunidad, ocupaciones colectivas y bienestar/malestar psicosocial. Con jóvenes transgresores de territorios Populares*. Universitat de Vic; Universitat Central de Catalunya, Chile. http://repositori.uvic.cat/bitstream/handle/10854/5286/tesdoc_a2017_palacios_monica_acerca_sentido.pdf?sequ%20ence=1&isAllowed=y

Tolvett, M. P., & Dreyer, C. S. (2014). Significados de la ocupación en jóvenes infractores de la ley, participantes de programas de inclusión social en Chile. *Ocupación Humana*, 14(2), 5–22. https://doi.org/10.25214/25907816.46

Twinley, R. (2013). The dark side of occupation: A concept for consideration. *Australian Occupational Therapy Journal*, 60(4), 301–303. https://doi.org/10.1111/1440-1630.12026

Twinley, R. (2020). The dark side of occupation: An introduction to the naming, creation, intent, and development of the concept. In R. Twinley (Ed.), *Illuminating the dark side of occupation: International perspectives from occupational therapy and occupational science* (pp. 1–14). Routledge.

Valderrama Núñez, C. M. (2019). Terapias ocupacionales del sur: Una propuesta para su comprensión. *Cadernos Brasileiros de Terapia Ocupacional*, 27(3), 671–680. https://doi.org/10.4322/2526-8910.ctoARF1859

Valderrama Núñez, C. M., & Riquelme, P. L. (2013). Cuestionamientos sobre el carácter beneficioso para la salud y el bienestar de la ocupación: La emergencia de la ocupación como fenómeno social. *Revista Terapia Ocupacional Galicia*, 10(18), 1–15. https://www.revistatog.com/num18/pdfs/original9.pdf

Valderrama Núñez, C. M., Sepúlveda Hernández, S., & Hermosilla Alarcón, A. (2021). Collective occupations and nature: Impacts of the coloniality of nature on rural and fishing communities in Chile. *Journal of Occupational Science*, 29(2), 252–262. https://doi.org/10.1080/14427591.2021.1880264

Van Aswegen, J., & Shevlin, M. (2019). Disabling discourses and ableist assumptions: Reimagining social justice through education for disabled people through a critical discourse analysis approach. *Policy Futures in Education*, 17(5), 634–656. https://doi.org/10.1177/1478210318817420

White, T. (2020). *Representation of parenting in occupational science and therapy literature: A critical interpretative*. Faculty of Graduate Studies Online Theses, Dalhousie University. http://hdl.handle.net/10222/79940

Whiteford, G. E. (2020). Practice-based enquiry, practice transformation, and service redesign. In *Sage research methods cases: Medicine and health.* https://doi.org/https://dx.doi.org/10.4135/9781529740363

Wilcock, A. (1993). A theory of the need for human occupation. *Occupational Science: Australia, 1*(1), 17–24. https://doi.org/10.1080/14427591.1993.9686375

CHAPTER 14

Creativity, Hope, and Collective Emancipatory Experimentation

Tools for Social Transformation through Occupational Therapy

Vagner Dos Santos and Gelya Frank

Abstract

This chapter discusses a growing body of theoretical and practical work by occupational therapists interested in developing practices around social transformation. A corresponding interest is also developing around the concept of collective occupations. Our intended audience is students and entry-level professionals in occupational therapy who will most likely find themselves in mainly corporatized health care systems. The chapter introduces Occupational Reconstruction Theory to students and practitioners of occupational therapy. Occupational Reconstruction Theory grows out of interdisciplinary scholarship in occupational science, social anthropology, 20th-century pragmatism, narrative studies, social movement studies, and occupational therapy. The purpose of Occupational Reconstruction Theory is to identify the key underlying principles guiding social transformation practice in occupational therapy. The chapter also discusses why practitioners need some familiarity with philosophical frameworks of thought to justify changes they may wish to make to theory and practice, as well as to adequately evaluate and critique changes proposed or enacted by others. Finally, the chapter discusses the Occupational Reconstruction Theory, which identifies a set of elements that appear to be common among documented instances of transformative social action. It also discusses how an occupational therapist could use Occupational Reconstruction Theory as a practical framework for social transformation practice.

Authors' Positionality Statement

Vagner Dos Santos (b. 1982) is a Brazilian occupational therapy clinician, educator, and scholar. Gelya Frank (b. 1948) is an American social and medical anthropologist who co-founded the discipline of occupational science. Vagner's native language is Portuguese; he is also fluent in English and Spanish, and proficient in French.

Vagner was born on the lands of the Guarani people, along the banks of the Uruguay River, in the territory known as São Borja, Brazil. He currently lives in, and has written this piece on, the land of the Birpai people, known as Port Macquarie, Australia.

He is dedicated to designing and advancing critical projects in occupational therapy, while recognizing that professional knowledge is deeply entangled with colonial projects. He has made extensive contributions to promoting southern perspectives, including leading edited publications on occupational therapy in South America.

Gelya's native language is English with some proficiency in French, Spanish, and Yiddish. Gelya was born and raised in New York City on Lenape land and lives in Santa Monica, California on unceded land of the Tongva people. Since 1972, she has consulted on indigenous history, land claims, and water rights to the Tule River Tribe of central California (Yowlumne, Yaudaunchi Yokuts, and Western Mono tribes). See Gelya Frank and Carole Goldberg, *Defying the odds: The Tule River Tribe's struggle for sovereignty in three centuries* (Yale University Press, 2010). Gelya is also founder of the occupation-based Tule River Tribal History Project and the NAPA/OT Interdisciplinary Field School in Guatemala (www.napotguatemala.com).

As colleagues since 2017, Vagner and Gelya are committed to developing conceptual frameworks to address problematic situations in a community's lived experience through collective occupation. Their work together emphasizes human and cultural rights, local experience and agency, the role of narrative in community building, and experimentation.

Objectives

This chapter:

- Reviews the notion of collective doings in occupational therapy and occupational science.
- Reviews recent arguments for social approaches in occupational therapy and defines the specific goals of social transformation practice.
- Discusses the interdisciplinary and philosophical sources contributing to Occupational Reconstruction Theory as a description of and guide to social transformation practice.
- Describes seven principles of Occupational Reconstruction Theory and suggests a practice framework for occupational therapists when applying them to practice.

Key terms

- **shared situations**
- **collective occupations**
- **social reconstructions**
- **occupational reconstructions**
- **social transformation practice**
- **Occupational reconstruction theory**

CREATIVITY, HOPE, AND COLLECTIVE EMANCIPATORY EXPERIMENTATION

14.1 Introduction

Social transformation refers to the process of change in a society's social structure and cultural norms. This change can occur through cultural diffusion, reform, revolution, or other means, mainly through collective engagement, to alter power dynamics, values, beliefs, and behavior patterns (Dos Santos, 2022; Dos Santos et al., 2020; Frank & Muriithi, 2015; Godoy et al., 2020). Examples of social transformations, specifically through social movements, include the Women's Suffrage Movement (Crawford, 2000), the Civil Rights Movement (Frank & Muriithi, 2015; Morris, 1986), and the LGBTQIAS+ rights movement (Terriquez, 2015). When aligned with justice, social transformation can inform professional development, advance equality, and promote inclusion and participation (Farias et al., 2016; Godoy et al., 2020).

A growing body of literature in occupational therapy and the discipline of occupational science argues for greater commitment to social transformative practices dealing with social-structured problems (van Bruggen et al., 2020; Cunningham et al., 2022; Dickie & Frank, 1996; Farias & Laliberte Rudman, 2016; Frank & Dos Santos, 2020; Galheigo, 2011; Hammell, 2020a; Lopes & Malfitano, 2020; Pollard et al., 2008). In this sense, occupational therapy and occupational science emerge as privileged to produce knowledge and apply social transformative practices.

Occupational therapy has historically been a profession concerned with individual independence (Bonikowsky et al., 2012). However, as indicated by critical scholars, this reflects normative views and toxic ableist ideology, and consequently limits the profession's scope of practice with disabled people (Grenier, 2021; Hammell, 2021, 2022, 2023). This individualist view aligns with the neoliberal common sense that celebrates independence and self-reliance as the core of individual productivity in the marketplace (Dos Santos, 2022). In this sense, occupational therapists' role is reduced to ensuring that individuals can work and become productive members of a capitalistic society while ensuring that those labeled unproductive are controlled and confined to the client role of the helping professions. This (arrested) professional development made occupational therapy a worthwhile project for health systems concerned with efficiency, time, and cost reductions, within a context focused on austerity measures and profit (Hayes et al., 2023a, 2023b).

In parallel, there is growing awareness that the profession has to face its contradictions and potentially overcome what the American sociologist Joseph Gusfield, writing about helping professions, called its benevolent repressive character in society (Gusfield, 1996). This means that support comes with a repressive nature, which aims to impose specific values and prevent personal and social emancipation. An example of overcoming the benevolent repressive nature of helping professions can be found in Dickie and Frank's (1996) discussion on artisan occupations as therapy and a form of collective resistance. Their argument moves craft beyond an individual experience of potential healing; instead, they placed craft as part of a social experience with the potential to challenge dominant structures. This demonstrates that a critical understanding of occupation can promote a shift in how knowledge is produced and applied. Indeed, they argue, in the early days of occupational science, that "the new discipline may be poised to develop a better understanding of resistance to domination by bringing patterns of everyday activities themselves to the foreground" (Dickie & Frank, 1996, p. 46).

Similarly, other disciplines and professions have been calling for a shift toward changes in cultural and social processes, expressing their social transformative aspirations. For instance, public health researchers and medical anthropologists envision a "fifth wave" in public health and call for nothing less than a paradigm shift in culture (Hanlon et al., 2011). They argue that a new wave will similarly require a shift in human consciousness. The new wave is in the realm of culture and experience: shared symbols, meanings, values, beliefs, and aspirations. Cultures are not merely beliefs and values but, as anthropologists and sociologists – for example, Pierre Bourdieu – have amply demonstrated, they are also embodied dispositions (Bourdieu, 1977).

More recently, many critical scholars are engaged in promoting epistemological and practical shifts in the profession (Emery-Whittington, 2021; Frank & Dos Santos, 2020; Galvaan, 2021; Galvaan & Peters, 2014; Godoy et al., 2020; Hammell, 2020b; Iwama, 2006; Leite Junior et al., 2021; Lopes & Malfitano, 2020; Pereira, 2017). This critical approach reflects a professional commitment to those vulnerable, neglected, and oppressed individuals, groups, communities, and populations. By challenging the *status quo* that reflects culturally specific, ableist, White, Anglophone, Judeo-Christian, Western, middle-class norms and values, the profession aims to increase its social relevance by addressing social-structured problems (Hammell, 2022b). Current evidence shows that social structure and dynamics determine health, well-being, participation, income, and education (Marmot, 2004, 2005; Venkatapuram, 2013). Thus, this shift from individual toward collective actors is necessary.

Yet, the effort to build theories and frameworks to reflect this change in education, research, and practice is still required. For instance, since the 1980s, Brazilian occupational therapists have been working to deal with social questions (Barros et al., 2002), i.e., social-structured problems that often can be presented as individual issues (e.g., unemployment, violence, and education). The propositions of Social Occupational Therapy reflect a commitment to social transformation through inclusion, participation, and autonomy (Lopes & Malfitano, 2020).

This chapter takes this critical approach to deal with collective actors and social-structured problems. Drawing from empirical data and theoretical formulations, we present the Occupational Reconstruction Theory to inform practice, education, and research. Occupational Reconstruction Theory contributes to the growing body of theoretical and practical discussions to advance the profession and the discipline's commitment to work with collective actors, deal with social issues, and promote justice. We therefore present the philosophical influences of the Occupational Reconstruction Theory and its potential use as a framework for practice with collective actors.

14.2 Philosophical Influences of Occupational Reconstruction Theory

The social anthropologist and occupational scientist Gelya Frank developed the Occupational Reconstruction Theory (Frank & Muriithi, 2015; Frank & Santos, 2020). The initial formulations of Occupational Reconstruction Theory come from Frank's interpretation of the pragmatic philosopher John Dewey's work. The focus on collective reconstructions of problematic situations by means of occupations comes from Dewey's interest in social reconstruction. Dewey saw the community as a culture that pre-exists individuals and continually reconstructs itself as a self-organizing and evolving entity. Dewey's view of education and democracy in the United States follows a model that focuses on cooperative problem-solving in response to challenges from, or in, the environment (Dewey, 1958). As a pragmatist, Dewey's philosophy deviated radically from its 19th-century antecedents in its approach to truth. Instead of a universal, timeless, abstract, and absolute principle, the pragmatist framing of truth held it to be emergent.

Dewey holds that truth is emergent through "situations," also called "problematic situations" (Dewey, 1958). Thus, truth, in the traditional pragmatic sense, of the "right" way to do things, adheres in the individual in the form of habits and in the culture the form of traditions. The two, habit and tradition, exist in a mutual relationship of transaction. A situation in this Deweyan sense refers to a noticeable hitch in the smooth flow of living, a disruption of habit and tradition that must be addressed. The usual ways of doing and thinking about the problem cannot solve it. Consequently, the (problematic) situation may prompt creative experimentation to devise an alternative way to do the desired thing. Reflection on the usefulness of the new way of doing things can result in a new, provisional truth about the situation and, by extension, the nature of reality. Thus, the pragmatic tradition informs us that something needs to be done.

Yet, the last century pragmatic philosophers cannot inform us about the inequalities of human life that we currently face, including but not limited to neoliberal politics and governance (Chomsky & Waterstone, 2021), Indigenous dispossession (Simpson, 2017), economic inequality (Sen, 1997), violence (Abrahams et al., 2014), and racism (Bailey et al., 2017), among other social-structured problems. Indeed, it has been argued that significant figures of Pragmatism were not committed to the injustices of the most vulnerable groups in their time. For instance, the most liberal democratic philosopher, Dewey, was not convinced that the world was in need of great social transformation (James, 2017). This is not to say that he was oblivious to the racism and inequality exacerbated by the Jim Crow Era and the Great Depression during his time in the United States, but he certainly neglected the critically examined racial, economic social-structured problems (James, 2017; Koopman, 2017).

In this sense, we build from Frank's initial pragmatic influences and combine other philosophical and practical influences. A theory founded on Pragmatism can, and should, be flexible and dynamic to capture changes in society, advances in science, and maintain its cross-cultural and cross-social relevance. Indeed, it has been argued that "Pragmatism's empirical methodology and its focus on concrete practical problems supposedly makes it the perfect mediator to connect people, ideas and practices" (Williams, 2019, p. 236).

Here we take seriously the professional pragmatic commitment to do something, to engage in diverse forms of doing to make life better, as articulated by Unger to pursue a "never-ending quest for social transformation and self-development" (West, 1989, p. 214). However, we recognize that we need to account for political and social struggles that systematically oppress individuals and groups. In this sense, we present Occupational Reconstruction Theory influenced by critically interpreting its application in occupational therapy work with/in collective actors and aiming to promote emancipatory experimentalism. Emancipation as a process of freeing individuals and collectives from their social, political, and economic oppressions. According to Gramsci, society's dominant ideologies often serve to maintain the *status quo* and reproduce the existing power relations, while obscuring the underlying conflicts and inequalities (Gramsci, 2011). This emancipatory perspective aligns with the growing social commitment of the profession, and it aims to create and expand from the traditional Pragmatism of Dewey.

The theory assumes that we share and (arguably) create problematic situations together. Consequently, the responsibility lies beyond individuals, to be located in collectives. Here interdependence emerges as a core element in informing our understanding of collective actions and actors. Interdependency refers to the interconnectedness of individuals, where actions and events in one social sphere affect others (Elias, 2001; Malfitano et al., 2021). This interconnectedness, or connection of actors and interactions, is also found in Bourdieu's notion of social fields, which refers to the interconnected network of social relations and institutions within which individuals and groups interact and compete for diverse forms of capital (Bourdieu, 1977). According to Bourdieu, the accumulation and distribution of cultural and economic capital are shaped by the relationships between agents and the structures of the social field, and it reflects and reinforces existing power relations. Taking these influences into account, we introduce below Occupational Reconstruction Theory, emphasizing its seven key principles.

14.3 Occupational Reconstruction Theory: Overview and Principles

Occupational reconstructions are forms of social experientialism and involve conscious engagement in concrete action or focused doing by a collective. Occupational reconstructions are a temporary, intermittent kind of social organization aimed at dealing with a problematic situation. They are hopeful experiments by collective actors to improve a problematic situation. A criterion for testing the truth of the new doing-thinking is its ability to improve or "ameliorate" the situation.

The process of occupational reconstruction always starts with a problematic situation and/or social constructed problems. Occupational reconstructions require people to unite and converge in collective action to improve a problematic situation. Members of this community of concern organize themselves around some focused kind of doing, and their organization is focused on "doing something" within an anticipated timeframe. This timeframe has an event structure or dramatic arc, i.e., it follows a narrative structure with a beginning, middle, and end. This structure will guide us when interpreting Occupational Reconstruction Theory as a practice framework. Because they are non-routine and hopeful experiments, occupational reconstructions involve risks and open spaces for creativity. This process engages emotions such as anger, grief, exhilaration, and joy.

Doing is a mind-body experience; thus, Occupational Reconstruction Theory considers how people come together to ameliorate problematic situations through doing. It is a social theory from and for occupational scientists and occupational therapists as it is grounded and focused on the potential of occupations. It is committed to understanding and answering consequential questions concerned with collective experimentation, a process of making hopeful improvements by means of occupations. The process requires reflection on how the doing affects the situation or changes the social-structured problems so that the results promote the desired social transformation. By its nature, it promotes transformative experiences at the individual and societal levels. Figure 14.1 presents the major constructs/elements of Occupational Reconstruction Theory.

Below, the seven principles of Occupational Reconstruction Theory are presented:

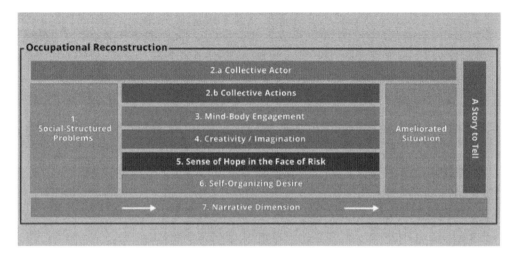

Figure 14.1 All elements and the seven principles of Occupational Reconstruction Theory.
Source: Credit for the digital artwork: Gareth Smart.

14.3.1 Addressing Social-structured Problems: Beyond Wicked Problem
Here we present two forms of interpreting problematic situations. The first refers to the traditional sense of the problematic situation, as explained before. In the pragmatic tradition, problematic situations refer to something that is not working well and consequently needs to be addressed. It can also be understood and dealt with as a wicked problem, a non-linear situation (Coyne, 2005). Rittel and Webber, design theorists, introduced the concept of "wicked problems" in the 1960s, as a mean to criticize the linear logic typically used in designing interventions to solve problems (Rittel & Webber, 1973). The typical approach looked to analyze all the components of a problem and then, step-by-step, move in a straight line from problem definition to problem solution. Under the influence of 20th-century pragmatist philosophy, two main weaknesses became evident: (i) in actual practice, designers noticed that their own design thinking and decision-making process was not simple and linear; and, (ii) they realized most design problems cannot actually be defined by linear analysis or solved by a step-by-step synthesis of the parts (Rittel & Webber, 1973). The wicked-problems approach suggests that there is a fundamental indeterminacy except in the most trivial design problems. Every wicked problem is particular and unique. In this pragmatic sense, solutions are not right or wrong, only good or bad.

The second sense of the problematic situation is not in opposition to the first one. However, it goes beyond the traditional understanding and, more specifically, places social-structured problems at the core of our attention about what is problematic. In the pragmatic tradition, problematic situations refer to something that is not working well and consequently needs to be addressed. However, drawing from critical scholars' work, we argue that some social-structured problems are neglected and hidden in society (Fassin, 2018). For instance, it was noticed that most of the occupational therapy practices in rural areas, including work with/in Indigenous communities, were a mere extension of neoliberal, hegemonic, and biomedical practices (Hayes et al., 2023a). Consequently, they reproduced normative views of society by identifying "situations" through their lens and neglecting the structural issues affecting those communities. Instead of only doing something to address "problematic situations," we argue the need for a critical take on understanding the situations that create the inequalities of human life and, consequently, their occupational implications. The profession is moving beyond its pragmatic aspirations, but it is using its influences to deal with specific social-structured problems, e.g., exclusion, racism (Grenier, 2020), oppression, violence, poverty, inequality, and so on. In this sense, the use and interpretation of Occupational Reconstruction Theory is not only aimed at recognizing and lamenting the inequalities of life, but also committed to addressing social-structured problems.

14.3.2 The Collective Actors and Collective Occupations: Sharing Desires and Efforts
Traditionally, occupational therapy is concerned with working with individuals (Bonikowsky et al., 2012; Malfitano et al., 2021). Several scholars have challenged this, and there is a call to advance the science and practice when working with collective actors (Barros et al., 2002; Cunningham et al., 2022; Frank & Dos Santos, 2020).

We highlight interdependence as a central concept to demonstrate the relevance of collective actors and occupations. Considering humans from the individual organism's standpoint would be an error for while each individual and their development plays a role in the survival and continuity of the species, humans did not survive and evolve as individuals but in groups. For instance, John Dewey (1859–1952) was never interested in education solely for the individual's development but in how to elicit, through a curriculum designed around carefully selected occupations, the growth of individuals as cooperating members of their specific culture with its very particular social organization and natural environment. Collective occupations are shared observable human behaviors. They consist of recognizable things people do together or in the aggregate in response to a problematic situation. Similarly, Ramugondo and Kronenberg (2015) argue that collective occupations are:

> occupations that are engaged in by individuals, groups, communities and/or societies in everyday contexts; these may reflect an intention towards social cohesion or dysfunction, and/or advancement of or aversion to a common good. Collective occupations may have consequences that benefit some populations and not others.
>
> *(p. 10)*

In Occupational Reconstruction, collective actors and occupations emerge as a response to deal with the shared problems. Examples can be found within occupational science and therapy literature (Frank & Muriithi, 2015; Frank & Dos Santos, 2020), as well as the social and political sciences (Hardin, 1982).

14.3.3 Mind-Body Engagement
The history of the mind-body concept in Western medicine and education suggests that we can view occupation – doing – as a transformational mind-body technology. Part of this inquiry must delve into the nature of human beings as curious, exploratory beings

that have intelligent capacities for mobility, tool use, language, and foresight. Doing consists of mind-body experiences. The elements of mind-body practices relate to the nature of human beings as curious, exploratory beings with diverse capabilities. These elements are present when investigating the mind-body notions developed at the start of the 19th century, as well as those developed by Dewey and his fellow liberal socialist and feminist thinkers and reformers at the start of the 20th. Despite significant digital development in the 21st century, to rightly interpret occupations there is a need to focus on them as mind-body practices.

14.3.4 Creativity and Imaginative Experimentation to Disrupt Routine Habits of Thinking and Doing

Participation may be loosely scripted but the doing itself opens spaces for innovation, improvisation, and transformation. There may be opportunities for play, new experiences of the self and other, and changes in the composition and structure of the group and collective identity. This is similar to the theatrical experimentalism of Augusto Boal developed in Brazil in the 1950s. Boal began a series of experiments now embraced by the term "Theatre of the Oppressed," one of the world's best-known, most effective and democratic forms of anti-spectatorial, public, and participatory art (Boal, 1994, 2002, 2013). Theatre of the Oppressed puts into performative venues Marxist humanist Paulo Freire's "pedagogy of the oppressed," a liberatory form of learning-by-doing developed with unschooled adults in Brazil by working directly with issues that they faced in their lives as impoverished farmers.

Boal's methodology – first "Arena Theatre," later "Forum Theater" – evolved as a workshop format in which participants are called to volunteer to narrate actual situations of powerlessness from personal experience. With volunteers in the workshop, they re-enact the oppressive situation on stage. The method next calls for volunteers to take the original actor's place to attempt to reverse, offset, or ameliorate the oppression by re-scripting the actor's previous lines and actions. Re-enactments continue introducing changes that imagine new possibilities for remedying the power relations, using reframing of the actor's response.

The heart of Boal's method is an anti-Aristotelian view of drama. Aristotle's Poetics treats the function and structure of drama as a progression of events that lead to a test of character for the tragic hero. This test comes from a fateful decision that arises from circumstances beyond the hero's control. In classic tragedies, the hero suffers. A character flaw prevents him (often a male figure) from seeing the truth, resulting in his making a choice that brings down the wrath of the gods, resulting in his punishment. The experience of the spectator is one of purification through catharsis – an experience of the passions (hatred, love, pride, etc.) that occur because of the audience's emotional identification (empathy) with the hero. The principle aim of tragedy in the poetics is catharsis – an experience of pity and fear. Boal argues that this Aristotelian system is repressive in that the spectators' aggressive and transgressive emotions are to be purged through the fate of the tragic hero who dared to go against the laws of a divinely sanctioned social order. Thus, Boal re-invented a poetics of revolution that empowers spectators to become "spectators" – that is, empowered agents of change. Similarly, to Boal's theater, occupational reconstruction requires creativity and imaginative experimentation to disrupt routine habits of thinking and doing.

14.3.5 The Sense of Hope in the Face of Risk and Indeterminate Outcomes When Claiming Authority and Power

Occupational reconstructions are hopeful experiments. They arise from the desire to make a change and call upon the knowledge and skills of the participants. But the desired change cannot be guaranteed. This is an important aspect to consider, as hope can be a driving force in the face of risk. An example to illustrate this can be found in Chile during the 1970s, when, under the military dictatorship in Chile, a group of women members of the *Agrupación de Familiares de Detenidos Desaparecidos* (AFDD) began to make *arpilleras* with political themes and statements in workshops under the Vicarate of Solidarity. *Arpilleras* are a kind of pictorial folk art traditionally produced by poor women in South American countries, particularly in Chile, to sell as a supplement to their income. They are decorative panels sewn using scrap materials to depict scenes of everyday life. They feature colorful appliques, patchwork, and embroidery (Adams, 2013).

Women, many of them members of the AFDD, transformed the rural folk imagery of this craft to two main types of scenes – on the one hand, scenes of disappearances, repression, and protest and, on the other, scenes of daily life under the regime. Again, the workshops built upon previously established models for organized women's activities, such as *Centro de Madres para Artesanía* (CEMA) a social welfare program initiated in the 1950s. Operating under the presidency of Eduardo Frei, from 1967 to 1970, it trained disadvantaged women from marginal neighborhoods in weaving, ceramics, knitting, and needlework. When Frei's Christian Democratic Party lost to Allende in 1971, CEMA was transformed to teach members at the neighborhood level how to organize to solve basic problems and to include welfare offices, health centers and clinics, and child-care centers. The example of non-party affiliated women in the neighborhoods organizing to solve basic problems was already in place.

The democratic nature of CEMA was quickly subverted when the wife of the military dictator August Pinochet was installed as director, introducing a top-down assembly line approach to crafts production in its workshops and promoting a discourse of women's dependency and loyalty to the Fatherland (Adams, 2013). However, the Vicarate assisted in the production and marketing of the *arpilleras*, providing scrap materials, purchasing the finished panels, and smuggling them out of the country for distribution and sale abroad. In this way, with help from the Vicarate, Chilean women dramatically repurposed a traditional woman's folk art into a tool of protest and survival (Adams, 2013).

The *arpilleras* were graphic and carried great specificity. Adams describes the work of one *arpillerista* ("Irma") who depicted the arrest of her son and daughter-in-law "on a downtown street in Santiago by three men dressed completely in black and carrying submachine guns." This exemplified mothers' sense of hope in the context of a political repression, facing risks and indeterminate outcomes when denouncing the injustices.

14.3.6 The Self-organizing Desire to Do Something about Something

A choice must be made and participation in the collective occupation is voluntary, not coerced. Participation arises through a desire and expresses freedom and solidarity. To exemplify how this individual desire aligns with collective action we compare two high-profile solidarity rallies held at the start of the 21st century: the "Unite the Right"

CREATIVITY, HOPE, AND COLLECTIVE EMANCIPATORY EXPERIMENTATION

rally in Charlottesville, Virginia on August 11, 2017, and the "Je Suis Charlie" rally in Paris on January 10–11, 2015. Both were organized voluntarily around doing something about a problematic situation. Using the lens of occupational reconstructions, the two rallies share the structural element of a group massing together to address a shared problematic situation. Both mediate between individual experiences of racial, social, and political identities and collective discourses about society itself. Both solicited members by means of face-to-face communication, social media, and widespread broadcast media; the desire and motivation were intrinsic – not imposed.

14.3.7 Narrative Dimensions

Narrative runs through occupational reconstructions and are metaphorical products. Stories about personal experiences express people's values and motives for participating in a shared effort to change a situation. As people act and interact to change the situation, alignments occur between their personal stories and stories about their collective experience. Narrative structure concerns the processes of doing things that anchor us in our realities in time and space. In the guise of routines and habits, narrative structures coordinate our activities with other people. But to leave it at that would fail to do justice to life. As with Mattingly's idea of prospective story-making, narrative structures also propel us forward through time toward our desired outcomes (Mattingly, 1991), which is intertwined with the hopeful characteristic of occupational reconstruction.

Lastly, occupational reconstructions have a narrative structure because they consist of events that take place in time with a beginning, middle, and anticipated end, which we also call Introduction (pre-experimentalism), Emancipatory experimentalism (happenings), and *Denouement* (post-experimentalism) when we present the theory as a practice framework. This event structure has a dramatic arc, a sequence of actions that begins with a problematic situation and a collective actor with a desire to transform it.

14.4 Occupational Reconstructions Theory as a Practice Framework

Similar to other professional practice frameworks, the Occupational Reconstruction Theory is organized in three phases when used as a practice framework. However, it does not use the traditional phases of assessment, intervention, and outcomes. The framework phases are Introduction (pre-experimentalism), Emancipatory experimentalism (happenings), and *Denouement* (post-experimentalism) (see Figure 14.2). This language is deliberately used to distance itself from traditional clinical language and reasoning, and the event structure, expressing a dramatic arc, has a sequence of actions that begins with a problematic situation, followed by actions, and ends with a narrative.

Below, the three phases of Occupational Reconstruction Theory as a practice framework are presented.

14.4.1 Introduction (Pre-experimentalism)

As occupational reconstructions are observable social events, occupational therapists can engage at any phase of the process and with different outcomes. It might be the case that occupational therapists want to support collective actors in identifying a shared problem, i.e., addressing inequality or occupational injustices. Or it might be the case

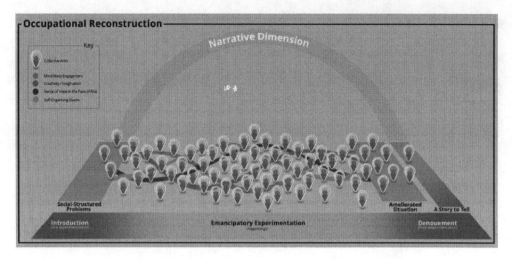

Figure 14.2 The elements and phases of Occupational Reconstruction as a practice framework.
Source: Credit for the digital artwork: Gareth Smart.

that an occupational therapist working in a catchment area identifies a common problem from individuals' narratives and works to connect people to create a cohesive collective actor.

The elements present in the Introduction phase are the problematic situation, i.e., the social-structured problem and a collective actor. Investing time to understand people's interpretation of the problematic situation is essential. Occupational therapists are encouraged to engage with people in their contexts to determine what sort of social-structured problem can be dealt with by diverse collective actors. It is important to note that each country will have a specific jurisdiction of occupational therapy practice; however, less privatized and profit-driven services will enlarge the possibilities of professional engagement with collective actors.

Collective actors for occupational reconstructions are somehow similar to Pichón Rivière's operative group (Rivière, 1975). There is a central axis on intentional and interconnected actions. The group's interactions are permeated by sharing of feelings, thoughts, understanding, and potential individual and social healings, but organized under the premise of action that transcends the mere acquisition of information and the development of skills, resulting in a change in participants' personalities and interpersonal and social relations and structures. This highlights the therapeutic or caring potential of Occupational Reconstruction Theory as a practice framework.

14.4.2 Emancipatory Experimentalism (Happenings)

The enactment of shared desires is a key element in guiding collective actions. If occupational therapists are not present in the Introduction phase, they can join the process in the second phase, Emancipatory experimentalism (happenings), by bringing dynamics and a critical stance about social processes and outcomes. We call the reader's attention to this phase, as occupational therapists can have a central role in interpreting and enacting the happenings. It can include diverse processes, including creative and artistic approaches. For instance, occupational scientists, using a theatrical method with homeless people, argue that "the transformational possibilities of theatre" arise from the idea of theater "as a subjunctive reality" (Fox & Dickie, 2010). For them, Boal's theatrical method called Theatre of the Oppressed becomes a liberating "as if" space "where unrealized human potential and hypothetical possibilities can be explored without the constraints of known situations and settled facts" (Horghagen & Hocking, 2017, p. 30). Occupational therapists in Brazil (Alves et al., 2013; Côrtes et al., 2011; Leão & Renó, 2021) and elsewhere (Horghagen & Josephsson, 2010) have largely used the Theatre of the Oppressed as a dynamic resource to produce hopeful, body-mind experimentations. These examples highlight that hope, creativity, and imagination are central to dealing with problems.

14.4.3 Denouement (Post-experimentalism)

In the final stage, collective actors and occupations start to dissolve. An occupational reconstruction allows for forming new networks of people and communities bound by shared meanings and purpose; making sense of every end is important. In the final phase, it is important to make sense of the story. We can call this process narrative alignment. It is the process by which people get on the same page to facilitate acting together with a common purpose. Not only does a new collective story – a story of "us" – emerge but this story of "us" also aligns with other discourses about the situation seen in histories, oral traditions, arts, public records, news, and other media.

Narrative alignment is also a process. It concerns the making of shared meanings – collective identities and collective experiences – through shared engagements in social contexts. As put by theorist of grass-roots activism, Marshall Ganz, community activists use the elicitation of personal stories as an effective tool to achieve "a story of us" to support collective action (Ganz, 2011). Marshall Ganz gives the name "public narrative" to the process, here called "narrative alignment." This story, Ganz cautions, is not the same as taking a posture through public speaking, messaging, or image-making. Instead, it is a personal account in which each individual shares the lived experiences and concerns that motivate his or her participation in the team and its goals. As team members participate in a public narrative session, they readily and spontaneously find the common threads among their experiences and concerns. As they continue to talk and act together, "story of us" emerges as a collective narrative. The "story of us" ultimately ties the participants to overarching stories – histories, songs, news accounts – of the situation that they desire to transform, putting their own contribution in perspective.

14.5 Conclusion

This chapter discussed a growing body of theoretical and practical work by occupational therapists interested in developing the area of "social transformation" and the concept of "collective occupations." An argument was put forward to mobilize the use of theory in practice; thus, the chapter presented the Occupational Reconstruction Theory, which identifies a set of seven principles that appears to be common among documented instances of transformative social action. Finally, we introduced the use of Occupational Reconstruction Theory as a guide to social transformation practice.

14.6 Summary
- Practices are developing around the area of social transformation as a means to respond to social-structured problems.
- Collective occupations are shared observable human behaviors. They consist of recognizable things people do together or in the aggregate in response to a problematic situation.
- Participation in a collective occupation is a choice and is voluntary, not coerced. Participation arises through a desire and expresses freedom and solidarity.
- Occupational Reconstruction Theory can provide a guide to social transformation practice.
- Occupational reconstructions arise from the desire to make a change and call upon the knowledge and skills of the participants.
- Occupational reconstructions have a narrative structure because they consist of events that take place in time with a beginning, middle, and anticipated end, which we also call Introduction (pre-experimentalism), Emancipatory experimentalism (happenings), and Denouement (post-experimentalism).
- The seven principles of Occupational Reconstruction Theory are (1) Social-structured problems; (2a) Collective actor; (2b) Collective actions; (3) Mind-body engagement; (4) Creativity/imagination; (5) Sense of hope in the face of risk; (6) Self-organizing desire; and (7) Narrative dimension.
- Narrative structure concerns the processes of doing things that anchor us in our realities in time and space.

14.7 Review Questions
1. Why is social transformation relevant to occupational therapists?
2. What is the relevance of theory to informing social transformative practices?
3. What is Occupational Reconstruction Theory?
4. How is it possible to apply the theory of occupational reconstruction in the practice of occupational therapy?

References
Abrahams, N., Devries, K., Watts, C., Pallitto, C., Petzold, M., Shamu, S., & García-Moreno, C. (2014). Worldwide prevalence of non-partner sexual violence: A systematic review. *The Lancet, 383*(9929), 1648–1654. https://doi.org/10.1016/S0140-6736(13)62243-6

Adams, J. (2013). *Art against dictatorship: Making and exporting arpilleras under Pinochet.* University of Texas Press.

Alves, I., Gontijo, D. T., & Alves, H. C. (2013). Teatro do oprimido e terapia ocupacional: Uma proposta de intervenção com jovens em situação de vulnerabilidade social/Theater of the oppressed and occupational therapy: A proposed action with youth in social vulnerability. *Cadernos Brasileiros de Terapia Ocupacional, 21*(2), Article 2. https://www.cadernosdeterapiaocupacional.ufscar.br/index.php/cadernos/article/view/819

Bailey, Z. D., Krieger, N., Agénor, M., Graves, J., Linos, N., & Bassett, M. T. (2017). Structural racism and health inequities in the USA: Evidence and interventions. *The Lancet, 389*(10077), 1453–1463. https://doi.org/10.1016/S0140-6736(17)30569-X

Barros, D. D., Lopes, R. E., & Galheigo, S. M. (2002). Projeto Metuia – Terapia ocupacional no campo social. *Mundo saúde (Impr.),* 365–369.

Boal, A. (1994). *The rainbow of desire: The Boal method of theatre and therapy.* Routledge.

Boal, A. (2002). *Games for actors and non-actors* (2nd ed.). Routledge.

Boal, A. (2013). *Theatre of the oppressed* (C. A. McBride, Trans.). Tcg ed. edition. Theatre Communications Group.

Bonikowsky, S., Musto, A., Suteu, K. A., MacKenzie, S., & Dennis, D. (2012). Independence: An analysis of a complex and core construct in occupational therapy. *British Journal of Occupational Therapy, 75*(4), 188–195. https://doi.org/10.4276/030802212X13336366278176

Bourdieu, P. (1977). *Outline of a theory of practice. Cambridge Studies in Social and Cultural Anthropology (16)*. Cambridge University Press.

Chomsky, N., & Waterstone, M. (2021). *Consequences of capitalism: Manufacturing discontent and resistance*. Haymarket Books.

Côrtes, C., Gontijo, D. T., & Alves, H. C. (2011). Ações da terapia ocupacional para a prevenção da violência com adolescentes: Relato de pesquisa. *Revista de Terapia Ocupacional da Universidade de São Paulo, 22*(3), Article 3. https://doi.org/10.11606/issn.2238-6149.v22i3p208-215

Coyne, R. (2005). Wicked problems revisited. *Design Studies, 26*(1), 5–17. https://doi.org/10.1016/j.destud.2004.06.005

Crawford, E. (2000). *The women's suffrage movement: A reference guide 1866–1928*. Routledge. https://doi.org/10.4324/9780203031094

Cunningham, M., Warren, A., Pollard, N., & Abey, S. (2022). Enacting social transformation through occupation: A narrative literature review. *Scandinavian Journal of Occupational Therapy, 29*(8), 611–630. https://doi.org/10.1080/11038128.2020.1841287

Dewey, J. (1958). *Experience and nature*. Dover Publications.

Dickie, V. A., & Frank, G. (1996). Artisan occupations in the global economy: A conceptual framework. *Journal of Occupational Science, 3*(2), 45–55. https://doi.org/10.1080/14427591.1996.9686407

Dos Santos, V. (2022). Social transformation on the neoliberal university: Reconstructing an academic commitment. *Journal of Occupational Science, 29*(4), 482–486. https://doi.org/10.1080/14427591.2022.2110660

Dos Santos, V., Frank, G., & Mizue, A. (2020). Candangos: Teoria da reconstrução ocupacional como uma ferramenta para a compreensão de problemas sociais e ações transformativas na utópica cidade de Brasília. *Cadernos Brasileiros de Terapia Ocupacional, 28*(3), 765–783. https://doi.org/10.4322/2526-8910.CTOAO2061

Elias, N. (2001). *Society of individuals*. Bloomsbury Publishing USA.

Emery-Whittington, I. G. (2021). Occupational justice: Colonial business as usual? Indigenous observations from Aotearoa New Zealand. *Canadian Journal of Occupational Therapy, 88*(2), 153–162. https://doi.org/10.1177/00084174211005891

Farias, L., & Laliberte Rudman, D. (2016). A critical interpretive synthesis of the uptake of critical perspectives in occupational science. *Journal of Occupational Science, 23*(1), 33–50. https://doi.org/10.1080/14427591.2014.989893

Farias, L., Laliberte Rudman, D., & Magalhães, L. (2016). Illustrating the importance of critical epistemology to realize the promise of occupational justice. *OTJR: Occupation, Participation and Health, 36*(4), 234–243. https://doi.org/10.1177/1539449216665561

Fassin, D. (2018). *Life: A critical user's manual*. Polity.

Fox, V., & Dickie, V. (2010). "Breaking in": The politics behind participation in theater. *Journal of Occupational Science, 17*(3), 158–167. https://doi.org/10.1080/14427591.2010.9686690

Frank, G., & Dos Santos, V. (2020). Occupational reconstructions: Resources for social transformation in challenging times. *Cadernos Brasileiros de Terapia Ocupacional, 28*(3), 741–745. https://doi.org/10.4322/2526-8910.ctoED2802

Frank, G., & Muriithi, B. A. K. (2015). Theorising social transformation in occupational science: The American Civil Rights Movement and South African struggle against apartheid as "occupational reconstructions." *South African Journal of Occupational Therapy, 45*(1), 11–19.

Galheigo, S. M. (2011). What needs to be done? Occupational therapy responsibilities and challenges regarding human rights. *Australian Occupational Therapy Journal, 58*(2), 60–66. https://doi.org/10.1111/j.1440-1630.2011.00922.x

Galvaan, R. (2021). Generative disruption through occupational science: Enacting possibilities for deep human connection. *Journal of Occupational Science*, 28(1), 6–18. https://doi.org/10.1080/14427591.2020.1818276

Galvaan, R., & Peters, L. (2014). *Occupation-based community development framework*. https://vula.uct.ac.za/access/content/group/9c29ba04-b1ee-49b9-8c85-9a468b556ce2/OBCDF/index.html

Ganz, M. (2011). Public narrative, collective action, and power. In S. Odugbemi & T. Lee (Eds.), *Accountability through public opinion: From inertia to public action*. The World Bank. https://doi.org/10.1596/978-0-8213-8505-0

Godoy, A., Cordeiro, L., & Soares, C. (2020). Emancipatory occupation: Labour as the conceptual basis for occupation-based social practices. In H. van Bruggen, S. Kantartzis, & N. Pollard (Eds.), *'And a Seed was Planted...' Occupation based approaches for social inclusion: Volume 1: Theoretical views and shifting perspectives* (pp. 61–74). Whiting & Birch Ltd.

Gramsci, A. (2011). *Prison notebooks volume 2*. Columbia University Press.

Grenier, M.-L. (2020). Cultural competency and the reproduction of white supremacy in occupational therapy education. *Health Education Journal*, 79(6), 633–644. https://doi.org/10.1177/0017896920902515

Grenier, M.-L. (2021). Patient case formulations and oppressive disability discourses in occupational therapy education. *Canadian Journal of Occupational Therapy*, 88(3), 266–272. https://doi.org/10.1177/00084174211005882

Gusfield, J. R. (1996). *Contested meanings: The construction of alcohol problems*. University of Wisconsin Press.

Hammell, K. (2020a). Ações nos determinantes sociais de saúde: Avançando na equidade ocupacional e nos direitos ocupacionais. *Cadernos Brasileiros de Terapia Ocupacional*, 28(1), 387–400. https://doi.org/10.4322/2526-8910.ctoARF2052

Hammell, K. (2020b). *Engagement in living: Critical perspectives on occupation, rights, and wellbeing*. Canadian Association of Occupational Therapists.

Hammell, K. (2021). Building back better: Imagining an occupational therapy for a post-COVID-19 world. *Australian Occupational Therapy Journal*, 68(5), 444–453. https://doi.org/10.1111/1440-1630.12760

Hammell, K. (2022). Editorial: Occupational therapy and the right to occupational participation. *Irish Journal of Occupational Therapy*, 50(1), 1–2. https://doi.org/10.1108/IJOT-05-2022-031

Hammell, K. (2023). A call to resist occupational therapy's promotion of ableism. *Scandinavian Journal of Occupational Therapy*, 30(6), 745–757. https://doi.org/10.1080/11038128.2022.2130821

Hanlon, P., Carlisle, S., Hannah, M., Reilly, D., & Lyon, A. (2011). Making the case for a "fifth wave" in public health. *Public Health*, 125(1), 30–36. https://doi.org/10.1016/j.puhe.2010.09.004

Hardin, R. (1982). *Collective action*. Resources for the Future.

Hayes, K., Dos Santos, V., Costigan, M., & Morante, D. (2023a). Extension, austerity, and emergence: Themes identified from a global scoping review of non-urban occupational therapy services. *Australian Occupational Therapy Journal*, 70(1), 142–156. https://doi.org/10.1111/1440-1630.12844

Hayes, K., Dos Santos, V., Costigan, M., & Morante, D. (2023b). Profile of occupational therapy services in non-urban settings: A global scoping review. *Australian Occupational Therapy Journal*, 70(1), 119–141. https://doi.org/10.1111/1440-1630.12835

Horghagen, S., & Hocking, C. (2017). Shout out who we are! How might engagement in cultural activities enhance participation in everyday occupations for people in vulnerable life situations? In A. H. Eide, S. Josephson, & K. Vik (Eds.), *Participation in health and welfare services: Professional concepts and lived experience* (pp. 128–140). Taylor & Francis.

Horghagen, S., & Josephsson, S. (2010). Theatre as liberation, collaboration and relationship for asylum seekers. *Journal of Occupational Science*, 17(3), 168–176. https://doi.org/10.1080/14427591.2010.9686691

Iwama, M. K. (2006). *The Kawa Model: Culturally relevant occupational therapy*. Elsevier Health Sciences.

James, V. D. (2017). Pragmatism and radical social justice: Dewey, Du Bois, and Davis. In S. Dieleman, D. Rondel, & C. Voparil (Eds.), *Pragmatism and justice* (pp. 163–1787). Oxford University Press. https://doi.org/10.1093/acprof:oso/9780190459239.003.0010

Koopman, C. (2017). Contesting injustice: Why pragmatist political thought needs Du Bois. In S. Dieleman, D. Rondel, & C. Voparil (Eds.), *Pragmatism and justice* (pp. 176–196). Oxford University Press. https://doi.org/10.1093/acprof:oso/9780190459239.003.0011

Leão, A., & Renó, S. R. (2021). What is the Oppressed Theater a powerful strategy for? An experience of the "Education through Work Program for Health" at the Psychosocial Care Center for Alcohol and other Drugs. *Cadernos Brasileiros de Terapia Ocupacional*, 29. https://doi.org/10.1590/2526-8910.ctoRE2088

Leite Junior, J. D., Farias, M. N., & Martins, S. (2021). Dona Ivone Lara e terapia ocupacional: Devir-negro da história da profissão. *Cadernos Brasileiros de Terapia Ocupacional*, 29, e2171. https://doi.org/10.1590/2526-8910.ctoarf2171

Lopes, R. E., & Malfitano, A. P. S. (2020). *Social occupational therapy: Theoretical and practical designs*. Elsevier.

Malfitano, A. P. S., Whiteford, G., & Molineux, M. (2021). Transcending the individual: The promise and potential of collectivist approaches in occupational therapy. *Scandinavian Journal of Occupational Therapy*, 28(3), 188–200. https://doi.org/10.1080/11038128.2019.1693627

Marmot, M. (2004). Status syndrome. *Significance*, 1(4), 150–154. https://doi.org/10.1111/j.1740-9713.2004.00058.x

Marmot, M. (2005). Social determinants of health inequalities. *The Lancet*, 365(9464), 1099–1104. https://doi.org/10.1016/S0140-6736(05)71146-6

Mattingly, C. (1991). The narrative nature of clinical reasoning. *American Journal of Occupational Therapy*, 45(11), 998–1005. https://doi.org/10.5014/ajot.45.11.998

Morris, A. D. (1986). *The origins of the civil rights movement*. Simon and Schuster.

Pereira, R. B. (2017). Towards inclusive occupational therapy: Introducing the CORE approach for inclusive and occupation-focused practice. *Australian Occupational Therapy Journal*, 64(6), 429–435. https://doi.org/10.1111/1440-1630.12394

Pollard, N., Kronenberg, F., & Sakellariou, D. (2008). *A political practice of occupational therapy*. Churchill Livingstone.

Ramugondo, E. L., & Kronenberg, F. (2015). Explaining collective occupations from a human relations perspective: Bridging the individual-collective dichotomy. *Journal of Occupational Science*, 22(1), 3–16. https://doi.org/10.1080/14427591.2013.781920

Rittel, H. W. J., & Webber, M. (1973). Dilemmas in a general theory of planning. *Policy Sciences*, 4, 155–169.

Rivière, E. P. (1975). *El proceso grupal: Del psicoanálisis a la psicología social (I)*. Ediciones Nueva Visión.

Sen, A. K. (1997). From income inequality to economic inequality. *Southern Economic Journal*, 64(2), 384–401. https://doi.org/10.1002/j.2325-8012.1997.tb00063.x

Simpson, L. B. (2017). *As we have always done: Indigenous freedom through radical resistance*. University of Minnesota Press.

Terriquez, V. (2015). Intersectional mobilization, social movement spillover, and queer youth leadership in the immigrant rights movement. *Social Problems*, 62(3), 343–362. https://doi.org/10.1093/socpro/spv010

van Bruggen, H., Kantartzis, S., & Pollard, N. (Eds.). (2020). *'And a Seed was Planted...' Occupation based approaches for social inclusion: Volume 1: Theoretical views and shifting perspectives*. Whiting & Birch Ltd.

Venkatapuram, S. (2013). Health, vital goals, and central human capabilities. *Bioethics*, 27(5), 271–279. https://doi.org/10.1111/j.1467-8519.2011.01953.x

West, C. (1989). *The American evasion of philosophy: A genealogy of pragmatism*. Springer.

Williams, N. W. (2019). Pragmatism and justice. *Contemporary Political Theory, 18*(S4), 236–239. https://doi.org/10.1057/s41296-018-0261-0

CHAPTER 15

Social Occupational Therapy

Contributions to Design a Field of Knowledge and Practices

Roseli Esquerdo Lopes, Denise Dias Barros, and Ana Paula Serrata Malfitano

Abstract

This chapter is a narrative based on the interpretation of Brazilian occupational therapy history and seeks to situate dynamic and theoretical choices to contextualize the development of social occupational therapy as a specific field of knowledge and practice. This process has been influenced by the Brazilian political and economic contexts throughout the period of military dictatorship, and raises questions about the technical, ethical, and political roles of all professionals. Social occupational therapy is configured as a complex and borderline field derived from the questioning of two perspectives. The first regards the debate about the social responsibility of professionals in the development of social values that includes their political-ethical exercise from a critical and conscious practice, and active participation in society. The second investigates medical-psychological knowledge and its reductionist ways of understanding and dealing with social fabric. These two perspectives were highlighted in the late 1990s, when, in the face of neoliberalism, occupational therapists were/are facing new contemporary demands and asking themselves if they could/can contribute to society. In this context, social technologies have been constituted as a framework for action, namely workshops of activities, dynamics, and projects; individual and territorial follow-ups; articulation of resources in the social field; and dynamization of service networks. Continuous and critical reflection on professional experiences is proposed that seeks the possible integration of action and theory, experience and reflection, and aims to contribute to the conditions of vast social inequalities experienced worldwide.

Authors' Positionality Statement

The authors of this chapter belong to an occupational therapy academic group and have years of professional experience as educators and researchers in the higher education sector. Geographically, our experiences represent perspectives from South America, particularly from Brazil. The information contained in this chapter, although not all-inclusive, provides an overview of social occupational therapy. Moreover, we wish to clearly express our positionality: we are white, Portuguese-speaking, university-educated, professionally qualified, cisgender, locally economically privileged women who work as educators, researchers, and scholars. We recognize that the subject matter of this chapter represents the social, political, cultural, and Global South views on the theme. In the process of drafting this chapter, we have made a concerted effort to include evidence-based, scholarly, inclusive, culturally sensitive, and gender affirmative material in an attempt to embrace a diverse range of perspectives. However, we acknowledge that the contents of this chapter are not exhaustive, completely bias-free, or representative of every cultural, racial, gender, economic, political, or social reality. We hope that this text can foster critical, inclusive, respectful, and progressive debate among current and future occupational therapists, nationally and internationally.

> **Objectives**
> This chapter will support readers to:
>
> - Discuss ethical and political actions in occupational therapy.
> - Understand the social question and related social issues within contemporary neoliberalism.
> - Know about the history of social occupational therapy in Brazil.
> - Recognize the social responsibility of professionals actively participating in society.
> - Discuss processes of medicalization within the social fabric of society.
> - Know the Metuia Network – Social Occupational Therapy history and its propositions.
> - Apply social technologies in occupational therapy practices.

> **Key terms**
> - social occupational therapy
> - social question
> - politics
> - social responsibility
> - political-ethical professional role
> - social action

15.1 Introduction

In this chapter, we present a discussion on the historical development of occupational therapy in Brazil, with emphasis on the constitution of its theoretical and practical foundations to the design in its current configuration. This specific history can contribute to different dialogues in occupational therapy globally, especially considering the social challenges present in the contemporary world.

From a narrative based on the interpretation of the history of occupational therapy in Brazil, we seek to situate the dynamics and the theoretical, professional, educational, and institutional choices that contextualize the development of social occupational therapy as a specific field of action and reflection. The social question concept is determined in capitalist societies by the peculiar relationship between capital and labor: namely, exploitation (Castel, 2003). Discussions about the social question refer to the necessary understanding of social cohesion possible within the capitalist structure and what agreement could be collectively reached to try to avoid social fracture. Social fracture is understood as a rupture in society generated by unequal access to social goods, which can be minimized by social policies (Castel, 2003; Lopes, 2021) in areas where occupational therapists usually work, such as health, welfare/social services, education, and justice.

Based on the debate about the social question in the spheres of our profession, we focus on the experience of the Metuia Project, currently Metuia Network – Social Occupational Therapy, and on the development of social technologies[1] aimed at the production of knowledge and contributing to professional performance with the intention of designing work with macro- and micro-social scopes.

15.2 Historical Perspective of Occupational Therapy Education and Practice in Discourses About the Social Question

In Brazil, the first occupational therapy undergraduate courses date back to the mid-1950s (Soares, 1991). These courses were aimed at preparing the so-called "rehabilitation professionals", mainly physical therapists and occupational therapists, and were organized through agreements with the United Nations (UN) and the United Nations Children's Fund (UNICEF). This education was based on health rehabilitation, in a broad sense, but focused mainly on the rehabilitation of victims of work accidents and was associated with a perspective of dysfunction and physical disability. In the profession's prevailing configuration in countries of "the North", this approach was also present in the field of psychiatry education and the use of rehabilitation for life within the concept of "occupation" (Lopes, 1990; Soares, 1991).

The axis of rehabilitation has become important for Brazilian occupational therapists in the constitution of professional identity and actions, albeit a controversial one. Its focus was sometimes on the function itself, i.e., on the individual's bodily capacity/incapacity, and sometimes on their functional and/or occupational performance. It was only in the mid-1970s that occupational therapy interventions were developed in the context of social service institutions.[1] Initially, these professionals were inserted in the labor market in prison institutions and in those caring for poor, abandoned children and adolescents, or for those who were in conflict with the law for some "offence" – a term under discussion at the time (Pinto, 1990). It is important to point out that the first actions as understood in the field of social assistance occurred during the military dictatorship in Brazil (1964–1985) and in the context of "total institutions" (Goffman, 1961), under the hegemony of repressive public policies (Barros et al., 2007).

Thus, the context of the profession in the 1970s focused on the attitudes/behaviors of individuals and groups seen as deviant, maladjusted, and marginal, both at the psychosocial and macro-social levels. Although this perspective was challenged, contestation was completely repressed. It was in this social and political context that multi-professional teams were formed and their actions in the social field constituted – these teams included occupational therapists, although they were only lately incorporated (Barros et al., 2007).

Due to the lack of documentation, it is difficult to understand the history of occupational therapy in Brazil before the 1980s, since it was only in the late 1970s that the importance of registering and documenting the profession was effectively recognized. As the profession's history and methodologies in Brazil have yet to be studied systematically, it is not possible to confirm whether or not that no actions taken by the occupational therapy profession beyond the health care system in the social field. The first publication on social and non-therapeutic practice by an occupational therapist appeared in 1979, in a paper by Jussara de Mesquita Pinto in the annals of a regional occupational therapy event, V São Paulo Scientific Meeting of Occupational Therapists. Jussara Pinto used the term "social occupational therapy" in referring to her work in a public institution for juvenile offenders, describing her approach to working with girls who had been deprived of their freedom (Pinto, 1979).

In 1979, following interest and demands from supervisors and students, undergraduate students enrolled in the Occupational Therapy Course at the University of São Paulo (USP) were able to join professional internships in social occupational therapy. The emergence of social occupational therapy in Brazil therefore started with this group of new interns, some of whom had prior experience in the use of group activities and dynamics which could be applied to the social field. At the time, it was important for occupational therapists to integrate into being active members of multidisciplinary social teams which in turn facilitated the further development of the profession. However, there was no reflection on professional actions in these new spaces as the initial intention was to be present professionally in some way, and achieve recognition (Barros et al., 2007).

There were also occupational therapists working with poor children living in asylums/shelters of public or private institutions, most of which were religious and philanthropic. Occupational-therapeutic interventions with young, poor children had, on the one hand, a social perspective which focused on the provision of essentials for their material existence and development, such as access to schools, family financial benefits, and other social rights. On the other hand, their professional practice was informed predominately from the perspective of "typical" human development, based on a psycho-pedagogical contribution.

The provision of "asylum" was present for different societal groups, including for children and young people. It refers to a practice that combined "shelter" and control that has been socially acceptable in Brazil since the beginning of the 20th century, allied to education for and through work (Rafante & Lopes, 2009). While the effective care of young children in poverty has always been a hot topic in Brazil, the care of young adolescents, especially those who are young, brown/black, and poor, has been mostly linked to control and repression.

In this national context, in the mid-1970s, social occupational therapy began to acquire its own contours, under the aegis of an authoritarian regime which imposed a disciplinary and segregating system on social institutions, legitimized by rules and regulations. By granting power to technicians, the junta sought to ensure compliance through violence in a deeply unequal society. Criticism of this model, which was prominent in the political moment of the late 1970s and early 1980s, through civil society organizations and movements was accompanied by academic debate that re-established the issue of social marginality and the theories that developed from it. These were established from the perspective of social conflict in a society based on private property and exploitation of labor (Barros et al., 2007).

During the same period, an important agenda for Brazilian occupational therapy was discussion about the formal structures of professionalization (regulatory and supervisory bodies) and education (minimum curriculum required for undergraduate courses), which confirmed occupational therapy as an academic profession. Aligned with this open and procedural discussion involving different perspectives and fields of knowledge, was expansion within the discipline of space for understanding the need for a critical, "technical and political" education, which was drawn from a strand of Gramscian historical materialism[2] (Lopes, 1990). This was advocated by professionals who worked in the social and cultural spheres and/or who fought for a more just and democratic society.

In social occupational therapy, the debate was intense and often dissonant and comprised numerous components: the naming of the field and the demands inherent in this; the need for knowledge and critical posture in relation to certain ideological positions; the concepts of human being and society; and the definition of intervention models. At the core of curricular reforms were discussions about the naming of disciplines and/or undergraduate teaching programs that would host this body of knowledge: "social occupational therapy" or "occupational therapy in the social field"? What would it mean to speak about occupational therapy as applied to social conditions or social dysfunctions? And what are social dysfunctions? Do dysfunctions result from society? Do individuals in society have dysfunctions? Would occupational therapy applied to social conditions address the lack of social conditions or the given conditions? (Lopes et al., 2015).

Additionally, there was resistance to the proposition of social occupational therapy, especially from professionals in the field of mental health. Many in this group were involved in the struggle for human and citizenship rights, militating for the deinstitutionalization of total institutions, and debating social conditions as they related to mental health care. This amalgamation of institutions of social assistance, education, and culture and institutions of rehabilitation and psychosocial care is still present today. In addition to the strengthening of professionals' presence in undergraduate and graduate college education, there has been significant expansion of experiences in this area, with increasing numbers of professionals working in different regions of the country (Oliveira et al., 2019) and abroad.

The notion of "social rehabilitation" was relevant and pertinent for the critical analysis of, and search for, other paradigms that sought to distance themselves from, or break with, the notion of rehabilitation as functionality or return to work. From the perspective of social epidemiology, a series of problems were posed; for example, professionals from different fields were concerned about the social dimensions present in their daily practice. This was particularly important in the health sector and the discussions about deinstitutionalization and public health. There was, however, a need for more intense dialogue with the human and social sciences to understand the differences (cultural, racial, religious, gender, and class) between social phenomena and institutions, such as those intended to shelter children, pregnant women, "single mothers", older individuals, and prisoners. During the 1980s, the theoretical foundations were of macro-social analyses of assistance and social security policies were critically debated – these were informed by various disciplines, including history, anthropology, and sociology, and health sectors that promoted democratic psychiatry, anti-psychiatry, and health reforms (Lopes & Malfitano, 2021).

While the critique of occupational therapy approaches was still mostly focused on "recovery of function", another important debate was occurring in universities on the fundamentals of occupational therapy. Among other initiatives, a group of professors from two Brazilian universities organized a discussion on the methods and fields of intervention (Pinto, 1987). This resulted in Berenice Francisco (1988) and Jussara Pinto (1990) developing what they called "methodological trends in occupational therapy", which sought to outline occupational therapy and its practices from a perspective of knowledge production. According to the classification, occupational therapy could be positivist, humanist, or historical-materialist, and in this context actions and approaches aimed at social transformation were placed under the aegis of historical materialism.[2] It would therefore not be a social occupational therapy concerned with social conflicts, but rather a total social question through which occupational therapists' approach and view the individual and society (Pinto, 1990).

While some Brazilian occupational therapists suggested that social reality should be imposed on professional practice, paradoxically, for practitioners, both the discussion and emphasis on socially related questions made a definition of social occupational therapy redundant. All occupational therapists in any case were faced with the challenges imposed by living conditions and the need for change in Brazilian society. It is important to acknowledge there was identification with the debate on social transformation, particularly within the core of theorization on social marginality and class relations, and critiques of the social and political role of professionals in contemporary societies and so-called materialist-historical occupational therapy.

In some higher education institutions, this perspective led to the exclusion of social occupational therapy courses from undergraduate curricula, or the incorporation of their content into other disciplines of different backgrounds. For example, professional practices originated from the debate about the "social question" and their alignment with historical materialism, critical and transforming perspectives of society, and the historical foundations of occupational therapy. Occupational therapists and teachers who identified the most with this view embraced the disciplines within this spectrum. A further bias occurred among those who sought to include the perspective of full human development, where it could be worked for in a socially referenced way. However, this discipline remained in the curriculum of other courses.

By the early 1980s and 1990s, the demand for professionalized occupational therapy in Brazil had been met, with the establishment of curricula and academic institutions that adequately educated their professionals. During this period, professors in the area trained for research and occupational therapists called for the integration of public policies and re-introduction of democratic procedures in the social sphere. The perspective of a social field in occupational therapy resurfaced when concrete spaces were created to develop interventions in specific fields to produce knowledge, actions, and assistance.

In the 1990s, the questions asked were "what is the place of the social question in the constitution of occupational therapy?" and "what is the constitution of the social field in occupational therapy?" Despite variations on the discourse about the social question in occupational therapy, some professionals began to take on the matter of performance and the proposition of developing "social occupational therapy". At the end of the 1990s, the debate about the social question resumed among occupational therapists, creating an important movement for the constitution of the social field in occupational therapy. This movement problematized the medicalization and psychologization of social conflicts and the interpretation of diversity and culture and criticized the reduction of occupational therapy to a profession that was linked primarily with health and disease (Barros et al., 2002).

Taking social issues and their basic theoretical perspectives to reflect on professional actions, we move on to the defense and formulation of professional occupational therapy practice that is organized around diverse and complex dimensions of human activity engagement, with historical contributions and perspectives of acting in different sectors, fields, and social and political movements. Recognizing the permanence and hegemony of health and psychosocial perspectives, we sought to think, propose, develop, and discuss professional actions and epistemic bases grounded in the human sciences and the arts, emphasizing the relevance of understanding the coexistence of fields of knowledge.

In the 1990s the world and Brazil underwent a period of radical economic liberalism[3] in the management of the public sphere, with important repercussions for the capital-labor relationship. As solutions were sought for the reconfiguration of the social question at the end of the 20th century (Castel, 2003), there was aggravation of social problems and confrontation within the broad social and professional sectors, including occupational therapy in Brazil.

15.3 Social Occupational Therapy: A Complex Field Between Borders

Two complementary theoretical perspectives underlie social occupational therapy in Brazil. The first had the analysis of the social question as a parameter, especially from the late 1970s to the mid-1980s, a time of ebullition around the social demands in Brazil. This moment was understood not only as resulting from capital-labor relations, but also referred to the construction of the public sphere mobilized by civil society in a moment of "political openness" at the end of the dictatorship period, although it was still permeated by important restrictions. The State, which was undergoing transformation itself, was arranged under a democratic and legal perspective, even within the limits of capitalism. This process, which involved the review of professional postulates, reached different sectors, including occupational therapy. Within this, the social responsibility of professionals in the forming of social values was debated in the struggle for hegemony, moving from political exercise to conscious practice, balancing consensus and dissent, participation, practice and politics (Gramsci, 1971; Lopes, 1993/1996). This review of professional action fostered questions, propositions, and a theoretical perspective that underpinned social occupational therapy (Barros et al., 2002; Lopes & Malfitano, 2021).

The second perspective arises from another question: the one that referred to medical-psychological knowledge and its reductionist ways of understanding and dealing with phenomena that were placed under the "health-disease" binomial. This was based on the disciplining and institutionalization of social problems and treated from the point of view of certain dominant values that controlled and suppressed individual and collective freedom (Barros et al., 1999). The extent to which medical/psychological/clinical disciplines were imbued with these values was discussed, with strong contributions from psychiatry and psychology, resulting in a series of propositions that would shape the action of professionals.

It is therefore theoretically important for social occupational therapy to understand the inequalities that emerge from social contradictions in capitalist societies, resulting from the capital-labor relationship and the exploitation and precariousness inherent in it. In the mid-1990s, labor flexibility and deregulation in the world of automation deepened in Brazil with large populations subject to dissolution of social ties and vulnerability in social support networks (Castel, 2003). These varied in form and intensity and caused a reconfiguration of the social question.

It is noteworthy that this reconfiguration will be perceived by occupational therapists in the late 1990s as contemporary demands, and in relation to which it is possible to contribute, requiring, for that, the construction of specific social technologies (Lopes et al., 2021). Individuals and collectives who, through social transformation, were more directly exposed to the rupture of social support networks, cultural and/or identity disqualification, precarious work conditions became the target for social occupational therapy.

As Castel (2003) described, deprivation can be understood as a result of the conjunction of two axes: labor relations (with an array of positions, from stable employment to complete absence of work, and precarious, intermittent forms of work) and relational insertion (also with a range of positions from participation in solid social networks to social isolation). Approaches to these two axes circumscribe different zones of the social fabric: the zone of integration in which there are guarantees of permanent employment and where solid relational supports can be mobilized; the zone of disaffiliation, where absence of employment and social isolation are combined, implying the double rupture of social and participatory networks; and the zone of vulnerability in which work precariousness and relational fragility are associated. The borders between these zones are porous and disaffiliation feeds on the dynamic of vulnerability, which expands according to the economic situation and situations of war (declared or "silent", as in Brazil), misery, and scarcity (Castel, 2003).

The zone of social vulnerability is presented from the perspective of employment and networks, and includes those who in addition to being unemployed do not have social support networks, such as close social relationships with family, neighbors, and culture. This also includes those resulting from configuration and access to social protection goods and services (the latter being a part of what Castel (2003) defined as the zone of assistance). For those without "employment/work" access to social networks in the insertion axis – family, community, and protection services – can neutralize and even prevent the formation of "disaffiliation". From the point of view of social inclusion, having economic availability is fundamental but this can also present challenges due to the lack of primary sociability which cannot be accessed outside the "market", i.e., through consumption, and individuals' affective, personal, and cultural issues.

From this understanding, social occupational therapy is based on the following assertions:

- the profession is part of the process and theoretical and practical choices produced and legitimized by professionals who take a political stand on the social issues of their time
- approaches to practice are constructions based on the interpretation of problems perceived and incorporated as relevant, and on which possible solutions and/or cultural negotiations are organized
- inequality and poverty are relevant challenges at the core of the Brazilian social question, requiring configurations that demand a review of professionals' technical education and the relevance of their role
- occupational therapy must contribute to the resolution of issues associated with social and cultural contradictions, disputes, and struggles that mark certain historical moments and processes
- contradictions within a society marked by inequalities and difficulties in negotiating differences demand that occupational therapists seek education that enables them to cope with the problems that emerge from social and cultural conflicts.

Hence, there is a need for concepts that assist understanding of the dynamics involved in social negotiations and incorporate socio-anthropological and ethnographic knowledge (Barros & Galvani, 2021) and investment in individual, collective, transdisciplinary, interprofessional, and intersectoral actions. In essence, this provides the foundation for the development of action in the social field and social occupational therapy (Barros et al., 2007).

In the context of Brazilian social occupational therapy in the 1990s and early 21st century, we have highlighted the importance of education in sociology, anthropology, and public health. These disciplines have made fundamental theoretical contributions, and even though they have not been rolled out at a national level, they have referenced concerted efforts to build bases for new territorial action. Actions are culturally sensitive to the complexities of the real world and the languages and expressions of a multicultural and poly cultural context (Barros & Galvani, 2021).

Intervention methodologies based on dialogues, dialogicity,[4] and social policies – across cultural, education, social assistance, health, housing, and social judicial contexts – have been created and developed through the construction of social occupational therapy. This has been led by the Metuia Project – an inter-institutional group for studies, education, and actions directed at Brazilian children, adolescents, and adults who are subject to the rupture of social support networks. Initially formed in 1998 by a group of Brazilian occupational therapy scholars from three universities, the Metuia Project has since built a theoretical-methodological framework, with different nuances, that have supported and added complexity to social occupational therapy (Barros et al., 2011). In late 2019, with the expansion of social occupational therapy in higher education institutions in Brazil, it was renamed the Metuia Network – Social Occupational Therapy.

In this process of collective construction of its meanings, we now turn to the strengthening of social occupational therapy, which is at the core of contemporary challenges. The Metuia Network comprises seven active centers established in universities in different regions of Brazil, in addition to collective projects or initiatives outside the universities. For example, the *Casa das Áfricas Amanar* (Pastore & Sato, 2018) in São Paulo and other Brazilian cities, action in Africa focused on human rights, education, aesthetic expressions, and migration, and the *Practs em Neuilly Sur Marne* Program in France which is dedicated to assisting migrants seeking asylum (Courtois, 2022; Marques & Morestin, 2020). Social occupational therapy, as understood by the Metuia Network, develops territorial and community actions aimed at socially vulnerable people and populations undergoing processes of disaffiliation, as well as fostering the recognition of rights, expansion of expressive possibilities, and life alternatives.

This plurality stems from growing sensitivity to territorial insertion, within both local and global approaches. Initially implemented by the founding centers of the former Metuia Project, the programs have expanded in number as have the different modalities of social action, which are conducted in urban, rural, and community spaces and involve economic, educational, artistic, and collective identities. Actions are aimed at both public policies and social movements in the defense of human, cultural and artistic, political, and social rights, i.e., the struggle for redistribution and recognition, and combating processes of subordination and oppression (as defined by Fraser (2000)). It is important to emphasize that other initiatives within the social field coexisted with those of the Metuia Project, and continue to do so alongside the Metuia Network, through actions in the fields of the arts, human rights, migration, the fight against racism and gender violence, cultural diversity, rurality, and traditional societies.

Since the beginning of the 21st century, social problems arising from changes in protective systems in the most economically and socially developed world, in terms of the construction of the public sphere and social protections, have prompted several other initiatives led by occupational therapists. The "Occupational Therapy without Borders" project is one such example. As a non-governmental organization which brought together occupational therapists with different experiences in the field, it has provided important visibility through the publication of *Occupational therapy without borders: Learning from the spirit of survivors* (Kronenberg et al., 2005) (later published in Spanish (Kronenberg et al., 2007).

There has been a strengthening of the idea that occupational therapy practice cannot be dissociated from political, technical, social, and cultural action. As the social question is reconfigured and social problems are no longer restricted to peripheral countries, it is evident that there is a growing tendency for occupational therapists from central countries[5] to start worrying about it within their own territories.

15.3.1 Propositions, Actions, and Dynamics

Metuia Network – Social Occupational Therapy projects have been conducted by occupational therapy researchers, educators, clinicians, and students. These projects have used different approaches, acquired characteristics, and developed diversified action proposals. Most of these promote the constant dialogue between practice (through projects developed by the university in partnership with the community, government, and/or non-governmental organizations), theory (research, publications, and seminars), and teaching (at undergraduate and graduate levels). Interventions and actions derive from research and extension university projects carried out in partnership with public institutions, social movements, and non-governmental organizations. Actions occur in urban or rural areas, public and community spaces, and social institutions such as schools, shelters, community centers, housing projects, libraries, cultural centers, and other social organizations that target populations experiencing rupture of social support networks and/or promote networks of interpersonal and community relationships (Lopes & Malfitano, 2021).

The plurality of the Metuia Network originates from the autonomy of its centers and initiatives, which formulate and carry out social, cultural, and educational projects with different theoretical orientations. They have in common spaces for debate and the challenge of creating social action technologies within the scope of activities that encompass economic, artistic, cultural, social assistance and educational life. Accumulated experiences have produced social technologies that can promote new interventions which integrate and combine macro- and micro-social actions. Several stand out resources arising from these experiences have been developed: workshops of activities, dynamics, and projects; individual territorial follow-ups; articulation, creation, and distribution of resources in the social field; activation of the social support network (Lopes et al., 2021).

15.3.1.1 Workshops of Activities, Dynamics, and Projects

Social occupational therapy uses activities as a mediating resource to approach, monitor, apprehend demands, and strengthen the individuals and collectives assisted by its actions. In our experience, the focus is on the use of activities in group and/or collective spaces. Through this work instrument, once mastered by the occupational therapists who use it, it is possible to know the immediate universe of the individuals, which significantly increases the chances of creating ties and thereby generating opportunities for professional performance that contribute to the joint construction of plans and projects. Through these activities, people learn about and recognize their needs, and develop the ability to seek their own creative solutions to their problems.

In potentially creating spaces for experimentation and learning, each participant is an active being in the process of building subjectivity – a being of praxis, action, and reflection. This, in turn, enables closer contact with individuals and collectives and more comprehensive reading of their needs, while also promoting greater contact and coexistence between the participants themselves. The setting both facilitates experimentation within a pleasant social space and the transference of exchanges from the physical space of the workshop to a broader context (Lopes et al., 2011).

The workshops (activities, projects, products, and dynamics) enable a powerful range of actions that can be classified, understood, and applied with different purposes in dealing with intrinsic techniques: using and producing materials and resources; transiting through different sectors (culture, art, sports, leisure, work, etc.); using previously prepared proposals with pre-established themes and objectives (e.g., debates about everyday life, life perspectives, exchanges and information about the world of work, educational processes, rights and duties, the protection network for children and adolescents in the city, among others); discussing the needs and possibilities of everyday life, as well as the different senses and meanings that the individuals in action can designate or realize according to their personal experiences. Even if proposals have previous indications or directions, the interest is in the participant's singular perception of that experience.

15.3.1.2 Individual Territorial Follow-ups

Individual territorial follow-ups are used in social occupational therapy as an intervention strategy to enable more realistic perception of an individual's life context and interactions in their everyday lives. Follow-ups interconnect their histories and trajectories, current situation, and network of relationships, and are initiated by listening attentively to the demands of individuals, groups, or collectives. Most of these demands are influenced by situations of vulnerability, social inequality, and lack of access to social services and essential goods (Lopes, Borba et al., 2011; Malfitano et al., 2011).

15.3.1.3 Articulation of Resources in the Social Field

Articulation of resources in the social field comprises a range of actions conducted at individual, group, and collective levels, and at policy and management levels. The strategy is to manage practices at different levels of assistance working toward common goals and using available resources, including financial, material, relational and affective components at the micro- or macro-social level to develop interventions. Intervention methodologies are also applied at these different levels to ensure the identification, negotiation, and effective contribution of these resources (Lopes et al., 2021).

15.3.1.4 Dynamization of the Support Network

Dynamization of the support network is aimed at mapping, disseminating, and consolidating all programs, projects, and actions from which a particular population and/or their community can benefit, with the intention of fostering interaction and integration between them, combining the different sectors and levels of intervention, facilitating effectiveness, and strategy targeting (Lopes et al., 2021).

15.4 Conclusion

This chapter sought to bring a historical understanding of the theoretical and practical contributions that have led to the development of social occupational therapy in Brazil. Historical events have been highlighted and discussed in relation to the set of procedures and resources that produced the foundations and parameters for social occupational therapy. Actions based on the territorial and community dimensions, locally contextualized professional contributions, and the challenges faced by those working in the social field were explored.

The chapter also reflected on the theories behind social occupational therapy and the practices implemented to gain a better understanding of the multiple dimensions of the themes within the projects. Finally, we emphasized that intervention requires reflection on the contexts, time, and historical spaces of the experience, since thinking, doing, and experience and reflection are inseparable. Paulo Freire's legacy (1979a, 1979b) continues to inspire and guide transformations which go beyond activism and rhetoric by linking action and theory, experience, and critical reflection.

15.5 Summary

- In capitalist societies, the social question concept is determined by the relationship between capital and labor, which today is shaped by neoliberalism.
- Occupational therapists should work with the social question, and design interventions that have macro- and micro-social scope.
- Social occupational therapy proposes dealing with the social question. Developed in Brazil in the late 1970s, it highlights the political-ethical role of the profession.
- The historical debate in Brazil has been whether the social question is in the scope of occupational therapy or if it is a specific field. On the one hand, it is necessary for all in the profession to reflect on social issues and its basic theoretical perspectives; on the other, it is necessary to advocate for social specificity that problematizes the medicalization and psychologization of the social fabric, and instead favors attention to difference, inequality, diversity, and culture.
- Social technologies proposed include workshops of activities, dynamics, and projects; individual territorial follow-ups; articulation of resources in the social field; and dynamization of the support network.
- Occupational therapists must reflect on current contexts and adopt a critical, situated, and horizontal perspective.

15.6 Review Questions

1. Why is the social question important to occupational therapists' actions?
2. In which contexts could occupational therapists apply social occupational therapy?
3. Why does social occupational therapy propose social technologies instead of "treatments"?
4. What is the connection between everyday life and workshops of activities, dynamics, and projects; individual territorial follow-ups; articulation of resources in the social field; and dynamization of the support network?

Notes

1 Considering the relevance of the discussion about vocabularies in the occupational therapy field (Malfitano, 2022), we propose the use of "social technologies" rather than models, treatments, or assessments, and highlight social approaches and the methodologies to develop it. Social technologies can be defined by the management of the social process, constructed in partnership with the community, through methodologies that can be reproduced in other contexts, representing actions aimed at social transformation (Dagnino, 2011).

2 Antonio Gramsci (1891–1937), an Italian philosopher, was imprisoned in the jails of Mussolini's fascist regime. He was an original follower of Marxism, which he preferred to call the Philosophy of Praxis. The proposition of historical materialism is based on Marx's formulation about the contradictions involved in life material reproduction. The concept is associated with the idea of *dialectic*, and considers all movements, changes, and interconnections involved in the social process, including contradictories and opposite movements.

3 "'Economic liberalism', sometimes called Neo-liberalism or 'big-L Liberalism' advocates a *laissez faire* economic regime, i.e., the right of property-owners to exercise the power of money unhindered by regulations, redistributive taxes and so on. Economic liberalism therefore easily makes common cause with the traditional sources of conservative politics – the landed aristocracy and Christian fundamentalists. Neo-liberalism ('Economic rationalism' in Australia) favours reliance on market forces to resolve social problems, rather than methods of state regulation" (Marxists Internet Archive Encyclopedia, 2022, n. p.).

4 *Dialogicity* is a concept developed by Paulo Freire (1921–1997), a well-known Brazilian international educator, which affirms the practice process as based on freedom and associated with conscientization. Dialogical practice in social occupational therapy is based on "the investment in relationships and the encounter to build the bond" (mediated by "doing / thinking / building / formulating / projecting with the individuals" and "Professional action articulated in the territorial, community, and cultural dimension" (Farias & Lopes, 2020, pp. 1352–1353).

5 "At the global level the center consists of those nations with high consumption levels, highly developed economic structures, and sophisticated technologies. The periphery consists of those dependent nations whose economies are tightly integrated with those of the center" (Simon, 2011, p. 149). It is necessary, however, to consider the dependence between peripherical and central countries, with economic predominance and maintenance of socioeconomic inequalities (Simon, 2011).

References

Barros, D. D., & Galvani, D. (2021). Occupational therapy: Social, cultural? Diverse and multiple! In R. E. Lopes & A. P. S. Malfitano (Eds.), *Social occupational therapy: Theoretical and practical designs* (pp. 29–47). Elsevier.

Barros, D. D., Ghirardi, M. I. G., & Lopes, R. E. (1999). Terapia ocupacional e sociedade. *Revista de Terapia Ocupacional da Universidade de São Paulo*, 10(2/3), 69–74.

Barros, D. D., Ghirardi, M. I. G., & Lopes, R. E. (2002). Terapia ocupacional social. *Revista de Terapia Ocupacional da Universidade de São Paulo*, 13(3), 95–103. https://doi.org/10.11606/issn.2238-6149.v13i3p95-103

Barros, D. D., Lopes, R. E., & Galheigo, S. M. (2007). Terapia ocupacional social: Concepções e perspectivas. In A. Cavalcanti & C. Galvão (Eds.), *Terapia ocupacional: Fundamentação e prática* (pp. 347–353). Guanabara Koogan.

Barros, D. D., Lopes, R. E., Galheigo, S. M., & Galvani, D. (2011). Research, community-based projects, and teaching as a sharing construction: The Metuia Project in Brazil. In F. Kronenberg, N. Pollard, & D. Sakellariou (Eds.), *Occupational therapy without borders – Volume 2: Towards an ecology of occupation-based practices* (pp. 321–327). Elsevier.

Castel, R. (2003). *From manual workers to wage laborers: Transformation of the social question* (R. Boyd, Trans.). Transaction.

Courtois, M. (2020). L'ergothérapie sociale au chevet des demandeurs d'asile. ASH Actualités Sociales Hebdomadaire. https://www.ash.tm.fr/hebdo/3148/focus/lergotherapie-sociale-au-chevet-des-demandeurs-dasile-547822.php

Dagnino, R. (2011). Tecnologia social: Base conceitual [Social technology: Conceptal basis]. *Ciência & Tecnologia Social*, 1(1). https://periodicos.unb.br/index.php/cts/article/view/7794

Farias, M. N., & Lopes, R. E. (2020). Social occupational therapy: Formulations by Freirian references. *Brazilian Journal of Occupational Therapy*, 28(4), 1346–1356. https://doi.org/10.4322/2526-8910.ctoEN1970

Francisco, B. R. (1988). *Terapia ocupacional*. Papirus.
Fraser, N. (2000). Redistribution, recognition and participation: Towards an integrated concept of justice. In United Nations. *World culture report 2000: Cultural diversity, conflict and pluralismo* (pp. 48–57). https://unesdoc.unesco.org/ark:/48223/pf0000121068
Freire, P. (1979a). *Pedagogia do oprimido* (7a ed.). Paz e Terra.
Freire, P. (1979b). *Educação como prática da liberdade* (9a ed.). Paz e Terra.
Goffman, E. (1961). *Asylums: Essays on the social situation of mental patients and other inmates*. Anchor Books Doubleday & Company, Inc.
Gramsci, A. (1971). *Selections from the prison notebooks*. International Publishers.
Kronenberg, F., Pollard, N., & Pollard, N. (2005). *Occupational therapy without borders: Learning from the spirit of survivors*. Elsevier.
Kronenberg, F., Simó Algado, S., & Pollard, N. (2007). *Terapia ocupacional sin fronteras: Aprendiendo del espíritu de supervivientes*. Médica Panamericana.
Lopes, R. E. (1990). Currículo mínimo para terapia ocupacional: Uma questão técnico-ideológica. *Revista de Terapia Ocupacional da Universidade de São Paulo, 1*(1), 33–41.
Lopes, R. E. (1993/1996). A direção que construímos: Algumas reflexões sobre a formação do terapeuta ocupacional. *Revista de Terapia Ocupacional da Universidade de São Paulo, 4/7*, 27–35.
Lopes, R. E. (2021). Citizenship, rights, and social occupational therapy. In R. E. Lopes & A. P. S. Malfitano (Eds.), *Social occupational therapy: Theoretical and practical designs* (pp. 1–11). Elsevier.
Lopes, R. E., Borba, P. L. O., & Cappellaro, M. (2011). Acompanhamento individual e articulação de recursos em terapia ocupacional social: Compartilhando uma experiência. *O Mundo da Saúde, 35*(2), 233–238. https://bvsms.saude.gov.br/bvs/artigos/acompanhamento_individual_articulacao_recursos_terapia.pdf
Lopes, R. E., Borba, P. L. O., Trajber, N. K. A., Silva, C. R., & Cuel, B. T. (2011). Oficinas de atividades com jovens da escola pública: Tecnologias sociais entre educação e terapia ocupacional interface. *Rede de Revistas Científicas da América Latina, Caribe, Espanha e Portugal, 15*(36), 277–288. https://www.redalyc.org/articulo.oa?id=180119115022
Lopes, R. E., & Malfitano, A. P. S. (2021). *Social occupational therapy: Theoretical and practical designs*. Elsevier.
Lopes, R. E., Malfitano, A. P. S., Silva, C. R., & Borba, P. L. O. (2015). Historia, conceptos y propuestas en la terapia ocupacional social de Brasil. *Revista Chilena de Terapia Ocupacional, 15*(1), 73–84. https://doi.org/10.5354/0719-5346.2015.37132
Lopes, R. E., Malfitano, A. P. S., Silva, C. R., & Borba, P. L. O. (2021). Resources and technologies in social occupational therapy: Actions with poor youth. In R. E. Lopes & A. P. S. Malfitano (Eds.), *Social occupational therapy: Theoretical and practical designs* (pp. 164–176). Elsevier.
Malfitano, A. P. S. (2022). An anthropophagic proposition in occupational therapy knowledge: Driving our actions towards social life. *World Federation of Occupational Therapists Bulletin, 78*(2), 70–82. https://doi.org/10.1080/14473828.2022.2135065
Malfitano, A. P. S., Adorno, R. C. F., & Lopes, R. E. (2011). A life story and an institutional path: Youth, medicalization and social distress. *Interface (Botucatu), 15*(38), 701–714. https://doi.org/10.1590/S1414-32832011005000042
Marques, A., & Morestin, F. (2020). La santé mentale des demandeurs d'asile confinés et le programme FASDA. *Les cahiers de l'espace éthique d'Ile de France*, hors série, pp. 41–42. https://www.espace-ethique.org/sites/default/files/hors-serie_ee_covid19.pdf
Marxists Internet Archive Encyclopedia. (2022). *MIA: Encyclopedia of Marxism: Glossary of Terms*. https://www.marxists.org/glossary/terms/l/i.htm
Oliveira, M. L., Pinho, R. J., & Malfitano, A. P. S. (2019). Occupational therapists inclusion in the 'Sistema Único de Assistência Social' (Brazilian Social Police System): Official records on our route. *Brazilian Journal of Occupational Therapy, 27*(4), 828–842. https://doi.org/10.4322/2526-8910.ctoAO1742

Pastore, M. N., & Sato, M. T. (2018). The patterns of socio-cultural diversity: Dialogues among occupational therapy, Africa and ethnography. *Brazilian Journal of Occupational Therapy, 26*(4), 952–959. https://doi.org/10.4322/2526-8910.ctoarf1240

Pinto, J. M. (1979). *Relato de uma experiência de terapia ocupacional no campo social*. Anais do V Encontro Científico Paulista de Terapeutas Ocupacionais.

Pinto, J. M. (1987). *De terapeuta ocupacional para terapeuta ocupacional: Os métodos de terapia ocupacional e suas elaborações na UFSCar (1983–1987)*. UFSCar.

Pinto, J. M. (1990). *As correntes metodológicas em terapia ocupacional no Estado de São Paulo (1970–1985)*. UFSCar.

Rafante, H. C., & Lopes, R. E. (2009). Helena Antipoff e a educação dos excepcionais: Uma análise do trabalho como princípio educativo. *Revista HISTEDBR On-line, 33*, 228–252. https://doi.org/10.20396/rho.v9i33.8639565

Simon, W. O. (2011). Centre-periphery relationship in the understanding of development of internal colonies. *International Journal of Economic Development Research and Investment, 2*(1), 148–156.

Soares, L. B. T. (1991). *Terapia ocupacional. Lógica do capital ou do trabalho?* Hucitec.

CHAPTER 16

Pragmatism

Current and Future Influence on Occupational Therapy and Occupational Science

Jacob Østergaard Madsen, Rodolfo Morrison, Vagner Dos Santos, and Tim Barlott

Abstract
This chapter presents a review and discussion of pragmatism's philosophical foundations, including the current and possible future influences on occupational therapy and occupational science. The chapter begins with an introduction to how philosophy can influence professional practice and research approaches, followed by a description of pragmatism as a philosophical and theoretical position and a description of relevant philosophers within pragmatism. The chapter further contains a presentation of how and in what ways pragmatism as philosophy and theoretical frame has affected both occupational therapy and occupational science until now, including a presentation of relevant concepts used. The chapter ends with a presentation and discussion of the use of a pragmatic temperament within occupational therapy practice and occupational science, and how this may foster a moral commitment to critically understand and deal with inequalities of life, generating action toward emancipatory ends.

Authors' Positionality Statement
This chapter has been written by four occupational therapists with histories and experiences from Australia, Brazil, Chile, Canada, Denmark, and Sweden. Each of these contexts influences the chapter presented and creates a framework for the authors' common reasoning on the chapter's topic, perspectives, and messages. Jacob's native language is Danish. He was born and lives in the northern part of Denmark. His academic journey and approach to pragmatism have been shaped by a Scandinavian approach, through his education at master's and doctoral level in both Denmark and Sweden. He is motivated by studying philosophical approaches to the understanding of humans as active beings and how this can create a theoretical ground for occupational therapy. Rodolfo's native language is Spanish. He was born in Chile (the territory also known as Wallmapu, ancestral land of the Mapuche people) and is Afro-Chilean-Panamanian. He did his masters and doctoral work in Spain, where he began to investigate pragmatism. Initially, his approach to pragmatism was from "translation" of documents, so

part of his understanding of the subject has to do with his own experience of being a Latin American man. Vagner's native language is Portuguese. He was born on the lands of the Guarani people, along the banks of the Uruguay River in the territory known as São Borja, Brazil. He currently lives in Port Macquarie, Australia, and has written this piece on the land of the Birpai people. He is dedicated to critical projects in occupational therapy, while recognizing that professional knowledge is deeply entangled with colonial projects. Tim's native language is English. He is a white, cisgendered settler living in Amiskwacîwâskahikan (also known as Edmonton, Canada), which is part of Treaty 6 and the traditional and ancestral territory of the Nehiyawak (Cree), Dene, Blackfoot, Saulteaux, Nakota Sioux, a diversity First Nations, and also the home to the Métis people. Tim is drawn to the ways philosophy (including pragmatism) and social theory can help to surface what is taken for granted and catalyze action.

We recognize that our social position has given us opportunities to thrive in life and a starting point for seeking to be critical of the understanding of the world, including social forces, in our work. We share the understanding that this opportunity can be used to create a more affirming world for and with people who experience a life of marginalization and inequality. We hope that this chapter will serve as a framework for reflection on how, when, and why pragmatism influences occupational therapy and occupational science.

> **Objectives**
> This chapter will allow the reader to:
>
> - Understand how philosophy can influence professional practice and research.
> - Describe pragmatism as a philosophical and theoretical position.
> - Account for how pragmatism has affected occupational therapy and occupational science.
> - Reflect on possible future application of pragmatism within occupational therapy practice and occupational science.

> **Key terms**
> - philosophy
> - pragmatism
> - pragmatic temperament
> - transaction
> - transactional perspective
> - situation
> - inquiry
> - context
> - end-in-view
> - functional coordination
> - habit
> - meliorism

16.1 Introduction

Philosophy, and the use of philosophical perspectives, has the potential to facilitate the discussion of existing knowledge, values, and actions, and frame a professional discipline's basic assumptions and dispositions in practice and research. This is also the case with occupational therapy and occupational science. Pragmatic philosophy is embedded in the contemporary fabric of the vocabulary, terminology, and theoretical ways of understanding occupation in Western/Northern practices of occupational therapy and occupational science. Because this embedding of pragmatism in some areas is taken for granted, this chapter presents pragmatism as a philosophical and theoretical position, including old and new directions, and how it has influenced occupational therapy and occupational science through time. Based on a historical overview of the development of pragmatism, from the perspective of relevant philosophers and their specific theoretical notions on human occupation and context, key concepts and definitions applied in occupational therapy and occupational science are exemplified. Other works within pragmatism that have not yet been explored from an occupational therapy and occupational science perspective may, however, inspire possible future application. In particular, societal- and health-relevant topics can be explored, enlivened, and brought to understanding using pragmatism. On this basis, a description of possible "future directions" and an alternative application of "a pragmatic temperament" that may inform how occupational therapy and occupational science deal with inequalities of our time is described and discussed.

16.2 Value and Potential of Philosophy in the Context of Professional Disciplines and Sciences

Philosophy can be defined as an activity that consists of "forming, inventing, and fabricating concepts" that respond to and represent the world as we know it (Deleuze & Guattari, 1994). Philosophy is, through this response and representation of the world, deeply connected with our experience as human beings and it expresses this through the creation of concepts.

Philosophy is inspired by and lived out in life and is therefore closely connected to our everyday experience as human beings. Philosophy can make sense of lived experiences, uncover and make sense of social phenomena, and has the potential to also set life in motion. Furthermore, philosophy also holds the potential to influence professional practice and research approaches. First, philosophy's constantly questioning approach is a kind of systematized doubt or wonder, where one does (or attempts to) not take anything for granted. Philosophy does not stop at concrete explanations, but constantly seeks further new horizons of knowledge. As such, philosophy is interested in what words and concepts we use about various topics and phenomena, i.e., how we comprehend, understand, apply, and live our everyday lives in which we commit ourselves as human beings. Second, philosophy is often preoccupied with an in-depth analysis of the answers we find, suggesting new concepts or pointing to new connections between concepts. This undertaking contributes to a new or improved understanding of the world. Philosophy is therefore, third, also critical, in the sense that it is not satisfied with a normal "stagnant" practice or understanding. On the contrary, philosophy seeks to challenge what is taken for granted (Chia, 2002).

Philosophy shows its value and potential in the context of professional disciplines and sciences, and makes it possible to challenge ingrained notions and assumptions.

As such, philosophical inquiry is an open and explicit activity in which the answer to "how might things be otherwise" is sought. An application of philosophical perspectives can thus contribute to illuminating existing knowledge, values, and actions, which form the basis for broader considerations, discussion, and potential rethinking of a professional discipline's basic assumptions and dispositions in practice (Taff, 2021).

16.3 Pragmatism as a Philosophical Position

Pragmatism is commonly used to describe a particular way of addressing and solving problems – a way of acting. The word "pragmatism" originally comes from the Latin pragmaticus and the Greek pragmatikos meaning "deed", and can be defined as a *pragmatic attitude or procedure*. In many ways, being pragmatic refers to elements of everyday life such as "being practical", "getting things done", and "doing things step by step" (Ormerod, 2006).

Pragmatism is based on a basic belief in changeability, in the sense that it regards the world as emergent and never final, and understands knowing the world as inseparable from agency within it. Pragmatism takes the meaning of a concept to depend upon its practical bearings. The upshot of this maxim is that a concept is meaningless if it has no practical or experiential effect on the way we conduct our lives or inquiries. An essential assumption in pragmatism is therefore that acquisition of knowledge in the world is presupposed by the fact that all philosophical concepts must be tested through experimental acting. This means that (1) a claim is only true if it is useful, (2) experience consists in dealing with nature, and (3) the articulated language rests on shared human practices reflected in the context in which we operate, which can never be completely "made explicit" due to the changeability of the world (Scheffler, 2013).

16.3.1 The History of Pragmatism

Pragmatic philosophy originated around 1870 in the United States, and its first generation was initiated by the so-called "classical pragmatists" (Morrison, 2021). Throughout history, various prominent figures have contributed to the development of pragmatism, and the following sections describe and characterize some of these individuals.

16.3.1.1 Charles Sanders Peirce

Charles Sanders Peirce (1839–1914) was an American polymath, born in Cambridge, Massachusetts. He grew up in an academic and intellectual environment, which helped shape his own view of life and approach to knowledge. Peirce was educated as a chemist and worked as a scientist for 30 years. Today, however, he is regarded by many as a philosopher and as one of the most original and versatile American philosophers and logicians. As a reformer in areas such as mathematics, research, philosophy of science, epistemology, and metaphysics he considered himself primarily a logician (examining statements to decide whether they are true) and a semiotician (studying the meaning and use of signs and symbols) (Burch, 2008).

Peirce is considered the first person who, together with his close friend and colleague William James, defined, formulated, and defended pragmatism. At the heart of Peirce's pragmatism is the notion that for a statement to be meaningful, it must have meaning in practice. This viewpoint is seen by many as the original maxim of pragmatism and suggests that the meaning of ideas lies in the actions that unfold these, rather than in their causes. Based on this approach, Peirce therefore saw the pragmatic description of meaning as a method for supporting scientific inquiry. Peirce's first published attempts at formulating pragmatism in the 1870s and the maxim he advanced is often considered not only a prototype in the development of pragmatist ideas, but an essential change in the philosophy of human thought and reasoning, which dominated American philosophy for the ensuing half-century or so (Scheffler, 2013).

16.3.1.2 William James

William James (1842–1910) was born in New York City and was a professor of psychology and philosophy at Harvard University. James turned out to be one of the most famous American psychologists and later the most famous living American philosopher of his time. James is described as an original thinker in and between the disciplines of physiology, psychology, and philosophy. His work was grounded in pragmatism and phenomenology, and influenced and inspired generations of thinkers in Europe and America (White, 2010).

James named Charles Sanders Peirce as pragmatism's originator and made the theory common philosophical knowledge. Both Peirce and James considered pragmatism to have its roots in works older than Peirce's theory from the late 19th century. James, in particular, viewed pragmatism as a method (the pragmatic method) that seeks a probable and temporary truth, guiding humans on a path forward, and adapting to different aspects of life and our experiences. Pragmatism as a method, as described by James, does not pronounce judgments of truth and falsity; rather, it is a matter of praxis – of doing and ordering (White, 2010).

16.3.1.3 John Dewey

John Dewey (1859–1952) was an American philosopher, educator, psychologist, and socialist social critic, born in Burlington, Vermont. He was a professor of philosophy and pedagogy in Chicago and philosophy at Columbia University. Dewey became a central figure within the pragmatic approach, and with his specific focus on politics, education, and social improvements, his thoughts are particularly interesting for pedagogical professionalism (Hildebrand, 2017).

Dewey viewed humans as continuous, internal to, inseparable from, and part of the world because of their actions. He argued that a human being or community is like a highly complex natural organism that must function within its environment and the pragmatic application of human knowledge in one's interaction with his or her environment is crucial to this functioning (Scheffler, 2013). He thus regarded the world as a place of change and becoming through problem solving, and the basic ontological entity that shaped Dewey's pragmatic attitude was consequently not "object" or "substance", but "event". An important element within Dewey's pragmatic reasoning is therefore that knowledge is effective action; it is doing (Kirby, 2005).

16.3.1.4 Jane Addams

Jane Addams (1860–1935) was an American feminist, sociologist, and social worker, born in Cedarville, Illinois. Addams was considered to be the forewoman of the American profession of "social work" based on pragmatic philosophy. In this regard, her views are also central in the understanding of pedagogical professionalism. She co-founded Hull House, a social settlement considered to be at the heart of feminist reform at the time, where the first Henry B. Favill School of Occupations (directed by Eleanor Clarke Slagle) was founded. Addams was different to the stereotypical "philosopher" as she held conferences in open spaces and put her ideas into action through her work at Hull House. Her theoretical work was intertwined with practice in an inextricable way, and she practiced one of the main maxims of pragmatism, i.e., philosophy is integrated into everyday life and it should not be distant from other parts of life (Morrison, 2022).

16.3.1.5 William Edward Burghardt Du Bois

Du Bois, commonly known as W. E. B. Du Bois, was known as a social activist for racial and economic equality. He was born into a working-class family in Great Barrington, Massachusetts. In June 1884, he was the first African-American to graduate from high school, and between 1888 and 1895, he completed his bachelor's, master's, and doctoral education at Harvard University.

His philosophical thinking and personal life intersected with the most influential pragmatic thinkers. For instance, William James was his professor at Harvard University and Du Bois' contributions align with Dewey's commitment to a socially engaged philosophy and a focus on education (Campbell, 1992). Du Bois' ideas are often labeled as radical or revolutionary and this interpretation of his work was potentially linked to his alignment with the Marxist critique of capitalism and his engagement in overcoming racism in the United States.

16.4 Current Influence on Occupational Therapy and Occupational Science

Pragmatism has influenced many of the historical and contemporary practices of occupational therapy and occupational science. Much of the vocabulary, terminology, and theoretical ways of understanding people and their occupations come from pragmatist foundations. This recognition, however, has not always been present in the history of occupational therapy. In the 1980s, Estelle Breines (1986) proposed the need to return to "lost principles" as part of occupational therapy's heritage, indicating how pragmatism allowed the distinctive installation of a way of being, doing, looking, and thinking in the profession. Thus, maxims related to the conception of the human being were consolidated such as, among others: human development comes from life experiences; knowledge – like the sciences – constantly changes as well as interpretations regarding the truth; and it is essential for the profession to have a holistic view (Breines, 1986).

Breines (1986) indicated that several of Adolf Meyer's perspectives are eminently pragmatist, although this was never explicitly stated in his writings. Meyer was a psychiatrist and is considered one of the founders of occupational therapy. Similarly, Eleanor Clarke Slagle (although she did cite pragmatists such as Addams and James in her writing), when preparing the first curriculum for occupational therapists, never explicitly articulated the ways that pragmatism shaped the centrality of occupation within the discipline (Morrison, 2022). On this point, Ikiugu (2001) has shown that various pragmatic terms have been used in the occupational therapy literature, e.g., adaptation, environment, balance, evolution, habits, routines, holism, and occupation. Ikiugu concluded that, following Breines' (1986) proposal, pragmatism is the basis of most of the concepts used in the occupational therapy profession.

In recent years, the literature referencing pragmatism in both occupational therapy and occupational science has increased notably (Morrison, 2021). One recommendation is the integration of pragmatism into the education curriculum for occupational therapy students as a relevant measure to align with the current paradigm, and to meet challenges within the profession (Ikiugu, 2001). New evaluation instruments and professional intervention models that are guided by pragmatism have also been proposed (Ikiugu & Smallfield, 2015).

Another of Dewey's pragmatist perspectives was the concepts of transaction and transactionalism which have been identified as having significant potential and use (Dickie et al., 2006). A transactional perspective, described more fully in the next section, offers a way of thinking about the inseparability of people and context – what we conventionally see as separate from the other is really part of the other (Dickie et al., 2006). A transactional perspective on occupation can contribute to expansion of occupational therapy interventions in the face of natural disasters, which have serious repercussions for people's occupations (Rushford & Thomas, 2016). It also assists in thinking about the transition of occupational science from an individualistic stance to a more global and contextualized one (Cutchin & Dickie, 2013), and facilitates the analysis of relationships between technology and people with disabilities (Barlott et al., 2021).

Although the pragmatist perspective is bound up in conceptualizations of occupational therapy and occupational science, it is important to maintain a situational perspective in the understanding of different problems (Madsen & Josephsson, 2017; Madsen et al., 2021). In Latin America, commentators have pointed out how, from a pragmatic perspective, situated occupational science can be understood by refraining from the use of theoretical models that are inconsistent with the specific problems of the region (Morrison et al., 2021). There is also an urgent need to look critically at the different possibilities that pragmatism provides in more complex and transactional understandings of occupation. For example, understanding that engagement in occupation and thus living an everyday life is dependent on knowledge; whoever knows is part of what they are knowing; and there is no independent knower (Madsen & Josephsson, 2017). From this perspective, occupation occurs in a situation formed by aspects of experience. Therefore, research should move away from dualistic perceptions of occupation and knowledge and toward a more holistic approach, thereby correcting a tendency to fracture transactional experience from the study of engagement in occupation.

Research on pragmatism in relation to the concept of occupation highlights Dewey's proposals that occupation is (a) a form of natural and social experience; (b) a primary means of fostering and structuring inquiry that allows people to practice and hone their habits and skills related to other research; and (c) a good way to have aesthetic experiences and thus a way to learn to live more meaningfully in the future (Cutchin, 2013).

Occupation is therefore considered to have practical importance, since it is conceived as a means by which people experience and put into practice their skills in order to improve their lives in particular situations, and to project those improvements into the future. Occupation also has theoretical value because it can be scientifically investigated to generate understandings and ideas about how to improve lived experience.

Other contributions include the revival of meliorism, which is an aspect of pragmatism that focuses on the belief that society can move forward, a core value within occupational science (Baranek et al., 2020); research on concepts related to pragmatism such as "occupational reconstruction" which considers approaches to social problems (Frank & Muriithi, 2015); and considerations of transactionalism within occupational science from a community perspective (Lavalley, 2017).

16.4.1 Concepts from Pragmatism Used within Occupational Therapy and Occupational Science

The application of pragmatism as a philosophical and theoretical framework has resulted in the application of certain concepts in occupational therapy and occupational science, particularly within the exploration of occupation as a phenomenon. The following sections describe and exemplify the concepts of situation, transaction, and inquiry.

16.4.1.1 Situation

According to pragmatism all human action is situated, meaning that individuals change their way of acting in everyday life in response to situations. Dewey (1998) named the circumstances that surround human actions the "situation". In pragmatism, the world is seen as a place of change and becoming through problem solving. Dewey described situations as basically uncertain and unstable and therefore unfinished, thus shaping a context of overcoming problems in everyday life through experimental action. From this perspective, situations are either indeterminate or determinate, characterized by certain challenges and needs.

An indeterminate situation is "open to inquiry" in the sense that its constituents are not a coherent and unified whole and, therefore, shaped by a problematic nature. Indeterminate situations are those in which an individual finds conflict between current needs and realities; for example, feeling cold or forgetting one's keys when arriving at work. The indeterminacy is then the driving force of inquiry, causing the individual to put on a coat or ask a colleague to unlock the office door. In each case, the inquirer seeks to establish a unified whole. In contrast, a determinate situation is a closed and unproblematic situation – that is, the inquiry (if successful) has transformed the situation into a determinate one. As such, human life is all about bringing stability and form to its incompleteness. Pragmatism, and Dewey in particular, was therefore concerned with processes used to create stability in life (Kirby, 2005).

Following this line of thought provides a theoretical understanding of occupation, as what we do as purposive organisms, in the larger context of uncertain and changeable situations. From Dewey's pragmatic approach to human action, a situation can be defined as a dynamic and unfinished feeding source for experimental actions toward stability. This perspective may entail a way of understanding occupation as a natural process of inquiry, providing a procedural perspective on occupation (Madsen & Josephsson, 2017).

16.4.1.2 The Theory of Transaction

Dewey emphasized the term "transactional" to describe his theories of knowledge and experience (Bentley & Dewey, 1949). A transactional perspective of human action forms the viewpoint that situational elements can be specified apart from the specification of all other elements and that no prior knowledge of the individual or environment alone and apart is adequate. According to Dewey, there are not organisms and environments but organisms-in-environments-as-whole. The concepts of functional coordination, habit, context, and end-in-view are central components of the complex character of transaction. These are to be understood as essential elements when observing human action as a situationally dependent phenomenon.

- *Functional coordination* is a constantly active process, dependent on the relationship of constructs formed and defined by situations. People are continually coordinating with the context and the situations they find themselves in. A person who realizes he or she forgot their office keys when arriving at work must coordinate with the context, such as calling a colleague or taking a bus back home to get their keys, meaning that the individual and the context co-constitute one another through their mutual relationship. The aim of this process is to maintain, enhance, and obtain an overall harmonic functioning within indeterminate or determinate situations (Aldrich, 2008; Cutchin et al., 2008; Madsen et al., 2021).
- *Habits* form and dominate transactions on a subconscious level and nurture a basic functional coordination of the inseparable person-context relationship. Habits continuously exist and work as predispositions to modes of response, becoming specific when applied in everyday life situations. Habits are necessary to functionally coordinate, meaning that situations become problematic when the habits are not well suited to the situation. As such, habits are inseparable from context in both their form and manner of acquisition and change (Aldrich, 2008; Cutchin et al., 2008; Madsen et al., 2021).
- *Context* is a spatial and temporal background affecting all thinking and thus action. Hence, it is to be seen as an overall condition affecting functional coordination. Objective conditions of context such as physical and social constraints or opportunities for education or employment influence the development and enactment of habits by shaping the situations in which habits function (Aldrich, 2008; Cutchin et al., 2008; Madsen et al., 2021).
- The *end-in-view* is the force that drives transaction through the support of habit and context. Ends-in-view are described by Dewey as forever incomplete and constantly developing manifestations, representing the aim as a transaction. Opposite to having a goal, ends-in-view represent a basic drive toward functionally coordinated relationships (Aldrich, 2008; Cutchin et al., 2008; Madsen et al., 2021).

Bentley and Dewey (1949) further argued that transaction should be regarded not as a theory but as a method allowing situational observation and description of action as always preliminary.

Dewey's theory on transaction highly influenced the development of a "transactional perspective on occupation". This perspective was spurred by Dickie et al.'s (2006) critique of individualism in occupational science and has been presented as important for achieving a more comprehensive understanding of occupation, because of its focus on the relations among constructs, rather than on isolated experiences within constructs. It facilitates a relational understanding of occupation from a context- and situation-dependent perspective (Cutchin & Dickie, 2013).

16.4.1.3 The Theory of Inquiry

Dewey stated that humans change in response to their current situation, meaning that life requires experimental action as a way of overcoming any problem in everyday life (Kirby, 2005). Dewey's theory on inquiry is about how to investigate, improve, and stabilize problematic situations through a transactional process (Kirby, 2005). Basically, Bentley and Dewey (1949) described transaction as an "inquiry in which existing descriptions of events are accepted only as tentative and preliminary, and where new descriptions of the aspects and phases of events based on inquiry may be made at any time" (Bentley & Dewey, 1949, p. 113).

Dewey explained inquiry as a controlled transformation of the indeterminate into determinate, turning the situation into a unified contextual whole. Inquiry is accordingly to be understood as a mode of thinking and acting (Dewey, 1998). As such, situation and inquiry are inseparable. The uncertain and continuously changing character of situations was therefore viewed by Dewey as generating an always developing inquiring point of departure for human action (Cutchin & Dickie, 2013; Dewey, 1998).

An example of the application of the Inquiry concept is Mattingly and Fleming's (1994) research on clinical reasoning. Inquiry is understood as an essential tool in the therapeutic process, and it is part of the resolution of problems. The authors follow Dewey in thinking about inquiry as a mental attitude and process at the same time, and a way of understanding how unintelligible processes become intelligible. Also inspired by Dewey's theory of inquiry, Madsen and Josephsson (2017) suggest that separating knowledge creation from engagement in occupation becomes problematic. They present the idea that occupation is "enacted situated inquiry", which is what happens within situations when people gain knowledge through engagement in occupation as transformative acts on how to live life.

16.5 The Future of Pragmatism in Occupational Therapy and Occupational Science

The influence of pragmatism in occupational therapy and occupational science is clear and ongoing, and this section discusses further considerations on its future relevance to a global profession in a fast-changing and unequal world. We support Frank's (2022) assertion that "pragmatist ideas are necessary – but not sufficient –resources for occupational science [and, we add to occupational therapy] in the 21st century" (p. 9). Using a hotel-corridor metaphor, we consider where our future interest and commitment lie.

16.5.1 Creating Spaces and Exploring "Corridors"

The corridor metaphor was first presented by Giovanni Papini, who deployed James' (1906) description of pragmatism as like a corridor in a hotel, from which 100 doors open into 100 chambers. In one room, you may see a man on his knees praying to regain his faith; in another, someone eager to destroy all metaphysics sitting at a desk;

in a third, a laboratory with an investigator looking for new footholds from which to advance upon the future. Yet, the corridor belongs to all, and all must pass through there. Pragmatism is, in short, a great "corridor theory" (p. 339). This metaphor was also used by James in 1907, when arguing that pragmatism can connect diverse philosophical projects.

These connections using pragmatism offer an opportunity to create new "professional territories". Brazilian social scientist and geographer Milton Santos' traditional view of territory as "spatial circuits of production and circles of cooperation" (Santos, 1996), helps us envision the corridors as spaces of cooperation for enhancing the social relevance of global occupational therapy and occupational science. Milton Santos coined the concept of "territory" which presents his preoccupation (both epistemological and praxis) with the functioning of society, places, and dynamics. It is a concept that can be used to reflect on these metaphorical corridors.

Within occupational therapy, a feature of the profession's momentum over the last two decades has been increasing international collaboration to expand the discipline's scope of practice. In this context, pragmatism can be used as a corridor to host professional and intellectual knowledge and experiences that benefit the profession and increase its disciplinary scope. For example, the four authors of this chapter reside in different countries and time zones and speak and think in different languages; yet, we communicated, met, and exchanged ideas and tasks in dealing with a specific "situation" that contributes to the profession's knowledge base, i.e., producing this chapter.

It is important, however, that pragmatic perceptions and the internationalization of professional dialogue are not limited to elite intellectual exchanges. We argue that professional momentum is also characterized by more substantial moral and political commitment (Hammell, 2020; Dos Santos et al., 2022). Professional dialogue in the early 21st century has resulted in enlargement of our professional engagement on issues related to inequalities of human lives, such as democratic participation, justice, environmental sustainability, racial equality, and social inequality in health. In this regard, the "situation" of writing a book chapter as previously presented becomes an issue of social relevance. The encounter in the corridor – the circle of cooperation – in this case is a symbolic one where ideas transit and should not be limited to completion of a chapter on pragmatism. It is about pushing a discussion further and presenting pragmatism as a tool in dealing with the situation of inequalities of human life. We do not invite you to subscribe to a specific way of thinking; rather, we aim to create a radical invitation to apply a *pragmatic temperament* instead of a pragmatic theory(ies) when walking through the corridors, e.g., physical and symbolic professional spaces.

16.5.2 Pragmatism Beyond Pragmatism: The Pragmatic Temperament

A pragmatic temperament reorients us to be open to possible futures rather than confined to a dogmatic image of pragmatism or specific pragmatic theory. Nicholson (2013) argued that a pragmatic temperament is characterized by "a flexible habit of mind that is not committed to any ideology or philosophical system and is compatible with a variety of philosophical approaches" (p. 43). Here, we imply that a pragmatic temperament, instead of only a commitment to pragmatic theory, can help us to produce practice and, consequently, knowledge to deal with diverse forms of inequalities of human life. With this alternative take on pragmatism, we bring our aspirations to deal with inequalities of human life and keep our reconstructive commitments to transform the agenda and practice of the discipline and the profession.

In the following section, we discuss projects as encounters on the metaphorical corridors that carry both a pragmatic temperament and moral commitment to critically understand and deal with inequalities of life. By using these examples, we suggest a way forward that encourages people's corridors of exploration to expand the professional scope of dealing with further aspects of inequalities of human life.

16.5.3 A Pragmatic Temperament to Understand Inequalities of Life

As we have articulated earlier in this chapter, "pragmatism is often characterized in terms of its emphasis on the practicability of getting things done over adherence to ideal principles" (Koopman, 2017, p. 179). However, the lack of principles can drive a social, and professional, project to morally questioned positions. Pragmatic thinkers have elaborated and invested their scholarship on democracy and contributed to important political-philosophical debates (see Chapter 6 for further details). Yet, pressing moral and political inequalities that result in specific forms of inequalities of life are too often neglected.

Similarly, the pragmatic stance and occupational therapy and science's focus on humans' capacity to do and live. However, we often do not engage with the philosophical question of what characterizes life and its inequalities. The epistemics of life (and how life is known and understood) is not new among philosophers, but this debate has been neglected among occupational therapists and scientists. There are different implications on what we do based on how we understand life, including how we shape and frame helping professions, such as the service, education, research (scope), and regulation (jurisdiction) of occupational therapy.

In this sense, the future of occupational therapy and occupational science, as well as pragmatism within the profession and the discipline, relies on our imaginative and collaborative efforts to make it globally relevant to deal with issues of our historical time. The non-pragmatic, French critical sociologist and philosopher, Didier Fassin (2018) acknowledges how we can envision two specific forms of inequalities of life based on this understanding. The first, natural and physical, relates to differences in age, illness, abilities, muscular strength, and qualities of spirit/soul. The second, moral and political, relies on a sort of convention (or *status quo*) and consists of different privileges possessed by some to the detriment of others; some become more honored than others.

Fassin's framework goes further and presents these as intertwined inequalities to reveal the troublesome treatment of human beings by contemporary society. To overcome these categories, his critical take of combining normative with genealogical views aims to reconcile the "social critique: our task is to change the world" with the "cognitive critique: our task is to change our view of the world". The different understandings of inequality will depend on our understanding of life. To this end, we explore some of the possible doorways that might be opened – opening possibilities for (future) action.

16.5.4 Exploring Doorways to Deal with Inequalities of Our Time

With a pragmatic temperament and critical eye, we can approach pragmatism as a corridor to deal with inequalities of our time. Applying this metaphor to a specific temperament allows us to deal with the promises of pragmatism and the contradictions of our time, using Roberto Mangabeira Unger's (2007, 2021) ideas to gain insight into the actual and imagination of the possible. To illustrate this, we present two examples of possible doorways.

The first example is American philosopher and political activist Cornel West's interpretation of pragmatism. In his prophetic project, he brings some of the pragmatic tradition, e.g., concerns with meliorism, to a radical interpretation of social realities and human life. As West (1989) indicates, his project focuses on "the emancipatory social experimentalism" (p. 249) which contains two central elements: emancipation and social experiment. While traditional pragmatism is concerned with the latter, the former is a core requirement for West's proposition of individual freedom through social life. Indeed, the project consists of "emancipatory experimentalism that promotes permanent social transformation and perennial self-development toward ever increasing democracy and individual freedom" (West, 1989, p. 241).

He takes pragmatism as the mediator (the corridor) to articulate his preoccupation with the human quest for freedom and the place of humans' qualities to think, reason, love, and act in society. To articulate his ideas, West uses the discursive space created by Roberto Mangabeira Unger that brought together traditional American pragmatism for social experimentation (e.g., Jefferson, Emerson, and Dewey) with traditions present in the work of emancipatory philosophers (e.g., Rousseau, Marx, and Gramsci). At the core of emancipatory experimentalism is justice and experimentation as actions that imagine a way out of economic, political, cultural, and social oppression. In this sense, West's project has a clear vision of why things need to be done and he expresses his preoccupation with "Promethean [rebelliously creative and innovative] human powers, the recognition of the contingency of the self and society, and the audacious projection of desires and hopes in the form of regulative emancipatory ideals for which one lives and dies" (West, 1989, p. 215).

The second example is the work of Boaventura Souza Santos on "epistemological pragmatism" in the field of Southern epistemologies (Nunes, 2008, p. 46). As with West's prophetic pragmatism, Boaventura Santos' emphasizes the experience and knowledge of oppressed people when thinking about promoting their quality of life. In doing so, Santos proposes his ecology of knowledge that implies thinking of knowledge (including traditional epistemology) within a field of non-hierarchical knowledge. To use our corridor metaphor, Santos created safe spaces, i.e., non-hierarchical corridors, for encounters. In this context, knowledge is not only abstractions, but also expressions of practice that facilitate or restrict certain experiences in the real world. This form of understanding – epistemological pragmatism – places the life experiences of the oppressed as intelligible in an epistemology of the consequences. In this process, emphasis is placed on the resolution of immediate problems from the point of view of the oppressed.

16.6 Conclusion

The value and potential of philosophy is demonstrated in the context of professional disciplines and sciences, such as occupational therapy and occupational science, and enables the challenging of rooted notions and assumptions. Pragmatism's influence in the development of occupational therapy and occupational science is demonstrated in the ideas and concepts of different pragmatists embedded in several of the basic foundations of the disciplines. Although a philosophy more than a century old, pragmatism remains current and relevant both in the reflections that it facilitates and as a useful tool for thinking about practice and research in occupational therapy and occupational science. Exercising a pragmatic temperament allows us to develop a practice of permanent doubt in which we question the "truths" given and question them based on the inequalities and problems people face in life. Pragmatism is a practical tool that makes it possible to contribute to solving inequalities of our time through professional practice and research.

16.7 Summary

- Philosophy can facilitate the discussion of existing knowledge, values, and actions of a professional discipline's practice and research.
- Philosophy forms, invents, and fabricates concepts that respond to and represent the world as we know it.
- Pragmatism is based on a belief in changeability and regards the world as emergent and never final.
- Pragmatism has been highly relevant in the development of occupational therapy and occupational science.
- The ideas and concepts of different pragmatists are current in several of the basic foundations of occupational therapy and science.
- Use of a pragmatic temperament may foster a moral commitment to critically understand and deal with inequalities of life.

16.8 Review Questions

1. What is the relationship between pragmatism and occupational therapy and occupational science?
2. Who are the main proponents of pragmatism that contributed to the development of occupational therapy and occupational science?
3. In which ways, in terms of thinking and acting, does pragmatism contribute to occupational therapy and occupational science?
4. In which ways do ideas from pragmatism show up across the disciplines of occupational therapy and occupational science?
5. What are the future possibilities of applying pragmatism in occupational therapy and occupational science?

References

Aldrich, R. M. (2008). From complexity theory to transactionalism: Moving occupational science forward in theorizing the complexities of behavior. *Journal of Occupational Science, 15*(3), 147–156. https://doi.org/10.1080/14427591.2008.9686624

Baranek, G. T., Frank, G., & Aldrich, R. M. (2020). Meliorism and knowledge mobilization: Strategies for occupational science research and practice. *Journal of Occupational Science, 28*(2), 274–286. https://doi.org/10.1080/14427591.2020.1824802

Barlott, T., MacKenzie, P., Le Goullon, D., Campbell, L., & Setchell, J. (2021). A transactional perspective on the everyday use of technology by people with learning disabilities. *Journal of Occupational Science, 30*(2), 218–234. https://doi.org/10.1080/14427591.2021.1970616

Bentley, A. F., & Dewey, J. (1949). *Knowing and the known*. Beacon Press.
Breines, E. (1986). *Origins and adaptations: A philosophy of practice*. Geri-Rehab.
Burch, R. W. (2008). Charles Sanders Peirce: 10. Mind and Semeiotic. *Stanford Encyclopedia of Philosophy*. Stanford University. https://plato.stanford.edu/entries/peirce/#mind
Campbell, J. (1992). Du Bois and James. *Transactions of the Charles S. Peirce Society*, 28(3), 569–581. http://www.jstor.org/stable/40320376
Chia, R. (2002). The production of management knowledge: Philosophical underpinnings of research design. In D. Partington (Ed.), *Essential skills for management research* (pp. 1–19). SAGE. http://doi.org/10.4135/9781848605305.n1
Cutchin, M. (2013). The art and science of occupation: Nature, inquiry, and the aesthetics of living. *Journal of Occupational Science*, 20(4), 286–297. https://doi.org/10.1080/14427591.2012.744290
Cutchin, M., & Dickie, V. (2013). Transactional perspectives on occupation: An introduction and rationale. In M. Cutchin & V. Dickie (Eds.), *Transactional perspectives on occupation* (pp. 1–10). Springer.
Cutchin, M. P., Aldrich, R. M., Bailliard, A. L., & Coppola, S. (2008). Action theories for occupational science: The contributions of Dewey and Bourdieu. *Journal of Occupational Science*, 15(3), 157–165. https://doi.org/10.1080/14427591.2008.9686625
Deleuze, G., & Guattari, F. (1994). *What is philosophy?* Columbia University Press.
Dewey, J. (1998). The place of habit in conduct (from *Human nature and conduct*). In L. Hickman & T. Alexander (Eds.), *The essential Dewey* (2nd ed., pp. 24–49). Indiana University Press.
Dickie, V., Cutchin, M. P., & Humphry, R. (2006). Occupation as transactional experience: A critique of individualism in occupational science. *Journal of Occupational Science*, 13(1), 83–93. https://doi.org/10.1080/14427591.2006.9686573
Dos Santos, V., Calvacante Bezerra, W., Godoy, A., & Terra, E. (2022). A terapia ocupacional de um Brasil democrático e livre. In V. Dos Santos, I. Muñoz, & M. Farias (Eds.), *Questões e práticas contemporâneas da terapia ocupacional na América do Sul* (2nd ed., Vol. 1, pp. 41–52). CRV.
Fassin, D. (2018). *Life: A critical user's manual*. John Wiley & Sons.
Frank, G. (2022). Occupational science's stalled revolution and a manifesto for reconstruction. *Journal of Occupational Science*, 29(4), 455–477. https://doi.org/10.1080/14427591.2022.2110658
Frank, G., & Muriithi, B. A. K. (2015). Theorising social transformation in occupational science: The American Civil Rights Movement and South African struggle against apartheid as 'Occupational Reconstructions'. *South African Journal of Occupational Therapy*, 45(1), 11–19. https://scielo.org.za/pdf/sajot/v45n1/03.pdf
Hammell, K. W. (2020). *Engagement in living: Critical perspectives on occupation, rights, and wellbeing*. Canadian Association of Occupational Therapists.
Hildebrand, D. L. (2017). Dewey, Rorty, and Brandom: The challenges of linguistic neopragmatism. In S. Fesmire (Ed.), *The Oxford handbook of Dewey* (pp. 99–130). https://doi.org/10.1093/oxfordhb/9780190491192.013.5
Ikiugu, M. N. (2001). *The philosophy and culture of occupational therapy* [Doctoral dissertation, Texas Woman's University]. https://hdl.handle.net/11274/11334
Ikiugu, M. N., & Smallfield, S. (2015). Instructing occupational therapy students in use of theory to guide practice. *Occupational Therapy Health Care*, 29(2), 165–177. https://doi.org/10.3109/07380577.2015.1017787
James, W. (1906). G. Papini and the pragmatist movement in Italy. *The Journal of Philosophy, Psychology and Scientific Methods*, 3(13), 337–341. https://www.jstor.org/stable/2011869
James, W. (1907). Pragmatism's conception of truth. *The Journal of Philosophy, Psychology and Scientific Methods*, 4(6), 141–155. https://doi.org/10.2307/2012189
Kirby, C. C. (2005). *Experience and inquiry in John Dewey's contextualism* [Graduate thesis, University of South Florida Tampa]. https://digitalcommons.usf.edu/etd/725

Koopman, C. (2017). Contesting injustice: Why pragmatist political thought needs Du Bois. In S. Dieleman, D. Rondel, & C. Voparil (Eds.), *Pragmatism and justice* (pp. 179–96). Oxford Academic. https://doi.org/10.1093/acprof:oso/9780190459239.003.0011

Lavalley, R. (2017). Developing the transactional perspective of occupation for communities: "How well are we doing together?" *Journal of Occupational Science, 24*(4), 458–469. https://doi.org/10.1080/14427591.2017.1367321

Madsen, J., & Josephsson, S. (2017). Engagement in occupation as an inquiring process: Exploring the situatedness of occupation. *Journal of Occupational Science, 24*(4), 412–424. https://doi.org/10.1080/14427591.2017.1308266

Madsen, J., Josephsson, S., & Kanstrup, A. M. (2021). Presenting an analytic framework facilitating a situationally oriented analysis of the use of digital technology for engagement in occupation. *Scandinavian Journal of Occupational Therapy, 28*(8), 631–642. https://doi.org/10.1080/11038128.2020.1829038

Mattingly, C., & Fleming, M. H. (1994). *Clinical reasoning: Forms of inquiry in a therapeutic practice*. F. A. Davis.

Morrison, R. (2021). Pragmatism in the initial history of occupational therapy. *Cadernos Brasileiros de Terapia Ocupacional, 29*, e2147. https://doi.org/10.1590/2526-8910.ctoARF2147

Morrison, R. (2022). The contributions of Jane Addams on the development of occupational therapy. *History of Science and Technology, 12*(2), 262–278. https://doi.org/10.32703/2415-7422-2022-12-2-262-278

Morrison, R., Silva, C. R., Correia, R. L., & Wertheimer, L. (2021). Why an occupational science in Latin America? Possible relationships with occupational therapy from a pragmatist perspective. *Cadernos Brasileiros de Terapia Ocupacional, 29*, e2081. https://doi.org/10.1590/2526-8910.ctoEN2081

Nicholson, C. (2013). Education and the pragmatic temperament. In A. Malachowski (Ed.), *The Cambridge companion to pragmatism* (Cambridge Companions to Philosophy, pp. 249–271). Cambridge University Press. https://doi.org/10.1017/CCO9781139022132.016

Nunes, J. A. (2008). Redeeming epistemology. *Revista Crítica de Ciências Sociais, 80*, 45–70. https://dialnet.unirioja.es/servlet/articulo?codigo=2763896

Ormerod, R. (2006). The history and ideas of pragmatism. *Journal of the Operational Research Society, 57*(8), 892–909. https://doi.org/10.1057/palgrave.jors.2602065

Rushford, N., & Thomas, K. (2016). Occupational stewardship: Advancing a vision of occupational justice and sustainability. *Journal of Occupational Science, 23*(3), 295–307. https://doi.org/10.1080/14427591.2016.1174954

Santos, M. (1996). *Metamorfosis del espacio habitado*. Oikos-Tau.

Scheffler, I. (2013). *Four pragmatists: A critical introduction to Peirce, James, Mead, and Dewey*. Routledge.

Taff, S. D. (Ed.). (2021). *Philosophy and occupational therapy. Informing education, research, and practice*. SLACK Inc.

Unger, R. (2021, March 6). *Losing and finding the way: The United States and Brazil* [Video]. YouTube. https://www.youtube.com/watch?v=sjdpBvaA94o&t=357s

Unger, R. M. (2007). *The self awakened: Pragmatism unbound*. Harvard University Press.

West, C. (1989). *The American evasion of philosophy: A genealogy of pragmatism*. Springer.

White, H. (2010). William James's pragmatism. Ethics and the individualism of others. *European Journal of Pragmatism and American Philosophy, II-1*. https://doi.org/10.4000/ejpap.941

CHAPTER 17

Gender and Human Occupation

Jens Schneider, Aiko Hoshino, Daniel Swiatek, Gunilla M. Liedberg, Mathilda Björk, Heather Baglee, Gustavo Artur Monzeli, and Ted Brown

Abstract
By the end of this chapter, the reader will be able to describe gender perspectives and concepts within historical and cultural contexts, and the relationship of those concepts to occupation and health. The reader will be able to explain factors that may impact cisgender occupational roles, habits, routines, identities, and repertoires, and discuss potential challenges related to cisgender occupational issues. The reader will be guided through an exploration of the relationship between transgender and gender-non-conforming people's experiences beyond gender norms and explore the subsequent impact on occupation. Heteronormative standards and gender stereotypes are also discussed, in order to provide recommendations for holistic and inclusive occupational therapy. The aim of the chapter is to develop a greater understanding of the dynamic relationship between human occupation and gender and to suggest measures to provide inclusive occupational therapy for individuals who experience occupational disadvantage due to their sexuality and/or gender identity.

Authors' Positionality Statement
The eight chapter authors are from diverse cultural backgrounds and geographies, including Australia, Brazil, Germany, Japan, Sweden, the United Kingdom, and the United States. Four of the authors identify as cisgender heterosexual females and four as cisgender gay males. All the authors have completed doctorates and are employed as university academics engaged in education and research and/or as practitioners. Their professional practice areas represented include geriatrics, adult mental health, neurology, pediatrics, chronic pain, and therapy interventions with gender and sexual minority groups. The authors have intentionally explored and provided both evidence-based and demographically diverse resources to illustrate a multitude of perspectives of gender and human occupation, e.g., queer, feminist, and masculine theories as well as pragmatist perspectives. Additionally, authors' views regarding the relation between gender and daily occupational performance are shaped, in part, by their life experiences

and reflect both the perspective of individuals from the Asia-Pacific, European, Latin, and North American regions of the world. Therefore, the authors are aware that the content is not exhaustive nor representative of every cultural and social reality. The authors also admit the cisgender privileges they have. They welcome the sociopolitical and sociocultural improvement in recognition of LGBTQIA+ issues (abbreviation for Lesbian, Gay, Bisexual, Transsexual/Transgender, Queer or Questioning, Intersexual, Asexual/Ally plus all other forms of gender and sexual identities), but recognize that this movement is in its infancy and requires continued attention through scholarly research and advocacy.

The authorship encourages readers to critically review the chapter and continue the discussion, enacting social and professional progress that represents a complex, diverse, and inclusive world of occupational opportunity for all people. In their view, a prerequisite for successful occupational therapy service is for occupational therapists to have an awareness and knowledge of gender and thus gender equality as a human right – both in interactions with the individual client and her/his/their human rights, but also in the profession's development of new knowledge. Being treated equally based on gender is a human right, and occupational therapists' and occupational therapy students' awareness of this fact is central to client- and person-centered care.

Objectives

- Describe gender perspectives and concepts in a historical and cultural perspective and the relationship to occupation and health.
- Explain factors that impact cisgender occupational roles, habits, routines, identities, and repertoires, and discuss potential challenges related to cisgender occupational issues.
- Explore the relationship between transgender and gender-non-conforming people's experiences beyond gender norms and the impact on occupation, and provide recommendations for holistic and inclusive occupational therapy service and research.
- Identify issues related to heteronormative standards and gender stereotypes, and suggest measures to provide inclusive service for individuals who experience occupational disadvantage due to their sexuality and/or gender identity.

Key terms

- **gender perspectives and concepts**
- **cisgender identities**
- **transgender and gender-non-conforming people**
- **gender inclusive services**
- **human occupation**

17.1 Traditional and Contemporary Understanding of Gender and Human Occupation

Gender operates at every level of human experience: global, cultural, societal, institutional, organizational, and individual (Connell, 2012). Today, the concept of gender is seen as broader than the traditional view of the female and male dichotomy of sex. It also considers sexual differences and less binary definitions of gender categorization (Heise et al., 2019). A wider example of a definition grounded in queer theories is presented by Riggs and Treharne (2017) and "suggests that all bodies and psyches are offered intelligibility through their relationship to a particular set of norms, ones that privilege the idealised white, heterosexual, middle-class, young, normatively sized, and abled body" (p. 102).

Analysis from a gender perspective specifies how a society handles sexuality, reproduction, child growth, motherhood, fatherhood, and aspects such as occupations socially connected with these processes. Individuals born biologically female or male develop into gendered beings and into a gender order. Connell (2012) defines the gender order as the way in which an individual identifies and how institutional structures intersect to produce the social arrangements that allow one gender to dominate socially, economically, and politically. A hierarchy of power and privilege is maintained by traditional gender norms which favor what is considered male or masculine over what is female or feminine. This perpetuates an inequality that weakens the rights of women and girls and reduces the opportunity for women, men, and gender minorities to express their genuine personality in non-traditional ways (Heise et al., 2019).

The ways in which historical (e.g., pre-industrial societal characteristics), cultural (e.g., marriage arrangements and family structures), social (e.g., attitudes toward women and men and their roles), economic (e.g., female labor force participation, financial autonomy), ethnic (e.g., family structures), religious (e.g., how different religious communities view the traditional male breadwinner conception), and political variables shape the role of gender in different societies varies and also differs over time (Giuliano, 2017).

Various theories also deepen the gender perspective. For example, feminist theories encompass the importance of questioning existing oppressive structures and systems, and whether or not these form obstacles for individuals. The aim is to enable discovery of how people interact within systems and possibly offer solutions to confront and eradicate oppressive systems and structures. Some of these theories do not refer to excluding men or only promoting women's conditions. They instead describe that women and men should be equal socially but also politically and economically. These theories emphasize that when oppression and power are recognized and opposed, understanding increases and change can take place (Biana, 2020). "Masculine [theories], like feminist [theories], opens up the possibility of examining how gender is scripted in text and in life, with the hope of transforming the social scripts and their enactments" (Bean & Harper, 2007, p. 13).

Gender operates to produce and reproduce gendered expectations and behaviors that become part of everyday occupations. Gender is often internalized in individual women and men, contributing to their gendered identity and how they interact with other people according to the gender order of their historical time and geographical place (Connell, 2012). Women and men are actors/doers in these socially constructed relationships and are in that way "doing gender". Further, because gender is "done" or constructed, it can also be "undone" or deconstructed. One way in which gender is undone is through women's presence in previously traditional male dominated work areas; for instance, the information and communications technology area. This sector is strongly dominated in the West by men due to their assumed closeness to technology (Kelan, 2010).

"Doing gender" in encounters with clients has been investigated in 17 occupational therapists who expressed insufficient theoretical knowledge of gender (Liedberg et al., 2010). The concept of gender was seen as value-loaded and placed outside occupational therapy as part of general mainstream theory. Hence, in assessments occupational therapists were found to focus their questions to clients on different spheres: for female clients, their household and family, and for male clients, their paid work situation. As such, the occupational therapists followed a societal tradition of "doing gender" (Liedberg et al., 2010). Further, in suggesting occupations to clients, 107 occupational therapy students made choices based on traditional gender roles (Liedberg & Hensing, 2011). The use of a client-centered and holistic approach was seen as a guarantee against gender stereotyping and the potential risk of treating women and men unfairly, and was recommended as a strategy to avoid a gendered perspective. Thus, it is important to combine individualized client-centeredness with an appropriate way to deal with the potential stereotypes that might occur in encounters between people (Sakellariou & Pollard, 2009).

Gender has been neglected in discussions of meaningful or purposeful occupation, but these factors should be considered since they are elements of assessments and interventions (Sakellariou & Pollard, 2009). If people are obliged to conform to societal expectations, rather than meet their individual needs, this gender role stereotyping can lead to occupational injustice (Bailliard et al., 2020), a situation that is in direct conflict with the profession's code of ethics (World Federation of Occupational Therapists, 2016). A gender-conscious approach results in all people receiving treatment based on their specific needs and allows the occupational therapist to disregard their own values and notions of traditional gender roles. Otherwise, communication, intervention, the rehabilitation process and, by extension, the clients' perceived health and well-being might be affected.

17.2 Cisgender People and Human Occupation

To contextualize how daily occupations relate to cisgender people, it is important to define key terms. Cisgender refers to people's gender identity that corresponds to their sex assigned at birth and can include heterosexual, homosexual, bisexual, asexual, and pansexual individuals (Saltzburg, 2015). Cisnormativity is the belief that the majority of individuals are cisgender while cissexism is the conviction that transgender people are inferior to cisgender people (Worthen, 2016). Cisgender privileges denote the advantages and benefits that cisgender people receive as a result of societal preferences for cisgender female-male relationships and sexuality above same-sex relationships. It can also relate to the alignment between a cisgender person's gender and perceived identity, e.g., "I perceive myself as male, and society recognizes me as being a male".

Cisgender roles impact the daily occupations individuals engage in and also which societal norms are considered appropriate or inappropriate for cisgender females and males (Cumming-Potvin & Martino, 2018). For example, child rearing and meal preparation may still be viewed as occupations that mainly cisgender females engage in. In some parts of the world cisgender roles are strict and prescribed, whereas in other societies cisgender roles are more fluid, flexible, and diverse. For example, in some religiously conservative countries, the range and type of clothing that cisgender people wear can be restricted, e.g., requiring women to wear a hijab head scarf, or a niqab and burka to cover the face and body. In liberal democratic countries, women and men can wear a much wider range of clothes and fashion items, e.g., both women and men can wear jewelry and make-up.

A number of traditional cisgender roles exist and these traditional female and male cisgender roles are often affiliated with certain daily occupations. It is recognized, however, that there has been a remarkable shift in traditional cisgender roles and identities compared to previous decades. Women now work full time outside the home, more men are taking on an active role raising children, and both groups are working in fields traditionally aligned with the other sex, e.g., women working in engineering and men working in nursing professions and occupational therapy. Despite these changes, cisgender women are still disadvantaged in comparison to their cisgender male counterparts, particularly in relation to salaries and career advancement (Karlsen, 2012; Schwiter et al., 2021). This inequity is called the cisgender gap and refers to disparities in economics, social and educational levels, and political participation that result from differences between the implicit and explicit status that society creates for women and men (World Economic Forum, 2017).

One notable example of cisgender inequity is male privilege. It has been reported that cisgender men are often unaware of their inherent societal privileges and that they may be unconsciously supported, economically and racially, by other privileged cisgender men. Cisgender male privilege is also bolstered via the economic, social, legal, religious, cultural, and educational systems and structures that reinforce patriarchal behaviors (Gruys & Munsch, 2020). As a result, in many countries there exists a notable cisgender gap between cisgender women and men that has a variety of impacts beyond traditional roles. For example, in the 38 member countries of the Organisation for Economic Co-operation and Development (OECD), cisgender women earn on average 13.9% less than men (OECD, 2015).

A further illustration of cisgender male privilege is the percentage of cisgender women in management positions. In Japan, for example, less than 20% of management positions are held by women (Japanese Ministry of Health, Labour and Welfare, 2021). Some experts also suggest that traditionally male-dominated academic fields in the STEM disciplines (STEM = science, technology, engineering, mathematics) have a significant impact on the career choices of female students (Froehlich et al., 2022; Ikkatai et al., 2021).

A number of change agents have contributed to the evolution of cisgender roles, including social, legal, ethical, moral, and human rights. These change agents include the gender equality, women's liberation/feminism, and diversity and inclusivity movements, and represent an evolution that has led to cisgender role fluidity, equality, and cross over. Changes in traditional cisgender occupational roles have contributed to new, emerging cisgender occupational roles, examples of which include workplace activities, housework, childcare, sports and recreation, arts and crafts, and food preparation. While there may now be more equity and equality between women and men in daily occupations related to work, self-care, education, and leisure activities, cisgender women in the end bear greater responsibility for the completion of domestic occupations (Cumming-Potvin & Martino, 2018; Park et al., 2013).

Furthermore, one must consider aspects of masculinity and gender norms that contribute to cisgender standards that are associated with cisgender males themselves. It has been reported that men are more likely than women to socially isolate because they are hesitant to express their feelings and less likely to actively seek out medical support; thereby maintaining their masculine guise and the appearance of being emotionally strong and self-contained, courageous, independent, dominant, and assertive (Galdas et al., 2005). Likewise, when considering cisgender-based occupations and their impact on occupational social norms, there are a variety of differences that go beyond the cisgender gap and can be considered disadvantageous or inequitable. For example, men may be expected and required to do more physical labor, e.g., required to be able to lift certain weights as part of a job, or be drafted into mandatory military service when they reach a certain age. In most countries, however, mandatory military service for women is not expected.

Gendered occupations may also be influenced by cisnormativity and heteronormativity. Social structures constituted by gender dualism and heterosexism-based norms impact the daily occupational performance of all people. Based on cisnormativity, for example, public documents or public services in some countries still allow cisgender women or men to be promoted over others and discriminate against non-cisgender individuals, e.g., transgender and gender-non-conforming people. People who identify as gender diverse or gender expansive may therefore be underprivileged. Additionally, from the perspectives of heterosexism, in many countries, including Bangladesh, Malaysia, Egypt, Jamaica, Uzbekistan, and Saudi Arabia, same-sex relations and marriage are legally banned. As a result, people may be subject to restrictions, social sanctions, and legal action since they are not privy to the same occupational rights and privileges when renting a place to live, parenting and adopting children, accessing education, reporting offenses to police, or receiving medical services.

In occupational therapy service, it is important to recognize cisgender women's and men's occupations not as a one-sided view, but as individual experiences. It is also key to understand that social structures and invisible norms still exist and are often covert, implicit, unstated, and veiled instead of overt, transparent, explicit, and visible. Practicing occupational therapists need to be aware of these issues when working with clients and their families.

17.3 Transgender and Gender-non-conforming People and Human Occupation

A number of studies in the fields of occupational therapy and occupational science have highlighted the use of occupation in expressing authentic gender identity, coping with challenging situations, and living a contented life for individuals who identify as transgender within and outside the binary gender system (Avrech Bar et al., 2016; Beagan et al., 2012; Dowers et al., 2019; McCarthy et al., 2022; Monzeli, 2022; Schneider et al., 2019; Schneider, 2022; Swenson et al., 2022). Findings from a study by Schneider et al. (2019) have shown that gender normative restrictions on transgender people's occupations may start in childhood. Some transgender people have reported that they were not allowed to dress according to their authentic gender identity, or to play with toys of their choosing. As a consequence, they attempted to adapt to the occupational expectations of their cisnormative environment, and sometimes this practice extended into adulthood.

Beagan et al. (2012) and Swenson et al. (2022) reported on examples in which transgender women were family fathers in their earlier lives before coming out, or took up professions typically considered overtly masculine, e.g., working as a soldier. Narratives of transgender youth illustrate how terrified some were by the transformation of their child body into an adult female or adult male during puberty. Hiding occupations such as binding female breasts or removing male body hair were carried out in response to unwanted bodily changes (Schneider et al., 2019; Schneider, 2022).

The disclosure of one's transgender identity is a pivotal life challenge and accompanied by the performance of many subsequent occupations such as looking for information about transgender issues, experimenting with alternative styles of clothing at home, and trying to connect with peers (Beagan et al., 2012; Schneider et al., 2019; Schneider, 2022). Dowers et al. (2019) and Monzeli et al. (2015) pointed out that individuals who identify in a more gender expansive or fluid manner, thereby challenging gender-normative boundaries, are in even more danger of suffering exclusion, discrimination, harassment and violence, and experiencing difficulties in accessing social rights such as education, health, leisure, work, and more. Transgender and gender-non-conforming people are restricted, or feel restricted, in their performance of occupations.

Before transgender people undergo gender-affirming interventions such as hormone treatment or surgeries, they may be recognizable as their authentic transgender selves by their physical features, dress, style, and behavior. The same may apply to gender-non-binary people whenever they publicly adopt a non-cisgender role and presentation. McCarthy et al. (2022) and Swenson et al. (2022) explored how the environment in which gender-non-binary people live affects their occupations. Participants in their studies reported that a cisgender normative environment negatively affected their feelings and created anxiety, and, as a result, they dressed and behaved according to cisgender normative expectations in spaces where they felt unsafe, or avoided these places. To live out their authentic gender identity, non-binary people prefer to place themselves in environments in which they feel comfortable and safe (McCarthy et al., 2022; Swenson et al., 2022).

Transgender people who identify within the binary gender system and who wish to transition from their gender assigned at birth to their authentic gender may face many challenges with which they try to cope through occupations (Beagan et al., 2012; Schneider et al., 2019; Schneider, 2022). Individuals may embark on a long-lasting gender transition process with goals connected to control of their lives and full expression of their gender identity. Consequently, they may need to perform meaningful occupations with long-term goals in mind, e.g., taking hormones or undergoing different gender-affirming surgeries to change their bodily appearance. Since some of these occupations can be fraught with hardship, transgender people may turn to occupations that are psychologically rewarding in order to create identity and to increase well-being (Beagan et al., 2012; Schneider, 2022). One such example is drawing. Sam, a transgender man participant in Schneider's study (2022), carried out the occupation of drawing at a time when he did not yet know himself that he identified as transgender. They describe this occupation as follows:

> [As part of the therapy ... I was supposed to describe my feelings] and because I can't do that very well verbally – I can do that better on paper when I draw ... [Drawing was a way of expressing myself.] I wasn't able to verbalize all that at that time ... When I'm at a loss for words – I'm still well able to say something with the coloured pencils. (p. 179)

Schneider (2022) found that various occupations performed by transgender men possess a transformative capacity and proposed that this practice may be generalizable to other transgender and gender-non-conforming people. These occupations play a central role during the gender transition process as they enable transgender people to perform the next occupation in their gender transition process, toward the aim of living a contented life (Schneider, 2022). For this reason, it is useful to develop occupational therapy interventions that support transgender and gender-non-conforming people to achieve their long-term goals. In addition, interventions that enable these individuals to overcome short-term hardships are required in order to stay on track toward their long-term goals (cf. Beagan et al., 2013; Daly & Hynes, 2020; Schneider, 2022; Swenson et al., 2022).

Authors of the aforementioned studies have called for further research into the occupations of transgender and gender-non-conforming people. In their study of transgender and gender-non-binary people, Dowers and Eshin (2020) posed the question of whether research with these groups is best performed by "insider" or "outsider" researchers. Researchers who are transgender or gender-non-binary may have a better understanding of the feelings and attitudes of, and the challenges faced by, this group and be better placed to more accurately interpret data. The risk of insider bias could be counterbalanced by cisgender researchers as allies of transgender and gender-non-conforming people. Given the vast array of un-researched transgender and gender-non-conforming topics, and the potential limited number of researchers who identify as transgender or gender-non-conforming, it may be challenging for these topics to be studied by inside researchers only.

In light of this, a commitment is necessary from cisgender researchers to practice honest self-reflection and reflexivity as a prerequisite for research with transgender and gender-non-conforming people (Dowers & Eshin, 2020). Schneider (2022) emphasized a number of ways to deconstruct the binary between researchers as insiders versus outsiders – being an "insider-outsider", e.g., belonging to the LGBTQIA+ community and having experience of providing services for transgender and gender-non-conforming people, but not identifying as transgender or gender-non-conforming. These recommendations have the advantage of creating common ground with transgender and gender-non-conforming people while also allowing researchers to retain a certain amount of distance. This assumption could also be applied to all LGBTQIA+ people and to occupational therapy services.

17.4 Challenging Heteronormative Binary Standards and Providing Inclusive Occupational Therapy Services

While well-being is accepted as being linked to the ability to partake freely in occupations of choice, the societal impact of gender on occupation where occupations are either gendered as feminine or masculine is undeniable (Almeida, 2022). One need only consider childrens' tools of play, where dolls are traditionally marketed to girls and play trucks to boys. These binary expectations continue into adulthood where women and men have traditionally been assigned leisure interests and work occupations depending on gender (Almeida, 2022). Recognizing gender as a learned activity, not a biologically-driven construct (Brennan & Gallagher, 2017), it can even be considered a performance (Butler, 1990).

People use occupations to act out gender-based traditional expectations of being female or male and to avoid occupations incongruent with gender. In Brennan and Gallagher's (2017) study on the occupational preferences of adolescents aged 11–14, the occupations of family and friends were found to be influential, along with available opportunities for community participation. In addition, participants' subjective interpretation of community expectations also influenced their willingness to pursue, or not pursue, occupations. Interpretation of community expectations also influenced the expectations they had for themselves, leading to Brennan and Gallagher's (2017) conclusion that occupational choice is negotiated with the environment. As occupation is intricately tied to standards for gender, it is therefore necessary to discuss the experiences of individuals who deviate from traditional binary occupational standards.

When occupation is broadly used as a means to empower or disempower a gender, it is referred to as a gendered occupation (Huff et al., 2022). The meaning of "gendered" is different to the meaning of "gender", which has traditionally been inclusive of only female or male. Gendered describes how sociopolitical forces have historically manipulated occupation for advantage and oppression, and gendered discrimination can overlap, or intersect with, other factors, such as disability status, socioeconomic class, ethnicity, race, and sexual identity (Gerlach, 2015; Huff et al., 2022). The concept of intersectionality recognizes that an individual can experience marginalization in multiple ways, such as LGBTQIA+ discrimination overlaid with racial discrimination and more (Gerlach, 2015).

The intersection LGBTQIA+ people experience is significant and the struggle for LGBTQIA+ equality has called for not only recognition and protections for LGBTQIA+ people, but challenges to occupational stereotypes. For example, child rearing and nurturing have traditionally been allocated to women. In countries where same-sex marriage and adoption are illegal, male co-parents face discrimination on at least two levels. First, two men co-parenting deviates from gendered norms for child rearing, and the male parents may experience various levels of stigmatization and unfair treatment. Second, restrictions are built into the legal framework of the country which prohibit same-sex couples from being recognized as legal co-parents. Such restrictions of occupational access have been called occupational apartheid (Morrison et al., 2020), and LGBTQIA+ people face a host of occupational difficulties across the lifespan even in countries where legal protections are in place. One occupation that can present significant challenges is work.

The workplace has been called an enforcer of heteronormative binary standards (Swenson et al., 2022) and is an environment where individuals will spend a great deal of their lives. Here, transgender and gender-non-conforming people are potentially at greatest risk of occupational deprivation or alienation. Research has indicated that they may feel compelled to refrain from authentic identity expression for fear of repercussions. Entering a public toilet or gym locker room are anxiety producing, and peacefully and productively engaging at work may not be possible without sacrifices to being one's authentic self (Phoenix & Ghul, 2016; Schneider et al., 2019; Swenson et al., 2022). Some feel it necessary to participate in traditional gendered roles to fit in, or to wear uniforms in conflict with their gender identity. While this assimilation provides safety and security, it ultimately detracts from work performance and creativity. Non-binary people may be more heavily impacted than transgender people who identify within the binary gender system because their outward presentation is fluid and less conforming to binary standards for traditional female or male workplace presentation (Swenson et al., 2022).

Transgender people who transition in the workplace face additional challenges. In a review of previous research, Phoenix and Ghul (2016) found that employers often lack policies and procedures related to employees' transitioning, and this caused uncertainly and confusion about expectations. Many transgender employees faced discrimination, particularly in male-dominated fields, and some opted to defer full-time transitioning until retirement rather than suffer workplace discrimination. Others reported the need to quickly meet traditional binary standards for female and male workplace presentation in order to better fit in (Phoenix & Ghul, 2016). One noteworthy finding was that expectations for tasks changed during transitioning. Transgender men were now asked to complete more physical occupations like moving furniture, and transgender women were given more traditional female tasks such as pruning plants. Misogynistic repercussions also appeared. Transgender men reported improved respect and more opportunities for advancement, while the skills of transgender women faced new, harsher scrutiny (Phoenix & Ghul, 2016), illustrating the role of intersectionality in discrimination.

Finally, recommendations for gender inclusive services are outlined. For example, approximately 12–13 million adults in the United States (US) identify as LGBTQIA+ (Conron & Goldberg, 2020). Of those adults, 1.3 million identify as transgender (Herman et al., 2022) and 1.2 million as non-binary (Wilson & Meyer, 2021). Individuals who identify as non-binary are recognized as a growing segment of the US LGBTQIA+ population, particularly among young people (Wilson & Meyer, 2021). As emphasized in this chapter, one tool occupational therapists must utilize to lessen the risk of implicit bias instilled by cisgender and heteronormative standards is the use of client-centered practice. As practitioners, researchers, and educators we must consider as best practice the use of holistic, individualized services and draw on the *LGBT+ Awareness and Good Practice Guidelines for Occupational Therapists* (AOTI, 2019), in which all the roles of the occupational therapist are considered as services, including client assessment and intervention, educating students/therapists, and conducting research (AOTI, 2019).

The AOTI utilizes the "4 Ps Model" in transforming services to become more LGBTQIA+ friendly through its "Framework for LGBT+ Inclusive Occupational Therapy". The 4 Ps are relevant for providing inclusive services for people who identify as LGBTQIA+ and, from the perspective of the chapter authors, for gender inclusive services in general. The 4 Ps are outlined below, supported with examples for better understanding:

1. **Public profile:** The organization's official website and related documents should clearly express that the occupational therapists welcome clients of all genders and sexualities, provide inclusive care, and prioritize gender equality.

2. **Policy and procedures:** Organizations should have a policy in place to ensure equal treatment and inclusion of all genders and sexualities. In addition, procedures for dealing with discriminatory behavior, such as sexism, homophobia, or transphobia, should be in place and trained for.
3. **Programs:** Actions should be taken and programs developed to improve services for gender inclusivity. The site should ask itself: What can be done to ensure that all people, regardless of their gender or sexual identity, experience a positive service environment?
4. **Professional development:** Education and training on the client's multifaceted needs, including gender identity, and how to interact with the LGBTQIA+ population overall are essential for inclusive services. Demonstrating respect and inclusivity for all genders and sexual identities must be a priority. It is recognized, however, that true inclusivity must go further. As presented earlier in this chapter, queer theories indicate that societal norms privilege Caucasian, heterosexual, young, middle-class, able-bodied people (Riggs & Treharne, 2017). There is a related concern in the field of occupational therapy, with Hammell (2015) suggesting that occupational therapy theory has largely been driven by a similar, homogenous group, and a call for greater focus on a variety of global contexts and perspectives. Organizations must be aware of professional groups that advocate for gender inclusivity and diversity in general, such as the International Network on Sexualities and Genders within Occupational Therapy and Occupational Science (SexGen-OTOS) and its national spinoffs, as well as the Coalition of Occupational Therapy Advocates for Diversity (COTAD).

17.5 Conclusion

Gender is understood as a significant factor in the daily occupations that people choose to engage in and should therefore be recognized as a necessary component in occupational therapists' world view. An assessment of occupational performance without consideration of a client's gender and whether gender has had an impact on occupational choice and performance would be incomplete and, therefore, not meet the profession's standards for client-centered practice.

It can be easy to see headline topics: cisgender experience through discrimination against cisgender females; privilege for cisgender males; displacement for transgender people; and a lack of understanding of the non-binary experience. It is essential, however, to look beyond the headlines to gain an understanding of the individual and to ask about the experience of discrimination or assumptions in their life.

Understanding of the ways that gender impacts everyday life and occupational choice is emerging, but research within the occupational therapy and occupational science disciplines continues to be limited. It is imperative to grow a body of empirical knowledge about the relationship between gender and occupation and this will, in turn, facilitate gender inclusive occupational therapy practice and expand research efforts in this area.

17.6 Summary

- This chapter explored the relationship between gender and occupation from the perspectives of people who are cisgender, transgender, and gender-non-conforming.
- There are a number of factors that may impact cisgender occupational roles, habits, routines, identities, and repertoires, and this chapter discussed potential challenges related to cisgender occupational issues.

- There is a dynamic relationship between transgender and gender-non-conforming people's experiences and this impacts their daily occupational performance; they may experience occupational disadvantage due to their sexuality and/or gender identity.
- To provide holistic and inclusive services to clients and their families, occupational therapists need to be aware of heteronormative standards and gender stereotypes.
- The expectation is that this focus will start a conversation among occupational therapy students and practitioners, and as research into this area develops so will understanding of the life experiences of people not previously considered in practice.

17.7 Review Questions

1. Review statements from the United Nations and World Health Organization in relation to gender equality worldwide to gain the broadest perspective of the impact of gender upon occupational choice.
2. Consider previous experiences and whether gender was encouraged as an aspect of assessment and intervention. Reflect on your experience and consider how you might approach this differently in the future.
3. Using this chapter as a starting point, develop your understanding of the life experience of transgender and gender-non-conforming people. Create prompts for new research in this area and read current research as it evolves.
4. The Association of Occupational Therapy of Ireland (AOTI) (2019) utilized the "4 Ps Model" to transform services in becoming more LGBTQIA+ friendly through its "Framework for LGBT+ Inclusive Occupational Therapy". What are the four 4Ps that make up this model?
5. Think about the daily occupations you engage in. What are two examples of the impacts of heteronormativity, cisnormativity, and cisgender privilege on those occupations?

References

Almeida, D. (2022). Night-time leisure: Gender and sexuality intersected by generation, style, and race in the Sao Paulo pop LGBTQ+ scene. *Journal of Occupational Science, 29*(1), 52–67. http://doi.org/10.1080/14427591.2022.2038248

Association of Occupational Therapists of Ireland. (2019). *LGBT+ awareness and good practice guidelines for occupational therapists*. Association of Occupational Therapists of Ireland. https://www.aoti.ie/news/AOTI-LGBT-Awareness-and-Good-Practice-Guidelines-for-Occupational-Therapists

Avrech Bar, M., Jarus, T., Wada, M., Rechtman, L., & Noy, E. (2016). Male-to-female transitions: Implications for occupational performance, health, and life satisfaction. *Canadian Journal of Occupational Therapy, 83*(2), 72–82. https://doi.org/10.1177/0008417416635346

Bailliard, A. L., Dallman, A. R., Carroll, A., Lee, B. D., & Szendrey, S. (2020). Doing occupational justice: A central dimension of everyday occupational therapy practice. *Canadian Journal of Occupational Therapy, 87*(2), 144–152. htpps://doi.org/10.1177/0008417419898930

Beagan, B. L., Chiasson, A., Fiske, C. A., Forseth, S. D., Hosein, A. C., Myers, M. R., & Stang, J. E. (2013). Working with transgender clients: Learning from physicians and nurses to improve occupational therapy practice. *Canadian Journal of Occupational Therapy, 80*(2), 82–91. https://doi.org/10.1177/0008417413484450

Beagan, B. L., De Souza, L., Godbout, C., Hamilton, L., MacLeod, J., Paynter, E., & Tobin, A. (2012). "This is the biggest thing you'll ever do in your life": Exploring the occupations of transgendered people. *Journal of Occupational Science, 19*(3), 226–240. https://doi.org/10.1080/14427591.2012.659169Bean, T. W., & Harper, H. (2007). Reading men differently: Alternative portrayals of masculinity in contemporary young adult fiction. *Reading Psychology, 28*(1), 11–30. https://doi.org/10.1080/02702710601115406

Biana, H. T. (2020). Extending Bell Hooks' feminist theory. *Journal of International Women's Studies, 21*(1), 13–29. https://vc.bridgew.edu/jiws/vol21/iss1/3

Brennan, G., & Gallagher, M. (2017). Expectations of choice: An exploration of how social context informs gendered occupation. *Irish Journal of Occupational Therapy, 45*(1), 15–27. https://www.emerald.com/insight/content/doi/10.1108/IJOT-01-2017-0003/full/html

Butler, J. (1990). *Gender trouble: Feminism and the subversion of identity.* Routledge, Chapman & Hall, Inc.

Connell, R. W. (2012). Gender, health and theory: Conceptualizing the issue, in local and world perspective. *Social Science & Medicine, 74*, 1675–1683. https://doi.org/10.1016/j.socscimed.2011.06.006

Conron, K. J., & Goldberg, S. K. (2020). *Adult LGBT population in the United States.* The Williams Institute, UCLA School of Law.

Cumming-Potvin, W. M., & Martino, W. (2018). Countering heteronormativity and cisnormativity in Australian schools: Examining English teachers' reflections on gender and sexual diversity in the classroom. *Teaching and Teacher Education, 74*, 35–48. https://doi.org/10.1016/j.tate.2018.04.008

Daly, V., & Hynes, S. H. (2020). A phenomenological study of occupational participation for people who identify as transgender. *Annals of International Occupational Therapy, 3*(3), 127–135. https://doi.org/10.3928/24761222-20200309-04

Dowers, E., & Eshin, K. (2020). Subjective experiences of a cisgender/transgender dichotomy: Implications for occupation-focused research. *OTJR: Occupation, Participation and Health, 40*(3), 211–218. https://doi.org/10.1177/1539449220909102

Dowers, E., White, C., Kingsley, J., & Swenson, R. (2019). Transgender experiences of occupation and the environment: A scoping review. *Journal of Occupational Science, 26*(4), 496–510. https://doi.org/10.1080/14427591.2018.1561382

Froehlich, L., Tsukamoto, S., Morinaga, Y., Sakata, K., Yukiko, Y., Keller, M. M., Stürmer, S., Martiny, S. E., & Trommsdorff, G. (2022). Gender stereotypes and expected backlash for female STEM students in Germany and Japan. *Frontiers in Education, 6.* https://www.frontiersin.org/articles/10.3389/feduc.2021.793486

Galdas, P. M., Cheater, F., & Marshall, P. (2005). Men and health help-seeking behaviour: Literature review. *Journal of Advanced Nursing, 49*(6), 616–623. https://doi.org/10.1111/J.1365-2648.2004.03331.X

Gerlach, A. (2015). Sharpening our critical edge: Occupational therapy in the context of marginalized populations. *Canadian Journal of Occupational Therapy, 82*(4), 245–253. https://doi.org/10.1177/0008417415571730

Giuliano, P. (2017). *Gender: An historical perspective.* The IZA Institute of Labor Economics. No. 10931.

Gruys, K., & Munsch, C. L. (2020). "Not your average nerd": Masculinities, privilege, and academic effort at an elite university. *Sociological Forum, 35*(2), 346–369. https://doi.org/10.1111/socf.12585

Hammell, K. W. (2015). Respecting global wisdom: Enhancing the cultural relevance of occupational therapy's theoretical base. *British Journal of Occupational Therapy, 78*(11), 718–721. https://doi.org/10.1177/0308022614564170

Heise, L., Greene, M. E., Opper, N., Stavropoulou, M., Harper, C., Nascimento, M., Zewdie, D., & Gender Equality, Norms, Health Steering Committee. (2019). Gender inequality and restrictive gender norms: Framing the challenges to health. *Lancet, 393*, 2440–2454. https://doi.org/10.1016/S0140-6736(19)30652-X

Herman, J. L., Flores, A. R., & O'Neill, K. K. (2022). *How many adults and youth identify as transgender in the United States?* The Williams Institute, UCLA School of Law.

Huff, S., Laliberte Rudman, D., Magalhães, L., & Lawson, E. (2022). Gendered occupation: Situated understandings of gender, womanhood and occupation in Tanzania. *Journal of Occupational Science, 29*(1), 21–35. https://doi.org/10.1080/14427591.2020.1852592

Ikkatai, Y., Inoue, A., Minamizaki, A., Kano, K., McKay, E., & Yokoyama, H. M. (2021). Masculinity in the public image of physics and mathematics: A new model comparing Japan and England. *Public Understanding of Science (Bristol, England), 30*(7), 810–826. https://doi.org/10.1177/09636625211002375

Japanese Ministry of Health, Labour and Welfare. (2021). *Basic survey on equal employment opportunities.* https://www.mhlw.go.jp/toukei/list/71-r03.html

Karlsen, H. (2012). Gender and ethnic differences in occupational positions and earnings among nurses and engineers in Norway: Identical educational choices, unequal outcomes. *Work, Employment and Society, 26*(2), 278–295. https://doi.org/10.1177/0950017011432907

Kelan, E. K. (2010). Gender logic and (un)doing gender at work. *Gender, Work and Organization, 17*(2), 174–193. https://doi.org/10.1111/j.1468-0432.2009.00459.x

Liedberg, G., & Hensing, G. (2011). Occupational therapy students' choice of client activities: Does patients' gender matter? British Journal of Occupational Therapy, 74, 277–283. https://doi.org/10.4276/030802211X13074383957904

Liedberg, G. M., Björk, M., & Hensing, G. (2010). Occupational therapists' perceptions of gender: A focus group study. *Australian Journal of Occupational Therapy, 57,* 331–338. https://doi.org/10.1111/j.1440-1630.2010.00856.xMcCarthy, K., Ballog, M., Carranza, M. M., & Lee, K. (2022). Doing nonbinary gender: The occupational experience of nonbinary persons in the environment. *Journal of Occupational Science, 29*(1), 36–51. https://doi.org/10.1080/14427591.2020.1804439

Monzeli, G. A. (2022). Social occupational therapy, social justice, and LGBTI+ population: With whom we produce our reflections and actions? *Brazilian Journal of Occupational Therapy, 30*(spe), e3095. https://doi.org/10.1590/2526-8910.ctoARF234130952

Monzeli, G. A., Ferreira, V. S., & Lopes, R. E. (2015). Among protection, exposure and conditioned admissions: Travestilities and sociability spaces. *Brazilian Journal of Occupational Therapy, 23*(3), 451–462. https://doi.org/10.4322/0104-4931.ctoAO0518

Morrison, R., Araya, L., Del Valle, J., Vidal, V., & Silva, K. (2020). Occupational apartheid and human rights: Narratives of Chilean same-sex couples who want to be parents. *Journal of Occupational Science, 27*(1), 39–53. https://doi.org/10.1080/14427591.2020.1725782

OECD Family Database. (2015). *LMF1.5: Gender pay gaps for full-time workers and earning differentials by educational attainment.* http://www.oecd.org/els/family/LMF_1_5_Gender_pay_gaps_for_full_time_workers.pdf

Park, A., Bryson, C., Clery, E., Curtice, J., & Phillips, M. (2013). Gender roles. In A. Park, C. Bryson, E. Clery, J. Curtice, & M. Phillips (Eds.), *British social attitudes: The 30th Report* (pp. 115–138). NatCen Social Research. https://library.bsl.org.au/jspui/bitstream/1/3523/1/British%20Social%20Attitudes%2030_full_report_final.pdf

Phoenix, N., & Ghul, R. (2016). Gender transition in the workplace: An occupational therapy perspective. *Work, 55*(1), 197–205. http://doi.org10.3233/WOR-162386

Riggs, D. W., & Treharne, G. J. (2017). Queer theory. In B. Gough (Ed.), *The Palgrave handbook of critical social psychology* (pp. 101–122). Palgrave Macmillan. https://doi.org/10.1057/978-1-137-51018-1

Sakellariou, D., & Pollard, N. (2009). Three sites of conflict and cooperation: Class, gender and sexuality. In N. Pollard, D. Sakellariou, & F. Kronenberg (Eds.), *A political practice of occupational therapy* (pp. 61–91). Churchill Livingstone Elsevier.

Saltzburg, S. (2015). Pedagogy for unpacking heterosexist and cisgender bias in social work education in the United States. In J. Fish & K. Karban (Eds.), *Lesbian, gay, bisexual and trans health inequalities: International perspectives in social work.* Policy Press Scholarship Online. Bristol University Press. https://doi.org/10.1332/policypress/9781447309673.003.0012

Schneider, J. (2022). *Narratives on meaningful occupations of transmen during their gender transition process* [Doctoral dissertation, University of Brighton]. The University of Brighton research portal (accessible to the public from January 2024). https://research.brighton.ac.uk/en/studentTheses/narratives-on-meaningful-occupations-of-transmen-during-their-gen

Schneider, J., Page, J., & van Nes, F. (2019). "Now I feel much better than in my previous life": Narratives of occupational transitions in young transgender adults. *Journal of Occupational Science*, 26(2), 219–232. https://doi.org/10.1080/14427591.2018.1550726

Schwiter, K., Nentwich, J., & Keller, M. (2021). Male privilege revisited: How men in female-dominated occupations notice and actively reframe privilege. *Gender, Work & Organization*, 28(6), 2199–2215. https://doi.org/10.1111/gwao.12731

Swenson, R., Alldred, P., & Nicholls, L. (2022). Doing gender and being gendered through occupation: Transgender and non-binary experiences. *British Journal of Occupational Therapy*, 85(6), 446–452. http://doi.org/10.1177/03080226211034422

Wilson, B. D. M., & Meyer, I. H. (2021). *Nonbinary LGBTQ adults in the United States*. The Williams Institute, UCLA School of Law.

World Economic Forum. (2017). *Education, skills and learning. What is the gender gap (and why is it getting wider)?* https://www.weforum.org/agenda/2017/11/the-gender-gap-actually-got-worse-in-2017

World Federation of Occupational Therapists. (2016). *Code of ethics*. www.wfot.org/checkout/1221/2110

Worthen, M. G. F. (2016). Hetero-cis-normativity and the gendering of transphobia. *International Journal of Transgenderism*, 17(1), 31–57. https://doi.org/10.1080/15532739.2016.1149538

CHAPTER 18

Technology and Human Occupation

Emma M. Smith, Christopher Trujillo, Stephanie Lancaster, Caroline Fischl, Rosalie H. Wang, and Ted Brown

Abstract
This chapter discusses the history and role of technology in human occupation. In particular, it explores the increasing role of technology in our daily lives, across all occupational domains. Through the use of theories of occupation and occupational therapy, case studies, and globally relevant examples, it addresses not only the ways in which technology has the potential to enhance our occupational performance and engagement, but also the ways in which our reliance on technology may lead to occupational disruption, challenges to occupational justice, and questions of ethics.

Authors' Positionality Statement
Emma Smith is an occupational therapist and assistive technology researcher who grew up in Canada but has since immigrated to Ireland. Christopher Trujillo is an occupational therapist and assistive technology professional residing in Arizona in the United States. His paternal grandparents migrated to the United States from Mexico. Stephanie Lancaster is an occupational therapist and assistive technology specialist who lives and works in Memphis, Tennessee (USA). She holds a speciality certification in assistive technology and is a member of the leadership team of the Coalition of Occupational Therapy Advocates for Diversity (COTAD) as well as President Elect of the Tennessee Occupational Therapy Association (TNOTA). Caroline Fischl trained as an occupational therapist in the Philippines and as an ergonomist in Sweden. She is currently working as a university lecturer, program manager, and researcher in Sweden. Rosalie Wang is an occupational therapy researcher and educator and immigrant to Canada from China at an early age, now a settler in Toronto, Ontario, Canada, which is covered by Treaty 13 with the Mississaugas of the Credit. Ted Brown is a Western-trained occupational therapist who was raised, educated, and worked in Ontario, Canada, until the age of 39. In 2002, he migrated from Canada to Australia where he settled on the traditional lands of the Bunurong Boon Wurrung and Wurundjeri Woi Wurrung

peoples of the Eastern Kulin Nation. He acknowledges the impacts of colonial hegemony on the First Nation peoples of Canada and Australia. All authors support decolonization, equality of all people, and social justice. All authors support occupational justice as well as equitable healthcare and education which are inclusive and respectful of all individuals, regardless of individual characteristics.

Objectives
This chapter will allow the reader to:

- Define *technology* and related terms relevant to occupation and occupational therapy practice.
- Describe the general history of technology and human occupation.
- Discuss where technology fits within theoretical models and frameworks.
- Discuss the complex relationship of technology in human occupation (habits, rituals, routines, roles) as a facilitator and barrier.
- Discuss the use and implications of technology as it relates to human occupation at the individual, group, community, and societal or population levels.
- Critically analyze issues in the use and integration of technology in daily life and society, including marginalized and historically excluded populations.

Key terms
- assistive products
- assistive technology
- high tech
- internet
- low tech
- occupation
- occupational performance
- occupational therapy
- Occupational Therapy Practice Framework-4
- smartphones
- technology

18.1 Introduction

Technology is all around us. Throughout every moment of our days, whether we are waking or sleeping, we are interacting with various technologies – some more complex than others – as we go about our day. Technologies are present in everything, from the clothes we wear to the way we prepare our food, and are integral to our work, school, and leisure pursuits. Regardless of where we are in our lives, where in the world we live, technology, and what abilities we have, technology has an influence on what we do, and how we do it. In this chapter, we discuss the complex relationship between occupation and technology. We begin with definitions of *technology* and related terms, followed by a brief history of technology and its relationship to occupation. Next, we explore where technology fits in several occupation and technology relevant theoretical models, helping to situate technology in our core understanding of occupation across the lifespan. Finally, we invite the reader to consider issues in technology and occupation – hopefully prompting further thought and debate. In this chapter, you will also be introduced to three case studies, which we invite you to consider when reading the text. These help to situate the conversation in the context of the occupational experiences of groups of people and allow for the questioning of the complex meaning of the intersection of technology and occupation.

Case Study 18.1
The Diné people, who live on the Navajo Nation, were at risk of occupational apartheid during the peak of the COVID-19 pandemic. Due to limited internet access and energy infrastructure obstacles, many families had to drive to and use the Wi-fi hotspot in their school's parking lot; others who relied on a generator for electricity but were unable to travel to purchase gas because of the "stay-at-home" orders resorted to calling in and listening to their online class, which meant they were unable to see their teacher or peers (Gewertz, 2021). Entities like the Navajo Native American Research Center for Health Partnership (Navajo NARCH) offered educational workshops and supported technology access to a limited number of high school and undergraduate students on the Navajo Nation. They were, however, unable to fully address the social isolation associated with mandated quarantine conditions using technology, and they had to adapt their programs to prevent the stress and strain associated with prolonged computer usage (Kahn et al., 2021). In the fall of 2022, it was announced that the Navajo Nation would receive federal grant (CARES Act and American Rescue Plan Act) funding to build 63 new broadband infrastructure projects, including 11 new telecommunication towers that will provide high speed access to 20,000 homes (U.S. Department of Commerce, 2022).

Case Study 18.2
Over the past seven years, the number of secure internet servers rose dramatically in the nation of Lesotho. Current data indicates that there are now 150 servers per 1 million people, which sharply contrasts with the 9 servers that were available to the entire population in 2016 (The World Bank, n.d.). During the COVID-19 crisis, many educational institutions were closed, requiring students to attend online education. Had it not been for the increase in internet access, the opportunity for online education would not have been an option. This option for education can still be considered a double-edged sword, as several students who participated in online university education reported that the digital conditions were not conducive to quality learning (Makafane & Chere-Masopha, 2021).

Case Study 18.3
The vision for eHealth in Sweden, first adopted in 2006 but replaced in 2016, is to

> use the opportunities offered by digitalization and eHealth to make it easier for people to achieve good and equal health and welfare, and to develop and strengthen their own resources for increased independence and participation in the life of society.
>
> *(https://ehalsa2025.se/english/; Swedish Ministry of Health and Social Affairs, & Swedish Association of Local Authorities and Regions, 2016)*

Within a decade, there was an increase in internet users among Swedes 76 years and older from 23% in 2010 to 69% in 2019 (https://svenskarnaochinternet.se/english/). During the COVID-19 pandemic, technologies for eHealth, including health information and booking appointments for COVID-19 vaccinations, rapidly developed. Health, welfare, and other public services online which required the use of e-identification increased. However, during this period and prior to 2022, the percentage of internet users 76 years and older remained less than 70% (https://svenskarnaochinternet.se/english/). Without social networks and support, approximately 30% of Swedes 76 years or older could be at risk of marginalization and lack of access to eHealth services, with limited opportunities to achieve good health and maintain their independence and participation in society.

18.2 Technology Terms and Definitions

Technology is "the application of scientific knowledge for practical purposes, especially in industry" (Oxford English Dictionary, 2022). In common language, the word technology is often used to refer to digital technology such as computers, smartphones, and the Internet, though by definition, technology includes products, infrastructure, processes, and services. While debatable, distinctions are often made between "low tech" and "high tech". Low tech often refers to products that are simple and involve few processes in their production and use, while high tech often refers to products that involve complex infrastructure, include digital electronics, and have advanced functions or features. Generally, technology may be used by individuals as part of their daily occupations, without additional classification. Technology applications may be specifically classified as assistive technology, but they may also be rehabilitative (capacity building) or used in service delivery (Wang et al., 2021).

According to the World Health Organization, *assistive technology* is "an umbrella term for assistive products and their related systems and services" (p. xi). Assistive technology is of fundamental importance for persons with permanent or temporary functional difficulties as it improves their functional ability and enables and enhances their participation and inclusion in all domains of life.

The International Organization for Standardization has created ISO 9999:2022 *Assistive products for persons with disability – Classification and terminology* to outline products based on their primary functions. The standard defines *assistive products* in line with the International Classification of Functioning, Disability, and Health (ICF) (WHO, 2002), as a "product that optimizes a person's functioning and reduces disability", where assistive products comprise "devices, instruments, equipment and

Table 18.1 Classes of Assistive Products Based on Functions, from ISO 9999:2022(E)

- Assistive products for measuring, stimulating, or training physiological and psychological functions.
- Orthoses and prostheses.
- Assistive products for self-care activities and participation in self-care.
- Assistive products for activities and participation relating to personal mobility and transportation.
- Assistive products for domestic activities and participation in domestic life.
- Furnishings, fixtures, and other assistive products for supporting activities in indoor and outdoor human-made environments.
- Assistive products for communication and information management.
- Assistive products for controlling, carrying, moving, and handling objects and devices.
- Assistive products for controlling, adapting, or measuring elements of physical environments.
- Assistive products for work activities and participation in employment.
- Assistive products for recreation and leisure.

software". The classes of assistive products are listed in Table 18.1. Services typically involve assessment, training, maintenance, and follow up related to the delivery of assistive products.

There has been substantial discussion and debate regarding the need for a common language for assistive technology. Considering the various related terms that are being used in different fields, sectors, and regions around the world, it has been challenging to arrive at a standardized terminology. Standardized terminology is further complicated by global language differences, which result in different translations of similar terms. Standardized terminology facilitates documentation and analysis of outcomes data, communication between people, groups, and populations, and clarity in both practice and policy (Elsaesser et al., 2022). Various technology-related terms and applications that may be encountered when discussing occupation and occupational therapy are detailed in Table 18.2.

18.3 The History of Technology and Human Occupation

"Technology, whether rehabilitative, adaptive, occupation-related, or as a means to assess or deliver therapy, is a constant in occupational therapy practice" (Canadian Association of Occupational Therapists, n.d.). Technology has existed since humans began to think, reason, and solve the challenges of everyday life. From the ancient people who developed innovative solutions like using a stone to crack a nut, or the more complex axe which combined two elements to chop, technology has always accompanied or aided occupational participation and performance. Technology enables the human species to survive by helping them to access food, shelter from the weather, achieve health, and enjoy life. This was confirmed by the United Nations Secretary General who recognized the potential for new and emerging technologies to advance human welfare (Canadian Association of Occupational Therapists, n.d.).

Technological advancement is built on innovation driven by occupational need. As early as 679 BC, the early Mesoamerican people used innovative mathematical concepts, such as zero, and symbolic representation to create complex calendars that tracked and predicted astronomical events and seasons. This ancient agriculturally dependent people created new technology to aid them in the occupation of survival.

Table 18.2 Technology-related Terms and Applications in Occupational Therapy

Adaptive technology	The definition of adaptive technology was originally developed by non-profit organizations and disability associations; adaptive technology is a subset of assistive technology and is any object or system *specifically designed* for the purpose of increasing or maintaining the capabilities of people with disabilities. Things classified as adaptive technology are not generally used by persons without disabilities.
Alternative and augmentative communication (AAC) technology	AAC falls under the broader category of assistive technology and includes strategies and tools to help support persons with disabilities in communicative exchanges. AAC, which may be used temporarily or on a permanent basis, is considered augmentative when it is used to supplement a person's communication or alternatively when it functions as a substitute for speech that is non-functional or absent (Elsahar et al., 2019).
Consumer technology	Technology that is created and marketed for the general public, such as smartphones, tablet computers, mobile applications, home automation devices, or virtual assistants. Because consumer technologies are available to the mass market and used by anyone, their use by persons with disabilities may be viewed as less stigmatizing than assistive products that may tend to appear medicalized.
Digital technology/information and communication technology	Digital infrastructure, tools, and media that can be used or applied in various life areas. Examples include personal computers, smartphones, and tablets – including applications that accompany these devices – combined with the Internet and the World Wide Web (Fischl, 2020).
Disruptive technology	Also called disruptive innovation, it refers to products or services that are introduced into society, improving the way things work and thereby replacing existing systems. This impacts the way a population or market functions (Christensen, 1997) which demonstrates how technology and its use shape occupations.
Everyday technologies	"Technological, electronic and/or mechanical devices and services that are commonly used in daily life at home and in public spaces" (Nygård & Starkhammar, 2007).
Emerging technology	Technology which is novel and growing quickly, and while these technologies have potential future impact their capacities are often not yet known (Rotolo et al., 2015).

(Continued)

Table 18.2 (Continued)

Gerontechnology	Technology designed to support older adults, and also an interdisciplinary field dealing with technology for older adults (Bouma et al., 2007).
Intelligent technologies	Technologies with in-built capability for computation and networked information communication, often involving sensors that collect data about environments (and users), algorithms that process the information and learn about the environment and users, and execution of responses that are adaptive to the situation to achieve user goals (Ienca et al., 2017).
Welfare technology	Digital technology that is intended to maintain or increase safety, activity, participation, or independence for a person who has, or is at increased risk of having, a disability (Swedish National Board of Health and Welfare, 2015).

The ancient Greeks created technology to support their cherished occupation of learning and astronomy. To this day, scientists are continuing to learn about planetary cycles by studying the hand-powered Antikythera Mechanism, which was invented in ancient Greece, 2,000 years ago. Even the ancient Han Dynasty tax collectors utilized the Saunpan (abacus) to master the occupation of tax collecting.

Technological devices can assist people with daily activities and occupational performance but they can also become an integral part of the occupation itself. Technology can organize daily occupations and influence our daily habits, roles, routines, and rituals. It could be argued that all technology exists to "assist" humans as they engage in an occupation or activity; assistive technology, however, is a term that is used to strategically describe specific products, related systems, and services.

As people and occupations shape the environment, so are people and their occupations shaped by the environment (Townsend & Polatajko, 2013). Disruptive technologies demonstrate how technology shapes occupations and when a disruptive technology is adopted by the majority, the old technology it replaces loses its place in daily life. From an occupational perspective, such technologies dramatically change the way people would traditionally perform a certain activity.

Consider the example of how disruptive technologies have changed acquiring and listening to music over time. With vinyl records, people would sit around a turntable to listen to music but with the development of cassette tapes and compact discs (CDs), each with portable players, people did not have to stay at home to listen to music. Additionally, people could listen alone while in the presence of others with the help of head- or earphones although, as with vinyl records, people still had to purchase cassette tapes and CDs in stores. The notion of purchasing and storing music changed, however, with the advent of online streaming which meant that people didn't need to be in a store physically to buy music nor store music in physical form. The earlier technologies (vinyl records, tapes, and CDs), although still available in the market to a limited extent, have become less available because of newer technologies that enable more contemporary occupational forms.

For the adopters of a disruptive technology, the new technology is perceived as matching one's needs and preferences, while the old technology is perceived as less convenient. As a newer technology pushes the older technology out of the market, access to the older technology and possibilities for its maintenance, as well as services offered with it, decrease. In turn, people who do not adopt the newer (disruptive) technology are at risk of marginalization.

18.4 Understanding the Relationship between Technology and Human Occupation

18.4.1 Technology within Theoretical Models and Frameworks

In this section, we discuss theoretical models and frameworks specific to occupational therapy or used in occupational science and how they have conceptualized and positioned technology in various ways. We have presented a practice framework used in occupational therapy (the Occupational Therapy Practice Framework-4), a model which helps us to understand how the body works for activity and participation (the International Classification of Functioning, Disability, and Health), and two models of assistive technology use (the Human Activity Assistive Technology (HAAT) Model and Student Environment Tasks and Tools (SETT) Framework). We also examine a model that describes how people integrate and accept technology in their lives (Technology Acceptance Model (TAM)). With each of these, we discuss the role technology plays in the model, and its relationship to occupation. These are not the only models which exist, and we encourage readers to consider the role of technology and occupation in the other models they may use every day.

18.4.1.1 Occupational Therapy Practice Framework-4th edition (OTPF-4) (AOTA, 2020)

The OTPF-4 comprises two components: (i) the Domain, which is made up of Occupations, Contexts, Performance Patterns, Performance Skills, and Client Factors; and (ii) the Process, which includes Evaluation, Intervention, and Outcomes (AOTA, 2020). According to the OTPF-4, nine specific categories of occupation are contained within the Domain:

- Activities of Daily Living (ADLs)
- Instrumental Activities of Daily Living (IADLs)
- Health Management
- Rest and Sleep
- Education
- Work
- Play
- Leisure
- Social Participation.

Similarly, as part of the Domain, contexts include environmental and personal factors while performance patterns take in habits, routines, roles, and rituals. Performance skills incorporate motor, process, and social interaction skills, while client factors include values, beliefs and spirituality, body functions, and body structures (AOTA, 2020).

TECHNOLOGY AND HUMAN OCCUPATION

Technology is included as an integral part of our everyday occupational lives, and it is integrated with the occupations we engage in, the daily environments where we live, work, and play, and the routines, roles, and rituals we take part in. For example, a tablet can be used in the execution of ADLs, IADLs, health management, education, work, play, leisure, and social participation occupations. Different technologies can be part of our life roles, routines, habits, and rituals and require specific motor, process, and social performance patterns as well as body functions, and structure client factors to be utilized effectively. The OTPF-4 provides a comprehensive framework for occupational therapy students, practitioners, educators, and researchers to refer to when they engage in learning, service provision, teaching, and investigation of aspects of technology and its relationship to daily human occupation. It also provides a point of reference for occupational therapy practitioners when providing occupation-focused service to clients and families.

18.4.1.2 International Classification of Functioning, Disability, and Health (ICF) (WHO, 2022)

The ICF was created as a framework to be used in clinical, research, and policy-related applications, and is the international standard for the description and measurement of individual and population health and disability. The framework includes terminology and a classification system for health and health-related domains, describing body function and structure, capacity (what someone is able to do in a standardized environment), and performance (what someone does in their own environment). With its foundation in a biopsychosocial model, the ICF deliberately reorients focus on a diagnosis or personal impairment perspective of disability to emphasize health and functioning in environments. Functioning and dysfunctioning (disability) are considered at three levels: (1) body functions and structures (body level); (2) activities (person level); and (3) participation (social context level). Functioning or disability results from dynamic interactions between health conditions and contextual factors, which include environmental and personal factors.

Classification domains within the framework comprise five broad categories: (1) body functions; (2) body structures; (3) activities and participation; (4) environmental factors; and (5) person factors, each of which include detailed lists of components. The environmental factors category includes products and technology as items, and classifications are broadly based on purposes such as for personal consumption, personal use in daily living, personal indoor and outdoor mobility and transportation, communication, education, employment, culture, recreation and sport, practice of religion and spirituality, and in relation to buildings for public and private use among other purposes that are more general in nature. Other environmental factors such as environmental modifications and services, systems, and policies may be considered as technology in the broadest definition. Person factors include age, gender, socioeconomic status, culture, ethnicity, religious beliefs, educational level, political beliefs, location of residence, and life roles.

18.4.1.3 Human Activity Assistive Technology (HAAT) Model

The HAAT model demonstrates the relationship of assistive technology to the human, context, and activity. In the HAAT model, the human, activity, and assistive technology work together within a specific context or contexts. The HAAT model aligns well to occupational therapy concepts of Person, Environment, and Occupation, specifically the Canadian Model of Occupational Performance and Engagement. The *human* component of the HAAT includes physical, cognitive, somatosensory, and affective subcomponents, and describes the attributes of the person which contribute to their use of technology to engage in activities in their contexts. These are linked to body structures and functions concepts in the ICF. Furthermore, the HAAT approaches the human from a lifespan perspective, understanding the changes that occur within the person over the course of their life.

The *activity* component of the HAAT Model comprises sub-concepts linked to the activity and participation domains of the ICF: three participation sub-concepts (self-care, productivity, and leisure) and four activity outputs (mobility, manipulation, communication, and cognition). Among the participation sub-concepts, self-care is understood to include ADLs; productivity includes activities at work, school, or other means of contribution to society; and leisure is defined as activities which are done for recreation. The four activity outputs are the human activity outputs which, together, are required for participation in one or more of the three domains of participation.

The *assistive technology* component of the HAAT is divided into four subcomponents: the human technology interface, processors, environment sensors, and activity outputs. These describe how the person interacts with the technology, how the technology integrates information from the human and the environment, and how the technology contributes to activity through an activity output. Each of these components may be identified regardless of the complexity of the technology.

In the HAAT model, the human, activity, and assistive technology all come together to produce an activity or participation outcome (occupation) within a particular context. Context is further subdivided into physical, social, cultural, and institutional contexts. Contexts are very important as they may influence whether or how the assistive technology is used, depending on the spaces in which they are used (physical), the attitudes, beliefs, and values of the person(s) using or engaging with the technology (social and cultural), and the rules and regulations surrounding the technology and access to it (institutional).

18.4.1.4 Student Environment Tasks and Tools (SETT) Framework

The SETT framework is designed to help us understand how technology and tools are used in an educational context (Zabala, 2002). Although primarily considered a framework for assessment, it also offers guiding principles for implementation planning and ongoing re-evaluation of effectiveness by helping professionals to identify the characteristics of a Student, the Environment(s) in which the assistive technology will be used, the Tasks the user will need to accomplish to be successful in those settings, and the Tools necessary for that to be accomplished. This framework was originally designed for collaborative decision making when developing assistive technology services for students in schools.

18.4.1.5 Technology Acceptance Model (TAM)

According to the TAM (Davis, 1989), the most important determinants in people's inclination to adopt and use technology are its *perceived usefulness* and *perceived ease of use* in occupations. *Perceived usefulness* refers to "the degree to which a person believes using a particular system would enhance his or her [job] performance" (Davis, 1989, p. 320). From an occupational perspective, perceived usefulness is the meaning or value a person assigns a technology in a particular occupation. Thus, a person who does not see the relevance of a technology is less likely to perform occupations that use that technology (Fischl, 2020). *Perceived ease of use* pertains to "the degree to which a person believes that using a particular system would be free from effort" (Davis, 1989, p. 320). A person who perceives a technology as easy to use is more likely to use it in occupations; conversely, a person who does not find a technology easy to use would be less likely to use that technology in occupations (Fischl, 2020). Studies related to the TAM have resulted in its adaptation to other population-specific TAMs.

An overarching principle across all the theoretical models and frameworks discussed is that to support the performance of occupational habits, routines, roles, and rituals in life by diverse individuals, environmental factors including technology may be needed. While not within the scope of this chapter, environments that are accessible and inclusive (including universally designed) may be essential elements to maximize the benefits of technology to achieve individuals' occupational goals.

18.4.2 Technology and Occupation across the Lifespan

We have previously discussed nine specific categories of occupation found in the OTPF-4 (AOTA, 2020) and the use of technology across the lifespan is relevant to each of these categories. In many ways, technology has become more essential to occupational performance than it has ever been in the past. Table 18.3 provides an overview of human occupations in each of the OTPF-4 categories of occupation, across seven lifespan stages from infancy to older adulthood.

As Table 18.3 illustrates, technology is used by people throughout the lifespan and across all areas of occupation. This can both facilitate development and impede it depending on the degree and context of use, as well as other factors. While various health agencies may provide specific recommendations for technology use with developmental considerations in mind, these guidelines are often not followed by those using the technologies. As an example, screen time, which is defined as activities completed with visual engagement using an electronic device with a screen such as a television, computer, or smartphone, is significantly more prevalent across the lifespan than advised by public health agencies and healthcare providers. The American Academy of Pediatrics (AAP) recommends no screen time except for occasional video chatting for children under two years old and an hour or less per day for children aged 2–5 (Ashton & Beattie, 2019). This aligns with the World Health Organization's (WHO) advice for abstinence from sedentary screen time for children under the age of two and for daily maximum sedentary screen time of an hour for children aged 3–4 (WHO, 2019). However, usage among children in these age groups is consistently above those guidelines (Laing et al., 2022). The challenge we face is how to balance the benefits of technology use with the risks, particularly in children and adolescents whose brains are still developing. The impact of high levels of technology use among young people and adults has yet to be fully realized.

Table 18.3 Human Occupation and Technology across the Lifespan

Occupations	Stages of life					
	Infants & toddlers (age 0–2)	Young children (ages 3–5)	Children (ages 6–12)	Youth & adolescence	Young adults	Adults	Older adults
Activities of Daily Living (ADLs)	Diapers with color-coding to indicate dryness; suction-cup plates; bottles with features to decrease spillage and air intake	Velcro shoe and clothing closures	Electric toothbrush	Microwave	Hairdryer	Air fryer and other kitchen devices	Wheelchairs, walkers, and other mobility devices
Instrumental Activities of Daily Living (IADL)	Video monitors; child safety gait	Car seat	Bicycle	Smartphones	Car; washer and dryer	Web-based software for budgeting and money management	
Health management	Nasal suction devices; online resources to monitor development	Digital thermometers	Eyeglasses	Treadmill	Cell phone and/or video conferencing for telehealth visits	Electronic medication management system	Blood pressure, blood sugar monitoring
Rest and sleep	White noise machines	Light-up stuffed animal or night light	Digital music player	Meditation app on a smart phone	Listening to podcasts to go to sleep		
Education Work	Electronic toys, videos, digital/talking books; online music sources	Educational games on tablets; educational TV programming	Computers; smart boards in classrooms	Computers	Audio books Computers		
Play Leisure			Voice recognition systems like Siri and Alexa	Video gaming system	Audio books		
Social participation	Video communication with family members		Watching a movie with friends	Playing video games with others	Social media		

18.4.3 How Technology Interfaces with Our Everyday Lives

As technology continues to advance, its impact, integration, and uptake continues at a rapid pace. Digital assistants now answer us in our homes, driverless automobiles are being developed, robots are replacing humans in manufacturing, and watches provide us with feedback on our bodily functions. Indeed, more than any other factor technology has revolutionized our daily occupational performance and impacted the ways we interact with our daily living environments (AOTA, 2020).

We use an electric toothbrush to clean our teeth at different speeds and we use a microwave to warm up, thaw, or cook food (e.g., ADLs). We use tablets and mobile phones to schedule our daily activities and watches to monitor our movement, blood pressure, and respiration rate (e.g., IADLs and health management). We use tablets and laptops for learning and studying purposes, to stay in contact with friends and peers, and to play electronic computer games (e.g., education, social participation, and play/leisure). We use smartphones, digital clocks, and other electronic devices to assist with our sleep and rest as well (e.g., setting an alarm to get up or adjust bedroom temperature). We interact with technology in our daily living environments at home, work, and school and within communities. Technology is integral to our occupational performance patterns including habits, routines, roles, and rituals.

Since the early days of the occupational therapy profession, technology has been an essential element of what people do and how they do it. Even the tools used for evaluation and intervention at the inception of the profession were part of what is classified as technology, from weaving looms to woodworking tools and cooking utensils. Throughout this evolution, "technology has redefined occupation forever" (Smith, 2017, n.p.). In 1992, technology was identified as a modality of occupational therapy (Pedretti et al., 1992), and since that time it has become an essential element of occupation for individuals of all ages and from all walks of life. As such, "Technological progress has changed what we do in practice because it has changed the way people function in their daily lives" (Pedretti et al., 1992; Smith, 2017).

The tools and strategies we use to engage in occupations as a society have changed drastically over time because of technological advances – as have the processes we use to participate in those occupations. For example, our social interactions are increasingly virtual, through the use of text, video, and voice messages, live chats, or interactions on social media. In many ways, having access to these options has increased options for engagement; however, it is also important to consider the potential negative impacts of technology on occupational performance and the health and wellbeing of society as a whole. While smartphones allow us to engage with others in contexts and ways not previously available, they also create dozens of interruptions in our daily routines. This type of "screen time" has also been shown to impact the quality and quantity of sleep in humans of all ages (Przybylski & Weinstein, 2017; Rosen et al., 2016; Sanders, 2017).

18.4.4 How Technology Interfaces with Occupation

There are many ways in which technology interfaces with occupation including its use as a tool to accomplish a task or occupation, either by replacing or augmenting human function. Here are some examples of technology interfacing with occupation:

Integral: There are some occupations in which technology is integral to participation in the occupation itself. For example, playing a video game requires technology and without the technology it would not be possible to engage in the occupation, regardless of the individual's function.

Augmentation: Technology may augment our ability to do certain occupations. In this case, the person may have the necessary function to engage in the occupation, but it is made easier or more efficient using technology. For example, while an individual may be able to ambulate in moving from one location to another, the use of technology, like a bicycle or train, allows them to move further and more efficiently.

Compensation: In cases where a person experiences functional limitations technology may compensate for those limitations and allow the person to complete the activities which are important to them. Technologies which compensate for functional limitations may support a function which is difficult or replace a function which is otherwise impossible for a person. For example, a person who has difficulty speaking or is unable to speak may use a communication board or dedicated device to communicate with those around them.

Remediation: When a person has sustained an injury or illness, but is expected to regain function, technology may be available to help that person in remediating the lost function. In this case, the technology use may be temporary, until the person has regained function. For example, a person who has had surgery on their hand may use a robotic glove to help them regain range of motion and strength.

When we think about the use of technology within occupational therapy practice, we may prescribe or suggest technologies for any of these functions. We may also use technologies ourselves to complete tasks like assessment and measurement, or as tools for service delivery.

18.5 Implications of the Use of Technology on Occupation

The pervasive use and transformational impact of technology on occupational performance, habits, routines, roles, and rituals have multi-level and intersecting implications for individuals, groups, communities, and populations. Furthermore, the rapid evolution of technology and deployment of technological applications have ethical, social, and legal implications, which may be positive, neutral, negative, or unknown.

Technology is often positioned as a universal enabler, or something that can benefit individuals and populations of all ages, abilities, and contexts across every functional domain (see Table 18.1). Nevertheless, technology can also be a disabler, especially if not implemented at the right time and place. We have previously presented some of the concerns regarding the use of technology on lifespan development. In the next section, we explore additional topical issues related to the use and integration of technology in human occupation.

18.5.1 Equitable Access to Technology

Access to technology is considered a fundamental human right which can promote equal social, educational, economic, and civic opportunities for all, and protect individuals' abilities to exercise their rights. From the perspective of occupational justice, lack of access and therein absence of the ability to fully participate in occupations can result in occupational deprivation. For example, globally equitable access to assistive technology is a critical issue. It is estimated that over 2.5 billion people worldwide can benefit from assistive products and that number is expected to increase to 3.5 billion by 2050 given the increasing population of older people and people living with non-communicable diseases (WHO & UNICEF, 2022).

Multiple technology divides exist – geographical, cultural, socioeconomic, and educational – that contribute to inequitable access. Access to technologies is most restricted in low-income countries, though higher income countries also experience inequities, and communities that have been historically marginalized are also highly impacted. As we become increasingly reliant on technologies – an issue we will discuss in the next section – this technology divide, between those who can and cannot access technologies, serves to increase inequity between groups.

18.5.2 Technology Dependence or Overreliance on Technology

When technology becomes accessible and integrated as part of everyday life, the potential exists for occupational disruption. This refers to times when there is a temporary disturbance to a person's usual pattern of occupational performance and occupational engagement (Nizzero et al., 2017). With the recent changes in performance patterns that came about during the COVID-19 pandemic in mind, we can see the cycle that exists when something happens to cause occupational disruption. As increased use of specific technologies in daily life becomes the norm, we have also seen people's reliance on technology as a tool. This is illustrated by the integration of Zoom and other video-conferencing technologies in education and business which became the standard and helped facilitate participation in occupations for many during the COVID-19 pandemic. However, this technology has also caused occupational disruption, resulting from the rapid change over to online learning and engagement. Further, occupational disruption may be experienced when a technology that is relied upon malfunctions and suddenly cannot be used in the way we have become accustomed to.

18.5.3 Digital Literacy and Keeping Up with Technology Developments

The increased use of technology in society and rapid pace of technological development raises questions of digital literacy. Digital literacy refers to

> the awareness, attitude and ability of individuals to appropriately use digital tools and facilities to identify, access, manage, integrate, evaluate, analyse and synthesize digital resources, construct new knowledge, create media expressions, and communicate with others, in the context of specific life situations, in order to enable constructive social action; and to reflect upon this process.
>
> *(Martin, 2006, p. 155)*

A lack of digital literacy can contribute to poor participation and inclusion in society for those who do not have the skills or knowledge required to effectively integrate technology into their lives. Older adults are often cited as an example of people who may not have the necessary digital literacy and are therefore constrained in their participation in daily life activities. However, as the gap in digital literacy for older adults narrows, we should also look to other populations who may be left behind, including those who live in lower resourced areas without access to the same technological advances as those in higher resourced environments. We must also consider when and how we teach digital literacy skills. It is increasingly apparent that children require training in digital literacy as they interact more and more with technologies from a very young age. However, children are not the only ones who require training in this area, and we must consider all groups who might benefit.

18.5.4 Technology and the Future of Work

Advancements in and deployment of technologies such as information and communication technologies, robotics, and artificial intelligence, along with enhanced computing power, have the potential to enhance productivity across all sectors, thereby facilitating greater economic advantage. Examples include robots for restocking merchandise or manufacturing, artificial intelligence to adjudicate insurance claims, chatbots for online assistance, or self-service checkout stations at retailers.

For some people with disabilities, technology has demonstrated potential to broaden opportunities for employment. These opportunities were highlighted during the COVID-19 pandemic, where working from home became increasingly mainstream. This societal shift emphasized the potential effectiveness of many job activities in virtual work environments, which can present significant advantages for individuals who find it challenging to mobilize to workspaces that may not be accessible.

Nevertheless, there are perceived and real concerns about technology replacing people and, indeed, therapists have voiced concern that the use of robotics in rehabilitation may take away their jobs. A seminal report by Frey and Osborne (2013), which examined the likelihood of work being computerized, found that 47% of jobs in the United States were at risk.

As work is a fundamental occupational domain, the loss or absence of employment for individuals and groups presents many difficulties. Employment is essential not only for securing monetary resources for living, but is meaningful in facilitating occupational habits and routines, and contributing to occupational roles with which people identify and develop. Consequently, occupational therapists have important roles to play in supporting people to access education or training for employment and acquiring, maintaining, or transitioning employment in the context of shifting job demands, or elimination of redundant or emergence of new jobs.

18.6 Reflection on the Relationship between Technology and Human Occupation

In this chapter, we have presented an overview of the relationship between technology and occupation from both theoretical and practical perspectives. We have explored some current issues in the application of technology to occupation and invited the reader to consider not only how technology may be used as an enabler, but also as a disruptor to occupation. As we are unable to address all potential issues relevant to technology and occupation, we invite the reader to consider some of the thought-provoking questions in the box below – either on your own or in discussion with others. Critically evaluating the role of technology in human occupation is an important part of how we continue to engage with technology in the future.

Critical Conversations in Technology and Occupation

- What is the role of emerging technologies such as artificial intelligence and biotechnologies in human occupation?
- How do we address issues of safety and privacy for intelligent technologies? Are there specific risks to health and wellbeing?
- What are the risks inherent in technology use, particularly those which track individuals such as facial recognition? What does this mean for occupational safety?
- As technologies collect more and more data about us and the groups and populations to which we belong, what are the impacts of the lack of ownership of that data?
- Can technologies be used for social good to improve our occupational performance as a society?
- How do virtual and augmented realities change our understanding of the context of human occupation?

18.7 Conclusion

Human occupation and technology are inextricably linked. Technology is present in all aspects of our daily lives and thus in all our occupations. While this is not a new phenomenon – humans have been using tools to accomplish tasks for thousands of years – the tools themselves have become more complex over time, and our use of them has become more integral to our occupations. There are significant benefits to the use of technology for occupation; they help us to complete tasks with efficiency, improve our quality of life, and help us to be more productive. However, the use of technology also comes with challenges, including issues of overreliance, ethical challenges, and equitable access. Careful consideration of the benefits and challenges of technology use in occupation will ensure we move into the future considering the needs and rights of all.

18.8 Summary

- Technology has always accompanied or aided occupational participation and performance, and technological advancement is built on innovation driven by occupational need.
- Technological devices can assist people with daily activities and occupational performance as well as organize daily occupations and influence our daily habits, roles, routines, and rituals.
- There are several theoretical models and frameworks that have conceptualized and positioned technology in various ways including the OTPF-4, ICF, HAAT Model, SETT Framework, and TAM.
- Technology is used by people across the lifespan and across all areas of occupation; this can both facilitate development and impede it depending on the degree and context of usage, as well as other factors.
- The increased use of technology in society and the rapid pace of technological development raises questions of digital literacy.

18.9 Review Questions

1. What is the difference between technology and assistive technology?
2. Where does technology fit into the OTPF-4, ICF, HAAT, and SETT models?
3. How can technology be used to engage in occupations across the lifespan?

4. List three risks of technology use in human occupation.
5. What are the differences between augmentative, compensatory, and remediative technologies?

References

American Occupational Therapy Association. (2020). Occupational therapy practice framework: Domain and process (4th ed.). *American Journal of Occupational Therapy, 74*(Suppl. 2), 7412410010p1–7412410010p87. https://doi.org/10.5014/ajot.2020.74S2001

Ashton, J. J., & Beattie, R. M. (2019). Screen time in children and adolescents: Is there evidence to guide parents and policy? *The Lancet: Child & Adolescent Health, 3*(5), 292–294. https://doi.org/10.1016/S2352-4642(19)30062-8

Bouma, H., Fozard, J. L., Bouwhuis, D. G., & Taipale, V. T. (2007). Gerontechnology in perspective. *Gerontechnology, 6*(4), 190–216. https://journal.gerontechnology.org/archives/721-723-1-PB.pdf

Canadian Association of Occupational Therapists. (n.d.). *Technology for occupation and participation network*. CAOT. https://caot.ca/site/prac-res/otn/technology

Christensen, C. M. (1997). *The innovator's dilemma: When new technologies cause great firms to fail*. Harvard Business School Press.

Davis, F. D. (1989). Perceived usefulness, perceived ease of use, and user acceptance of information technology. *MIS Quarterly, 13*(3), 319–340. https://doi.org/10.2307/249008

Elsaesser, L. J., Layton, N., Scherer, M., & Bauer, B. (2022). Standard terminology is critical to advancing rehabilitation and assistive technology: A call to action. *Disability and Rehabilitation: Assistive Technology, 17*(8), 986–988. https://doi.org/10.1080/17483107.2022.2112985

Elsahar, Y., Hu, S., Bouazza-Marouf, K., Kerr, D., & Mansor, A. (2019). Augmentative and alternative communication (AAC) advances: A review of configurations for individuals with a speech disability. *Sensors, 19*, 1911. https://doi.org/10.3390/s19081911

Fischl, C. (2020). *Ageing in a digital society: An occupational perspective on social participation*. Umeå University. http://urn.kb.se/resolve?urn=urn:nbn:se:umu:diva-169583

Frey, C. B., & Osborne, M. A. (2013). *The future of employment: How susceptible are jobs to computerisation?* Machines and Employment Workshop. Oxford University Engineering Sciences Department. https://www.oxfordmartin.ox.ac.uk/downloads/academic/The_Future_of_Employment.pdf

Gewertz, C. (2021). Sitting on the roof at night for Internet: Pandemic learning in the Navajo Nation. *Education Week*. https://www.edweek.org/teaching-learning/sitting-on-the-roof-at-night-for-internet-pandemic-learning-in-the-navajo-nation/2021/02

Ienca, M., Fabrice, J., Elger, B., Caon, M., Scoccia Pappagallo, A., Kressig, R. W., & Wangmo, T. (2017). Intelligent assistive technology for Alzheimer's disease and other dementias: A systematic review. *Journal of Alzheimer's Disease: JAD, 56*(4), 1301–1340. https://doi.org/10.3233/JAD-161037

Kahn, C. B., Dreifuss, H., Teufel-Shone, N. I., Tutt, M., McCue, K., Wilson, J., Waters, A. R., Belin, K. L., & Bauer, M. C. (2021). Adapting summer education programs for Navajo students: Resilient teamwork. *Frontiers in Sociology, 6*, 617994. https://doi.org/10.3389/fsoc.2021.617994

Laing, K., Machin, T., Adamson, M., & Lovric, K. (2022). Technology use of children 0–6 years of age: A diary study. In T. Machin, C. Brownlow, S. Abel, & J. Gilmour (Eds.), *Social media and technology across the lifespan. Palgrave studies in cyberpsychology* (pp. 9–26). Palgrave Macmillan. https://doi.org/10.1007/978-3-030-99049-7_2

Makafane, D. T., & Chere-Masopha, J. (2021). COVID-19 crisis: Challenges of online learning in one university in Lesotho. *African Perspectives of Research in Teaching & Learning, 5*(1), 126–138. https://www.proquest.com/scholarly-journals/covid-19-crisis-challenges-online-learning-one/docview/2542473916/se-2

Martin, A. (2006). A European framework for digital literacy. *Nordic Journal of Digital Literacy, 1*(2), 151–161. https://doi.org/10.18261/ISSN1891-943X-2006-02-06

Nizzero, A., Cote, P., & Cramm, H. (2017). Occupational disruption: A scoping review. *Journal of Occupational Science, 24*(2), 114–127. https://doi.org/10.1080/14427591.2017.1306791

Nygård, L., & Starkhammar, S. (2007). The use of everyday technology by people with dementia living alone: Mapping out the difficulties. *Aging & Mental Health, 11*(2), 144–155. https://doi.org/10.1080/13607860600844168

Oxford English Dictionary. (2022). *Oxford English Dictionary*. Oxford University Press. https://www.oed.com/

Pedretti, L., Smith, R. O., Hammel, J., Rein, J., Anson, D., & McGuire, M. J. (1992). Use of adjunctive modalities in occupational therapy treatment. *American Journal of Occupational Therapy, 46*, 1075–1081. https://doi.org/10.5014/ajot.46.12.1075

Przybylski, A. K., & Weinstein, N. (2017). A large-scale test of the Goldilocks hypothesis. *Psychological Science, 28*, 204–215. https://doi.org/10.1177/0956797616678438

Rosen, L., Carrier, L. M., Miller, A., Rokkum, J., & Ruiz, A. (2016). Sleeping with technology: Cognitive, affective, and technology usage predictors of sleep problems among college students. *Sleep Health: Journal of the National Sleep Foundation, 2*, 49–56. https://doi.org/10.1016/j.sleh.2015.11.003

Rotolo, D., Hicks, D., & Martin, B. R. (2015). What is an emerging technology? *Research Policy, 44*(10), 1827–1843. https://doi.org/10.1016/j.respol.2015.06.006

Sanders, L. (2017). Smartphones may be changing the way we think. *Science News, 191*(6), 18. www.sciencenews.org/article/smartphones-may-be-changing-way-we-think

Smith, R. O. (2017). Technology and occupation: Past, present, and the next 100 years of theory and practice (Eleanor Clarke Slagle Lecture). *American Journal of Occupational Therapy, 71*, 7106150010. https://doi.org/10.5014/ajot.2017.716003

Socialstyrelsen [Swedish National Board of Health and Welfare]. (2015). Välfärdsteknik [Welfare technology, Swedish]. Socialstyrelsen. https://termbank.socialstyrelsen.se/?TermId=385&SrcLang=sv

Swedish Ministry of Health and Social Affairs, & Swedish Association of Local Authorities and Regions. (2016). *Vision for eHealth 2025 – common starting points for digitisation of social services and health care*. https://ehalsa2025.se/english/

The World Bank. *Secure internet servers – Lesotho*. The World Bank. https://data.worldbank.org/indicator/IT.NET.SECR?locations=LS

Townsend, E., & Polatajko, H. J. (2013). *Enabling occupation II: Advancing an occupational therapy vision for health, well-being & justice through occupation: 9th Canadian occupational therapy guidelines* (2nd ed.). Canadian Association of Occupational Therapists.

U. S. Department of Commerce. (2022). Press release: Biden-Harris Administration award more than $105 million in grants to expand high-speed internet access on tribal land in Arizona. https://www.commerce.gov/news/press-releases/2022/08/biden-harris-administration-awards-more-105-million-grants-expand-high

Wang, Q., Sun, W., Qu, Y., Feng, C., Wang, D., Yin, H., Li, C., Sun, Z., & Sun, D. (2021). Development and application of medicine-engineering integration in the rehabilitation of traumatic brain injury. *BioMed Research International, 2021*, 9962905. https://doi.org/10.1155/2021/9962905

World Health Organization. (2002). *Towards a common language for functioning, disability and health: The International Classification of Functioning, Disability, and Health*. WHO. https://cdn.who.int/media/docs/default-source/classification/icf/icfbeginnersguide.pdf?sfvrsn=eead63d3_4&download=true

World Health Organization. (2019). *Guidelines on physical activity, sedentary behaviour and sleep for children under 5 years of age*. WHO. https://www.who.int/publications/i/item/9789241550536

World Health Organization, & United Nations Children's Fund (UNICEF). (2022). *Global report on assistive technology*. WHO. https://apps.who.int/iris/handle/10665/354357

Zabala, J. S. (2002). *SETT framework. Assistive technology*. http://assistedtechnology.weebly.com/sett-framework.html

CHAPTER 19

Human Occupation and Environmental Sustainability

Lisa C. Lieb, Tenelle Hodson, and Camille Dieterle

Abstract
Unsustainable patterns of human occupation have detrimentally affected the natural world, disrupted ecosystems, and placed the long-term health of humanity at risk, making environmental sustainability a topic of paramount importance to occupational therapists. To minimize damage to the natural environment and promote human health, well-being, and justice, occupational therapists should develop knowledge of environmental sustainability and human occupations. This chapter aims to provide readers with a basic understanding of the impact that human occupation has on the environment, the effects of climate change on human occupation, and the ethical dimensions of sustainability. Additionally, this chapter will introduce readers to the application of occupational therapy theory to environmental sustainability concepts, as well as initiate a discussion of environmental sustainability in occupational therapy practice settings, treatment, and education.

Authors' Positionality Statement
The authors of this chapter reside in the USA and Australia, both countries that have profited from industrialization and who remain large contributors to climate change. While our countries have been impacted by climate change-fueled disasters (e.g., wildfires and flooding), we acknowledge that the impact of such events has been far less than those in countries which are less economically advantaged. The authors would also like to acknowledge that while we all have tertiary qualifications in occupational therapy, none of the authors possess formal education in environmental sustainability or climate change. Our knowledge in this area has been developed through research, personal studies, and curiosity. While expressed differently, all authors have a great respect for their relationship with nature and the environment, with a commitment to ensuring that it can be sustained for generations to come. Finally, all authors are non-Indigenous and wish to acknowledge and pay respect to the Traditional Custodians of our respective countries.

We acknowledge that climate change has disproportionately impacted the Traditional Custodians of our countries and that the Traditional Custodians hold knowledge of more sustainable practices.

> **Objectives**
> This chapter will allow the reader to:
>
> - Critically examine the relationship between human occupation, environmental sustainability, and climate change.
> - Engage in ethical reasoning related to human occupation and environmental sustainability.
> - Identify strategies for integrating environmental sustainability into occupational therapy practice.
> - Identify opportunities to increase knowledge of environmental sustainability in occupational therapy.

> **Key terms**
>
> - **environmental sustainability**
> - **climate change**
> - **environmentally sustainable lifestyle**
> - **environment**
> - **health**
> - **occupational justice**

19.1 Introduction

Climate change has been described as one of the most pressing issues of the 21st century and requires global efforts directed at minimizing greenhouse gas emission (Intergovernmental Panel on Climate Change [IPCC], 2021). As human activity, and likewise human occupation, has been identified as the primary cause of climate change, occupational therapists have an important role in addressing this issue. This chapter serves as an introduction to the topic of human occupation and environmental sustainability. Within the context of sustainable development, it is acknowledged that sustainability more broadly relates to ensuring that actions that provide benefits today do not sacrifice future environmental, social, economic, and personal health (United Nations, 2015). While the authors wish to acknowledge that each of these elements of sustainability is equally as important, this chapter will focus solely on environmental sustainability. It aims to provide readers with the necessary knowledge to understand this complex topic and integrate environmental sustainability concepts into practice.

The first section provides the reader with a general overview of the relationship between human occupation and climate change, while also highlighting guidance from the World Federation of Occupational Therapists (WFOT) and the ethical dimensions of environmental sustainability in occupational therapy. Additionally, a brief review of core occupational therapy theories will be presented, along with ways in which these theories may be interpreted and applied through an environmental sustainability lens. Readers will then examine concepts of environmentally sustainable health systems and policy and explore how to implement environmental sustainability in practice settings. The last section provides examples of ways that environmentally sustainable concepts could be implemented in occupational therapy graduate education and professional development.

19.2 Human Occupation and Climate Change

19.2.1 Human Occupation and Its Contribution to Climate Change

It is now understood that human activity has directly impacted the earth's climate, warming the atmosphere, ocean, and land (IPCC, 2021). Occupational therapists view such human activity through the lens of "occupation," the mechanism through which people interact with the environment. Occupations can either contribute to environmental degradation or preservation (Lieb, 2020). An environmentally sustainable lifestyle is one in which the individual mindfully takes into account how they and their community contribute to climate change and environmental degradation, making changes when possible to ameliorate these harms (e.g., engaging in gardening and planting trees to remove carbon from the atmosphere). Unfortunately, many societies, especially those in which occupational therapy is most prolific, engage in unsustainable lifestyles that are driven by a consumerist culture, one where mass production, consumption, and disposal of resources is prevalent (Aoyama, 2014).

Therefore, occupations that have a degrading impact on the environment (i.e., those that are dependent on or produce fossil fuels) are more often engaged in than occupations that preserve it. Consequently, to mitigate the effects of climate change, people will need to alter the type of occupations they engage in, and how. As experts in occupation, it can be suggested that occupational therapists and occupational scientists are well positioned to assist in this change process. The WFOT (2018) supports this notion and encourages occupational therapists and occupational therapy students to actively participate in the development of solutions to the current climate crisis.

19.2.2 Climate Change and Its Impact on Human Occupations

While human occupations may be contributing to climate change, the effects of climate change will continue to impact our ability to engage in occupations. Direct links have been made between climate change and extreme weather events, and as the earth continues to warm, the frequency and severity of these events will increase (IPCC, 2021). Extreme weather events can alter the environment in which humans live and consequently alter the interaction between people and the environment, disrupting how occupations are engaged in. Weather events such as flooding and bushfires can destroy homes and communities, changing the way people go about their daily life due to the need to relocate, take time off work, and find new schooling. Smith and Matthews (2011) provide an exemplar of such impacts through their exploration of the experiences of people who lived through Hurricane Ike. The authors highlighted that one year on, people reported occupational and role losses because of the changed environments they found themselves in due to relocation, facilities remaining closed, and diminished water quality.

Increased stress from extreme weather events can have an impact on mental and physical health, as does the prospect of climate change and what it could mean for future generations. For instance, "Climate Anxiety" is a phenomenon increasingly observed in children and young people, and in creating pessimistic beliefs about the future it is reported as having a functional impact (Hickman et al., 2021). What is clear is that climate change is, and will continue to, impact human health and people's ability to participate and engage in occupations.

19.2.3 Guidance from the WFOT

The WFOT recommends addressing environmental sustainability in occupational therapy education, practice, and scholarship by helping individuals and communities perform occupations in a sustainable way, shifting health care systems to deliver care more sustainably, meeting immediate needs through disaster preparedness and response, and including environmental sustainability in education and research (WFOT, 2018). The WFOT defines five principles to help occupational therapists integrate environmental sustainability into their work by (1) increasing their understanding of environmental sustainability issues and how they relate to occupational therapy; (2) working with interested individuals and communities to mitigate environmental damage from unsustainable lifestyles; (3) helping clients to adapt to climate change and environmental damage; (4) developing competencies for empowering communities to increase the environmental sustainability of their occupations in an equitable way; and (5) developing competence in delivering interventions that address environmental sustainability issues (WFOT, 2018).

19.2.4 Occupational Justice and Environmental Sustainability

A major impetus for the development of WFOT's environmental sustainability recommendations was the awareness that climate change, borne out of unsustainable occupational engagement, generates occupational injustices (WFOT, 2018). Occupational justice is an ethic in which all persons are afforded occupational rights that ensure equal opportunity for engagement in meaningful occupations (WFOT, 2018). Occupational rights include the right to participate in a variety of occupations, the right to choose which occupations to engage in, and the right to freely engage in occupations (WFOT, 2018). A violation or compromise of a person's occupational rights constitutes an occupational injustice (WFOT, 2018). Climate change and environmental degradation have negative effects on the occupational rights of individuals, communities, and populations.

Furthermore, climate change threatens the occupational rights and opportunities for future generations as well, creating occupational injustice, while the overuse of occupational rights in current generations threatens the ability of future ones to meet their basic occupational needs (Drolet et al., 2020). Therefore, when providing occupational therapy services occupational therapists must now consider the rights of future generations as well as the health of ecosystems. Engagement in environmentally sustainable occupations can help to promote occupational justice by advocating for the health of one's lived environment, building relationships among community members, and ensuring that the occupational rights of individuals, both locally and globally, are respected (Drolet et al., 2020).

19.2.5 Environmental Justice and Human Occupation

Similarly, environmental injustice is an important consideration in relation to environmental sustainability and occupation. The environmental justice movement was a response to the recognition that certain communities, particularly people of color, Indigenous peoples, and low-income communities, systematically experience greater exposure to environmental hazards and toxins compared to wealthier white communities (Bullard, 2000). The movement seeks to ameliorate racial, socioeconomic, housing, and employment inequalities related to the environment in which people live. As with occupational therapy, the environmental justice movement recognizes that the environment directly affects how people carry out their daily occupations. Environmental injustices limit the variety of occupational choices, quality of occupational participation, and degree of occupational freedom afforded to individuals within a community (Blakeney & Marshall, 2009) and are therefore closely tied to the notion of occupational injustice. Also, as the health of the environment is associated with human health and well-being, environmental injustices are frequently linked to health disparities (Bullard, 2000). This means that outcomes such as health and wellness, quality of life, and well-being may not be fully realized in the context of environmental injustices (Hammell, 2021).

19.3 Implementing Sustainability Initiatives into Occupational Therapy Practice

19.3.1 Occupational Therapy Theory and Environmental Sustainability

While environmental sustainability may be an unfamiliar concept to some occupational therapists, traditional occupational therapy theories can be adapted to assist practitioners in integrating environmental sustainability into their practice.

19.3.1.1 Model of Human Occupation (MOHO)

When using MOHO to support engagement in sustainable occupations, the therapist must examine the interaction between the client's volition, habituation, performance capacity, and environment. Collectively, these factors shape the way in which an individual engages in occupation (Taylor, 2017). Volition encompasses the client's values, beliefs, and motivations to participate in occupations. An assessment of the client's volition will guide the therapist in identifying environmentally sustainable occupations in which the client is motivated to participate. Once client-centered environmentally sustainable occupations have been established, the therapist may present the client with opportunities to develop performance capacity, or a sense of competency, in environmentally sustainable occupations by structuring the tasks to promote successful participation.

Developing performance capacity is essential, as it has been shown that self-efficacy in environmentally sustainable occupations is positively associated with participation in such occupations (Yusliza et al., 2020). As the client's performance capacity increases, the therapist may encourage the client to integrate the environmentally sustainable occupation into their daily routine to facilitate habituation. Throughout this process the therapist may need to modify aspects of the client's environment to facilitate environmentally sustainable occupational engagement, as individuals may be more likely to engage in such occupations within a supportive environment (Dharmesti et al., 2020).

19.3.1.2 Person Environment Occupation Performance (PEOP) Model

The PEOP Model (Baum & Christiansen, 2005) can be applied to sustainable occupational performance and participation. Within this model, the occupational therapist must examine how personal factors and the environment impact occupational performance to facilitate environmentally sustainable occupational participation. Personal factors are intrinsic characteristics of an individual that impact occupational performance. These factors include the client's physiological, cognitive, spiritual, neurobehavioral, and psychological dimensions. Within the PEOP Model, the therapist examines each of these features and identifies how person-related factors may impact performance in the client's environmentally sustainable occupational goals. In conjunction with examining personal factors, the therapist must also investigate the impact of environmental factors on the client's environmentally sustainable occupational performance. Extrinsic factors, such as access to natural spaces within the built environment (Alcock et al., 2020) have been shown to affect engagement in environmentally sustainable occupations.

Treatment interventions are implemented to reduce the impacts of personal factors or environmental barriers on environmentally sustainable occupational performance. The occupational therapist may provide client-centered interventions aimed at modifying the environment to promote environmentally sustainable occupational performance, such as creating neighborhood green spaces to facilitate occupational participation (Alcock et al., 2020). Alternatively, the therapist may provide interventions aimed at establishing new skills, such as environmental advocacy, to prevent occupational performance issues caused by environmental degradation.

19.3.1.3 Canadian Model of Occupational Performance and Engagement (CMOP-E)

The CMOP-E may be applied to sustainable occupational therapy practice (Polatajko et al., 2007). The CMOP-E conceptualizes occupation as the medium through which the person interacts with the environment. Using the CMOP-E, an occupational therapist may consider how changes in the natural physical environment may be impacting an individual's ability to participate and engage in an occupation. For instance, if a client or community had been impacted by bushfires, an occupational therapist may focus on how this physical environment change has impacted their ability to engage in everyday occupations. Moreover, they may consider how self-care, productive, and leisure occupations that an individual engages in may be impacting the natural physical environment.

For example, with clients who have expressed a desire to undertake volunteering, an occupational therapist may discuss the prospect of engaging with an organization that restores wetland habitats. The CMOP-E centers the person around their Spirituality, which reflects the "essence" of the person, their values, motivations, and passions. This element of the CMOP-E can be particularly important to determine a client's readiness to engage in environmentally sustainable occupations. Therapists may be able to identify that a client has a passion for social justice or the environment and, therefore, their participation in sustainable occupations should be prioritized.

19.3.2 Health Care Systems and Environmental Sustainability

As occupational therapists adapt to work in the era of climate change, they must also focus on how their own practices contribute to climate problems. In industrialized countries health care is a primary employer of occupational therapists and a major contributor to climate challenges. Carbon emissions from the health care sector are significant (Sherman et al., 2020). Environmentally sustainable health care systems reduce greenhouse gas emissions and excessive use of materials, such as single use plastics, reduce excessive demand for services by promoting public health, and match the supply of health services to demand (MacNeill et al., 2021; Sherman et al., 2020). Measuring the sustainability of health care systems is currently sparse and sporadic, but it has started in several countries in Asia, Australasia, Europe, and North America. Promoting environmental sustainability as a quality and value improvement marker may encourage environmentally sustainable health care efforts, since addressing environmental sustainability impacts can lead to better health and less resource utilization (Sherman et al., 2020).

Addressing environmental sustainability in health care is now consistently and prominently featured in global conferences such as the annual United Nations (UN) conference on climate change. Health was selected as a priority area at the UN Climate Change Conference (COP26) in 2021 and a Health Programme was created to help global leaders place a stronger focus on health care. During the conference, 50 countries pledged to make changes in their health care systems to better address climate change; 45 countries committed to a reduction in system-level carbon emissions from their health care practices; and 14 made it a goal to have carbon neutral health care systems by 2050 (World Health Organization [WHO], 2021). In subsequent years, the WHO has hosted a Health Pavilion with extensive programing throughout the conference to continue this momentum (WHO, 2022).

As of 2023, the Greener National Health System (NHS) in the United Kingdom is the current global leader in environmentally sustainable health care. It has the most robust goals and actions in place and the most thorough system of measurement, education, and practice regarding environmentally sustainable health care. Progress has been made on emissions, efficiency in models of care, medicine and supply chains, transport, digital innovation, hospital architecture and design, heating and lighting and other facilities, food, waste management, resilience and adaptation, values, and governance (NHS, 2020). Occupational Therapists in OT Susnet, part of the Centre for Sustainable Healthcare (CSH) in the United Kingdom, has contributed to these gains and provided resources and opportunities for occupational therapists to add an environmental sustainability lens to their practice (CSH, n.d.).

19.3.3 Environmental Sustainability across Occupational Therapy Practice Settings

19.3.3.1 Hospitals and Medical Settings: Inpatient, Outpatient

In institutional health care facilities occupational therapists can collaborate with relevant stakeholders in shifting practices to become more environmentally sustainable, such as designing the physical environment to better promote both environmental sustainability and health. From the patient perspective, environmentally sustainable care can include more pleasant green architecture and green spaces in health care environments, utilizing products that create less waste, and reassuring patients that their care is not harming the environment (Sherman et al., 2020). There is evidence that clinical services and rehabilitation treatment occurring in pleasant outdoor settings can increase patient motivation for treatment and positively impact staff, especially when therapists are involved in designing the space (Winterbottom & Wagenfeld, 2015).

19.3.3.2 Schools: Primary, Secondary, Post-secondary

Within schools, occupational therapists have abundant opportunities to incorporate environmental sustainability in their practice. Crafts, games, and other therapeutic and educational activities can include environmental sustainability through both content and methodology. Occupational therapists can implement school-wide initiatives, such as re-using waste materials for craft projects or starting a garden, and integrate them with therapeutic outcomes. For instance, an occupational therapy garden program in elementary schools demonstrated better learning outcomes, along with a range of other health benefits (Wagenfeld & Whitfield, 2015). Engaging students in all levels of education to complete environmental sustainability projects in their sphere of influence can easily tie into therapy and educational goals, and create benefits for individuals and the school-wide community (Dieterle, 2020; Molitor et al., 2020). With mental health becoming a greater focus in school settings, creating health-promoting outdoor spaces and environmental sustainability-focused group projects that foster social inclusion, meaning, hope, and self-esteem may be especially relevant for occupational therapists to pursue.

19.3.3.3 Community-based Settings: Home Health, Community-based Programs

Community and home-based programs are primed for environmental sustainability efforts because so many daily occupations occur in the home and community. Occupational therapists can help clients perform occupations more sustainably, such as becoming more conscious of water use, reducing household waste, and selecting and preparing food in a way that is both healthy and sustainable. In the community, occupational therapists are well-positioned to influence groups to change their values, behaviors, and culture (Molitor et al., 2020; York & Wiseman, 2012). For example, an occupational therapy-led gardening program for people who have been socially isolated due to mental illness was able to shift participants from being passive consumers to active agents of change in their community (York & Wiseman, 2012).

19.3.4 Environmentally Sustainable Occupational Therapy Interventions
19.3.4.1 Nature-based Occupations

Occupational therapists have used gardening in their work with clients since the founding of the profession. Gardening is applied in a variety of settings to assist motor function, sensory processing, cognitive function, and socioemotional development, improve occupational performance and patterns, and foster a sense of social belonging, agency, self-esteem, and spiritual connection (Koch, 2019; Wagenfeld & Atchison, 2014; York & Wiseman, 2012). Evidence also demonstrates that gardening can lead to stress reduction, improved attention, reduction in symptoms of depression and anxiety, improvements in body mass index, and increases in life satisfaction, quality of life, and sense of community (Wagenfeld & Atchison, 2014).

More broadly, any nature-based occupation can promote similar health outcomes, with nature-based interventions providing opportunities for functional activity in a natural environment. Specific examples of nature-based interventions created by occupational therapists include a program utilizing surfing for post-traumatic stress disorder and depression in veterans (Rogers et al., 2014) and outdoor occupational therapy camps and other play interventions for children (Hanscom, 2016).

19.3.4.2 Lifestyle Redesign® as an Environmental Sustainability-focused Intervention

Behavior change in daily occupations has been identified as a key contributor in addressing environmental sustainability and can lead to numerous health co-benefits (WFOT, 2018). Lifestyle Redesign® (LR) is a behavior change intervention that increases clients' knowledge and skills to become more environmentally sustainable and integrate environmentally sustainable occupations into their daily habits and routines. An occupational therapist using LR guides clients through a process of occupational self-analysis to increase awareness of the environmental sustainability of their current habits and routines, and how these behaviors impact their health and well-being. Over weeks and months, the client discovers which environmentally sustainable habits and routines fit well with and enhance their quality of life and health (Dieterle, 2020). Examples of actions that could create co-benefits for various chronic health conditions include reducing meat consumption, incorporating active transportation into routines, and reducing landfill waste and household clutter by revising consumption choices.

19.4 Environmental Sustainability in Occupational Therapy Education
19.4.1 Current Status of Environmental Sustainability Within Occupational Therapy Education

Within occupational therapy tertiary education curricula there is a noted absence of environmental sustainability (Aoyama, 2014); therefore, without formal training or qualifications, occupational therapists may not feel able to incorporate environmental sustainability into their practice (Dunphy, 2014). Indeed, occupational therapists have stated that they felt their education has not provided them with the appropriate knowledge and awareness about sustainability issues (Chan et al., 2020). As many occupational therapists have a desire to learn more in this area, it is important this issue is addressed by occupational therapy associations and the education system (Chan et al., 2020). It is reported, however, that many academics also do not feel comfortable delivering this topic (Dunphy, 2014).

Few undergraduate occupational therapy programs explicitly address environmental sustainability in their curricula. Wagman and colleagues (2020), however, report on the Occupational Therapy Program at Jönköping University, where aspects related to the United Nations' (2015) Sustainable Development Goals (which include more than just environmental sustainability) were addressed in many courses (Wagman et al., 2020). In one course, students discussed how occupations aligned with sustainable development and how they could be made more sustainable while upholding the intrinsic meaning of the occupation itself (Wagman et al., 2020).

A more explicit example of how environmental sustainability is currently being taught in occupational therapy programs is the "Creating a Sustainable Lifestyle" course, taught by Associate Professor Camille Dieterle at the University of Southern California (USC). The course uses didactic and experiential learning methods to teach students about Lifestyle Redesign® and incorporates core occupational therapy concepts such as occupational self-analysis, narrative reasoning, and problem solving (Dieterle, 2020). Students complete an occupational analysis to identify their own habits, routines, and choices, and recognize how they could make them more environmentally sustainable (Dieterle, 2020). Occupational therapy programs elsewhere can draw upon these examples to integrate environmental sustainability concepts into their curricula.

In terms of professional development, the United Kingdom's CSH currently provides a range of multidisciplinary courses on sustainable health care. Similar organizations are located in several countries and are invaluable resources for administrators and clinicians seeking to address sustainability in all aspects of their care (CSH, n.d.). The WFOT also offers a Disaster Management for Occupational Therapists course which aims to provide knowledge and skills on risk reduction, how to respond to disasters, and how to build resilience. This course could assist occupational therapists to identify the role they can play when working with individuals affected by extreme weather events resulting from climate change.

19.4.2 The Future of Sustainability Within Occupational Therapy Education

Further environmental sustainability concepts should be incorporated into occupational therapy curricula and occupational therapy academics need to feel confident about their knowledge of environmental sustainability and how it relates to occupational therapy. Alongside the growth in the literature on occupational therapy and environmental sustainability, it is hoped that academics' knowledge of and confidence in these concepts will also grow. In the interim, it is suggested that co-teaching occurs with academics from other disciplines such as environmental science and environmental management (Smith et al., 2020). Occupational therapy academics can also draw upon the methods used in Dieterle's course at USC, as discussed above, and content already established in occupational therapy programs that relates, or can be easily linked, to environmental sustainability. For example, as core concepts that are taught in occupational therapy curricula, the theoretical models presented in this chapter can be used by educators to link with and relate to environmental sustainability.

Further professional development opportunities should be offered to better equip occupational therapists who are currently practicing and increase the number of occupational therapists well-versed in environmental sustainability. In this process we may need to call upon colleagues in the environmental science and management field. The creation and delivery of online courses that occupational therapists can access internationally would also assist development, transfers, and exchanges of knowledge and information on environmental sustainability, as would establishing special interest groups in this area (Chan et al., 2020).

19.5 Conclusion

Just as climate change influences all aspects of human occupation, human occupation has the potential to impact the natural world positively or negatively. The occupational choices made by humans today will shape the occupational opportunities available to others in the future. Given the significance of climate change for vulnerable populations and future generations, occupational therapists have a moral responsibility to respond within their practice. The holistic nature of our profession places occupational therapists in a unique position to act as catalysts of change in facilitating a shift toward environmental sustainability in human occupation.

Despite the novelty of this practice area, there are many accessible ways in which occupational therapists can implement sustainability principles in treatment programs. In the contexts in which occupational therapists learn and practice – occupational therapy education, health care systems, schools, and communities – increasing awareness of environmental sustainability will be crucial in supporting the widespread adoption of environmentally sustainable occupational therapy practice. As the profession evolves in response to the climate crisis, occupational therapists are encouraged to develop creative environmentally sustainable solutions within their own practices and lives. Using both top-down and grassroots initiatives, occupational therapists can help to shape a world that supports equitable and environmentally sustainable occupational participation for their clients and communities.

19.6 Summary

- This chapter has emphasized the relationship between occupational therapy and environmental sustainability.
- It is paramount that environmental sustainability is prioritized in occupational therapy to ensure that future generations can continue to engage in occupations that are meaningful to them.
- Occupational therapy models can help to identify the needs of those impacted by extreme weather events resulting from climate change.
- As a relatively new area of practice, further research and education is required.

19.7 Review Questions

1. Thinking about your local context, how could you apply environmental sustainability concepts in your practice?
2. From a service level perspective, how might you be able to advocate for the integration of environmental sustainability initiatives in your local context?
3. What barriers do you foresee to the integration of environmental sustainability initiatives into your local context? How might you overcome these?

References

Alcock, I., White, M. P., Pahl, S., Duarte-Davidson, R., & Fleming, L. E. (2020). Associations between pro-environmental behaviour and neighbourhood nature, nature visit frequency and nature appreciation: Evidence from a nationally representative survey in England. *Environment International*, 136, 105441. https://doi.org/10.1016/j.envint.2019.105441

Aoyama, M. (2014). Occupational therapy and environmental sustainability. *Australian Occupational Therapy Journal*, 61(6), 458–461. https://doi.org/10.1111/1440-1630.12136

Baum, C. M., & Christiansen, C. H. (2005). Person-Environment-Occupation-Performance: An occupation-based framework for practice. In C. H. Christiansen, C. M. Baum, & J. Bass-Haugen (Eds.), *Occupational therapy: Performance, participation, and well-being* (3rd ed., pp. 243–266). SLACK Inc.

Blakeney, A. B., & Marshall, A. (2009). Water quality, health, and human occupations. *American Journal of Occupational Therapy, 63*(1), 46–57. https://doi.org/10.5014/ajot.63.1.46

Bullard, R. D. (2000). *Dumping in Dixie: Race, class, and environmental quality* (3rd ed.). Westview Press.

Centre for Sustainable Healthcare (CSH). (n.d.). *Sustainability and health Organizations*. https://sustainablehealthcare.org.uk/who-we-are/sustainability-and-health-organisations

Chan, C. C. Y., Lee, L., & Davis, J. A. (2020). Understanding sustainability: Perspectives of Canadian occupational therapists. *World Federation of Occupational Therapists Bulletin, 76*(1), 50–59. https://doi.org/10.1080/14473828.2020.1761091

Dharmesti, M., Merrilees, B., & Winata, L. (2020). "I'm mindfully green": Examining the determinants of guest pro-environmental behaviors (PEB) in hotels. *Journal of Hospitality Marketing & Management, 29*(7), 830–847. https://doi.org/10.1080/19368623.2020.1710317

Dieterle, C. (2020). The case for environmentally-informed occupational therapy: Clinical and educational applications to promote personal wellness, public health and environmental sustainability. *World Federation of Occupational Therapists Bulletin, 76*(1), 32–39. https://doi.org/10.1080/14473828.2020.1717055

Drolet, M.-J., Désormeaux-Moreau, M., Soubeyran, M., & Thiébaut, S. (2020). Intergenerational occupational justice: Ethically reflecting on the climate crisis. *Journal of Occupational Science, 27*(3), 417–431. https://doi.org/10.1080/14427591.2020.1776148

Dunphy, J. L. (2014). Healthcare professionals' perspectives on environmental sustainability. *Nursing Ethics, 21*(4), 414–425. https://doi.org/10.1177/0969733013502802

Hammell, K. W. (2021). Occupation in natural environments: Health equity and environmental justice. *Canadian Journal of Occupational Therapy, 88*(4), 319–328. https://doi.org/10.1177/00084174211040000

Hanscom, A. (2016). *Balanced and barefoot: How unrestricted outdoor play makes for strong, confident and capable children*. New Harbinger Publications.

Hickman, C., Marks, E., Pihkala, P., Clayton, S., Lewandowski, R. E., Mayall, E. E., Wray, B., Mellor, C., & van Susteren, L. (2021). Climate anxiety in children and young people and their beliefs about government responses to climate change: A global survey. *Lancet Planet Health, 5*, e863–e873. https://doi.org/10.1016/S2542-5196(21)00278-3

IPCC. (2021). Summary for policymakers. In V. Masson-Delmotte, P. Zhai, A. Pirani, S. L. C. Connors, C. Péan, S. Berger, N. Caud, Y. Chen, L. Goldfarb, M. I. Gomis, M. Huang, K. Leitzell, E. Lonnoy, J. B. R. Matthews, T. K. Maycock, T. Waterfield, O. Yelekçi, R. Yu, & B. Zhou (Eds.), *Climate change 2021: The physical science basis. Contribution of Working Group I to the sixth assessment report of the intergovernmental panel on climate change* (pp. 3–32). Cambridge University Press. https://doi.org/10.1017/9781009157896.001

Koch, L. (2019). *The use of nature as a treatment modality in occupational therapy* [Honors thesis, Western Michigan University]. https://scholarworks.wmich.edu/honors_theses/3163

Lieb, L. C. (2020). Occupation and environmental sustainability: A scoping review. *Journal of Occupational Science, 29*(4), 505–528. https://doi.org/10.1080/14427591.2020.1830840

MacNeill, A., McGain, F., & Sherman, J. (2021). Planetary health care: A framework for sustainable health systems. *The Lancet, 5*(2), e66–e68. https://doi.org/10.1016/S2542-5196(21)00005-X

Molitor, W., Kielman, K., Cooper, J., Wheat, K., & Besons, A. (2020). Promoting environmentally sustainable occupational engagement on a college campus: A case study. *World Federation of Occupational Therapists Bulletin, 76*(1), 4–6. https://doi.org/10.1080/14473828.2020.1717056

National Health Service (NHS). (2020, October 1). *Delivering a net zero health service*. https://www.england.nhs.uk/greenernhs/publication/delivering-a-net-zero-national-health-service/

Polatajko, H. J., Townsend, E. A., & Craik, J. (2007). Canadian Model of Occupational Performance and Engagement (CMOP-E). In E. A. Townsend & H. J. Polatajko (Eds.), *Enabling occupation II: Advancing an occupational therapy vision of health, well-being, & justice through occupation* (p. 23). Canadian Association of Occupational Therapists.

Rogers, C., Mallinson, T., & Peppers, D. (2014). High-intensity sports for posttraumatic stress disorder and depression: Feasibility study of ocean therapy with veterans of Operation Enduring Freedom and Operation Iraqi Freedom. *American Journal of Occupational Therapy*, 68(4), 395–404. https://doi.org/10.5014/ajot.2014.011221

Sherman, J., Thiel, C., MacNeill, A., Eckelman, M., Dubrow, R., Hopf, H., Lagasse, R., Bialowitz, J., Costello, A., Forbes, M., Stancliffe, R., Anastas, P., Anderko, L., Baratz, M., Barna, S., Bhatnagar, U., Burnham, J., Cai, Y., Caseels-Brown, A., ... Bilec, M. (2020). The green print: Advancement of environmental sustainability in healthcare. *Resources, Conservation & Recycling*, 161, 104882. https://doi.org/10.1016/j.resconrec.2020.104882

Smith, D. L., Fleming, K., Brown, L., Allen, A., Baker, J., & Gallagher, M. (2020). Occupational therapy and environmental sustainability: A scoping review. *Annals of International Occupational Therapy*, 3(3), 136–145. https://doi.org/10.3928/24761222-20200116-02

Smith, A. B., & Matthews, J. L. (2015). Quantifying uncertainty and variable sensitivity within the US billion-dollar weather and climate disaster cost estimates. *Natural Hazards*, 77, 1829–1851. https://doi.org/10.1007/s11069-015-1678-x

Taylor, R. R. (Ed.). (2017). *Kielhofner's Model of Human Occupation: Theory and application* (5th ed.). Wolters Kluwer.

United Nations. (2015). *Transforming our World: The 2030 Agenda for Sustainable Development*. United Nations. https://sdgs.un.org/sites/default/files/publications/21252030%20Agenda%20for%20Sustainable%20Development%20web.pdf

Wagenfeld, A., & Atchison, B. (2014). Putting the occupation back in occupational therapy: A survey of occupational therapy practitioners' use of gardening as an intervention. *The Open Journal of Occupational Therapy*, 2(4), 1–19. https://doi.org/10.15453/2168-6408.1128

Wagenfeld, A., & Whitfield, E. (2015). Going, doing, gardening: School gardens in the underrepresented communities of Lake Worth, Palm Springs, and Greenacres, Florida. *Children, Youth and Environments*, 25(1), 119–131. https://doi.org/10.7721/chilyoutenvi.25.1.0119

Wagman, P., Johansson, A., Jansson, I., Lygnegård, F., Edström, E., Björklund Carlstedt, A., Morville, A., Ahlstrand, I., & Fristedt, S. (2020). Making sustainability in occupational therapy visible by relating to the Agenda 2030 goals – A case description of a Swedish university. *World Federation of Occupational Therapists Bulletin*, 78(1), 7–14. https://doi.org/10.1080/14473828.2020.1718266

Winterbottom, D., & Wagenfeld, A. (2015). *Therapeutic gardens: Design for healing spaces*. Timber Press.

World Federation of Occupational Therapists, Shann, S., Ikiugu, M. N., Whittaker, B., Pollard, N., Kahlin, I., Hudson, M., Galvaan, R., Roschnik, S., & Aoyama, M. (2018). *Project report: Sustainability matters: Guiding principles for sustainability in occupational therapy practice, education, and scholarship*. WFOT. https://wfot.org/resources/wfot-sustainability-guiding-principles

World Health Organization (WHO). (2021, November 9). *Countries commit to develop climate-smart health care at COP26 UN climate conference*. https://www.who.int/news/item/09-11-2021-countries-commit-to-develop-climate-smart-health-care-at-cop26-un-climate-conference

World Health Organization (WHO). (2022, November 18). *COP27 Health Pavilion*. https://www.who.int/news-room/events/detail/2022/11/06/default-calendar/cop27-health-pavilion

York, M., & Wiseman, T. (2012). Gardening as an occupation: A critical review. *British Journal of Occupational Therapy*, 75(2), 76–84. https://doi.org/10.4276/030802212X13286281651072

Yusliza, M. Y., Amirudin, A., Rahadi, R. A., Athirah, N. A. N. S., Ramayah, T., Muhammad, Z., Mas, F. D., Massaro, M., Saputra, J., & Mokhlis, S. (2020). An investigation of pro-environmental behaviour and sustainable development in Malaysia. *Sustainability*, 12(17), 1–21. https://doi.org/10.3390/su12177083

SECTION THREE

Principal Concepts

CHAPTER 20

Key Occupational Concepts

Occupational Engagement, Occupational Balance, Occupational Adaptation, and Participation

Jane A. Davis, Carita Håkansson, and Kim Walder

Abstract

With occupation as the core domain of concern for occupational therapy, key occupational concepts need to be explored to discern their relevance in informing and delineating occupational therapy practice. This chapter will present definitions and descriptions of the key concepts of occupational engagement, occupational balance, and occupational adaptation, highlighting their key attributes, theories, and models. Then, these three concepts will be integrated through an intersectional lens in a discussion of the concept of participation, demonstrating their important connections. Readers will be challenged to expand their current understandings and application of the presented concepts through an intersectional lens to bring forward critiques in relation to systemic oppression, such as ableism, ageism, classism, racism, and gender discrimination. This serves as an introduction to the subsequent chapters in this section. An occupational narrative is presented to illustrate how these concepts hold relevance to clients' occupational lives and can inform occupational therapy practice.

Authors' Positionality Statement

As authors of this chapter, we acknowledge that our positionality and experiences have shaped our worldview. Our Western minority-world perspective is not a reflective representation of our diverse profession and the individuals, groups, and communities we work alongside. In the spirit of self-reflexivity, we recognize our positions of privilege as white cisgendered middle-aged women who received postgraduate education and have worked as occupational therapists, researchers, and educators for over 30 years in Canada, Sweden, and Australia. While we seek to understand and address systemic racism, ableism, ageism, and other biases experienced by marginalized groups, we cannot speak on behalf of other groups or individuals. However, it is our intention within this chapter to represent widely the global community, highlight cultural and intersectional considerations, and provide diverse examples.

Objectives
This chapter will define for readers the key concepts of:

- Occupational engagement, outline its attributes, and contrast it with the concepts of occupational performance and participation.
- Occupational balance, outline its attributes, and present key research on occupational balance and well-being.
- Occupational adaptation, outline its attributes, and its link to occupational identity and competence.
- This chapter will describe for the reader how these key concepts relate to participation through an intersectional lens.
- This chapter will conclude by providing the reader with an occupational narrative integrating the key concepts to illustrate their application to occupational therapy practice.

Key terms
- intersectionality
- occupational adaptation
- occupational balance
- occupational performance
- occupational engagement
- occupational identity
- occupational pattern
- participation

20.1 Introduction

This chapter presents three key occupational concepts: occupational engagement, occupational balance, and occupational adaptation. Each concept is defined and described in relation to its historical development and related concepts and perspectives. The main attributes of each concept, consistent with its stated definition, are outlined, and theories, models, and research are presented, as relevant. These three occupational concepts are integrated within a brief discussion of the concept of participation using an intersectional lens – how each person uniquely views the world through their own multiple identities – demonstrating their important connections and general significance to a critically reflexive understanding of occupation. Last, an occupational narrative is provided to illustrate how these concepts interact within a situation relevant to occupational therapy practice.

20.2 Key Concepts
20.2.1 Occupational Engagement
20.2.1.1 Definitions

Since its first mention in the literature, occupational engagement has been discussed as conceptually related to, yet distinct from, occupational performance. As Yerxa (1980) argued, "engagement in occupation encompasses not only the observable performance of individuals, but also their subjective reactions to the activity and objects with which they are occupied" (p. 534). Occupational engagement is the life energy of occupational beings as it maximizes the potential of performance and participation, and supports health, well-being, and justice (AOTA, 2020; Polatajko et al., 2007). When people are occupationally engaged, they are more likely to remain involved in that occupation because of the significance they ascribe through their engagement to mind-body-spirit or inner connections, as well as environmental contexts (AOTA, 2020; Kennedy & Davis, 2017; Polatajko et al., 2007).

As with all aspects of occupational behavior, how occupational engagement is perceived and defined has been shaped by issues of equity, diversity, and inclusion.

In the years since Yerxa's initial statement about occupational engagement, its definition has been debated and refined (Black et al., 2019; Cruz et al., 2023). In this chapter, a more equitable definition of occupational engagement is used: the subjectively perceived connection to an occupation demonstrated through cognitive, emotional, or attitudinal involvement in the occupation of interest. While many authors and organizations, such as the AOTA (2020), define occupational engagement as requiring an observable or performance component, others argue that occupational engagement moves beyond including an observable or performance component from essential to optional (Cruz et al., 2023; Kennedy & Davis, 2017; Polatajko et al., 2007). This key delineating feature broadens the application of this concept to more diverse groups whose connection to occupation is often not physical or performance related. Instead, the focus of the concept is on its specific significance, as demonstrated through cognitive, emotional, or attitudinal involvement, to individuals, groups, or their communities.

Two related concepts, occupational performance and occupational participation, have some attributes that are consistent with those of occupational engagement; however, they are not to be confused with it (Cruz et al., 2023; Kennedy & Davis, 2017). Individuals may perform some occupations and participate in others, but in all we strive to be occupationally engaged. Unlike occupational performance, occupational engagement does not require observable performance – although it may include it – as the specific attributes that support one to be engaged in occupations are beyond the performance of an occupation. Unlike participation, occupational engagement does not require a social location where the significance of an occupation is necessarily related to being with others or feelings of belonging.

20.2.1.2 Attributes

Occupational engagement is typically viewed as a subjective experience supported by aspects of motivation, interest, meaning, purpose, and self-efficacy (Black et al., 2019; Kennedy & Davis, 2017; Polatajko et al., 2007). Polatajko and colleagues discuss how occupational engagement is developed through individuals' perceived motivation, meaning or interest, and self-efficacy, and how these attributes fit with the occupation and environment.

Kennedy and Davis (2017) present two types of attributes for occupational engagement: essential elements (a sense of readiness to engage, purpose or meaning, participation, and motivation and interest) and influencers (mental health status and cognitive capacity, challenge and feedback, environmental elements). A sense of readiness was found to be important to support continued engagement and ongoing occupational changes or adaptation, as required. Significance of the occupation within individuals' lives, often discussed as perceived purpose, meaning, or value, is viewed as the "inner connection" to the occupation that supports ongoing engagement (AOTA, 2020; Black et al., 2019; Kennedy & Davis, 2017). For example, Cruz et al. (2023) present a narrative case study about Joana engagement in revisiting a Brazilian beach, that held strong inner connections to past experiences with her mother.

Some level of active (performing or directing) or passive participation (attending) is discussed as required for occupational engagement; however, individuals can participate, or be involved socially, without any indication of engagement or with only minimal engagement (Black et al. 2019; Kennedy & Davis, 2017). While the requirement of performance is optional, being cognitively, affectively, or attitudinally involved in the occupation is essential for engagement. Having an interest in an occupation could support becoming engaged in that occupation. Intrinsic task-specific motivation is typically viewed as supporting increased engagement, although an individual may be engaged in an occupation through extrinsic motivation only (AOTA, 2020; Kennedy & Davis, 2017; Kielhofner, 2008). Having the choice of occupations is also viewed as supporting occupational engagement, which is consistent with the arguments of the importance of client-centered practice. However, within collectivist cultures, often choice and intrinsic motivation are not viewed as influencers of occupational engagement. Instead, understanding one's cultural connection to the occupations may support occupational engagement (Yazdani, 2023).

Influencers of occupational engagement are described as cognitive abilities and mental health status, which may shape the level of occupational engagement attained (Kennedy & Davis, 2017; Sutton et al., 2012). External support, such as positive feedback, just-right challenge, and a supportive environment, promote engagement, while negative feedback, unmatched occupational challenge to skills, and environmental barriers decrease occupational engagement (AOTA, 2020; Black, et al., 2019; Kennedy & Davis, 2017).

Kennedy and Davis (2017) found that when they asked occupational therapists to define occupational engagement, they would often start their discussion with the importance of therapeutic engagement or a client's level of engagement in therapy or therapeutic activities. Therapeutic engagement was viewed by therapists as a necessary pre-cursor within the practice process for a client to develop and maintain occupational engagement in the community (Kennedy & Davis, 2017). Thus, understanding clients' past and desired occupational repertoires and using them for goal setting in practice may be crucial to support occupational engagement long term.

20.2.1.3 Theories/Models

The Canadian Model of Occupational Performance and Engagement (Polatajko et al., 2007) was the first model to explicitly present the concept of occupational engagement when it was added to the updated version of the model. This addition is viewed as extending the core purpose of the profession to include engaging individuals occupationally as performers *or* directors (Cruz et al., 2023; Polatajko et al., 2007). Kielhofner

(2008) mentions occupational engagement in his description of the theoretical underpinnings of the Model of Human Occupation (MOHO). However, he does not include occupational engagement as a component of the MOHO and positions occupational engagement as involving performance of a task, as well as the subjective experience associated with that task performance.

Csíkszentmihályi's (1990) Flow Theory offers additional understandings to the concept of occupational engagement. Flow is defined as a state of full concentration in an activity within a specific situation. Csíkszentmihályi argues that internal motivation is important for achieving flow, where time and context are ignored, and your whole being is engaged. To be in flow, a high-level skill must match one's capacity, as one cannot achieve flow in tasks that are too easy or too difficult. Being in flow speaks to an extreme of engagement in an occupation, where individuals may be so focused on that one occupation that they neglect other occupations, i.e., excessive engagement. Thus, although being engaged in one occupation may support optimal performance or participation, such as with elite sports, work, or drug use, when engagement in one occupation impacts engagement in others, the resulting constrained occupational repertoire may lead to occupational imbalance and negative well-being. Instead, ideally people's lives involve times of full occupational engagement to times of disengagement and all modes in between (Sutton et al., 2012), which affords people the capacity to navigate occupational transitions, restructuring, imbalance, and disruptions. Diverse needs for engagement at different points in time may be an important consideration for supporting well-being and meaning in relation to occupational engagement outcomes.

In occupational therapy, full occupational engagement can be perceived as positive or negative. Occupational engagement can lead to individual and social flourishing (i.e., fairness, equity, inclusion, health, and well-being); however, occupational engagement does not necessarily result in flourishing, as one can be engaged in occupations, possibly to excess, that do not support flourishing, and instead may be unhealthy, risky, or lead to social exclusion (Polatajko et al., 2007; Stewart et al., 2016). Individual and social flourishing is the main indicator of whether occupational engagement supports health, well-being, and justice. Occupational disengagement, or pulling back from full engagement, may be needed if an occupation is too engaging, i.e., engagement in it is overwhelming other aspects of one's life, leading to an imbalanced repertoire or impacting health or well-being (Cruz et al., 2023; Sutton et al., 2012).

Although occupational engagement is often confused with occupational balance – through discussions of the imbalances of the extremes of disengagement and engagement – they are distinct concepts (Black et al., 2019). Engagement in occupations is fluid and will vary across days, months, and years in relation to personal and environmental contexts (AOTA, 2020) leading to fluctuations of balance and imbalance depending on life needs, wants, and expectations (Yazdani, 2023).

20.2.2 Occupational Balance
20.2.2.1 Definitions

The core dimensions implied in most definitions of occupational balance are time use, harmonic mix, meaningfulness, equilibrium, and congruence between what the individual is doing and wants to do. In this chapter, of the several definitions that exist, occupational balance is defined as a subjective perception of having the right amount and variation of occupations in the occupational pattern (Wagman et al., 2012). Occupational balance is associated with health, well-being, and life satisfaction, which makes it central to occupational therapy and occupational science.

20.2.2.2 Attributes

Occupational balance has a long history in occupational therapy, first described 100 years ago (Meyer, 1977/1922). Occupational balance is subjectively defined by the individual and focuses on the amount and variation of occupations, regardless of what they are. However, occupational balance is not about spending the same amount of time in each occupation. The individual needs to perceive having the just-right amount of each occupation, as well as the just-right total number of occupations in the occupational pattern. That is, the design of an individual's occupational pattern in time and space must have neither too many nor too few occupations in relation to the individual's abilities and available resources. Further, occupational balance means a variation between different occupations, meaning that individuals have a mix of different occupations in their occupational pattern. Thus, a prerequisite for the perception of occupational balance is not having too much engagement in only one occupation.

Occupational balance differs among individuals and across an individual's life course. The amount, variation, and degree of occupational balance an individual perceives as contributing the right balance among their occupations varies over both the short and long terms. In research, we often want to understand what is occurring at the extremes because individuals who perceive extremely low (i.e., occupational imbalance) or high occupational balance can tell us something about health and well-being. As examples, one study demonstrated that high occupational balance may be associated with well-being (Håkansson & Lexén, 2021), while an earlier study showed that low balance may be associated with increased stress (Håkansson et al., 2016). In this study, insufficient time for relaxation was associated with stress in working parents with small children. Among the mothers, stress was associated with insufficient time for children, friends, and physical exercise. Fathers often perceived better occupational balance than mothers, which may be due to the demands placed on women as a result of perceived gender roles (Håkansson et al., 2016).

Women more often need to balance work, instrumental activities of daily living, leisure, rest, and sleep to experience occupational balance, while men, to a greater extent, perceive occupational balance if they can balance work and recovery (Uthede et al., 2022). Similarly, parents with children living at home were found to score significantly lower concerning time spent engaging in desired occupations compared with people without children (Wagman & Håkansson, 2014). Based on these results, it can be argued that all the occupations in the occupational pattern are important for the perception of the right amount and the right variation among the different occupations in daily life (i.e., occupational balance). Additionally, the right amount of and variation among the different occupations in the occupational pattern are important for the perception of well-being, and the social context appears to affect the perception of occupational balance.

20.2.2.3 Theories/Models

Occupational balance is a subjective perception, and the perception occurs from the dynamic transaction among the individual, their context, and their occupational pattern. An individual's perception of occupational balance is affected by their occupational pattern, and a satisfying occupational pattern is a prerequisite for the perception of a high occupational balance. Thus, occupational balance is also influenced by the context (i.e., physical, social, cultural, and institutional) in which the individual lives (e.g., family and work/school) and by various abilities and available resources. Research has demonstrated that factors in the psychosocial work context, such as workload, control, and reward, predict occupational balance (Håkansson & Lexén, 2023). However, another study showed that occupational balance is more important for health than psychosocial work environment factors (Håkansson & Lexén, 2021).

Further, Håkansson, Gard, et al. (2020) found that for both women and men, occupational imbalance was the most important predictor of impaired work ability when investigating perceived work stress, overcommitment, occupational imbalance, and individual factors. The working life of parents of young children has also been explored. Findings revealed those who experienced positive attitudes toward parenthood and parental leave among colleagues and managers were more likely to perceive their occupational balance as high than parents who were confronted with negative or neutral attitudes. Further, having strategies for handing over tasks in the event of absence was also associated with a high occupational balance (Borgh et al., 2018). Taken together, these examples demonstrate the importance of occupational balance and how factors in the work environment interact with the perception of occupational balance.

Individuals must also be afforded the resources and accommodations needed to support their equitable occupational engagement to perceive occupational balance. Research has shown that individuals with varying abilities experienced a sufficiently high occupational balance when they were aware of their own occupational needs (Sandqvist et al., 2012). Individuals experienced high occupational balance if they could meet those needs through the effective use of available resources and accommodations to enable them to adapt their work situation (i.e., reduced working hours and flexible working hours) and their life outside work (i.e., more rest and recreational occupations) (Sandqvist et al., 2012).

The COVID-19 pandemic can be seen as a contextual disruption, and disruptions can affect people's perceptions of occupational balance (Nissmark & Malmgren Fänge, 2020). Occupational balance of people with and without inflammatory arthritis was compared before and during the pandemic (To-Miles et al., 2022). The results showed that occupational balance of both groups increased during the pandemic compared to pre-pandemic. A possible explanation could be that slowing down the pace of life, not having to commute to work, and fewer social obligations may have made it possible to engage in meaningful occupations that are otherwise deprioritized. These changes could have contributed to improved occupational balance (To-Miles et al., 2022).

Occupational balance is a subjective experience derived from the transaction between the individual, context, and occupational patterns. Hence, an individual's perception of occupational imbalance is affected by their occupational patterns and their engagement in the occupations that compose those patterns. When imbalance occurs, individuals will attempt to adapt occupationally, as needed, to the perceived changes within the environment, the individual's capacities, or the occupation.

20.2.3 Occupational Adaptation
20.2.3.1 Definitions

Researchers have argued that occupational adaptation lacks clarity and consensus in definition (Grajo et al., 2019; Walder et al., 2021), which is reflected in several, distinct definitions of occupational adaptation that have been proposed. In this chapter, the authors define occupational adaptation as a response by an individual, group, community, or population, occurring due to an occupational challenge, which, if effective, enables occupational engagement, participation, and fulfillment of occupational roles in a satisfying manner (Kielhofner, 2008; Schkade & Schultz, 1992). The process of occupational adaptation is a personal one; however, it is shaped by the social, political, cultural, economic, and historic contexts in which it occurs.

As such, the unique personal context that individuals bring to the situation – including their values, preferences, and goals – will be directly impacted by any dominant societal considerations, such as opportunities (or lack thereof), prejudices, biases, and role expectations. Occupational adaptation is an everyday process that occurs alongside changes within the environment, the individual's capacities, or the occupational form, i.e., the directly observable aspects of occupation. For example, an individual may adapt how they perform different occupations depending on the weather or their level of fatigue. However, occupational adaptation is more pronounced at times of significant change or transition. This change may primarily be within the environment (e.g., resettlement in a new country), the person (e.g., following an acquired brain injury), and/or within the occupation/occupational role (e.g., retirement or becoming a first-time parent).

20.2.3.2 Attributes

A concept analysis by Walder et al. (2021) helped refine the understanding of occupational adaptation by identifying some commonly mentioned attributes: (a) internal process; (b) transactional process; (c) life-long cumulative process; (d) adaptation through occupation; (e) mastery and competence; and (f) occupational identity.

The internal processes that occur during occupational adaptation are arguably the most important part of the process to ensure effective adaptation (Schkade & Schultz, 1992). These processes involve gaining awareness, emotional regulation, problem-solving, cognitive reframing, sense-making, acceptance, value consolidation, and decision making (Walder et al., 2021). Motivation and a perception of personal agency are key determinants of successful occupational adaptation (Kielhofner, 2008; Schkade & Schultz, 1992). It is the individual's or group's desire for occupational engagement that drives the adaptive response, which is linked to a perception of choice, occupational possibilities, sense of competence, confidence, satisfaction, and ability to make decisions (Grajo et al., 2019; Walder & Molineux, 2017a). The experiences of the internal processes occurring during occupational adaptation following stroke were revealed in a study by Walder and Molineux (2017b): acceptance of altered occupational competence and the need for help; imagining a revised future; managing fatigue; becoming confident; and seizing control of decision making and goal setting. Interestingly, feeling one has a sense of control is important as both an enabler and an outcome of occupational adaptation. Stanley (2019) described occupational adaptation as involving "reconfiguring identity, choices and a sense of control" (p. 175), as it enables individuals or groups to re-establish their occupational identity and perception of occupational competence.

The transactional nature of occupational adaptation is well recognized. Schkade and Schultz (1992) described occupational adaptation as "the interaction of the person and the environment as they come together in occupation" (p. 831). Occupational adaptation occurs in response to demands from the environment and the individual's or group's desire to be occupationally engaged in the environment (Walder et al., 2021). The occupational adaptation process can involve the individual or group impacting their environment, e.g., installing bathroom handrails, advocating for change, or requesting support from others. Additionally, the physical, social, cultural, institutional, economic, and political environments can impact the occupational adaptation process positively or negatively.

Many authors, including Nayar and Stanley (2015), highlight the social context within which occupational adaptation occurs, including the role of social support systems and the importance of aligning with cultural and societal values and expectations. The environment provides feedback on the effectiveness of the individual's or group's adaptive response and occupational performance, either through presenting ongoing challenge or in providing direct feedback (Schkade & McClung, 2001). Examples of this challenge or feedback are a doorway a person bumps into as they are learning to mobilize in a wheelchair, or peers providing a child with nonverbal feedback about the effectiveness of their emotional regulation in the classroom. The environment can provide supports for occupational adaptation, such as others providing encouragement of an individual's attempts at trying revised ways to perform occupations. It can also present barriers, such as rigid workplace policy preventing a person experiencing auditory hallucinations from using an adaptive strategy of listening to music at work, resulting in decreased occupational performance and engagement.

Occupational adaptation is an ongoing, dynamic process that is cumulative and non-linear. People learn through their experiences of occupational adaption and this learning may be used to help with their process of occupational adaptation in future (Walder et al., 2021). Working with individuals and groups to build their adaptive capacity through embedding a range of occupational adaptation strategies will support them to navigate the process of occupational adaptation across the life course. Occupational therapists may work to enhance an individual's or group's repertoire of adaptive strategies by incorporating metacognitive training until the strategies become habitual.

Through occupational engagement and participation, people learn about their occupational performance, problem solve, modify their approach, and refine their occupational identity (Walder et al., 2021). In other words, occupational adaptation occurs through engaging in occupation as individuals consciously or subconsciously monitor and modify their adaptive response. For many people, this process occurs as part of daily life, whereas others may need support with the process.

Effective occupational adaptation provides an individual or group with a sense of occupational competence, control, and fulfillment (Walder et al., 2021) by achieving engagement and participation and meeting role expectations that are congruent with one's values and goals. Schkade and Schultz (1992) stressed the importance of self-evaluation in relation to the effectiveness of the adaptive response through three occupational measures that they called "relative mastery": effectiveness, efficiency, and satisfaction. They suggested that self-evaluation is critical for learning to occur, so the individual or group does not continue to make previous ineffective responses. They proposed that the effectiveness of occupational adaptation is identified by people's ability to meet their occupational challenge and the extent to which they can build an adaptive repertoire and generalize their adaptive response to other occupational challenges.

An important distinction exists between the external evaluation of skill mastery (someone else's judgment of competence) and one's self-evaluation of occupational mastery (Schkade & McClung, 2001). Further, even where systemic or other barriers appear insurmountable, an adaptive response, such as acceptance, is seen as effective if the individual or group is satisfied with the outcome. The perception of an adaptive response varies among individuals. For example, acceptance of environmental barriers to using public transport and opting to use a private vehicle may be seen as an adaptive response by a wheelchair user who is tired of fighting the issue. However, her response may be viewed as maladaptive by others whose adaptive response to that situation would be to advocate for changes at a local government level or to ableist policies.

Positive outcomes of occupational adaptation may include the actualization of one's potential, as facilitated through imagining possibilities and growth from occupational challenge (Walder et al., 2021). Indeed, opportunity has been identified as a trigger for occupational adaptation, where individuals or groups take advantage of opportunities, rather than outcomes being driven by circumstance (Nayar & Stanley, 2015). Occupational injustice and inequity in opportunity compound occupational challenge, impacting occupational adaptation.

The relationship between occupational identity and occupational adaptation is complex, dynamic, and bi-directional (Walder & Molineux, 2017a). A robust occupational identity enhances the ability to occupationally adapt. Conversely, the process of occupational adaptation can impact one's occupational identity. For some, the process of occupational adaptation leads to an ability to maintain one's occupational identity in the face of occupational challenge. For others, adaptation may be accepting an altered occupational identity through developing competence in new occupations and roles (Walder et al., 2021). For example, individuals may experience sudden occupational identity disruption following a stroke and may initially be committed to returning to their previous sense of self. However, through occupational adaptation they may develop a modified occupational identity based on different levels of competence, modified ways of engaging, altered roles, reviewed values, and cognitive reframing. It is important for occupational therapists to understand where individuals or groups are in their journey of occupational adaptation and identity re/construction to incorporate therapeutic approaches in a client-centered manner (Walder & Molineux, 2017a).

20.2.3.3 Theories/Models

Two theoretical models have occupational adaptation as a central construct: the Occupational Adaptation Model (Schkade & Schultz, 1992) and the MOHO (Kielhofner, 2008). Meyer (1977) first discussed a link between the two concepts of occupation and adaptation, but Rosenfeld (1989) was the first to use the term "occupational adaptation." Schkade and Schultz (1992) built on this earlier work together with other theories of adaptation (e.g., Llorens; Reed) to develop their model. They described occupational adaptation as an internal, normative process involving occupation to adapt to occupational challenge. Kielhofner's (2008) MOHO refers to occupational adaptation as an interaction between the person and environment to achieve occupational competence and a positive occupational identity. To date, much of the research on occupational adaptation has focused on exploring it within different practice or lived experience contexts, rather than consolidating a theoretical understanding (Walder et al., 2021), which would facilitate the development of practice resources and valid and reliable outcome measures (Grajo et al., 2019).

20.3 Understanding Participation as an Outcome of Engagement, Balance, and Adaptation as Applied through an Intersectional Lens

Participation, defined as the "involvement in a life situation" (World Health Organization, 2001, p. 10), is commonly viewed as the overarching outcome for occupational therapy. Meaningful participation is achieved when individuals, groups, and communities can maintain engagement in valued occupations through an ongoing process of occupational adaptation. Situations, such as prolonged occupational imbalance, when individuals, groups, and communities may be unable to occupationally adapt to maintain their occupational engagement, will negatively impact participation.

Participation is shaped by individuals' memberships in specific social groups based on one's characteristics. The intersection of these memberships often leads to the formation of complex identities that inequitably privilege some while many others experience oppression. Applying an intersectional lens to understanding participation requires occupational therapists to critically reflect on the inequities constructed and reproduced through interpersonal interactions and structural systems of oppression, such as ableism, ageism, racism, sexism, healthism, colonialism, and discrimination based on gender, citizenship, and socioeconomic status, that impact occupational engagement, balance, and adaptation for many equity-deserving groups (e.g., racism experienced by African Canadian women reported by Beagan and Etowa, 2009). In addition, sociocultural demands and expectations, often related to systemic inequities, impact occupational possibilities and participation, and are closely linked to how people and groups perceive their occupations, their capacity to adapt, and their occupational balance. As such, occupational engagement may be out of reach for some individuals, groups, and communities who experience ongoing disadvantage and discrimination.

Although occupational engagement is an individual's cognitive, emotional, or attitudinal involvement in the occupation of interest, systemic inequities constrain the composition of an individual's occupational repertoire, and thus the possibilities for engagement in occupations that are valued and hold significance for the individual and society. If an individual or group is not able to occupationally adapt to those inequities impacting their occupational engagement, participation restrictions and imbalance will occur (Davis & Polatajko, 2010).

20.4 Occupational Narrative: Judi Murdoch

Judi remembers, as a young child, playing with her three siblings. Those first few years of her life were happy ones; Judi has always longed to regain those feelings of family, security, and happiness. Judi's father worked consistently as a plumber after her parents married and started having children. Although financially stable, life changes resulting from parenting four small children all under five began to rupture her parents' marriage. Judi's parents, at that time in their mid-20s, began to drink alcohol and smoke marijuana daily to relax and manage their stress. Then, when Judi was 4 years old, her father abruptly left the family after starting a new relationship. Mostly, Judi remembers how her happy life changed after her father left, as her mother increased her drinking and began using crack cocaine to manage her sadness. Judi received some stability and support from her father's mother, Margaret Murdoch, who lived in the next town, but she remained living in her mother's home. Judi's life became erratic with her two older brothers staying out late, leaving her and her younger sister to care for each other.

Judi found school to be a reprieve from the neglect at home. She was very good at mathematics and engaged in learning to use a computer, which she did not have access to at home. To make sure that no one found out what was happening in her home, she kept to herself at school and did not make any friends. She did become close to a few teachers who nurtured her engagement in computers. With her feelings of loneliness and regular exposure to marijuana, Judi started smoking it at 9 years of age when she felt stressed. Judi managed to make it through primary school and two years of high school, using the adaptive strategies she learned. After finishing her second year of high school, she dropped out at 16 when she became pregnant with her first child and her life became more imbalanced. Judi gave birth to a healthy baby who was placed in her grandmother's custody. After this experience, Judi began drinking heavily and using crack cocaine when she could acquire it. Her occupational engagement shifted to using drugs and drinking, and she learned new adaptive strategies to maintain participation in substance use.

Currently, Judi's entire immediate family – her mother, two brothers, and sister – use crack. Judi has not seen her father since she was four years old; she does not know if he is alive and does not care. She has two children, Michaela, seven years old, and Jason, three years old. Her children have different fathers, and neither of the fathers are involved with the children or her and have never provided any support for the children. Judi did receive ongoing support from her grandmother, Margaret, who cared for both of Judi's children. Her grandmother was her biggest support and the only "clean and sober" person she had known. However, she died one year ago of cardiac arrest. After her death, Judi's children were placed in foster care. Judi found it very difficult to adapt to the changes as her life became increasingly imbalanced. She became extremely depressed and disengaged from all occupations outside of drug use. Her drug use increased as engagement in this occupation was the only adaptive response to managing her feelings that she knew.

KEY OCCUPATIONAL CONCEPTS

Judi, at 24 years of age and six months pregnant with her third child, was found in a crack house raid nine weeks ago. After detoxing within the hospital to ensure that she and the baby were safe, she completed one month of inpatient court-ordered rehabilitation for her substance use disorder. The nursing records indicate that she was extremely uncooperative regarding hospital rules for the first two weeks of treatment. She often refused to attend treatment sessions. The hospital records indicate that Judi had a breakthrough in week three of treatment. She began making friends with some of the other patients, which was a new experience for her. Judi stated that she had never trusted anyone enough to develop friendships before she came to inpatient drug rehabilitation. This adaptive response – not trusting – helped her when she was using crack and begging or exchanging sex for money to support her drug use, but was maladaptive when trying to build new healthy relationships. It was easier in the hospital because she knew that other people were not wanting to be friends with her just to get drugs, money, and sex. Judi began to understand that life could involve engaging in other occupations besides drug use.

During the first few weeks of her stay in the hospital, Judi did not understand what right people had to force her to stay off drugs. When the occupational therapist asked her about what she would do if she didn't use drugs, Judi stated, "drugs are my life and all I have known since I was young. I don't know what I would do without them." In speaking with her, the occupational therapist discovered that Judi had a strong occupational identity as a drug user and had been very competent in her performance in the occupations related to her drug use, which had intensified her engagement in using drugs. To continue drug use over the past decade, Judi had to occupationally adapt to barriers presented within her environment that would impact her participation. Before hospitalization, Judi's occupational pattern was dominated by engagement in drug use and performing the occupations and activities to obtain the drugs, leading to long-term occupational imbalance. This information helped the occupational therapist understand Judi's occupational engagement, repertoire, and the meanings she associated with her drug user identity, shaping her participation.

As Judi heard other people's stories about their lives, she began to understand that she had not really been happy with her life since she was very young. The occupational therapist asked Judi to complete the Occupational Balance Questionnaire (OBQ11) (Håkansson, Wagman, et al., 2020). The OBQ11, using 11 statements with four response alternatives, measures self-rated occupational balance in the present and is based on the definition of perceiving the right amount of and variation between different occupations in everyday life (Wagman et al., 2012). Judi obtained a low total score on the OBQ11 indicating that she had low occupational balance. The occupational therapist used these assessment findings to guide Judi in exploring how to restructure her occupational life to discover occupations beyond drug use that she found engaging and to improve her occupational balance.

With this new information and the support of the occupational therapist, Judi began to reframe her goals by reflecting on her values and priorities and current and desired occupational identity and roles. On discharge from the inpatient unit, Judi set her long-term goals as regaining custody of her two older children and keeping and caring for her third child. She wanted to establish a new occupational identity of mother and carer for her children by learning how to take care of herself and her children and support them financially. With the occupational therapist's support, Judi realized that achieving her desired identity and roles would enhance her ability to occupationally adapt, supporting improved competence and engagement in new occupations that would improve her occupational balance.

Judi has now been in the partial hospitalization program for pregnant individuals for one month following discharge from inpatient drug rehabilitation. This program is for those individuals who have recently given or will soon give birth, have or may be granted custody of their infant, and have a recent history of substance use disorder. The program is provided for one year, five days per week, eight hours a day. There is also 24 hour/7 days per week contact in case of emergency or crisis. The program provides rehabilitation services, including substance abuse counselling, and occupational therapy focused on educational support to complete high school, employment training, and parenting and life skills training.

Judi is currently sharing an apartment with two women in the program, one of whom gave birth seven months ago. In each apartment, there is one "senior" woman who has been in the program for over six months. Each senior woman is expected to act as a peer role model for the other two women sharing the same apartment. Judi is learning, with the support of an occupational therapist and her roommates, to cook, clean, care for her home, and budget the allowance she receives from the program to fulfil her long-term goals. She has continued the friendships that she began in the hospital especially with the women with whom she lives. They all realized they like dogs, so they began volunteering for a few hours every weekend at an animal shelter. In the past month in this community program, Judi has expanded considerably her engagement in diverse occupations, supporting improved balance in her life. While waiting for the birth of her third child, Judi will keep working with the occupational therapist to expand her learning of mothering occupations, such as bathing and dressing an infant.

For the first time, Judi is able to reframe how she sees her future and can see a different life for herself. As she always valued learning, she wants to finish high school and find a job. She would like to learn to become a good mother to her three children and eventually marry so that her children have a stable environment like she remembers when she was very young. Because of previous drug convictions and the possibility of her child being born addicted to drugs, Judi will have to demonstrate to child and family services that she can take care of herself and her new baby. Judi's occupational engagement in her past schooling in mathematics and computers may assist her in completing high school and obtaining a job to support her children. Expanding her occupational repertoire through engaging in new or previous occupations will improve her perceived occupational balance and feelings of health and well-being, which will support her ability to occupationally adapt to small or sudden changes in her daily life. Judi believes that she has a better occupational balance, feels better, and is on her way to the goal of being able to take care of her children again and participating in a broader social life.

20.5 Conclusion

This chapter defined and described three key concepts fundamental to occupational therapy practice: occupational engagement, occupational balance, and occupational adaptation. The understandings of these concepts have changed overtime and continue to shift as new knowledge pertaining to these concepts has been generated. A shift in how occupation is viewed in relation to health and well-being, and a greater focus on equity, diversity, and inclusion, has led to re-conceptualization of these concepts over the past decades. Additionally, the importance of the subjective experiences of individuals, groups, and communities, and the impact of systemic oppression on participation in occupation, are highlighted. The occupational narrative presented in this chapter illustrates the application of these concepts within this changing occupational therapy practice environment.

20.6 Summary

- This chapter presents three key concepts, occupational engagement, occupational balance, and occupational adaptation, to illustrate their potential for supporting participation, health, and well-being.
- As the core concern for occupational therapy, clarification of the definitions and attributes of occupation and its key concepts help to articulate the breadth of occupational therapy practice.
- Meaningful participation is achieved when individuals, groups, and communities can maintain engagement in valued occupations through an ongoing process of occupational adaptation.
- Situations, such as prolonged occupational imbalance, when individuals may be unable to occupationally adapt to maintain their occupational engagement, will negatively impact participation.
- Participation in life situations is shaped by the intersection of individuals' social characteristics that inequitably privilege some while others experience oppression.

20.7 Review Questions

1. What are the definitions and key attributes of occupational engagement, occupational balance, and occupational adaptation?
2. How does the definition of occupational engagement differ from occupational performance?
3. What does the Occupational Balance Questionnaire measure and how is it used?
4. How does occupational adaptation relate to transition and change of occupations in the everyday and in times of crisis?
5. What is the definition of participation and how do the concepts of occupational engagement, occupational balance, and occupational adaptation relate to participation?
6. Why is it important to consider intersectionality when speaking about occupation?

References

American Occupational Therapy Association. (2020). Occupational Therapy Practice Framework: Domain and process (4th ed.). *American Journal of Occupational Therapy*, 74(Suppl. 2), 7412410010p1–7412410010p87. https://doi.org/10.5014/ajot.2020.74S2001

Beagan, B. L., & Etowa, J. (2009). The impact of everyday racism on the occupations of African Canadian women. *Canadian Journal of Occupational Therapy*, 76(4), 285–293. https://doi.org/10.1177/000841740907600407

Black, M., Milbourn, B., Desjardins, K., Sylvester, V., Parrant, K., & Buchanan, A. (2019). Understanding the meaning and use of occupational engagement: Findings from a scoping review. *British Journal of Occupational Therapy*, 82(5), 272–287. https://doi.org/10.1177/0308022618821580

Borgh, M., Eek, F., Wagman, P., & Håkansson, C. (2018). Organisational factors and occupational balance in working parents in Sweden. *Scandinavian Journal of Public Health*, 46(3), 409–416. https://doi.org/10.1177/1403494817713650

Cruz, D., Taff, S., & Davis, J. A. (2023). Occupational engagement: Some assumptions to inform occupational therapy [Engajamento ocupacional: Alguns pressupostos para a terapia ocupacional]. *Brazilian Journal of Occupational Therapy*, 31, e3385. https://www.scielo.br/j/cadbto/a/Qd54RP6dqYkfqL9QVSK8tGF/

Csíkszentmihályi, M. (1990). *Flow: The psychology of optimal experience*. Harper and Row.

Davis, J. A., & Polatajko, H. J. (2010). Occupational development. In C. Christiansen & E. Townsend (Eds.), *Introduction to occupation: The art and science of living* (2nd ed., pp. 135–174). Pearson Education.

Grajo, L., Boiselle, A., & Dalomba, E. (2019). Defining the construct of occupational adaptation. In L. C. Grajo & A. Boiselle (Eds.), *Adaptation through occupation: Multidimensional perspectives* (pp. 3–18). Slack.

Håkansson, C., Axmon, A., & Eek, F. (2016). Insufficient time for leisure and perceived health and stress in working parents with small children. *Work*, 55(2), 453–461. https://doi.org/10.3233/WOR-162404

Håkansson, C., Gard, G., & Lindegård, A. (2020). Perceived work stress, overcommitment, balance in everyday life, individual factors, self-rated health and work ability among women and men in the public sector in Sweden: A longitudinal study. *Archives of Public Health*, 78, Article #132. https://doi.org/10.1186/s13690-020-00512-0

Håkansson, C., & Lexén, A. (2021). The combination of psychosocial working conditions, occupational balance and sociodemographic characteristics and their associations with no or negligible stress among Swedish occupational therapists: A cross-sectional study. *BMC Health Service Research*, 21, Article #471. http://doi.org/10.1186/s12913-021-06465-6

Håkansson, C., & Lexén, A. (2023). Work conditions as predictors of occupational therapists' occupational balance. *Scandinavian Journal of Occupational Therapy*, 30, 520–526. https://doi.org/10.1080/11038128.2022.2158928

Håkansson, C., Wagman, P., & Hagell, P. (2020). Construct validity of a revised version of the Occupational Balance Questionnaire. *Scandinavian Journal of Occupational Therapy*, 27(6), 441–449. https://doi.org/10.1080/11038128.2019.1660801

Kennedy, J., & Davis, J. A. (2017). Clarifying the construct of occupational engagement for occupational therapy practice. *OTJR: Occupation, Participation and Health*, 37(2), 98–108. https://doi.org/10.1177/1539449216688201

Kielhofner, G. (2008). *Model of Human Occupation: Theory and application* (4th ed.). Lippincott Williams & Wilkins.

Meyer, A. (1977). The philosophy of occupational therapy. *American Journal of Occupational Therapy*, 31, 639–642 (*Archives of Occupational Therapy*, 1922, 1, 1–10).

Nayar, S., & Stanley, M. (2015). Occupational adaptation as a social process in everyday life. *Journal of Occupational Science*, 22(1), 26–38. https://doi.org/10.1080/14427591.2014.882251

Nissmark, S., & Malmgren Fänge, A. (2020). Occupational balance among family members of people in palliative care. *Scandinavian Journal of Occupational Therapy*, 27(7), 500–506. https://doi.org/10.1080/11038128.2018.1483421

Polatajko, H. J., Davis, J., Stewart, D., Cantin, N., Amoroso, B., Purdie, L., & Zimmerman, D. (2007). Specifying the domain of concern: Occupation as core. In E. A. Townsend & H. J. Polatajko (Eds.), *Enabling occupation II: Advancing an occupational therapy vision for health, well-being, and justice through occupation* (pp. 13–36). CAOT Publications ACE.

Rosenfeld, M. S. (1989). Occupational disruption and adaptation: A study of house fire victims. *American Journal of Occupational Therapy*, 43(2), 89–96. https://doi.org/10.5014/ajot.43.2.89

Sandqvist, G., Hesselstrand, R., Scheja, A., & Håkansson, C. (2012). Managing work life with systematic sclerosis. *Rheumatology*, 51, 319–323. https://doi.org/10.1093/rheumatology/ker324

Schkade, J., & McClung, M. (2001). *Occupational adaptation in practice: Concepts and cases*. Slack.

Schkade, J., & Schultz, S. (1992). Occupational adaptation: Toward a holistic approach for contemporary practice: Part 1. *American Journal of Occupational Therapy, 46*(9), 829–837. https://doi.org/10.5014/ajot.46.9.829

Stanley, M. (2019). The lived experience of occupational adaptation: Adaptation in the wake of adversity, life transitions, and change. In L. C. Grajo & A. Boiselle (Eds.), *Adaptation through occupation: Multidimensional perspectives* (pp. 175–192). Slack.

Stewart, K., Fischer, T., Hirji, R., & Davis, J. A. (2016). Toward the reconceptualization of the relationship between occupation and health and well-being. *Canadian Journal of Occupational Therapy, 83*(4), 249–259. https://doi.org/10.1177/0008417415625425

Sutton, D. J., Hocking, C. S., & Smythe, L. A. (2012). A phenomenological study of occupational engagement in recovery from mental illness. *Canadian Journal of Occupational Therapy, 79*, 142–150. https://doi.org/10.2182/cjot.2012.79.3.3

To-Miles, F., Backman, C. L., Forwell, S., Puterman, E., Håkansson, C., & Wagman, P. (2022). Exploring occupations and well-being before and during the COVID-19 pandemic in adults with and without inflammatory arthritis. *Journal of Occupational Science, 29*(3), 368–385. https://doi.org/10.1080/14427591.2022.2057573

Uthede, S., Nilsson, I., Wagman, P., Håkansson, C., & Farias, L. (2022). Occupational balance in parents of pre-school children: Potential differences between mothers and fathers. *Scandinavian Journal of Occupational Therapy*. Advance online. http://doi.org/10.1080/11038128.2022.2046154

Wagman, P., & Håkansson, C. (2014). Exploring occupational balance in adults in Sweden. *Scandinavian Journal of Occupational Therapy, 21*(6), 415–420. https://doi.org/10.3109/11038128.2014.934917

Wagman, P., Håkansson, C., & Björklund, A. (2012). Occupational balance as used in occupational therapy: A concept analysis. *Scandinavian Journal of Occupational Therapy, 19*(4), 322–327. https://doi.org/10.3109/11038128.2011.596219

Walder, K., & Molineux, M. (2017a). Occupational adaptation and identity reconstruction: A grounded theory synthesis of qualitative studies exploring adults' experiences of adjustment to chronic disease, major illness or injury. *Journal of Occupational Science, 24*(2), 225–219. https://doi.org/10.1080/14427591.2016.1269240

Walder, K., & Molineux, M. (2017b). Re-establishing an occupational identity after stroke: A theoretical model based on survivor experience. *British Journal of Occupational Therapy, 80*(10), 620–630. https://doi.org/10.1177/0308022617722711

Walder, K., Molineux, M., Bissett, M., & Whiteford, G. (2021). Occupational adaptation: Analyzing the maturity and understanding of the concept through concept analysis. *Scandinavian Journal of Occupational Therapy, 28*(1), 26–40. https://doi.org/10.1080/11038128.2019.1695931

World Health Organization. (2001). *International Classification of Functioning, Disability and Health* (ICF). WHO.

Yazdani, F. (2023). *Occupational wholeness for health and wellbeing: A guide to re-thinking and re-planning life*. Taylor & Francis.

Yerxa, E. J. (1980). Occupational therapy's role in creating a future climate of caring. *American Journal of Occupational Therapy, 34*(8), 529–534. https://doi.org/10.5014/ajot.34.8.529

CHAPTER 21

Person Factors
Values, Beliefs, Spirituality, Body Functions, and Body Structures

Barbara M. Doucet and Carrie A. Ciro

Abstract
Occupational therapy practitioners are uniquely qualified to understand all the variables that affect occupational performance. This chapter will explore the role of *person factors* as potentially supporting or limiting performance and participation. The need to integrate approaches that focus solely on person factors with approaches that emphasize occupational performance is discussed. A holistic, integrated approach brings the best of what occupational therapy can offer to the clients, families, and communities we serve.

Authors' Positionality Statements
Dr. Doucet is a white, married, middle-aged female with a PhD and lives in the southern United States. She was brought up in a family with a strong Catholic faith which emphasized family values, love, and the importance of education. At the time of writing, she serves as an occupational therapy researcher and educator for a large, private university, and her career has focused on improving independence for people with neurological disorders. Dr. Ciro is a white, married, middle-aged female with a PhD who lives in the midwestern United States. At the time of writing, she serves as an administrator, educator, and researcher for a large public university. In her career, she has focused on improving occupational performance in people with chronic conditions or progressive neurological conditions such as dementia.

> **Objectives**
> This chapter will allow the reader to:
>
> - Describe person factors and how this impacts occupational performance.
> - Define approaches to intervention, including top-down, bottom-up, and integrated.

DOI: 10.4324/9781003504610-24

- Discuss the importance of using both patient-reported and therapist-reported measures in client assessment.
- Explore and apply the use of person factors through a case study.

Key terms
- person factors
- body structure
- body function
- patient-reported outcomes
- task and occupation-based outcomes

21.1 Introduction

From the inception of the occupational therapy profession, a core underpinning has been the belief that occupations and engagement in activities that hold inherent meaningfulness and purpose in life drive the health process (American Occupational Therapy Association, 2020). The unique value of the occupational therapy profession is that practitioners understand the complexity of human occupation and the significant role participation in daily activities can play in maintaining and improving physical and mental health. When disease processes or pathology interrupt the ability to engage and participate in desired activities, the occupational therapist is the most qualified healthcare practitioner to evaluate the loss of occupational performance and determine which variables impact performance.

Person factors are those human abilities, characteristics, and capabilities that support engagement in occupations. Physical and mental functions such as cognition, movement, vision, beliefs, emotions, joint function, pain, values, endurance, and spirituality all contribute to the ability to engage in activities. Client factors can be addressed at individual, group, and population levels. At an individual level, an occupational therapy practitioner could work with a person after tendon surgery to restore strength and range of motion. At a group level, an occupational therapist may create a weekly group class for a homeless shelter to review how to reestablish life skills using personal values, beliefs, and spirituality. At a population level, an occupational therapy practitioner may work with businesses to develop wellness programs to reduce visual, physical, and mental fatigue that can be incorporated into daily schedules.

A comprehensive approach to occupational therapy includes examining client factor abilities and impairments, along with occupations and environments, to produce a plan for optimal occupational performance and participation. Approaches to assessment and intervention in occupational therapy should be person-centered, using tasks grounded in real-life activities, and incorporate both top-down and bottom-up strategies (Meriano & Latella, 2016). A top-down approach implies that the occupational therapy practitioner evaluates occupational performance and participation, and then develops a treatment plan to address limitations and restrictions.

In a bottom-up approach, the occupational therapist evaluates foundational client factors and then develops a treatment plan to remediate or compensate for impairments. An *integrated approach* allows a comprehensive evaluation of individual daily functioning and client factors through direct observation by the occupational therapy practitioner who then can report data-driven objective results and measures. Additionally, important subjective data related to patient perceptions that can be obtained through patient-reported measures should be paired with the objective data to create a comprehensive, integrated intervention plan aimed at restoring or compensating for lost function.

Interventions in occupational therapy should be task-based and ecologically valid. Ecological validity is present when an intervention or an assessment possesses characteristics that are typically seen in a daily living environment and are contextually appropriate (Crist, 2015). Neuroscientists have demonstrated that tasks with meaning produce observable changes in the neurophysiology of the brain; however, performance of simulated or contrived functional activities without the use of real-world objects alter and disrupt the typical motor and sensory responses seen with human movement (Hubbard et al., 2009). An American Occupational Therapy Association (AOTA) taskforce, in collaboration with the American Board of Internal Medicine (ABIM), identified the use of non-purposeful activities in occupational therapy as a practice that should be questioned by providers (AOTA, 2022); therefore, therapeutic methods are most effective when they are realistic, functional, client-specific, and goal-directed.

21.2 Values, Beliefs, and Spirituality

21.2.1 Values

Values have been described as "…the unique preferences, concerns, and expectations that are brought by each patient to a clinical encounter and must be integrated into clinical decisions if the patient is to be served" (Institute of Medicine, 2001, p. 47). Kielhofner (2008) defined values as beliefs being derived from culture, thereby identifying what is appropriate, correct, and important to do. Values can impact not only specific healthcare decisions, but also other areas such as healthcare planning, communication, and the involvement of significant others (Armstrong & Mullins, 2017). Identifying patient values early on as well as throughout the occupational therapy process is recommended so that person-centered care and actions taken are aligned with client values. Examples of relevant assessments that incorporate values can be found in Table 21.1.

21.2.2 Why It Matters to Occupational Therapy Practitioners

Values inherently influence personal as well as healthcare outcomes, and while rehabilitation tends to focus on the treatment of disease and remediation of impairments, the lived experience of the person is often neglected (Fadyl, 2020). As healthcare professionals, we should understand that values can vary greatly between clients, that these need to be considered when designing plans for treatment, and that we are professionally bound to provide respect to all, especially in situations where our values do not align with those we serve.

Table 21.1 Non-Inclusive List of Client Factors Assessment

Functions	Chart review	Patient-report measures	Therapist-observed measure
Values, beliefs, and spirituality	Values and beliefs	Model of Human Occupation Screening[1] Pediatric Volitional Questionnaire[2] Volitional Questionnaire[3]	
	Spirituality Hospital chart	FICA Spiritual Assessment Tool[4] Spiritual Assessment Guidelines[5] The Multidimensional Measurement of Religiousness/Spirituality for Use in Health Research[6]	
Specific mental	Attention, memory, executive function Multi-disciplinary notes, caregiver report	Cognitive Failures Questionnaire[7] PROMIS Cognition Abilities Scale[8] Rivermead Post-Concussion Symptoms Questionnaire[9] FACT-Cog[10]	Test of Everyday Attention[11] Cognitive Assessment of Minnesota[12] Contextual Memory Test[13] Executive Function Performance Test (EFPT)[14] Neuropsychological Battery[15] ■ Attention ■ Memory ■ Executive functions Rivermead Behavioral Memory Test[16] Mini-Mental Status Exam (MMSE)[17] Montreal Cognitive Assessment (MoCA)[18] PASS[19]

(Continued)

Table 21.1 (Continued)

Functions		Chart review	Patient-report measures	Therapist-observed measure
Global mental	Emotional regulation	Multi-disciplinary notes, caregiver report	Cognitive Emotion Regulation Test[20] Vineland Adaptive Behavior Scales[21]	
	Praxis			Sensory Integration and Praxis Test[22]
	Conscious-ness Orientation	Multidisciplinary notes Multi-disciplinary notes and caregiver report		Glasgow Coma Scale[23] MMSE[17] MoCA[18]
	Psychological	Multi-disciplinary notes and caregiver report	Beck Depression Inventory II[24] Generalized Anxiety Disorder Assessment (GAD)[25] Eating Attitudes Test (EAT-26)[26]	
	Tempera-ment and personality	Psychology or neuro-psychology testing	Myers-Briggs Type Indicator[27]	
	Energy (cognitive)		Mental Fatigue Scale[28]	Psychomotor Vigilance Test[29] Four Choice Test of Serial Reaction Time[30]
	Sleep	Multi-disciplinary notes and caregiver report Sleep study report	Pittsburgh Sleep Quality Index[31]	
Sensory	Visual	Ophthal-mology or neuro-ophthalmology tests	Visual Function Questionnaire (VFQ-25)[32]	Visual Acuity Test[33] NSUCO Oculomotor Test[34]
	Hearing	Audiology assessment	Hearing Handicap Inventory[35]	
	Taste			Flour Waver Test[36]

(Continued)

Table 21.1 (Continued)

Functions		Chart review	Patient-report measures	Therapist-observed measure
	Smell		Odor Awareness Scale[37]	University of Pennsylvania Smell Identification Test[38]
	Touch			Sensory Tests[39]
	Pain	Multi-disciplinary notes and caregiver report	Wong-Baker Pain Scale[40] Functional Pain Scale[41]	Critical Care Pain Observation Tool[42]
	Vestibular	Reports of dizziness, near falls, and falls	Vestibular activities and participation	Vestibular Test Battery[43]
Neuro-musculo-skeletal and movement-related functions	Joint mobility and stability	Multi-disciplinary notes Functional range of motion		Dynamic Gait Index[44] Elderly Mobility Scale[45] Rivermead Mobility Index[46] Get-Up and Go Test[47]
	Muscle functions (power, tone, and endurance)	Observation during functional activity		Ashworth Scale/Modified Ashworth Scale[48] Motor Evaluation Scale[49] Motricity Index[50]
	Movement functions (motor reflex, voluntary and involuntary movement, and gait patterns)	Multi-disciplinary notes		Fugl-Meyer Assessment of Motor Recovery After Stroke[51] Motor Assessment Scale[52] Wolf Motor Function Test[53] Functional Gait Assessment[54]
Cardio-vascular	Blood pressure (BP) Heart rate Oxygen saturation levels	Multi-disciplinary notes	Health-Related Quality of Life Scale (HRQOL-14)[55] Short Form-36/Short Form-12 SF-36/SF-12[56]	Six Minute Walk Test[57]

(Continued)

Table 21.1 (Continued)

Functions		Chart review	Patient-report measures	Therapist-observed measure
Hemato-logical	Blood count	Complete blood count (CBC)	HRQOL-14[55] SF-36/SF-12[56]	
	Hormone	Hormone tests (thyroid, follicle stimulating, estrogen, progesterone, and testosterone)[34]		
Immuno-logical	Immune system	Immune function assays	HRQOL-14[55] SF-36/SF-12[56]	
Respiratory	Lung	Pulmonary function tests	HRQOL-14[55] SF-36/SF-12[56]	
	Exercise tolerance	Exercise stress test	Borg Perceived Exertion Scale[58] Multi-dimensional Dyspnea Profile[59]	
Voice and speech	Voice production Speech articulation	Speech-language pathology (SLP) assessments	Evaluating Voice Disability-Quality of Life (EVD-QOL)[60]	
Digestive	Eating, drinking	Multi-disciplinary notes and caregiver report		Functional Independence Measure (FIM)[61]
	Swallowing	SLP notes Bedside swallow Evaluation		Modified Barium Swallow Study[62]
	Defecation	Multi-disciplinary notes and caregiver report	Fecal Incontinence Severity Index[63] Fecal Incontinence Quality of Life Measure[64]	
Metabolic		Body mass index	HRQOL-14[55] SF-36/SF-12[56]	

(Continued)

Table 21.1 (Continued)

Functions		Chart review	Patient-report measures	Therapist-observed measure
Endocrine	Energy (physical)	Multi-disciplinary notes and caregiver report	HRQOL-14[55] SF-36/SF-12[56] Positive Associations with Energy: Depressive Symptoms[65]	Positive Associations with Energy: 400m Walk Test Time[65] Negative Association with Energy: Usual and Rapid Gait Speed, Time Spent in Intense Exercise[65]
	Stress	Cortisol levels and inflammatory markers	Perceived Stress Reactivity Scale[66] Adverse Childhood Experiences Questionnaire[67]	
Genito-urinary	Urination	Multi-disciplinary notes and caregiver report	Severity Index of Urinary Incontinence[68] HRQOL-14[55] SF-36/SF-12[56]	FIM[61]
Reproductive	Pelvic floor function	Multi-disciplinary notes and caregiver report	HRQOL-14[55]	Pelvic Floor Assessment[69]
Skin	Wound assessment	Multi-disciplinary anwd caregiver report	Cardiff Wound Impact Schedule[70]	Photographic Wound Assessment Tool[71]

1. Kramer, J., Kielhofner, G., Lee, S. W., Ashpole, E., & Castle, L. (2009). Utility of the Model of Human Occupation Screening Tool for detecting client change. *Occupational Therapy in Mental Health*, 25(2), 181–191. 2. Kiraly-Alvarez, A. (2015). Assessing volition in pediatrics: Using the volitional questionnaire and the pediatric volitional questionnaire. *The Open Journal of Occupational Therapy*, 3(3), 7. 3. Chern, J. S., Kielhofner, G., de las Heras, C. G., & Magalhaes, L. C. (1996). The volitional questionnaire: Psychometric development and practical use. *The American Journal of Occupational Therapy*, 50(7), 516–525. 4. Borneman, T., Ferrell, B., & Puchalski, C. M. (2010). Evaluation of the FICA tool for spiritual assessment. *Journal of Pain and Symptom Management*, 40(2), 163–173. 5. Schnorr, M. A. (1999). Spiritual assessment guidelines. In J. Greene & M. Walton (Eds.), *Fostering vital friends meetings* (pp. R2–53). QuakerPress of FGC. 6. Traphagan, J. W. (2005). Multidimensional measurement of religiousness/spirituality for use in health research in cross-cultural perspective. *Research on Aging*, 27(4), 387–419. 7. Broadbent, D. E., Cooper, P. F., FitzGerald, P., & Parkes, K. R. (1982). The cognitive failures questionnaire (CFQ) and its correlates. *British Journal of Clinical Psychology*, 21(1), 1–16. 8. Saffer, B. Y., Lanting, S. C., Koehle, M. S., Klonsky, E. D., & Iverson, G. L. (2015). Assessing cognitive impairment using PROMIS® applied cognition-abilities scales in a medical outpatient sample. *Psychiatry Research*, 226(1), 169–172. 9. Maruta, J., Lumba-Brown, A., & Ghajar, J. (2018). Concussion subtype identification with the Rivermead post-concussion symptoms questionnaire. *Frontiers in Neurology*, 9, 1034. 10. Costa, D. S., Loh, V., Birney, D. P., Dhillon, H. M., Fardell, J. E., Gessler, D., & Vardy, J. L. (2018). The structure of the FACT-Cog v3 in cancer patients, students, and older adults. *Journal of*

(Continued)

Pain and Symptom Management, 55(4), 1173–1178. 11. Robertson, I. H., Ward, T., Ridgeway, V., & Nimmo-Smith, I. A. N. (1996). The structure of normal human attention: The Test of Everyday Attention. *Journal of the International Neuropsychological Society, 2*(6), 525–534. 12. Rustad, R. A., Borowick, L. G., DeGroot, T. L., Freeberg, K. S., Jungkunz, M. L., Toglia, J. P., & Wanttie, A. M. (1993). *The Cognitive Assessment of Minnesota*. Therapy Skill Builders. 13. Toglia, J. P. (2004). *Contextual Memory Test*. Therapy Skill Builders. 14. Baum, C. M., Connor, L. T., Morrison, T., Hahn, M., Dromerick, A. W., & Edwards, D. F. (2008). Reliability, validity, and clinical utility of the Executive Function Performance Test: A measure of executive function in a sample of people with stroke. *American Journal of Occupational Therapy, 62*(4), 446–455. 15. Pulsipher, D. T., Stricker, N. H., Sadek, J. R., & Haaland, K. Y. (2013). Clinical utility of the Neuropsychological Assessment Battery (NAB) after unilateral stroke. *The Clinical Neuropsychologist, 27*, 924–945. 16. Moradi, A. R., Doost, H. T. N., Taghavi, M. R., Yule, W., & Dalgleish, T. (1999). Everyday memory deficits in children and adolescents with PTSD: Performance on the Rivermead Behavioural Memory Test. *The Journal of Child Psychology and Psychiatry and Allied Disciplines, 40*(3), 357–361. 17. Tombaugh, T. N., & McIntyre, N. J. (1992). The mini-mental state examination: A comprehensive review. *Journal of the American Geriatrics Society, 40*(9), 922–935. 18. Julayanont, P., Tangwongchai, S., Hemrungrojn, S., Tunvirachaisakul, C., Phanthumchinda, K., Hongsawat, J., Suwichanarakul, P., Thanasirorat, S., & Nasreddine, Z. S. (2015). The Montreal Cognitive Assessment-Basic: A Screening Tool for Mild Cognitive Impairment in Illiterate and Low-Educated Elderly Adults. *Journal of the American Geriatrics Society, 63*(12), 2550–2554. 19. Holm, M. B., & Rogers, J. C. (2008). The Performance Assessment of Self-Care Skills (PASS). In B. J. Hemphill-Pearson (Ed.), *Assessments in occupational therapy mental health* (2nd ed.). SLACK. 20. Garnefski, N., & Kraaij, V. (2007). The Cognitive Emotion Regulation Questionnaire: Psychometric features and prospective relationships with depression and anxiety in adults. *European Journal of Psychological Assessment, 23*(3), 141–149. 21. Yang, S., Paynter, J. M., & Gilmore, L. (2016). Vineland adaptive behavior scales: II profile of young children with autism spectrum disorder. *Journal of Autism and Developmental Disorders, 46*(1), 64–73. 22. Ayres, A. J. (1989). *The sensory integration and praxis tests*. Western Psychological Services. 23. Teasdale, G., Maas, A., Lecky, F., Manley, G., Stocchetti, N., & Murray, G. (2014). The Glasgow Coma Scale at 40 years: Standing the test of time. *The Lancet Neurology, 13*(8), 844–854. 24. Wang, Y. P., & Gorenstein, C. (2013). Psychometric properties of the Beck Depression Inventory-II: A comprehensive review. *Brazilian Journal of Psychiatry, 35*, 416–431. 25. Swinson, R. P. (2006). The GAD-7 scale was accurate for diagnosing generalised anxiety disorder. *Evidence-based Medicine, 11*(6), 184. 26. Garner, D. M., & Garfinkel, P. E. (1979). The Eating Attitudes Test: An index of the symptoms of anorexia nervosa. *Psychological Medicine, 9*(2), 273–279. 27. Pittenger, D. J. (1993). The utility of the Myers-Briggs type indicator. *Review of Educational Research, 63*(4), 467–488. 28. Johansson, B., & Rönnback, L. (2014). Evaluation of the mental fatigue scale and its relation to cognitive and emotional functioning after traumatic brain injury or stroke. *International Journal of Physical Medicine & Rehabilitation, 2*(1). 29. Basner, M., Mollicone, D., & Dinges, D. F. (2011). Validity and sensitivity of a brief psychomotor vigilance test (PVT-B) to total and partial sleep deprivation. *Acta Astronautica, 69*(11–12), 949–959. 30. Wilkinson, R. T., & Houghton, D. (1982). Field test of arousal: A portable reaction timer with data storage. *Human Factors, 24*(4), 487–493. 31. Buysse, D. J., Reynolds III, C. F., Monk, T. H., Berman, S. R., & Kupfer, D. J. (1989). The Pittsburgh Sleep Quality Index: A new instrument for psychiatric practice and research. *Psychiatry Research, 28*(2), 193–213. 32. Mangione, C. M., Lee, P. P., Gutierrez, P. R., Spritzer, K., Berry, S., Hays, R. D., & National Eye Institute Visual Function Questionnaire Field Test Investigators. (2001). Development of the 25-list-item National Eye Institute visual function questionnaire. *Archives of Ophthalmology, 119*(7), 1050–1058. 33. Feder, R. S., Olsen, T. W., Prum, B. E., Jr, Summers, C. G., Olson, R. J., Williams, R. D., & Musch, D. C. (2016). Comprehensive Adult Medical Eye Evaluation Preferred Practice Pattern(®) Guidelines. *Ophthalmology, 123*(1), 209–236. 34. Haddad, R. A., Giacherio, D., & Barkan, A. L. (2019). Interpretation of common endocrine laboratory tests: technical pitfalls, their mechanisms and practical considerations. *Clinical Diabetes and Endocrinology, 5*, 12. 35. Ventry, I. M., & Weinstein, B. E. (1982). The hearing handicap inventory for the elderly: A new tool. *Ear and Hearing, 3*(3), 128–134. 36. Hummel, T., Erras, A., & Kobal, G. (1997). A test for the screening of taste function. *Rhinology, 35*(4), 146–148. 37. Smeets, M. A., Schifferstein, H. N., Boelema, S. R., & Lensvelt-Mulders, G. (2008). The Odor Awareness Scale: A new scale for measuring positive and negative odor awareness. *Chemical Senses, 33*(8), 725–734. 38. Doty, R. L., Shaman, P., Kimmelman, C. P., & Dann, M. S. (1984). University of Pennsylvania Smell Identification Test: A rapid quantitative olfactory function test for the clinic. *The Laryngoscope, 94*(2), 176–178. 39. Ciro, C., & Doucet, B. M. (2021). Sensory assessment and intervention. In D. P. Dirette & S. A. Gutman (Eds.),

(Continued)

Occupational therapy for physical dysfunction (8th ed., pp. 176–196). Wolters Kluwer. 40. Wong, D. L., & Baker, C. M. (1988). Pain in children: Comparison of assessment scales. Pediatric Nursing, 14(1), 9–17. 41. Arnstein, P., Gentile, D., & Wilson, M. (2019). Validating the functional pain scale for hospitalized adults. Pain Management Nursing, 20(5), 418–424. 42. Zhai, Y., Cai, S., & Zhang, Y. (2020). The diagnostic accuracy of the critical care pain observation tool (CPOT) in ICU patients: A systematic review and meta-analysis. Journal of Pain and Symptom Management, 60(4), 847–856. 43. Wuyts, F. L., Furman, J., Vanspauwen, R., & Van de Heyning, P. (2007). Vestibular function testing. Current Opinion in Neurology, 20(1),19–24. 44. Whitney, S. L., Hudak, M. T., & Marchetti, G. F. (2000). The dynamic gait index relates to self-reported fall history in individuals with vestibular dysfunction. Journal of Vestibular Research, 10(2), 99–105. 45. Smith, R. (1994). Validation and reliability of the Elderly Mobility Scale. Physiotherapy, 80(11), 744–747. 46. Hsieh, C. L., Hsueh, I. P., & Mao, H. F. (2000). Validity and responsiveness of the Rivermead Mobility Index in stroke patients. Scandinavian Journal of Rehabilitation Medicine, 32(3), 140–142. 47. Mathias, S., Nayak, U., & Isaacs, B. (1986). Balance in elderly patients: The 'get-up and go' test. Archives of Physical Medicine and Rehabilitation, 67(6), 387. 48. Bohannon, R., & Smith, M. (1987). Interrater reliability of a modified Ashworth scale of muscle spasticity. Physical Therapy, 82(1), 25. 49. Johansson, G. M., & Hager, C. K. (2012). Measurement properties of the Motor Evaluation Scale for upper extremities in stroke patients (MESUPES). Disability and Rehabilitation, 34(4), 288–294. 50. Collin, C., & Wade, D. (1990). Assessing motor impairment after stroke: A pilot reliability study. Journal of Neurology, Neurosurgery and Psychiatry, 53, 576–579. 51. Fugl Meyer, A. R., Jaasko, L., & Leyman, I. (1975). The post stroke hemiplegic patient. A method for evaluation of physical performance. Scandinavian Journal of Rehabilitation Medicine, 7(1), 13–31. 52. Poole, J. L., & Whitney, S. L. (1988). Motor assessment scale for stroke patients: Concurrent validity and interrater reliability. Archives of Physical Medicine and Rehabilitation, 69, 195–197. 53. Wolf, S. L., Catlin, P. A., Ellis, M., Archer, A. L., Morgan, B., & Piacentino, A. (2001). Assessing Wolf motor function test as outcome measure for research in patients after stroke. Stroke, 32, 1635–1639. 54. Wrisley, D. M., Marchetti, G. F., Kuharsky, D. K., & Whitney, S. L. (2004). Reliability, internal consistency, and validity of data obtained with the functional gait assessment. Physical Therapy, 84(10), 906–918. 55. Centers for Disease Control and Prevention. (2017). Health-Related Quality of Life (HRQOL): CDC HRQOL-14 "Healthy Days Measure." CDCP. 56. Farivar, S. S., Cunningham, W. E., & Hays, R. D. (2007). Correlated physical and mental health summary scores for the SF-36 and SF-12 Health Survey, V. 1. Health and Quality of Life Outcomes, 5(1), 1–8. 57. Enright, P. L. (2003). The six-minute walk test. Respiratory Care, 48(8), 783–785. 58. Chen, M. J., Fan, X., & Moe, S. T. (2002). Criterion-related validity of the Borg ratings of perceived exertion scale in healthy individuals: A meta-analysis. Journal of Sports Sciences, 20(11), 873–899. 59. Banzett, R. B., O'Donnell, C. R., Guilfoyle, T. E., Parshall, M. B., Schwartzstein, R. M., Meek, P. M., & Lansing, R. W. (2015). Multidimensional Dyspnea Profile. An instrument for clinical and laboratory research. European Respiratory Journal, 45(6), 1681–1691. 60. Smith, E., Gray, S., & Verdolini, K. (1995). Effects of voice disorders on quality of life. Otolaryngology-Head and Neck Surgery, 113(2), 121. 61. UDSMR. (1993). Guide for the Uniform Data System for Medical Rehabilitation (Adult FIM), Version 4.0. UDSMR. 62. Martin-Harris, B., Canon, C. L., Bonilha, H. S., Murray, J., Davidson, K., & Lefton-Greif, M. A. (2020). Best practices in modified barium swallow studies. American Journal of Speech-Language Pathology, 29(25), 1078–1093. 63. Rockwood, T. H., Church, J. M., Fleshman, J. W., Kane, R. L., Mavrantonis, C., Thorson, A. G., & Lowry, A. C. (1999). Patient and surgeon ranking of the severity of symptoms associated with fecal incontinence. Diseases of the Colon & Rectum, 42(12), 1525–1531. 64. Rockwood, T. H., Church, J. M., Fleshman, J. W., Kane, R. L., Mavrantonis, C., Thorson, A. G., ... & Lowry, A. C. (2000). Fecal incontinence quality of life scale. Diseases of the Colon & Rectum, 43(1), 9–16. 65. Ehrenkranz, R., Rosso, A. L., Sprague, B. N., Tian, Q., Gmelin, T., Bohnen, N., ... & Rosano, C. (2021). Functional correlates of self-reported energy levels in the Health, Aging and Body Composition Study. Aging Clinical and Experimental Research, 33(10), 2787–2795. 66. Schlotz, W., Yim, I. S., Zoccola, P. M., Jansen, L., & Schulz, P. (2011). The perceived stress reactivity scale: Measurement invariance, stability, and validity in three countries. Psychological Assessment, 23(1), 80–94. 67. Murphy, A., Steele, M., Dube, S. R., Bate, J., Bonuck, K., Meissner, P., Goldman, H., & Steele, H. (2014). Adverse Childhood Experiences (ACEs) Questionnaire and Adult Attachment Interview (AAI): Implications for parent child relationships. Child Abuse & Neglect, 38(2), 224–233. 68. Hanley, J., Capewell, A., & Hagen, S. (2001). Validity study of the severity index, a simple measure of urinary incontinence in women. British Medical Journal, 322(7294), 1096–1097. 69. Dietz, H. P. (2009). Pelvic floor assessment. Fetal and Maternal Medicine Review, 20(1), 49–66. 70. Price, P., & Harding, K. (2004). Cardiff Wound Impact Schedule: The development of a condition-specific questionnaire to assess health-related quality of life in patients with chronic wounds of the lower limb. International Wound Journal, 1(1), 10–17. 71. Thompson, N., Gordey, L., Bowles, H., Parslow, N., & Houghton, P. (2013). Reliability and validity of the revised photographic wound assessment tool on digital images taken of various types of chronic wounds. Advances in Skin & Wound Care, 26(8), 360–373.

PERSON FACTORS

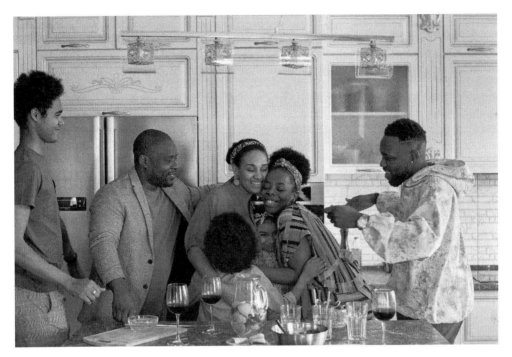

Figure 21.1 A client limited by a diagnosis of multiple sclerosis has a family ritual where her children and grandchildren congregate at her home for a family meal on Sundays.

Source: Photo by August de Richelieu, image used under license from pexels.com.

21.2.3 Occupational Performance Example

A client limited by a diagnosis of multiple sclerosis has a family ritual in which her children and grandchildren congregate at her home for a family meal on Sundays. As a value she holds family togetherness strongly and is very reluctant to give up her primary role as host (see Figure 21.1).

21.2.4 Interventions

Occupational therapy can be involved in helping people to explore, identify, and maintain occupations that support their values. In the case example, the occupational therapy practitioner could help the client create a plan whereby she identifies small components of the meal preparation in which she can engage without excessive fatigue.

21.3 Beliefs

Beliefs are individualistic and defined by the person. Belief in external drivers or internal will, belief in a higher power or absence of one, belief in a healthcare professional to heal, or the power of pharmaceuticals; these represent beliefs that may impact health, healing, recovery, and quality of life. Recognizing "whole wellbeing" and considering individual expression and beliefs not only at the start of care, but throughout the entire process, is central to providing person-centered care (Santana et al., 2018, p. 430). Additional consideration should be given to *practitioner beliefs* that will impact client–therapist relationships. Occupational therapy practitioners may find themselves focused on competent as well as compassionate care, but these characteristics can be restricted by the desire to "fix" or cure patients, practice according to prescribed and accepted methods, or meet financial or corporate productivity standards (Peloquin, 1993).

Examples of relevant assessments incorporating client beliefs can be found in Table 21.1.

21.3.1 Why It Matters to Occupational Therapy Practitioners

Occupational therapy can be involved in helping people to explore, identify, and maintain occupations that support their beliefs. A recent systematic review revealed that a person's beliefs regarding their physical condition, the associated symptomatology, and potential consequences of the disease can profoundly impact engagement in everyday activities, with negative beliefs being associated with poorer outcomes (Shi & Hu, 2020).

21.3.2 Occupational Performance Example

A client with rheumatoid arthritis who lives alone experiences difficulty and pain when caring for her two dogs and is frustrated by having to ask a neighbor to assist in the related care and feeding tasks. Because she values independence, she is beginning to carry the belief that her condition is making her useless.

21.3.3 Interventions

Occupational therapy practitioners can facilitate an understanding of the beliefs that support or hinder a person's occupational performance and quality of life. Task and environmental modifications can be recommended. Using health belief models, occupational therapy practitioners can show people how to embrace or rewrite the narrative of their disease process.

21.4 Spirituality

Spirituality intersects with beliefs. While spirituality is often defined as participation in organized, defined doctrines of specific faiths, many people feel that spirituality can be an individual definition that pertains to a relationship with a higher being or other entity. The role and extent that spirituality can play in persons faced with life-altering diagnoses or even minor injury can reinforce the frailty of the physical human body, and lead some to examine and seek external support in various forms. Spiritual practices can occur individually, such as a person whose routine involves daily reading of scripture to begin their day. Spirituality can be practiced in groups, such as home groups for bible study or a group of attendees at a worship service. Populations can also foster spirituality or spiritual practices as entire members of a denomination, such as Catholics or Protestants. It is important to note that spirituality does not need to be an organized religion or a structured practice of worship. Spirituality can exist individually, with a person focusing on self and one's own meaning and existence; interpersonally, where connections to others may be examined; and transpersonally, across beings with consideration of an external spirit, force, or energy (Griffiths et al., 2007). Examples of relevant assessments that address spirituality can be found in Table 21.1.

21.4.1 Why It Matters to Occupational Therapy Practitioners

Spiritual occupations such as prayer, bible study, private devotions, or reading sacred literature have been described as essential ways to understand suffering and to make meaning from life events (Beagan & Etowa, 2011). Patients will often rely on faith and their spiritual beliefs in a time of need. Expressions of gratitude for the help of others when needed, hope for the future, and awareness of one's own mortality have been observed in persons facing significant health issues (McColl, 2000).

21.4.2 Occupational Performance Example

An older adult client with Stage 2 Parkinson's disease (PD) is a devout Catholic. Rigidity in his arms and legs makes the required sacred movements during mass (kneeling, genuflecting, standing, etc.) difficult. His walking has slowed and he experiences daily fatigue that limits participation in church events; his wife feels isolated.

21.4.3 Interventions

The occupational therapy practitioner helps the person to explore, identify, and maintain tasks that support spirituality, a process that can also include remediation or improvement of client physical factors through exercise and physical activity programs. For example, the client could participate in a Lee Silverman Voice Treatment (LSVT) BIG (LSVT Global, 2019) program to retrain him to move with larger and more effortful amplitudes which can help offset the typical bradykinesia seen during walking and when performing daily tasks. This could improve gait speed and increase mobility to enable full participation in the Catholic mass when standing, sitting, kneeling, and genuflecting. Rock Steady boxing (http://rocksteadyboxing.org) is another program that uses power and momentum during boxing to improve gross motor skills and increase strength and endurance, with the aim of enabling the client to tolerate a full hour of mass and a return to participating in church community events. Activity modification, assistive devices, and environmental modifications should also be evaluated and provided as needed.

21.5 Mental Functions

Mental functions are used to describe different ways in which the brain functions. Specific mental functions describe the details of how our brain functions while global mental functions describe general functions of the brain. Both are foundational for occupational performance.

21.5.1 Specific Mental Functions

Specific mental functions include different aspects of cognition, including attention, memory, judgment, sensory perception, emotional regulation, and the sequencing of complex movement (WHO, 2001). *Cognition* is the action or process of acquiring knowledge and understanding through thought, experience, and the senses. The scope of this definition implies that cognitive processes are not just thoughts, but also how we understand the environment through experiences we have (e.g., movement and activities) and through the senses (e.g., hearing, seeing, smelling, and tasting) that interpret our experiences (Giles et al., 2013). Contemporary writers in occupational therapy further separate cognition from "functional cognition," which may help our profession better understand our unique role in cognitive assessment and intervention.

Functional cognition is defined as how an individual utilizes and integrates his or her thinking and processing skills to accomplish everyday activities (Giles et al., 2020). Although these are important distinctions, we must be able to integrate and analyze cognition through both lenses to serve our clients best. Dysfunction in cognition can occur due to acquired disorders such as traumatic brain injury (TBI), stroke, dementia, cancer, diabetes, or congenital disorders such as Down's syndrome, cerebral palsy, and autism (Giles et al., 2013).

21.5.2 Body Structures and Function

Based on our definition of cognition, the body structures involved in cognition or functional cognition include structures that support the central and peripheral nervous systems, movement, and hearing and vision. Specific body functions associated with cognition include cognitive processing (e.g., attention, memory, emotions, and energy), sensory functions (e.g., vestibular, proprioceptive, touch, and pain), and musculoskeletal and movement functions (e.g., joint mobility, muscle power, and gait) (WHO, 2001). Examples of relevant assessments related to body structures and function can be found in Table 21.1.

21.5.3 Why It Matters to Occupational Therapy Practitioners

Occupational performance is supported by the integrated and reiterative use of specific mental functions (cognition). In other words, we use attention, memory, and problem-solving skills simultaneously and repetitively. Cognition also supports the choice, initiation, sustainment, and ending of occupation (Giles et al., 2020). For a client to make a sandwich for the life-preserving occupation of eating, they must first choose the type of sandwich, be able to initiate the task cognitively and physically, and know when the sandwich is complete to begin eating. To accomplish this, the person must stay on task (attention), remember the steps of the task (requires underlying sustained attention and sequencing), appropriately use kitchen items (requires underlying memory), and potentially problem solve what to do when the kitchen does not have the preferred condiments (requires underlying attention, memory for other preferred condiments, and cognitive flexibility). Therefore, making a sandwich requires the integration of the cognitive processes of decision making, attention, initiation, sequencing, memory and problem solving.

21.5.4 Occupational Performance Example

A 67-year-old female with a diagnosis of early Alzheimer's disease is referred for problems with accurately taking medication. Because she lives alone and wants to age in her home for as long as possible, it is critical that she does this task independently. Using an integrated approach, the occupational therapy practitioner would first interview and observe her medication routine such as the use of a pill box and the use of alarms to remember when to take medicines. Second, the occupational therapy practitioner would complete a brief cognitive assessment to determine areas of limitation in cognitive processes (e.g., attention and memory), which together with skilled observation, can provide a full picture of the overall strengths and weaknesses of the client.

21.5.5 Interventions

Historically, occupational therapy practitioners have been taught to choose either appropriate restorative treatment and/or compensatory techniques that enable occupational performance. Restorative treatment implies that the underlying cognitive condition can be reversed or recovered and should be done early in the treatment of acute cognitive problems. Compensatory intervention implies that remediation may not be achieved and supporting performance with cognitive strategies is the best route, particularly in people with chronic or progressive cognitive problems (Giles et al., 2013). Both approaches can be used across a variety of diagnoses. In the example above, the occupational therapy practitioner may recommend a pill box with an alarm system to alert her to take medications (compensatory). Through practice, the client can reinforce and strengthen procedural memory for completing the task (remediation) (Ciro et al., 2013).

21.6 Global Mental Functions

Global mental functions include different aspects of general brain functioning involving consciousness, orientation, psychosocial processing, temperament and personality, and energy and sleep. Consciousness refers to a person's state of awareness and alertness. Orientation is the knowledge of who one is, where one is, the date and time of day, and who others are in relation to self. Psychosocial function includes evolving mental functions and abilities that support personal interactions with others. Energy functions regulate energy levels and motivation, and sleep functions include the physiological process of sleep, as well as the quality of sleep (WHO, 2001). Disruption in global mental functions can occur due to acquired brain disorders, mental health conditions, congenital disorders, and stress (Giles et al., 2013). Examples of relevant assessments related to global mental functions can be found in Table 21.1.

21.6.1 Body Structures and Function

Based on our definition of global mental functions, the body structures and functions involved include structures that support the central (e.g., arousal, consciousness, circadian rhythms, speech, and motivation) and peripheral (e.g., sensation and movement) nervous systems, sensory functions (e.g., eyes, ears, and sensory receptors), and neuromuscular and movement related functions (e.g., voluntary movement and involuntary reactions) (WHO, 2001). Examples of relevant assessments related to body structures that support global mental function can be found in Table 21.1.

21.6.2 Why It Matters to Occupational Therapy Practitioners

Successful occupational performance requires the use and maintenance of global mental functions, and a client must first be conscious to engage in occupations. Orientation is required for occupations that are completed on certain days of the week or at certain times, and optimal psychological state is foundational to appropriate activity choices and follow-through of occupational performance. Sleep and rest are crucial for maintaining appropriate energy levels to engage in the breadth and depth of occupational performance valued by individuals.

21.6.3 Example and Application

People with TBI can experience negative changes in global mental functions that affect occupational performance. The occupational therapist must assess arousal and alertness for everyday tasks, general orientation to self and environment, energy level and motivation for performance, the quality and quantity of sleep, and changes in personality and interpersonal skills that are commonly associated with brain injury.

21.6.4 Interventions

Implementing coma stimulation techniques, orienting clients with training and supports, conducting social skills groups, and providing meaningful daily activities for arousal are examples of activities that can stimulate mental functions and assist with client motivation (Burson et al., 2017; Giles et al., 2013).

21.7 Sensory Functions

Sensory functions include all the ways in which we are aware of and interpret different sensations (WHO, 2001). *Visual function* refers to the quality of what we can see across the environments in which we perform and includes visual acuity, visual perception (e.g., depth perception, and spatial awareness), and visual fields. *Hearing function* includes detecting, localizing, and discriminating between sounds. For example, a person who is driving would need to hear an ambulance (detection) behind them (locality) and recognize the type of siren (discriminate) in order to determine whether it is necessary to pull the car over to the side of the road. *Taste function* refers to our ability to detect and discriminate between sweetness, sourness, bitterness, and saltiness. *Smell functions* represent how we detect and discriminate between odors. *Touch function* is an important protective sensation so that we can feel differences in sharp versus smooth, heat versus cold, high pressure versus low pressure, moving versus stable touch, and detection of vibration. *Pain* is a feeling that alerts us to the possibility of or actual damage to a body structure. For example, pain in the wrist during activity may signal the diagnosis of carpal tunnel, while pain in the shoulder may represent arthritis or in the case of referred pain, it may indicate a heart attack.

Vestibular function is our awareness of where our body is in space so that we can adjust our movements around people and environments and maintain our balance (WHO, 2001). If we close our eyes, we can determine the location of our body parts (e.g., head and shoulders are in alignment facing a book) and the position of each joint such as flexion or extension. Detection and discrimination of sensory functions occur in both the central and peripheral nervous systems, and these systems also support the cognitive and motor responses (voluntary and involuntary) needed to react to sensory function. Natural aging or specific disorders can affect any of the sensory functions (Li & Lindenberger, 2002). Examples of relevant assessments related to sensory functions can be found in Table 21.1.

21.7.1 Body Structures and Function

The body structures involved in sensory functions include structures that support the central (e.g., brain and spinal cord) and peripheral (e.g., nerves and sensory receptors) nervous systems, sensory organs (e.g., eyes, ears, tongue, and nose), and neuromuscular and movement related structures (e.g., muscles and tendons). Body functions that support these structures detect and discriminate between sensory input that supports vision, hearing, taste, touch, and vestibular perception. Such body functions also drive voluntary and involuntary movement (WHO, 2001). Examples of relevant assessments related to body structures that support sensory function can be found in Table 21.1.

21.7.2 Why It Matters to Occupational Therapy Practitioners

Sensory functions support occupational performance by providing signals for the need for movement (e.g., hand on a hot stove), increasing enjoyment of occupations, and enhancing quality of life.

21.7.3 Occupational Performance Example

TBI can affect sensory function in profound ways and lead to dysfunction in occupational performance. For example, a 16-year-old female volleyball player who sustained a mild TBI may have difficulty with headaches (pain), appreciating the location of the volleyball (visual), knowing where she is in space to position her body correctly (vestibular), and choosing the appropriate pressure to hit the ball (touch) (see Figure 21.2).

21.7.4 Interventions

The occupational therapy practitioner must know if a person's sensory deficits lie in detection or discrimination of the sensory function to develop an appropriate treatment plan of remediation and/or compensation. For example, compensatory strategies may be the only solution to retinal damage, but ocular muscle weakness may be remediated through strengthening exercises (Below & Lewis, 2021). Practitioners can use remediation techniques such as sensory retraining, mirror therapy, and desensitization techniques to improve touch sensation and reduce pain; as well as sensory integration and sensory processing interventions (AOTA, 2021; Bissell, 2015; Gronski & Neville, 2017; Ismael et al., 2018; Turville et al., 2017).

21.8 Neuromuscular and Movement-Related Functions

Neuromuscular and movement functions allow performance of motor tasks, a central component in the ability to engage in occupations. This includes functions of the joints and bones, and the ability of muscles to produce power, maintain or vary tone, and sustain endurance of activity over time. Movement functions include motor reflexes, voluntary and involuntary movement, and gait patterns (AOTA, 2020).

21.8.1 Body Structures and Function

Motor activity occurs by way of the central nervous system, and because participation in many occupations involves movement, neuromuscular function will be a primary goal

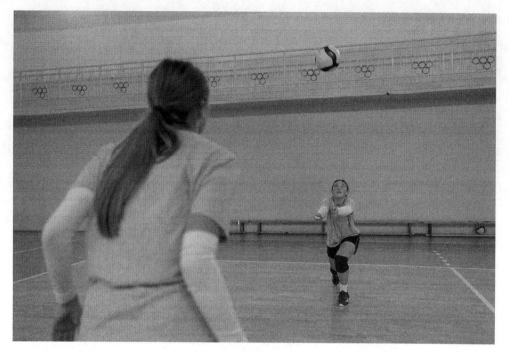

Figure 21.2 A 16-year-old female volleyball player who sustained a mild TBI may have difficulty with headaches (pain), appreciating the location of the volleyball (visual), knowing where she is in space to position her body correctly (vestibular), and choosing the appropriate pressure to hit the ball (touch).

Source: Photo by Pavel Danilyuk, image used under license from pexels.com.

for many patients. The brain and spinal cord, through a complex network of neural synapses, propagations, activations, and inhibitions, allow human movement. Coordinated actions of postural control, eye-hand coordination, gross motor skill, and fine-motor dexterity facilitate engagement in activities ranging from feeding abilities observable in the developing toddler to elite athletic abilities seen in professional athletes. Muscles within the human body perform through coordinated and synchronized variations in tension, power, or endurance to provide mobility or stability as tasks demand. Anatomically and physiologically, the body was created for movement; when movement cannot occur, body structures and functions far beyond just the neuromuscular system are impacted that can disrupt overall function, health, wellbeing, and quality of life. Examples of relevant neuromuscular assessments can be found in Table 21.1.

21.8.2 Why It Matters to Occupational Therapy Practitioners

Performance of tasks and activities typically require motor and sensory function of the neuromuscular system. Movement allows engagement in many occupations that are valuable to our patients and clients. Conditions such as stroke, brain or spinal injury, degenerative diseases, or chronic musculoskeletal debility can disrupt neuromuscular function and limit engagement in activity. Occupational therapists comprehensively assess neuromuscular function and are uniquely trained to perform task and activity analysis; consideration of person factors, task requirements, and environmental demands is a novel hallmark of occupational therapy practice and essential for restoring or enabling a client's occupational performance.

21.8.3 Occupational Performance Example

A young adult male experiences a mild stroke resulting in weakness on the right (dominant) side of his body. He is concerned about being able to perform his computing job duties and the physical appearance of his arm and face, which are moderately hypotonic.

21.8.4 Interventions

Functional movement assessment in the upper and lower extremities should be evaluated as well as sensory function which can also be impaired. Tone normalizing through weight-bearing, repetitive performance of available active movement patterns, neuromuscular contract-release methods, or neuromuscular electrical stimulation for impairment-level restoration or compensation can be incorporated. These can be followed by functional task performance such as handwriting, computing, fine-motor manipulating and grasping activities, making a sandwich or bag lunch, unloading a dishwasher, catching a bus, or navigating hallways or busy sidewalks for integration of neuromuscular and movement function.

Neuromuscular function should be assessed at a structural (or impairment) level through observation and evaluation (bottom-up); however, it is incumbent upon the occupational therapist to assess at a *task level* as well, evaluating the client's ability to perform simple or complex tasks using activity analysis, standardized assessment, and skilled observation (top-down).

21.9 Cardiovascular, Hematological, Immunological, and Respiratory Functions

Cardiovascular function is the efficiency with which the heart, blood vessels, and blood transport nutrients and oxygen-rich blood to all parts of the body and then return deoxygenated blood back to the lungs (WHO, 2001). Complications in cardiovascular function can lead to serious conditions often seen by occupational therapy practitioners, including stroke, heart attack, high blood pressure, and coronary artery disease. *Hematological function* refers to the speed and quality of efficient blood and blood cell production and coagulation (WHO, 2001). Difficulties in hematological function can lead to infections, cancers, and thinning/thickening of blood. Through healthy *immunological function*, our body can detect healthy cells from unhealthy invaders such as bacteria, viruses, and parasites (WHO, 2001). When the body cannot detect healthy cells from invading cells, people have auto-immune disorders such as rheumatoid arthritis, Type I diabetes, and celiac disease. Foreign invaders can cause a cold, flu, COVID-19, or Lyme's disease. *Respiratory function* is necessary for breathing and involves the healthy exchange of oxygen and carbon dioxide (WHO, 2001). Complications in breathing can contribute to asthma, bronchitis, chronic obstructive pulmonary disease, and pneumonia. In all these functions, people can experience temporary, long-term, or permanent changes in body structure and function that impact occupational performance.

21.9.1 Body Structures and Function
21.9.1.1 Cardiovascular System

Body structures include the heart, arteries, veins, blood vessels, heart valves, capillaries, and lungs; body functions include heart rate, heart rhythm, blood supply to heart, blood transportation, oxygenation of blood, maintenance of body temperature, and fluid levels (WHO, 2001).

21.9.1.2 Hematological System

Body structures include blood (plasma, red and white blood cells, and thrombocytes) and bone marrow. Body functions include production of blood, clotting, and forming and transporting cells that remove waste and transport gases, blood cells, immune cells, antibodies, and hormones throughout the body (WHO, 2001).

21.9.1.3 Immune System

Body structures include organs such as the thymus, spleen, bone marrow, and lymph nodes, as well as cells such as phagocytes and lymphocytes. Body functions include detection of external invaders, developing and transporting protective cells, sustained and appropriate response to unhealthy cells, and ending the immune response when appropriate (WHO, 2001).

21.9.1.4 Respiratory System

Body structures include organs such as the nose, sinuses, trachea, diaphragm, and muscles that support inspiration and exhalation, bronchial tubes, alveoli, and the lungs, as well as cellular structures such as cilia and capillaries. Body functions include respiration rate, rhythm and depth, exercise tolerance (e.g., endurance, aerobic capacity, fatiguability, and stamina), coughing, and mucous production (WHO, 2001). Examples of relevant assessments can be found in Table 21.1.

21.9.2 Why It Matters to Occupational Therapy Practitioners

The cardiovascular, hematological, immunological, and respiratory functions are not only critical for living but also complement and support one another for health function. Changes in body structure and function of these systems can lead to significant impairments in activities and restrictions in community participation.

21.9.3 Occupational Performance Example

COVID-19 is a virus that can affect all of the systems described in this section. A previously healthy 67-year-old man may now present with a cough and dyspnea (respiratory function), tachycardia (cardiovascular function), fever (immune function), and a blood clot in the right leg (hematologic). Each of these contributes to changes in energy and endurance that negatively affect occupational performance. Occupational therapy practitioners may be advised to monitor blood pressure, heart rate, blood oxygenation levels, and lab values as part of screening prior to, during, or after treatment.

21.9.4 Interventions

Clients with chronic conditions benefit from learning disease self-management, which can be tied to and become daily habits and routines. Self-management examples include vital sign monitoring, medication management, exercise, and stress management. Skilled and individualized education in activity simplification, energy conservation techniques, and diaphragmatic and pursed lip breathing may also be appropriate for people learning to manage chronic conditions. Prior to engaging in exercise, occupational therapists should prescribe or consult with other health professionals to individualize exercise and activity appropriate for specific metabolic equivalences as needed. The occupational therapist should consider environmental modification to reduce the burden of energy consumption and to promote safety. Palliative and end-of-life care are appropriate interventions for occupational therapy practitioners to provide to clients across the lifespan (Bradshaw, 2017; Pickens et al., 2016; Siebert & Schwartz, 2017).

21.10 Voice and Speech, Digestive, Metabolic, Endocrine, Genitourinary, and Reproductive Functions

Voice and speech functions represent how we produce sound and speech to interact with others in our daily lives. *Language*, the words (oral or written) and manual gestures we use to communicate with one another, relies on voice and speech function for oral production (WHO, 2001). Dysfunction can lead to stuttering and dysarthria. *Digestive functions* support the ingestion of food and liquid, the digestion and transportation of food for absorption and assimilation, and the removal of waste by defecation (WHO, 2001). Disorders caused by dysfunction in the digestive system include irritable bowel syndrome, lactose intolerance, gastroesophageal reflux disease, and food motility disorders. *Metabolic function* enables the body to process the proteins, carbohydrates, and fats ingested through eating and drinking, and convert it chemically into energy (WHO, 2001). Problems with metabolism can cause obesity, diabetes, and metabolic syndrome.

Endocrine function supports hormone production and delivery to control metabolism, energy, reproduction, growth, and response to stress (WHO, 2001). Disorders in the endocrine system can lead to hypo/hyperthyroidism, adrenal insufficiency, hypopituitarism, and polycystic ovary syndrome. *Genitourinary function* is necessary to filter blood and secrete waste products through urine (WHO, 2001). In men, disorders of this system can include issues with the prostate, erectile dysfunction, and urogenital cancer; in women, urinary tract, vaginal infections, and pelvic inflammatory disease. *Reproductive functions* serve to produce egg and sperm cells, transport and sustain reproductive cells, nurture the fetus and offspring, and produce hormones (WHO, 2001). Disorders in the reproductive system of women can cause endometriosis, cervical dysplasia, and pelvic floor prolapse, and in men, erectile dysfunction, prostate disease, and infertility.

21.10.1 Body Structures and Function

21.10.1.1 Voice and Speech

Body structures include the lips, teeth, tongue, palate, uvula, nasal and oral cavities, facial muscles, larynx, vocal cords, and ears. Language requires central and peripheral nervous system structures (e.g., brain and spinal cord) to produce appropriate language and convey through writing or manual signing. Body functions include the production and quality of voice, articulation, prosody, fluency, rhythm, speed and melody of speech, and alternative vocalizations such as production of notes (singing), and range of sounds (e.g., crying and cooing) (WHO, 2001).

21.10.1.2 Digestive System

Body structures of the digestive system include the mouth, pharynx, esophagus, stomach, small and large intestine, rectum, and anus. It also includes the organs that produce digestive enzymes to help the body digest food and liquids, such as salivary glands, liver, pancreas, and gallbladder. Body functions include chewing, sucking, swallowing, vomiting, peristalsis, nutrition absorption, elimination of feces, weight loss, gain, and maintenance, bloating, and gas production (WHO, 2001).

21.10.1.3 Metabolic System

The liver is the primary body structure involved in the body function of metabolism which is a chemical process. Inherent in metabolism is the basal metabolic rate, carbohydrate, protein, and fat metabolism, and water, mineral and electrolyte balance (WHO, 2001).

21.10.1.4 Endocrine System

Body structures involved in the endocrine system include the adrenal glands, hypothalamus, ovaries, parathyroid, pineal, thyroid, and pituitary glands, testes, and thymus. Body functions associated with the endocrine system are metabolism, reactions to stress, body temperature regulation, and pubertal processes (body, breast, penis, testes, and pubic hair development) (WHO, 2001).

21.10.1.5 Genitourinary System

Body structures involved include the kidneys, ureters, bladder, urethra, and genital organs. Body functions of these structures include collection and filtration of urine, urinary functions such as urination, sensation, frequency, and continence (WHO, 2001).

21.10.1.6 Reproductive System

Body structures include the penis, testes, ovaries, uterus, vagina, vulva, accessory glands, duct systems, and the endocrine structures involved in hormone production.

Body functions include but are not limited to sexual function, menstruation, procreation (e.g., fertility, pregnancy, and lactation) and discomfort associated with sexual intercourse, menstruation, and menopause (WHO, 2001). Examples of relevant assessments can be found in Table 21.1.

21.10.2 Why It Matters to Occupational Therapy Practitioners

Digestion, metabolic, endocrine, and genitourinary function is critical to support life, while voice and speech function and reproductive function are important to quality of life. Each of these systems support occupations that are primary to everyday life such as eating, drinking, urinating, speaking, and sexuality.

21.10.3 Occupational Performance Example

A cerebral vascular accident (CVA or stroke) can impact many of these systems. For example, a 72-year-old female post-left CVA can present with dysphagia (digestive), dysarthria (voice and speech), numbness on the right side of the body that affects vulva sensation (reproductive), and urinary incontinence (genitourinary). In this case, the occupational therapy practitioner will need to understand deficits in these body functions to optimize occupational performance.

21.10.4 Interventions

The occupational therapy practitioner should encourage the development of habits that support digestion, metabolism, continence, and sexuality; provide occupational adaptation, assistive technology, and environmental modification that optimize occupational performance; and provide exercises for pelvic floor strengthening (Clark et al., 2003).

21.11 Skin and Related Structure Functions

Skin functions are vital for protecting against germs, regulating body temperature, and enabling touch sensations (WHO, 2001). Disorders in skin include open wounds, pressure ulcers, acne, dermatitis, and excessive sweating. *Functions related to skin* include hair and nails. Hair provides protection and warmth for the head, while nails protect the sensitive tips of fingers and toes (WHO, 2001).

21.11.1 Body Structures and Function

Body structures involved with skin and related functions are skin (epidermis, dermis, hypodermis), hair shafts, follicles and bulbs, nails, nail plates, cuticles, and oil, sweat, mammary, and ear wax glands. The skin interacts with other systems to supply nutrients to skin, hair, and nails. Body functions of the skin include protection, repair of skin, skin sensation, Vitamin D absorption, cooling, and sweat secretion. Body functions that support hair and nail structure include processes that grow pigment, hair, and nails, and maintain the quality of both (WHO, 2001). Examples of relevant assessments that address skin issues can be found in Table 21.1.

21.11.2 Why It Matters to Occupational Therapy Practitioners

Skin is vital to living and therefore critical for optimal occupational performance. While hair and nails are not necessary for life, they play an important role with skin in how a person expresses themselves and the appearance they project to others. Routine care of hair, nails, and skin are part of everyday habits and routines.

21.11.3 Occupational Performance Example

A nerve injury to the hand can affect all these functions. A person with long-standing carpal tunnel syndrome may undergo surgery to relieve pressure on the nerve. In their first post-operative visit, the occupational therapy practitioner notices that the skin is red, and warm to and sensitive to touch. Because the skin was not fully closed, an infection set into the wound. The practitioner also notes changes in the texture of the skin due to limited nerve supply to the hand. Because of the occupational therapy practitioner's knowledge of these systems, the doctor will be alerted to the infection and the patient will be educated on strategies to close the wound.

21.11.4 Interventions

Occupational therapists should encourage the development of habits that support hair, nail, and skin functions which include washing and combing hair, trimming nails, and applying lotion for dry or fragile skin. In people with cancer diagnoses, occupational therapy practitioners provide education to prevent and treat lymphedema. People at risk of pressure ulcers, skin cuts, and burns related to poor sensation may require education and services for splinting, wound care, physical agent modalities, and appropriate positioning (Amini, 2018; Bondoc & Feretti, 2018).

21.12 Case Study

Mrs. Lyons is a 55-year-old female married for 30 years to "Les," a practicing dentist. She has three children and one grandchild and works as a dental hygienist in her husband's practice. She was recently diagnosed with a left frontal lobe brain tumor and is now status post-craniotomy to remove the tumor. She is currently receiving chemotherapy and has been referred to occupational therapy for evaluation and treatment. She complains of nausea and vomiting which began with chemotherapy. As per her medical records, she presents with right-side paresis, including right-foot drop and frequent falls. She feels "numb" on the right side of her body and although she can move her right hand, she is weak and uncoordinated. She complains of visual changes that make reading and seeing challenging. Her husband notes that her ability to pay attention, remember, and make decisions is different since her diagnosis. She also now has behavioral outbursts of anger and increased irritability, with signs of depression. He reports that she needs assistance with all self-care, is having trouble staying asleep through the night, is difficult to motivate, and he feels like she has just "given up."

Mrs. Lyons understands what is being said to her but has trouble articulating her words for people to understand what she is saying. She has told her surgeon that she fears she will not be able to return to work (see Figure 21.3).

PERSON FACTORS

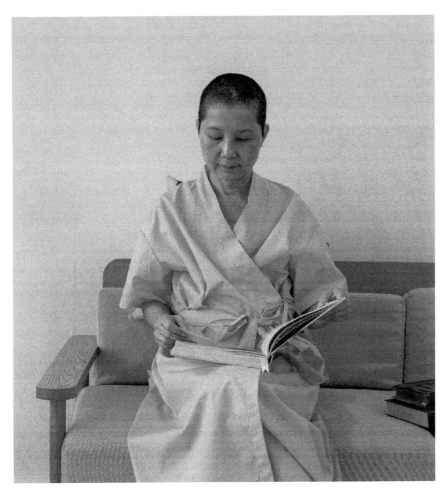

Figure 21.3 Mrs. Lyons is a 55-year-old female who was recently diagnosed with a left frontal lobe brain tumor and has undergone a craniotomy to remove the tumor. She is currently receiving chemotherapy and is referred to occupational therapy for evaluation and treatment.

Source: Photo by Michelle Leman, image used under license from pexels.com.

1. In the case of Mrs. Lyons, which body functions appear to be involved?
2. Prioritize five different body function assessments you would use in this case.
3. Identify five different task or occupation-based assessments you would use in this case.
4. What types of interventions may be relevant for Mrs. Lyons?

21.13 Conclusion

Occupational therapy practitioners are uniquely qualified to understand, evaluate, and provide intervention for variables that affect occupational performance. *Person factors* are human abilities, characteristics, and capabilities that support engagement in occupations, and depending on the individual, these can support or limit occupational performance.

The occupational therapy practice framework organizes person factors by values, beliefs and spirituality, and body structures/functions. Values, beliefs, and spirituality are individual, culturally derived, and potentially long-standing beliefs and actions. In a client-therapist relationship, both sides bring unique perspectives to perceived goals and valued outcomes. It is incumbent upon the occupational therapy practitioner to understand and serve the client using their values, beliefs, and spirituality as a motivator in therapy.

Person factors that affect occupational performance also include body structures and function. Body structures include a wide range of microscopic and visible body parts that underlie function. For example, body structures can range from a microscopic red blood cell to the visible hand and wrist. Body functions are the action element of the body parts, such as clotting for red blood cells or movement of the fingers. Impairments in body structure and function can have an impact on the type of occupations chosen, the time spent in preferred occupations, and how and where occupations are performed.

Occupational therapy practitioners can apply different approaches to evaluation and treatment of people with occupational performance dysfunction. For example, you can use a top-down approach by examining and treating only occupation-specific limitations and participation restrictions without significant knowledge of the underlying body structures/function. In contrast, a bottom-up approach implies that the occupational therapist evaluates body structure and function systems first, and then attempts to remediate deficits to enhance occupational performance. In this chapter, we have emphasized an integrated approach where both processes are used to gain a holistic understanding of the client's performance challenges and body structure/function strengths and limitations.

21.14 Summary
- *Person factors* are human abilities, characteristics, and capabilities that support engagement in occupations, and depending on the individual, can be supportive or limiting to occupational performance.
- Person factors include values, beliefs and spirituality that are individualized and culturally derived and should be used to guide the occupational therapy process.
- Cognitive processes, motor skills, sensory abilities, and psychological states are person factors affected by variation in development, acquired injury, or chronic condition.
- Internal body functions such as digesting, breathing, blood oxygenation, urinating, and wound repair are person factors that support quality of life and occupational performance.
- Person factors can be addressed at the individual, group, and population level.
- Optimal occupational performance and participation includes a comprehensive approach to patient factors, occupations, and environments.

21.15 Review Questions
1. What does it mean to say that occupational therapy interventions should ultimately be occupation based and ecologically valid?
2. Describe the differences and similarities between values, beliefs, and spirituality. What role should each play in the occupational therapy process?
3. What is the difference between body structures and function, and how might these both support and limit occupational performance?

4. Review the differences between a top-down, bottom-up, and integrated approach to evaluation and intervention in occupational therapy.
5. How does an integrated approach support optimal occupational performance?

References

American Occupational Therapy Association. (2020). Occupational therapy practice framework: Domain and process (4th ed.). *American Journal of Occupational Therapy, 74*(Suppl. 2), 7412410010p–17412410010p87. https://doi.org/10.5014/ajot.2020.74S2001

American Occupational Therapy Association. (2021). Role of occupational therapy in pain management. *American Journal of Occupational Therapy, 75*(Suppl. 3). https://doi.org/10.5014/ajot.2021.75S3001

American Occupational Therapy Association. (2022). *Ten things patients and providers should question.* https://www.choosingwisely.org/societies/american-occupational-therapy-association-inc/

Amini, D. (2018). Role of occupational therapy in wound management. *American Journal of Occupational Therapy, 72*(Suppl. 2), 7212410057p1–7212410057p9. https://doi.org/10.5014/ajot.2018.72S212

Armstrong, M. J., & Mullins, C. D. (2017). Value assessment at the point of care: Incorporating patient values throughout care delivery and a draft taxonomy of patient values. *Value Health, 20*(2), 292–295. https://doi.org/10.1016/j.jval.2016.11.008

Beagan, B. L., & Etowa, J. B. (2011). The meanings and functions of occupations related to spirituality for African Nova Scotian women. *Journal of Occupational Science, 18*(3), 277–290. https://doi.org/10.1080/14427591.2011.594548

Below, C. P., & Lewis, K. (2021). Visual function intervention. In D. P. Dirette & S. A. Gutman (Eds.), *Occupational therapy for physical dysfunction* (8th ed.). Wolters Kluwer.

Bissell, J. (2015). Occupational therapy for children and youth using sensory integration theory and methods in school-based practice. *American Journal of Occupational Therapy, 69*(Suppl. 3), 6913410040p1–6913410040p20. https://doi.org/10.5014/ajot.2015.696S04

Bondoc, S., & Feretti, A. M. (2018). Physical agents and mechanical modalities. *American Journal of Occupational Therapy, 72*(Suppl. 2), 7212410055p1–7212410055p6. https://doi.org/10.5014/ajot.2018.72S220

Bradshaw, M. (2017). Occupational therapy and complementary health approaches and integrative health. *American Journal of Occupational Therapy, 71*(Suppl. 2), 7112410020p1–7112410020p6. https://doi.org/10.5014/ajot.2017.716S08

Burson, K., Fette, C., & Kannenberg, K. (2017). Mental health promotion, prevention, and intervention in occupational therapy practice. *American Journal of Occupational Therapy, 71*(Suppl. 2), 7112410035p1–7112410035p19. https://doi.org/10.5014/ajot.2017.716S03

Ciro, C. A., Hershey, L. A., & Garrison, D. G. (2013). Enhanced task-oriented training in a person with dementia with Lewy-Bodies. *American Journal of Occupational Therapy, 67*(5), 556–563. https://doi.org/10.5014/ajot.2013.008227

Clark, G. F., Avery-Smith, W., Wolf, L. S., Anthony, P., Holm, S. E., Hertfelder, S. D., & Youngstrom, M. J. (2003). Specialized knowledge and skills in eating and feeding for occupational therapy practice. *American Journal of Occupational Therapy, 57*(6), 660–678. https://doi.org/10.5014/ajot.57.6.660

Crist, P. A. (2015). Framing ecological validity in occupational therapy practice. *Open Journal of Occupational Therapy, 3*(3). https://doi.org/10.15453/2168-6408.1181

Fadyl, J. K. (2020). How can societal culture and values influence health and rehabilitation outcomes? *Expert Review of Pharmacoeconomics & Outcomes Research, 21*(1), 5–8. https://doi.org/10.1080/14737167.2021.1848550

Giles, G. M., Edwards, D. F., Baum, C., Furniss, J., Skidmore, E., Wolf, T., & Leland, N. E. (2020). Making functional cognition a professional priority. *American Journal of Occupational Therapy, 74*(1), 7401090010p1–7401090010p6. https://doi.org/10.5014/ajot.2020.741002

Giles, G. M., Radomski, M. V., Champagne, T., Corcoran, M. A., & Gillen, G. (2013). Cognition, cognitive rehabilitation, and occupational performance. *American Journal of Occupational Therapy, 67*(6), S9–S31. https://doi.org/10.5014/ajot.2013.67S9

Griffiths, J., Caron, C. D., Desrosiers, J., & Thibeault, R. (2007). Defining spirituality and giving meaning to occupation: The perspective of community-dwelling older adults with autonomy loss. *Canadian Journal of Occupational Therapy, 74*(2), 78–90. https://doi.org/10.2182/cjot.06.0016

Gronski, M., & Neville, M. (2017). Vestibular impairment, vestibular rehabilitation, and occupational performance. *American Journal of Occupational Therapy, 71*(Suppl. 2), 7112410055p1–7112410055p13. https://doi.org/10.5014/ajot.2017.716S09

Hubbard, I. J., Parsons, M. W., Neilson, C., & Carey, L. M. (2009). Task-specific training: Evidence for translation to clinical practice. *Occupational Therapy International, 16*(3–4). 175–189. https://doi.org/10.1002/oti.275

Institute of Medicine. (2001). *Crossing the quality chasm: A new health system for the 21st century.* National Academy Press.

Ismael, N., Lawson, L. M., & Hartwell, J. (2018). Relationship between sensory processing and participation in daily occupations for children with autism spectrum disorder: A systematic review of studies that used Dunn's Sensory Processing Framework. *American Journal of Occupational Therapy, 72*(3), 7203205030p1–7203205030p9. https://doi.org/10.5014/ajot.2018.024075

Kielhofner, G. (2008). *The model of human occupation: Theory and application* (4th ed.). Lippincott Williams & Wilkins.

Li, K. Z., & Lindenberger, U. (2002). Relations between aging sensory/sensorimotor and cognitive functions. *Neuroscience & Biobehavioral Reviews, 26*(7), 777–783. https://doi.org/10.1016/S0149-7634(02)00073-8

LSVT Global. (2019). *Lee Silverman Voice Treatment BIG.* https://blog.lsvtglobal.com/research/big-reference/

McColl, M. A. (2000). Muriel Driver Memorial Lecture: Spirit, occupation, and disability. *Canadian Journal of Occupational Therapy, 67*(4), 217–228. https://doi.org/10.1177/000841740006700403

Meriano, C., & Latella, D. (2016). *Occupational therapy interventions: Functions and occupations.* Slack.

Peloquin, S. M. (1993). The patient-therapist relationship: Beliefs that shape care. *American Journal of Occupational Therapy, 47*(10), 935–942. https://doi.org/10.5014/ajot.47.10.935

Pickens, N., Chow, J. K., & McKay, H. (2016). Role of occupational therapy in end-of-life care. *American Journal of Occupational Therapy, 70*, 1–16. https://www.proquest.com/docview/2080984471?pq-origsite=gscholar&fromopenview=true

Rock Steady Boxing. (n.d.). http://rocksteadyboxing.org

Santana, M. J., Manalili, K., Jolley, R. J., Zelinsky, S., Quan, H., & Lu, M. (2018). How to practice person-centred care: A conceptual framework. *Health Expectations, 21*(2), 429–440. https://doi.org/10.1111/hex.12640

Shi, Y., & Hu, M. (2020). Do people's beliefs about their illness affect their engagement in daily routine activities? [Poster session]. *American Journal of Occupational Therapy, 74*(4_Supplement_1), 7411505172p1. https://doi.org/10.5014/ajot.2020.74S1-PO5723

Siebert, C., & Schwartz, J. (2017). Occupational therapy's role in medication management. *American Journal of Occupational Therapy, 71*(S2), 7112410025p1–7112410025p20. https://doi.org/10.5014/ajot.2017.716S02

Turville, M., Carey, L. M., Matyas, T. A., & Blennerhassett, J. (2017). Change in functional arm use is associated with somatosensory skills after sensory retraining poststroke. *American Journal of Occupational Therapy, 71*(3), 7103190070p1–7103190070p9. https://doi.org/10.5014/ajot.2017.024950

World Health Organization. (2001). *International Classification of Functioning, Disability, and Health: ICF.* WHO.

CHAPTER 22

Performance Skills
Motor, Process, and Social Interaction

Karina M. Dancza, Anita Volkert, Karen P. Y. Liu, and Louise Gustafsson

Abstract
Performance skills are the actions that are observable elements of an occupation. Occupational therapists analyze how people carry out their activities, often through observation, with the aim of enhancing their participation and satisfaction in life roles. When observing a person doing an occupation, occupational therapists look at performance skills – the smallest observable actions that people do, regardless of age or ability level. This chapter describes three categories of universal performance skills that are the observable elements within most occupations: motor, process, and social interaction. The chapter provides practical examples of observed occupations for each category of universal performance skills. It then explores how the universal performance skills fit into the three-phase occupational therapy process of evaluation, intervention, and outcome evaluation, using an illustrative example. The chapter emphasizes the importance of performance skills in occupation- and person-centered approaches.

Authors' Positionality Statement
The authors of this chapter have gained experience living and working in different countries, including Australia, Hong Kong, Singapore, and the United Kingdom. We are all female with a university education, and our work experiences have spanned clinical settings, policy roles, and occupational therapy education. Among us, three authors have been influenced by their backgrounds and training in the Assessment of Motor and Process Skills, which may have impacted the writing style of this chapter.

Objectives
This chapter will invite the reader to:

- Understand the importance of performance skills for occupational participation and occupational therapy.

- Describe each universal performance skill within the context of an occupation.
- Understand how performance skills are integrated within the occupational therapy process.

Key terms
- performance skills/universal performance skills
- motor skills
- process skills
- social interaction skills
- occupational performance analysis/occupation analysis/performance analysis

22.1 Introduction

Analyzing occupational performance is fundamental to our work as occupational therapists. By understanding how a person carries out their occupations, we can work together to enhance a person's participation and satisfaction in life roles. When analyzing occupational performance, we often use observations of the person doing an occupation, and it is through these observations that occupational therapists examine a series of discrete, observable, goal-directed actions that are called performance skills.

Performance skills can be collectively categorized as motor, process, or social interaction skills (Fisher & Marterella, 2019; Park et al., 1994). The term "universal performance skills" is often used because they are the smallest observable actions that people do as they undertake their occupations, regardless of age, ability level, or setting. Some occupations also have task-specific skills, such as kicking the ball when playing football. Although these can also be observed, the focus of this chapter is on universal performance skills as these are common to most occupations. Motor skills are how people move themselves and objects around. Process skills refer to how a person organizes objects, space, and time, and modify their actions in response to problems encountered. Finally, social interaction skills refer to how a person interacts with others in the performance of an occupation.

Universal performance skills focus our attention on what to observe so we can gauge how effectively, efficiently, and safely the occupation is carried out. These observations may be guided by using an occupational analysis (American Occupational Therapy Association [AOTA], 2020), an occupation performance analysis (Dancza et al., 2018), or during the conduct of a standardized performance analysis (Fisher & Bray Jones, 2014).

In this chapter, we first describe performance skills and provide definitions and illustrative examples of motor, process, and social interaction skills. Next, we situate performance skills within the occupational therapy process and consider their importance during evaluation (assessment), intervention, and outcome evaluation. Throughout the chapter, we will use illustrations and examples to highlight relevant points and explain how performance skills can be practically incorporated into our occupational therapy process when working with individuals and groups.

22.2 Performance Skills

Performance skills are a way of describing seen actions, and are the smallest observable elements of a person doing an occupation (Fisher & Marterella, 2019). There are universal performance skills that have been developed, described, and included in the *Occupational Therapy Practice Framework: Domain and Process – Fourth Edition* (OTPF-4) (AOTA, 2020). These are part of standardized performance analysis assessments such as the Assessment of Motor and Process Skills (AMPS) (Fisher & Bray Jones, 2012, 2014); the School AMPS (Fisher et al., 2007); and the Evaluation of Social Interaction (ESI) (Fisher & Griswold, 2018).

These universal performance skills can be seen in most daily tasks that involve interaction with objects or social interactions (Fisher & Marterella, 2019). For example, imagine a person picking up a glass of water and drinking it. We can observe the person moving their arm toward the glass (reaches), opening their fingers, wrapping them around the glass with enough force that it does not slip from their hand or break (grips and calibrates), lifting the glass smoothly and carefully to their mouth, and tipping it so they can drink (lifts, flows, and handles).

In this simple scenario, you can see that each step has one or more associated actions that are indicated in the brackets. These actions are the performance skills and are the smallest elements we can see. When they link together (e.g., reaching for the glass, gripping it, and lifting it) they form the steps of the occupational performance. To illustrate this point further, we invite you to consider Table 22.1 where we have given an example

Table 22.1 Steps and Actions When Buying Noodles and Juice from a Street Stall

Steps	*Actions*
Approach the street stall	*Walking* to the street stall
	Standing in front of the street stall
Check the menu	*Searching* for and locating the menu
	Reading the menu
Decide to buy a bowl of noodles and a bottle of juice	*Choosing* the type of noodles and juice
Place the order	*Moving* close to the cashier
	Taking turns including waiting to be first in the queue
	Greeting the cashier
	Speaking to the cashier
	Asking for noodles and juice
	Replying when asked additional questions by the cashier
Paying in cash for the bill	*Looking* at how much to pay
	Choosing enough money from wallet
	Giving out money to the cashier
	Waiting to receive the change
Wait for the order	*Placing self* at an appropriate distance from the queue but remaining close to the stall
	Waiting to be called
Collect the order	*Responding* when order is called
	Walking close to the stall to take the order
	Checking if the order is correct
	Transporting the noodles and juice
	Leaving the street stall
	Finding a place to sit and eat

of identifying the component steps and actions when buying a bowl of noodles and a drink from a street stall. This is a useful activity to try yourself to reinforce the detail of what we are looking for when observing a person doing an occupation.

Motor, process, and social interaction performance skills are considered "universal" as they can be seen in almost all occupational performances (Fisher & Marterella, 2019). It is possible, however, for us to observe other actions that are more specific to certain occupations. For example, if you are working with a child and they prioritize skipping with a rope, you may be observing the task-specific performance skills of *jumping* or *turning* (the rope). These are not listed in the universal performance skills, but they may still be important to your observation. You will also notice in Table 22.1 that we have included both universal and task-specific performance skills in describing how a person might buy noodles and juice from a street stall. If you are new to this form of observation, however, we suggest that you start by becoming familiar with the universal performance skills, which are explained in detail in the next section.

22.3 Motor Skills

Motor skills refer to how we observe the person move themself or objects as they are doing an occupation. We are looking for effective movements that enable the occupational performance and note any areas of awkwardness or increased effort (Fisher & Marterella, 2019). Examples of motor skills include a person *walking* to the bathroom, *reaching* for the door handle to open the door, *gripping* the pants to pull them down, *bending* to sit or squat on the toilet, etc. Table 22.2 lists the 15 universal motor skill items to look out for when observing a person doing a meaningful occupation in their typical setting.

Table 22.2 Motor Skills

Motor skills	*Description (during a task performance)*	*Example (toast with butter and jam)*
Effectively positioning the body		
Stabilizes	Maintain upright sitting or standing position	Stabilize (without propping) at kitchen counter when opening head-height cupboard to get jam jar out
Aligns	Sustain an upright sitting or standing position	Align body upright in a sustained position at kitchen counter when spreading jam on bread
Positions	Position body to facilitate efficient arm movement	Stand or sit on a stool of appropriate height to position self at kitchen counter when preparing toast with butter and jam
Effectively obtaining and holding objects		
Reaches	Extend the arm (and body if required) to grasp or place objects	Reach to grasp a small plate from kitchen cupboard

(Continued)

Table 22.2 (Continued)

Bends	Flex, rotate, or twist the trunk	Bend to move stool to an appropriate position if necessary, and be seated to eat breakfast
Grips	Pinch or grip objects	Grip plastic bag containing sliced bread
Manipulates	Use dexterous grasp and release and finger movements when handling objects	Manipulates plastic bag and small plastic clip/fastening to open plastic bag
Coordinates	Use two or more body parts to stabilize or manipulate objects	Coordinate two hands when getting bread from bag; one holding bag, one reaching in to manipulate bread slices
Effectively moving self and objects		
Moves	Push or pull objects	Move plastic bag of bread to side after getting bread out
Lifts	Raise or lift objects from one place to another	Lift bread slices to place in toaster
Walks	Ambulate on level surfaces	Walk to fridge to get butter out
Transports	Carry objects from one place to another	Transport butter from fridge to countertop
Calibrates	Regulate force and speed when interacting with objects	Calibrate force appropriately when spreading butter on the toasted bread
Flows	Use smooth and fluid arm movement when interacting with objects	Smooth arm movement when spreading jam on toast and butter
Effectively sustaining performance		
Endures	Persist and complete task	Endure and complete toast with butter and jam preparation and consumption

Source: Adapted from OTPF-4 [AOTA, 2020, pp. 43–44]

22.4 Process Skills

Process skills refer to how efficient or organized the person is observed to be as they are doing an occupation. We are looking for how well the person selects and uses required objects, how seamlessly and logically they carry out the steps of the task, and how they modify their performance if they experience problems (Fisher & Marterella, 2019). Examples of process skills include a person *searching for and locating* the knife in the cutlery drawer, *choosing* a knife to cut up a carrot (rather than a spoon), *gathering* the knife and carrot to the chopping board, *organizing* the chopping board and carrot on the work surface so that it is within reach and doesn't fall off the edge, etc. Table 22.3 lists the 20 universal process skill items to look out for when observing a person doing a meaningful occupation in their typical setting.

Table 22.3 Process Skills

Process skills	Description (during a task performance)	Example (supermarket shopping)
Effectively sustaining performance		
Paces (note this is both a motor and a process skill)	Maintain a consistent and effective tempo	Moves through supermarket aisles at a consistent pace to complete task effectively
Attends	Maintain focus	Attends to their shopping list and does not get distracted from task by other items, displays, and noises
Heeds	Action toward carrying out and completing a task	Purchases required items and completes task
Effectively applying knowledge		
Chooses	Select necessary and appropriate tools and materials	Selects shopping basket or trolley in accordance with the amount on shopping list
Uses	Use tools and materials appropriately and reasonably	Uses shopping basket or trolley to carry selected items
Handles	Support and hold tools and materials appropriately	Handles shopping basket or trolley with care, without dropping it or allowing it to roll away
Inquires	Seek information when necessary	Looks for information such as signs on aisles of supermarket shelves or asks staff for items that cannot be found
Effectively organizing timing		
Initiates	Start next action or step without hesitation	Initiates moving to next item on shopping list after one is found
Continues	Perform series of actions without hesitation	Continue to work through shopping list, locating required items
Sequences	Perform steps in practical or logical order	Pick up basket or trolley, start searching for items, proceed to checkout, pack items, pay, leave supermarket
Terminates	Stop next action or step readily and appropriately	Terminates search for item when it is picked up and put in shopping trolley
Effectively organizing space and objects		
Searches/locates	Look for and locate tools and materials in logical manner	Locates all similar items in respective section before moving to another section of supermarket (e.g., fresh vegetables from vegetable aisle)
Gathers	Collect needed tools and materials together	Gather all selected items to be brought to checkout for payment
Organizes	Orderly positioning of tools and materials	Organize items for packing, e.g., heavier items in bag first, all chilled items together, lighter weight/fragile items on top of bag

(Continued)

Table 22.3 (Continued)

Restores	Put away tools and materials or restore workspace	Restore basket or shopping trolley to original place or pick-up point
Navigates	Modify movement patterns around obstacles	Navigate self and shopping trolley to avoid bumping into others
Effectively adapting performance		
Notices/responds	Respond to environment regarding task progression	Notice an available checkout and move to that checkout during payment
Adjusts	Change work environment when a problem arises or to prevent problems from arising	Move items to available checkout
Accommodates	Modify actions or location of objects within workplace when a problem arises or to prevent problems from arising	Change where items are placed in shopping trolley when it is full to put in more items
Benefits	Anticipate and prevent undesirable outcomes	Relocate egg carton from middle of shopping trolley to side when adding large heavy items to basket or trolley

Source: Adapted from OTPF-4 [AOTA, 2020, pp. 44–47]

22.5 Social Interaction Skills

Social interaction skills refer to how effective a person is at doing an occupation that involves interacting with other people. We are looking at how a person engages and communicates with someone else, and if this interaction helps or hinders the performance of the occupation (Fisher & Marterella, 2019). Examples of social interaction skills include a person *turning toward and looking* at a cashier in a food stall, *starting a conversation by saying hello and smiling at the cashier* (*produces speech and gesticulates*), *speaking fluently* as the person asks for a coffee, *taking turns* as the cashier asks what type of coffee they want to buy, *replying* in a *timely way* with their order, etc. Table 22.4 lists the 27 universal social interaction skill items to look out for when observing a person doing a meaningful occupation that includes communicating with others in their typical setting.

One important point to note is that performance skills are *observable* and should not be confused with a body function. This is an important distinction to make as when we observe an action (performance skill), it is because of *many* body functions (like breathing, attention, muscle strength, and memory). To explain this point using our example of drinking water from a glass – we observed the person gripping the glass with enough force so that it did not slip or break (grips and calibrates); however, we did not observe the person's muscle strength which is a body function. We could *assume* that the person had sufficient muscle strength as they were able to pick up the glass, but we cannot see the muscles firing inside the body (Fisher & Griswold, 2019).

Table 22.4 Social Interaction Skills

Social interaction skills	Description (during a task performance)	Example (student group collaborating on a project in an online breakout room – first meeting)
Effectively initiating and terminating social interaction		
Approaches/ starts	Begins a social interaction with a partner in a socially appropriate manner	Starts by saying hello or similar greeting and saying their name and designation
Concludes/ disengages	Effectively ends a social interaction or brings closure to a topic being discussed	Concludes by saying goodbye
Effectively producing social interaction		
Produces speech	Produces spoken, signed, or augmentative messages that can be heard or clearly articulated	Speaks into microphone so others can hear
Gesticulates	Uses socially appropriate gestures that support communication	Waves goodbye at end of meeting
Speaks fluently	Speaks at an appropriate pace	Speaks in full sentences and paragraphs with limited hesitations, connecting words together meaningfully
Effectively physically supporting the social interaction		
Turns toward	Actively positions or turns body or face toward social partner	Positions self in front of camera so that their face is seen clearly on screen
Looks	Makes appropriate eye contact with social partner	Looks at camera to indicate they are making eye contact with social partner
Places self	Positions self at an appropriate location or distance from social partner	Positions in center of camera range so that head and shoulders are in frame
Touches	Responds to and uses touch or bodily contact with social partner in an acceptable way	Not applicable as communication is online
Regulates	Does not demonstrate irrelevant, repetitive, or impulsive behaviors during social interaction	Regulates facial expression and non-verbal body language to maintain sense of interest and connection in what is being said by others
Effectively shaping the content of the social interaction		
Questions	Requests relevant information and asks things that support intended purpose of social interaction	Asks questions to check understanding and progress the group's thinking on the project, "Do we want to approach the task like this, or like that?"

(Continued)

Table 22.4 (Continued)

Replies	Keeps conversation going by responding appropriately	Replies to questions from others to clarify understanding and contribute to group's thinking on the project. "Just to clarify, our hand-in date is…"
Discloses	Shares opinions, feelings, and private information about self or others in a socially acceptable and appropriate way	Discloses worries or concerns about the group's timeline, e.g., if too ambitious, "I'm worried we are trying to do too much in a short time frame"
Expresses emotions	Displays affect and emotions in a socially acceptable way	Expresses fear of failure, "I'm really scared of failing this task."
Disagrees	Expresses differences of opinion in a socially acceptable way	Expresses disagreement with overall direction project is taking. "I don't agree that we should focus on this – I have a different view…"
Thanks	Uses suitable words or gestures to acknowledge receipt of something	Thanks group members for participating, "Thanks everyone for today"

Effectively maintaining the flow of the social interaction

Transitions	Makes or handles changes in topic of conversation appropriately without disrupting social interaction	Transitions smoothly from one topic to the next, "Shall we move on to talking about…"
Times response	Replies to social messages without inappropriate delay or hesitation or interruption to social partner	Responds to others' contributions and questions in an appropriate, timely manner
Times duration	Speaks for a reasonable length of time given the complexity of message	Speaks for an appropriate amount of time when it is their turn
Takes turns	Speaks, in turn, and gives space for others to take their turn	Allows others to speak equally and uses hands up function appropriately

Effectively verbally supporting the social interaction

Matches language	Uses a tone of voice, dialect, level of language that are socially appropriate and acceptable to social partner	Matches language of the group, does not speak simplistically or in too complex language
Clarifies	Notices when a social partner is not understanding the message and makes changes to help them follow the conversation	Clarifies with questions anything unclear or not understood
Acknowledges/ encourages	Responds appropriately to let social partner know they have received the message or to encourage social partner to continue interaction	Responds to others with verbal acknowledgment and encourages development of ideas and/or quieter group members to speak

(Continued)

Table 22.4 (Continued)

Empathizes	Is supportive or understanding of a social partner's feelings or experiences	Empathizes with others' concerns, worries, and fears about the group task
Effectively adapting social interaction		
Heeds	Keeps focused on intended purpose of social interaction	Heeds time and keeps group working to task through the planned hour
Accommodates	Prevents ineffective or socially inappropriate social interaction	Suggests use of chat box when one member loses microphone
Benefits	Prevents problems from happening again	Suggests creation of an instant messaging group between members in case of technology issues

Source: Adapted from OTPF-4 [AOTA, 2020, pp. 47–49]

Another example is when we observe a person searching in the kitchen to locate a bowl and spoon. If they take a long time and open many drawers and cupboards, we may think that it is caused by a memory problem (e.g., they have forgotten where they store their bowl and spoon). However, we cannot observe a memory problem directly; we only see what is happening as they search many places and delay the task to find their bowl and spoon. While it is possible that what we observe is caused by a memory problem, we should keep an open mind and consider other elements that may have contributed. For example, if the person is using a hospital kitchen, they may be unfamiliar with the location of items, or if they have never needed to get their own bowl and spoon before, they may not know where it is kept. It is also possible that a person may have been asked to do a task that is not actually meaningful for them but based on standard practice or the policy of the setting. Therefore, their performance may be impacted by their frustration with the situation.

When you are using performance skills to guide your observations, you are systematically looking at the quality of a person doing an occupation and reporting findings using a common language. Then you can interpret what might be causing that quality of performance, considering multiple elements, including, but not limited to, underlying body functions, the context where the occupation was performed, the complexity of the task, and a wide range of other factors as guided by your chosen professional model (e.g., the Transactional Model of Occupation [Fisher & Marterella, 2019]). To further explain how to use performance skills and interpret what we observe, we need to place this within the occupational therapy process, and this is what we will explore next.

22.6 Performance Skills and the Occupational Therapy Process

There are a range of occupational therapy processes available. Each of them has a specific perspective on how to provide occupational therapy, although there are similarities too. For example, if we look at the OTPF-4 (AOTA, 2020, p. 17), this explains that occupational therapists move through a three-part process when working with people who access their services:

- evaluation
- interventions that are designed to achieve
- targeted outcomes.

Performance skills may feature in each of the three parts, although you may be most familiar using them in assessment (or evaluation) stages, where the priority occupations are identified and an analysis of occupational performance occurs. In the following sections, we consider each part of the occupational therapy process and explore the role and value of performance skills.

22.6.1 Performance Skills and Evaluation

Our work with people who access our services is largely about making and managing changes to enhance their experiences of occupations that contribute to them living their lives. When you begin your occupational therapy process, one of the first things you will do is find out about the person and the occupations that are important to them. When you know what their priority occupations are, doing an observation of those important occupations can enable you to see what is working well and what might require adjustment or change. This is where performance skills can guide how you observe.

Using the performance skills to guide your observation requires practice and critical reflection. To help you make sense of your observations in preparation for intervention, the occupational performance analysis guidance provided in a standardized or non-standardized tool is a useful resource (Dancza et al., 2018; Fisher & Marterella, 2019). In addition, we suggest three ideas we have found helpful.

Try to observe when the person typically does the occupation. For example, if mealtimes are a challenge, then try to observe during a time when the person is typically having their meal (e.g., during lunch). If it is not possible, negotiate with the person the best available time or consider being online or using video recordings if that is more convenient for everyone (adhering to any confidentiality requirements).

The most authentic and helpful place to observe is where the person typically does that occupation. For example, if a child is having challenges doing their schoolwork in class, then observing the classroom would provide the best opportunity for you to understand the contextual influences on the child's performance (e.g., teacher instructions, other children, layout of the classroom, and social expectations). If, however, that is not possible, try to replicate the context as closely as you can to the typical setting. For example, if you are observing a person make a hot drink in a hospital kitchen, find out where items are usually kept in the home kitchen and try to replicate it. While not ideal, it may be the only practical choice you have in your setting, and it can still offer some useful insights.

Keeping all 62 performance skills in mind while you observe the occupation would certainly be a bit much for us as authors and perhaps also a challenge for you. However, we know from our experience that taking good notes during the observation is critical as, despite good intentions, most of us cannot hold all the information in our heads. When taking notes during an observation, perhaps an easier way than trying to note all the performance skills is to record what happens as it happens. Figure 22.1 illustrates

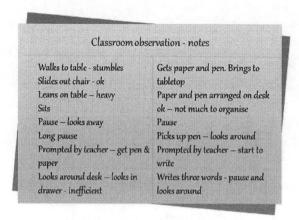

Figure 22.1 Example of observation notes.

how notes may be recorded, but you are likely to find your own way of doing this as you practice.

Once you have observed and gathered your rough notes, the next step is to make sense of them and consider what might be effective as an intervention. To illustrate how we might use our rough notes to make sense of our observations, we would like to share Eva's story.

Eva is a 56-year-old woman who is recovering from a respiratory infection that resulted in an Intensive Care Unit admission and extensive hospital stay. Eva has now returned home and would like to get back to her prior levels of occupational performance. In particular, she would like to reduce her reliance on other people for assistance. Her current focus is on meal preparation.

When we completed our evaluation, we observed Eva prepare and serve canned tomato soup and bread for herself in her own home kitchen. This was a typical meal she liked to eat. As we observed, we carefully noted down what Eva did in the order that she did it.

After the observation and session ended, we used the performance skills descriptions to help us make sense of what we observed. We completed the performance analysis systematically, referring as needed to our rough notes. The areas we thought most impacted Eva's occupational performance are listed in Table 22.5.

Analyzing occupational performance using the performance skills enables us to have a detailed understanding of how Eva performed the occupation. However, it is a complex process that requires practice, reflection, and feedback during supervision to develop. Next, we consider what may be impacting Eva's performance, thinking about personal, occupational, and environmental factors. This helps us to identify what could be a focus for intervention.

22.6.2 Performance Skills and Intervention

Following the steps of the occupational therapy practice process, we next had a discussion with Eva to share the outcomes of the evaluation and obtain her views. During this discussion, we spoke about the performance skills related to obtaining and

Table 22.5 Performance Skill Observations of Note for Eva

Motor performance skills	Observation
Stabilizes	Eva props on kitchen countertop when reaching for plate and bowl in above-head cupboards and when stirring soup.
Reaches	Effortful reach to gather items from cupboards and when placing saucepan on stove.
Bends	Effortful "stiff" bend when retrieving saucepan from cupboard under kitchen countertop.
Grips	Grip slipped when trying to stabilize soup can. Required assistance to open soup can.
Manipulates	Fumbles when using can opener. Fumbles when placing fastening back on bread bag.
Coordinates	Grip slip and fumble when using two hands to open soup tin – required assistance. Fumble when using two hands to place fastening back on bread bag.
Lifts	Slides soup tin along counter rather than lifts.
Endures	Eva voices that she feels tired and sits down several times in dining area adjacent to kitchen. She has some shortness of breath.
Paces	Eva started quickly and then gradually moved more slowly during task.

Process performance skills	Observations
Attends	Not watching saucepan while resting.
Handles	Delay to support saucepan when stirring, sliding on stovetop.
Terminates	Soup boiling to point of starting to boil over.
Notices/responds	Delay in noticing that soup was starting to boil over.

holding objects, moving self and objects, and sustaining performance, providing Eva with examples of how we had observed their impact on her occupational performance. Eva provided her perspectives of the performance and agreed that we had identified the important performance skills.

We then discussed each step and the associated performance skills, identifying how they may have been influencing occupational performance and what could potentially be changed. Together we decided that the soup started to boil over (attends, terminates, notices/responds) because of Eva's reduced endurance and her need to sit down in the dining area, away from the kitchen. We also noted that some of the items she needed were placed in high cupboards. Eva also shared how she would like to return to more complex meal preparation, and was keen to address some of these issues so she could sustain her performance for longer.

Based on the observations and the analysis that was completed together with Eva, the following ideas for intervention were agreed:

- Introduction of a kitchen stool so that Eva could rest for short periods but remain in the kitchen and monitor her cooking. Eva decided she would like to gradually increase her time standing when preparing meals, so she could build up her tolerance and potentially cook more complex meals.

- Rearrange commonly used items in the kitchen to her countertop or lower cupboards so Eva could more effectively reach for what she needed.
- Plan a range of meals that are graded by number of steps, options to take rest breaks during preparation, and effort to prepare, so that Eva can select the type of meal according to her energy levels for that day.

It is important to remember, when determining what is possible to change, that we must work closely with the individual and draw from our professional models (introduced in Chapter 5) and related knowledge to help us understand the multiple elements that contribute to someone doing their occupations. For example, many of our professional models highlight the importance of the person (e.g., priorities, interests, values, routines, and body functions), environment (e.g., social, physical, cultural, historical, political, and economic), occupational elements (e.g., tasks, steps, actions, duration, frequency, purpose, tools, and materials), and the interplay and effect these elements have on a person's occupational performance and participation (Fisher & Marterella, 2019; Liu & Ng, 2008). By considering this wide range of elements that contribute to a person's occupational performance, we can generate multiple possibilities for improving their performance and satisfaction with the activity.

22.6.3 Performance Skills, Monitoring, and Outcomes

Performance skills remain important for ongoing monitoring and outcome evaluation. If we return to the example of Eva, we may follow-up with Eva to ask about her current satisfaction with her performance and if there is anything new that she would like to discuss or work on. We may also want to complete another observation of her performance when cooking. We can then compare her original cooking performance with her performance following intervention and note any areas that are more effective and efficient, or if new challenges are experienced.

It will be important to remember that any improvements in Eva's performance and satisfaction may be the result of changes in several elements, such as Eva's body functions (e.g., her fitness and tolerance have increased for preparing a meal), environmental modifications (e.g., the kitchen is now easier to use with the changes in its organization), or the cooking task (e.g., the steps and complexity of the meal), or a combination.

By using performance skills to observe and analyze the situation, we can monitor the effectiveness of interventions and make necessary adjustments. And while there may be changes in the quality of the performance skills, the main outcome should always be focused on Eva's satisfaction and performance in cooking her meals, which was her original goal. This person-centered approach ensures that we remain focused on the person's goals and needs throughout the process.

22.7 Conclusion

In this chapter, we have described the techniques we use to closely observe a person performing an occupation, using performance skills as our guide. By carefully analyzing what we see, our observations can provide valuable insights that guide our interventions when we are working with someone to make changes to their occupational performance and participation. As occupational therapists, we need to have a thorough understanding of each element and how they interact with each other to form the overall occupational performance, as the combination of these elements is more significant than their individual parts.

22.8 Summary

- Performance skills are the observable actions of occupations; they are not body functions.
- Observations inform occupational therapy practice as they are the foundation assessment of occupational performance.
- Performance skills can be observed during standardized and non-standardized observational assessments.
- Performance skills can guide the development of occupation-centered, personalized interventions.

22.9 Review Questions

1. What value have I placed on performance skills in my experience as an occupational therapy student or practitioner?
2. How do I see observational assessment guided by performance skills being useful in my future practice?
3. What do I already know about doing observational assessments? Are there any new insights I might want to consider, enhancing what I do already? Do I need any development or support to do this?
4. How can I more clearly incorporate performance skills into my observational assessments and reporting?
5. How much do I involve and collaborate with people who access my services when planning what to observe, interpreting the observations, and planning interventions? Is there anything else I could do?

References

American Occupational Therapy Association. (2020). Occupational Therapy Practice Framework: Domain and Process – Fourth Edition. *American Journal of Occupational Therapy, 74*(Supplement_2), 7412410010p7412410011–7412410010p7412410087. https://doi.org/10.5014/ajot.2020.74S2001

Dancza, K., Head, J., & Mesa, S. (2018). Key tools of the occupational therapist: Occupational profiling, activity analysis and occupational performance analysis. In K. Dancza & S. Rodger (Eds.), *Implementing occupation-centred practice: A practical guide for occupational therapy practice learning* (pp. 49–79). Routledge. https://doi.org/10.4324/9781315297415

Fisher, A., & Griswold, L. A. (2019). Performance skills: Implementing performance analysis to evaluate quality of occupational performance. In B. A. Boyt Schell & G. Gillen (Eds.), *Willard and Spackman's occupational therapy* (13th ed., pp. 335–335). Wolters Kluwer.

Fisher, A. G., & Bray Jones, K. (2012). *Assessment of Motor and Process Skills. Vol. 1: Development, standardization, and administration manual* (7th ed.). Three Star Press.

Fisher, A. G., & Bray Jones, K. (2014). *Assessment of Motor and Process Skills. Vol. 2: User manual* (8th ed.). Three Star Press.

Fisher, A. G., Bryze, K., Hume, V., & Griswold, L. A. (2007). *School AMPS: School version of the Assessment of Motor and Process Skills* (2nd ed.). Three Star Press.

Fisher, A. G., & Griswold, L. A. (2018). *Evaluation of social interaction* (4th ed.). Three Star Press.

Fisher, A. G., & Marterella, A. (2019). *Powerful practice: A model for authentic occupational therapy*. Center for Innovative OT Solutions.

Liu, K. P., & Ng, B. F. (2008). Usefulness of the model of human occupation in the Hong Kong Chinese context. *Occupational Therapy in Health Care, 22*(2–3), 25–36. https://doi.org/10.1080/07380570801989333

Park, S., Fisher, A. G., & Velozo, C. A. (1994). Using the Assessment of Motor and Process Skills to compare occupational performance between clinic and home settings. *American Journal of Occupational Therapy, 48*(8), 697–709. https://doi.org/10.5014/ajot.48.8.697

CHAPTER 23

Performance Patterns

Habits, Routines, Rituals, and Roles

Heather Fritz

Abstract
Performance patterns influence the structure, rhythm, and meaning of everyday life as well as the distribution of occupational engagement through time, space, and across social networks. Performance patterns comprise habits, routines, roles, and rituals. Each of those components is influenced by context and all evolve and change across the life course. Together, habits, routines, rituals, and roles have a significant impact on what clients choose to do, how they choose to do, and how those choices contribute to identity, health, and well-being. In this chapter, we unpack the concepts of habits, routines, rituals, and roles. Using examples from the literature, we illustrate how those concepts are socially constructed and how they synergistically shape the form of human doing.

Author's Positionality Statement
The author of this chapter is an occupational therapist and educator with years of professional experience working with diverse clients and colleagues in clinical, community, and higher education settings. While the author has made a concerted effort to include evidence-based, scholarly, inclusive, and culturally intelligent material to embrace a diverse range of perspectives, the content and narrative of this chapter is inherently influenced by the author's geographical location in the United States, a Westernized, developed country. The narrative is also inherently influenced by the author's privileged position as a professionally qualified, European-American, cisgender, English-speaking individual.

Objectives
This chapter will allow the reader to understand:

- How habits develop, function, and support occupation.
- How societal structures shape routines and by extension opportunities for health.

- The role of rituals in occupation and their contribution to transformational experiences.
- How roles are socially constructed and why those constructions are important for occupational identity, engagement, health, and well-being.
- How habits, routines, ritual, and roles synergistically shape occupation, health, and well-being.
- How social inequalities shape habits, routines, rituals, and role to adversely impact health.

Key terms
- habits
- routines
- rituals
- roles
- performance patterns

23.1 Introduction

People do not just "do" – they do in regularly occurring patterns that are shaped by context and provide structure and meaning to their lives. The Occupational Therapy Practice Framework – 4th Edition refers to the habits, routines, rituals, and roles that shape the patterning of human doing as performance patterns (American Occupational Therapy Association, 2020, p. 12). Occupational therapy professionals should use their knowledge of performance patterns and how changes to those patterns can optimize the health and well-being of their clients. Performance patterns, however, are more than simply the sum of their parts, or a sequence of occupations performed in a particular order.

Performance patterns are complex, in part, because habits, routines, rituals, and roles are complex, and each is shaped by and performed in a myriad social and personal context. Even in cases where people share similarities in their performance patterns (e.g., members of a family eat breakfast together every day), each person's pattern comprises different habits of thought and action as well as different routines and rituals, and each person is enacting a differing set of roles. For those reasons, the phrase "performance patterns" is potentially problematic. The phrase is introduced here because of its use in official documents that guide occupational therapy practice in the United States. However, for the remainder of the chapter, the use of the term is avoided as it obfuscates the rich, overlapping, and synergistic interplay of habits, routines, rituals, and roles in everyday life. To illustrate the complex interplay of habits, routines, rituals, and roles, and their impact on occupational engagement, health, and well-being we discuss each concept below, in turn.

23.2 Habits

In this chapter, habits are presented first because habits have been referred to as the building blocks of all thought and action (Dewey, 1957), which by extension suggests habits are the building blocks of occupations. Of course, occupations are not solely the product of habit. It is commonly accepted that human behavior is the product of reflective as well as habitual thoughts and acts (Gawronski & Creighton, 2013). Nonetheless, each of us engages in a range of occupations every day, many of which are executed at least in part by relying on habitual thought and action. How we do and how our doing impacts health and wellness, therefore, has much to do with the constellations of habits that form the basis of our occupational engagement.

23.2.1 Defining Habit

Definitions of habit vary, but there is consensus that habits are behaviors operating largely below conscious awareness that develop over time as individuals repeat behaviors or are repeatedly exposed to thoughts and opinions in similar situations (Gardner, 2015). Numerous books, blogs, and podcasts focus on the topic of habits, and there are even mobile applications that use the scientific principles of habit formation (e.g., focusing on cues, cognitive load, and motivation) to help people change a range of behaviors. Many of those popular media do a commendable job of distilling the science of habit, which allows the public to understand the actions they can take to create or modify habits. Those media, however, fail to address the transactional and significant role of occupation in habit formation and change.

Since behaviors are enacted in the context of occupational performance and participation, occupation can be thought of as the seedbed of habits. When referring to habitual actions, social psychologists refer to "cue-contingent" behavior (Gardner, 2015) because over time a particular situation becomes a "cue" that elicits the habitual response. Stated another way, habit formation can be thought of as a mode of associative learning since cues are "associated" with a particular course of action. The hallmark of cue-contingent behavior is the predictable cause and effect sequence triggered by a particular situation. A situation could refer to a particular place, a sequence of events, or being around a particular person or group of people (Lally & Gardner, 2013).

There are other, numerous examples of cue-contingent behavior each of us experiences during occupational engagement every day. Entering a vehicle may cue someone to put on their seatbelt. Doing oral care may cue someone to take their daily medications. One of the benefits of habit is that because our habits operate largely below conscious awareness, we can function to some degree on autopilot and offload some of the cognitive load associated with our everyday doing. At the same time, since habits operate largely below our awareness, they are difficult to change.

Habits also are considered goal-dependent automatic behaviors (Wood & Neal, 2007), meaning that habits are activated by situational features associated with a goal (Sheeran et al., 2005). For example, many young children learn to lower their voices or whisper when in a place of reverence through observation and reinforcement of the behavior by those around them. There are arguably several possible goals related to why a young child would develop such a habit, including fitting in, being praised by one's parent for exhibiting good behavior, or simply not getting reprimanded for causing a disturbance. The child may not be aware of any of those goals. Parents, however, may be very aware of the desired goals and actively working to shape habits that lead to those goals. In this scenario, the habit of lowering one's voice is a function that develops over time because the situation (social context of such places) is frequently encountered, and the act is supported by social approval of parents and others. Over time, the behavioral response is triggered automatically upon entering the place of reverence.

23.2.2 Habit and the Social Good

In the context of habit formation, it is easy to fall into the trap of attributing value to certain habits. Health care discourse frequently emphasizes the importance of developing good habits and breaking bad habits. A more accurate way to characterize habit is as a "function". A habitual thought or action is enacted in response to a cue and its enactment is in the service of goal achievement. The thoughts/acts themselves are functions, devoid of intrinsic moral value. Any attribution of moral value is merely a social construction. The implications of attributing moral value to a habit are significant. For example, though the dynamics at play in colonization are complex, part of the mechanics of colonization involves colonizers privileging (ascribing a higher moral value) their own habits of thought and action. Evidence of the moral prioritization of habits can be seen as colonizers impose social structures and systems that work to reinforce and reproduce certain habits of thought and action while extinguishing others. An example of this can be seen in the historic use of boarding schools to acculturate indigenous youth. Removing indigenous youth from their familiar context and placing them in boarding schools allowed colonizers to create (and control) situations to foster the development of habits more highly valued by the dominant group (e.g., habits of language, dress, and social behavior). The moral privileging on certain habits over others was an underlying justification for such heinous acts.

While habits may be neither good nor bad, the environments that foster habit formation should be critically examined and judged as to whether they provide equitable possibilities for developing the types of habits that assist individuals in living a satisfying and healthy life, and for offering occupational possibilities. The American Pragmatist philosopher John Dewey contributed much to how contemporary social scientists understand habit. Dewey understood the role of the environment in habit formation and that not all environments were equally rich in terms of the possibilities for habit formation. He also understood that society has a moral responsibility to ensure environmental conditions are equitable so that all people can live well.

> The best we can accomplish for posterity is to transmit unimpaired and with some increment of meaning the environment that makes it possible to maintain the habits of decent and refined life. Our individual habits are links in forming the endless chain of humanity. Their significance depends upon the environment inherited from our forerunners, and it is enhanced as we foresee the fruits of our labors in the world in which our successors live.
>
> *(Dewey, 1957, p. 21)*

Unfortunately, the disparities in infrastructure, schools, opportunities, and social class that informed Dewey's thinking persist today and reduce the opportunities some groups and populations have to develop the habits to maintain a "decent" life. The two images in Figure 23.1 illustrate this point. The habits of thought and action that

PERFORMANCE PATTERNS

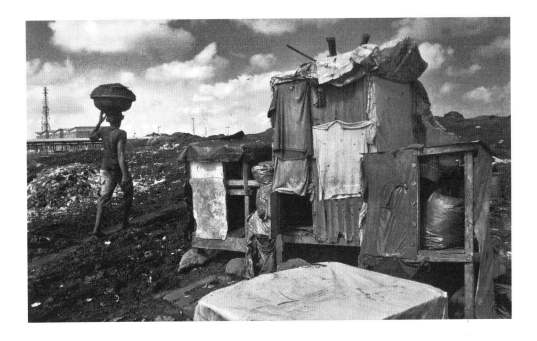

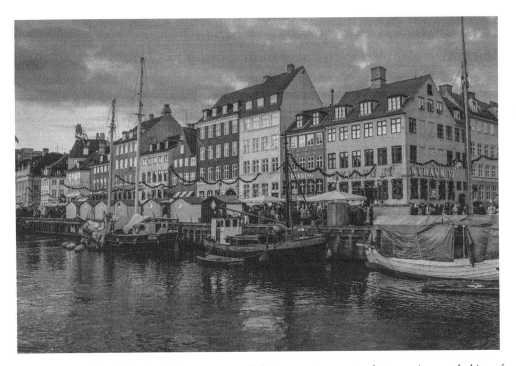

Figure 23.1 Disparities in infrastructure and living environments that can impact habits of thought and action of individuals.

develop in response to living in each of these environments can be expected to differ. Such habits can include habits of thought about oneself and possibilities in life, how one behaves socially, or how one engages in daily occupations (e.g., the motor habits of using outdoor versus indoor toileting facilities).

Based on an understanding of the role of environments on habit formation, occupational therapy professionals should both employ environments in intervention and advocate for the types of environments that foster habits of thought and action that are so fundamental to occupations and a healthy life across the life course. For example, when a practitioner advocates for improved infrastructure (e.g., sidewalks or bike lanes, safe lighting, or public transportation) they are working to create environments that may support habits related to exercise, leisure exploration, or employment, all of which may contribute directly or indirectly to health and well-being.

23.2.3 Extinguishing and Modifying Existing Habits

Occupational therapy professionals can play an important role in assisting individuals in modifying their habits. Doing so may benefit clients in a variety of ways. For example, clinicians may assist individuals in developing healthier "lifestyle" habits such as those related to diet, physical activity, or medication management. They may also help clients develop a host of other habits related to health maintenance, managing instrumental activities of daily living, the maintenance of social relationships, and so on. In practice however, clinicians often find themselves struggling to assist clients with habit formation and modification. One common pitfall that professionals make is to advise clients to simply stop doing something. However, one cannot develop a habit of not doing something.

Another common pitfall is to recommend a different course of action based on the desired health outcome without consideration of the function of the existing habit. Cigarette smoking is a helpful example. The reader should not confuse the concept of habit with addiction. Addictions are more difficult to manage than other behavioral habits due to the physiological dependency involved. However, behaviors at the heart of addiction, such as smoking, serve many functions (e.g., relieves stress and provides a moment for connection with co-workers). Whether the habit of concern is cigarette smoking or the consumption of sugary drinks, the practitioner should first use their skills in activity analysis to understand the function of the habit for the client so they can recommend substitutions that serve a similar function. In the case of smoking, if the primary function is for rapid stress relief, the practitioner could then work with the client toward developing new tobacco-free habits that address the need for rapid stress relief.

When developing new habits, the performance context must remain stable so that the individual has repeated opportunities to act in response to the cue (situation) to develop cue-contingent automaticity. The more stable the environment and the more frequently someone engages in the behavior, the faster a habit will form (Lally et al., 2010). Once established, it is the stability of the environment that allows the habit to be maintained. For those reasons, one of the most effective means of extinguishing a health-hindering habit or creating a new health-promoting habit is to modify the environmental context(s) (Verplanken & Wood, 2006). Modification can be made on micro- or macro-levels (Fritz & Cutchin, 2016). For example, having a client place their walking shoes in front of their couch may cue them to go for a walk before sitting down to relax after dinner.

Similarly, a habit of eating sweets at work could be extinguished if the person refrained from purchasing sweets and bringing them to the office. The change in context (no sweets available) disrupts the established habit. Naturally occurring and significant context changes brought about by serious illness or injury also disrupt daily habits. When practitioners help clients re-engage in daily occupations, they do so in part through helping their clients develop new habits of doing that allow them to function in their situations, which in many cases includes functioning within their changed physical capacities.

Context modifications are one tool to foster habit formation, but they do not guarantee the client will follow through with the behavior. Individuals must also be motivated to engage in the behavior and be able to exercise some degree of reflective control over their behaviors until they develop into habits. Implementation intentions are a proven strategy to aide with habit formation. Implementation intentions are essentially a "if–then" plan that articulates what a person will do in a situation (e.g., "If I want a snack, I will eat piece of cheeses instead of a chocolate bar") (Webb & Sheeran, 2008). The use of implementation intentions places the new course of action on more equal cognitive footing with the default course of action, whereby increasing the likelihood the new behavior is performed.

Habit stacking is a specific form of implementation intention where the individual pairs their new habit to an established habit. Intending to take one's medication while the coffee is brewing is an example of habit stacking. If the coffee-making habit is strong and done daily, then the person is more likely to also take their medications daily since the new medication-taking behavior would be anchored to a well-developed habit. It is important to note that no single approach to habit formation is guaranteed to be successful. Knowledge of how habits develop and their relationship with the environment, however, can assist practitioners in selecting appropriate interventions.

A discussion of habits would be incomplete without noting the interpenetration of habits. Though individuals may be accustomed to thinking of habits as individual behaviors, the behavior or occupation we "see" is the sum of numerous habitual and reflective thoughts and actions. Moreover, each occupation is also connected to other occupations and routines performed at other times of the day. For example, a habit of feeding the family takeaway food on the way home from work is related to other occupations (work, caregiving, shopping) each with its own constellation of habits. Each link in the chain of everyday occupations could be a possible point for intervention; however, knowing which area is best as a point of intervention requires a client-centered approach and an understanding of the functional role of habits in everyday life.

23.3 Routines

The occupational therapy profession has a rich history of attending to the patterning of daily life. For example, one of the most well-known occupational therapy theories, the Model of Human Occupation (MOHO), includes the concept of "habituation", which refers to the processes by which occupations are organized into patterns or routines (Kielhofner, 1980). Performing Salat (the five daily Muslim prayer times), watching a weekly television show, and selling one's crops monthly at the local market are examples of routines occurring on different timescales. However, because routines are both individual and collective and shaped by social structures and public institutions (as well as one's own wants and needs), individuals may vary in the control they have over the patterning of their everyday lives. Existing occupational therapy and occupational science research about routines has tended to focus on how people use their time, how routines are constructed and negotiated, and how the construction of one's routine may help or hinder health.

23.3.1 Time Use

How people use their time may be one of the most underappreciated influences on health and well-being. Most people can relate to feeling stressed because they have too much to do in too little time, or to being bored because they have too much time and nothing satisfying to do with it. How we plan out and use our time is theorized to contribute to one's perception of occupational balance or occupational imbalance. Although those terms are discussed in more depth in Chapter 20, we briefly discuss the concepts here as they relate to time use and daily routines. Occupational balance refers to one's perceived congruence between desired and actual patterns of occupation (Christiansen & Matuska, 2006; Wagman et al., 2012). Occupational imbalance, conversely, describes a state where the type and/or number of occupations and demands are unsatisfactory or overwhelming. Imbalance is believed to contribute to stress, burnout, and distress (Håkansson & Ahlborg, 2018).

What makes for "imbalance" is complicated, however. For some, it is the types of activities; for others, imbalance involves the number of activities; and in most cases, we presume the meaning of the activities that make up one's routine matter for balance. For instance, a study of 100 Swedish women who worked outside of the home examined the degree to which women had to shift between different types of occupations. Study results showed increasing routine complexity (defined as the frequency of shifting between categories of occupation) was associated with lower levels of self-rated health (Erlandsson & Eklund, 2006). The type and number of activities alone, however, do not fully explain how routines influence our sense of balance, health, and well-being. The meaning of the activities we engage in is equally important. It is possible someone could have a very complex routine, but if the activities and tasks that make up the routine are enjoyable and exciting, the individual may not experience burnout. Conversely, a less complex routine comprises unstimulating activities may lead to feelings of boredom and restlessness (Marshall et al., 2020).

23.3.2 Construction and Negotiation of Routines

As previously noted, though it is tempting to believe individuals have control over the construction of their own routines, all of us are tied to others either through kin, friendships, social networks, roles, and occupations. Our embeddedness in social networks and society at large means that routines are often a product of negotiation with and among other people. Families make an interesting case study for examining the intersection of individual and communal routines. Family routines have been considered in various ways (see Fiese, 2006) but can generally be defined as the sequences of occupations or activities that family members engage in. Though the form and meaning of participation may vary across family members, there is some shared component of experience. The literature on family routines is often focused on families of children with illness, disability, or injury. Those studies, however, provide important information about how routines are constructed and negotiated in the context of what are often very different abilities, preferences, and roles.

For example, while many individuals with Autism prefer structure in the form of daily routines, their desired structure may look very different to the desired structure of other members of their family. Specifically, some individuals with Autism may prefer to invest significant amounts of time in a narrow range of activities, which may make participation in more numerous, varied, and spontaneous routines more difficult for the rest of the family (Boyd et al., 2014). The sensory needs of individuals with Autism may also shape family routines as some activities, such as a trip to a crowded market, may be exciting for one member of the family and over-stimulating for another.

The social and economic situation of families and communities may also shape how routines are negotiated. Families who live in remote or impoverished areas with underdeveloped infrastructure may need to allocate most of their time to survival-related occupations such as harvesting or hunting food or searching out sources of clean water. Millions of children also engage in child-labor each year working in industries such as cacao production. In such cases, the imbalance of time spent in survival or work-related occupations decreases the time available to allocate to education, play, and leisure; taken-for-granted components of a weekly routine for many families in Westernized societies.

23.3.3 Changes in Routines Are Related to Changes in Habits

Routines change across the life course as individuals grow older, roles change, etc. Unexpected or dramatic changes in routines may pose unique challenges and opportunities, especially for health management occupations. In terms of challenges, since habits are cue-contingent behaviors, changes to a routine can disrupt existing cue-behavior associations thereby rendering established habits ineffective (Fritz, 2014), an undesirable result if the established habits supported health. An area of occupation that has significant implications for health and well-being is the area of work. The extensive literature on shift work and health provides insights into how changes in one's work routine impact health and well-being. For example, frequent changes in shifts worked are associated with worse health across almost every domain, including dietary quality, time spent in physical activity, sleep patterns, and mental health outcomes (Silva et al., 2020). One reason shift work is thought to have an ill-effect on health is because when one's routine frequently changes, it makes it difficult to develop or sustain health-promoting habits.

Another way one's routine can impact health is the degree to which the routine aligns with or disrupts ones' circadian rhythm. Circadian rhythms vary within a population and across age groups. For example, teenagers experience later signaling of wakefulness and alertness during the day than adults or young children. An individual's preferred timing of sleep and activity is referred to as their "chronotype". When we refer to people as "night owls" or "early birds" we are referring to chronotypes. A mismatch between one's chronotype and daily patterning of activity increases the risk for the development of neurologic, psychiatric, cardiometabolic, and immune disorders (Fishbein et al., 2021). Further complicating the matter, diseases, conditions, and medication may also disrupt circadian rhythms (Fishbein et al., 2021). Though a practitioner may not be able to address the impact of disease on circadian rhythm, they can suggest plausible modifications to behaviors and environment to bring one's daily routine and chronotype into better alignment.

Since the stability of one's routine is connected to one's habits, it is important to also note that not all people have the same level of control over their daily or weekly routines. Individuals differ in the occupations available to them and which make up their routines, as well as how much control they have over the patterning of occupations. A white-collar worker in the technology industry may have the ability, because of their profession, education level, and job prospects, to negotiate the ability to work at home and set their own schedule if projects get completed on time. A migrant worker employed in construction would likely not have such control and autonomy. Moreover, they may be expected to work very long hours in unsafe conditions, and because of their socioeconomic position or legal status, may feel powerless to advocate for a more stable and time-balanced routine. At the individual or family level, understanding the significance of routines to habit formation, health, and well-being can assist the occupational therapy professional in analyzing their client's routines and making recommendations for more health-promoting activity patterns. At the group, community, or population level, it is important for practitioners to understand how social institutions, policies, and practices provide different opportunities for the construction and control of routines. Understanding those dynamics, and their implications for inequality, would inform professional advocacy efforts.

23.4 Rituals

Rituals are defined as "symbolic actions with spiritual, cultural, or social meaning, the frequency and consistency of which vary greatly" (American Occupational Therapy Association, 2020, p. 12). Rituals are often the source of cultural transmission, be it through types that unite kin and close friends, such as holiday dinners; or those that mark major life events, such as birth and coming of age celebrations (e.g., baptisms, bar mitzvah, and quinceañeras), weddings, and funerals; or those that serve to preserve and pass on religious traditions. People are born into existing cultural milieus that shape us from the start – culture has us before we have it (Garrison, 2002) – therefore rituals also contribute to individual and shared identity in powerful ways.

23.4.1 Ritual as Re-working the Everyday

In his essay about the movie *The Feast*, which features the Yanomami tribe in Brazil, Moore (1996) presents an analysis of the video footage from the perspective that ritual is simply "the reworking of everyday events" (p. 6). The analysis focuses on a feast between neighboring tribes which is intended to promote an alliance. Moore identifies key dimensions of the ritual, namely, getting ready (where tribesmen clean the gathering hall and prepare food, and where members of the tribe paint and adorn their bodies), receiving the guests (when the neighboring tribes people enter), and talking and trading (which occurs after the feast). As Moore continues his analysis, he illustrates how each phase of the ritual comprises activities that are also done in everyday life (e.g., cleaning house, dressing, and eating) but that are "re-worked" in the context of ritual.

Reflecting on Moore's essay, it is easy to apply his argument to other rituals more familiar to readers such as weddings, funerals, and celebrations of religious or cultural holidays. Across cultures, those celebrations, while greatly varied, also include elements of the everyday, which are re-worked due to the symbolic meaning of the ritual. For example, it is not uncommon for a Hindi woman to wear a sari during everyday activities, but the type of saris or lehenga worn at one's wedding is typically more ornate to signal the significance of the occasion. Before hosting a Hanukkah, Christmas, or Karamu dinner hosts also typically engage in cleaning the home (or arrange to have others perform the task), preparing food, and donning festive attire. However, each of those activities is conducted differently to the everyday. Cleaning is likely deeper, food preparation likely involves special ingredients or complicated dishes, and dress may be more formal or festive than what one would typically wear on a Wednesday evening for dinner with the family. Such rituals also often differ from their everyday counterparts because of the individuals included. For example, during Iftar, the meal served at the end of the day during Ramadan to break the day's fast, it is common to invite less fortunate members of the community to one's table. Though eating breakfast may be a typical activity, and though an Iftar meal may include some typical breakfast foods, the makeup of those sharing in the meal may greatly differ from the everyday. These transformations of aspects of the everyday are what is special about ritual from an occupation perspective.

23.4.2 Ritual as Transformative

The International Classification of Functioning, Disability and Health defines participation as involvement in life situations (World Health Organization, 2001). Because rituals are special in terms of how one engages in what would otherwise be everyday activities (e.g., eating, dressing, and spending time with friends), the participation dimensions of rituals may be especially important to health, well-being, and one's sense of self and life coherence. Rituals often serve as a means through which individuals, families, groups, communities, and populations transform or transition among states more quickly than could be achieved otherwise. Thus, many rituals are performed with the explicit intention that performance will lead to some positive new state, however temporary.

Transformation through ritual may take many forms such as from states of solitariness to togetherness, from enemies to allies (as in the above example from The Feast), or from states of distress to ones of peace. For example, the form, function, and meaning of the Jewish Sabbath is for individuals and families to transition from the busyness, stress, and distraction of daily life to a state of respite, relationship, and community (Smith-Gabai & Ludwig, 2011). The ceremonial lighting of the Sabbath candles marks the transition to a more calm and peaceful state. The form of the Sabbath, which includes attendance at religious services, communal meals, and, perhaps most importantly, a lengthy list of occupations one is prohibited from engaging in during the Sabbath, serve to further ensure the time and space to transform to a state of calm, community, and introspection.

The above examples illustrate the enduring importance of ritual as it is transmitted across generations. Although rituals tend to stand the test of time, that is not to say that rituals remain static. Rituals continually evolve in form though the meaning and function may remain intact. The work of Shordike and Pierce (2005) on Christmas traditions in Kentucky, United States, provides an example of how rituals are adapted to new contexts. For example, women in the study discussed how Christmas traditions were adapted due to a range of factors, including death of elders, deteriorating health, special dietary needs, or geographic relocation (Shordike & Pierce, 2005). While the form of the Christmas meal may change over the years, the intentions of the ritual (e.g., religious observance and familiar bonding) remained salient. Rituals as occupational and transformational experiences are part of the human condition and its restoration.

23.4.3 When the Everyday Becomes Ritual

The emphasis on hallmark cultural rituals may distract from the everyday work of ritual making that occurs across the life course. At any stage of life, mundane everyday activities can be elevated to the role of ritual. For example, when a person dedicates extra time to make a bath and uses special bath care products, lights a candle, and reads a book in the tub rather than taking a quick shower, they are elevating the everyday to ritual. Though important across the life course, rituals may be especially important for those suffering from terminal illness (Pace & Mobley, 2016).

A case example from a client with advanced cancer serves to further illustrate this point. The client was seen by an occupational therapist during her inpatient treatment for a recurrence of an aggressive form of breast cancer. During the initial evaluation the client discussed the activities that were most important for her to participate in given her symptoms and prognosis. The client shared how important it was for her to maintain the ability to make a cup of tea each day. This client had been drinking tea her whole life and had never given the act much thought. However, in the context of illness, the act became ritual. She used a special tea set, one that was given to her by her sister many years ago. Though she had previously viewed the tea set as little more than a decorative item, finding it too "fussy" for daily use, she now took great care in preparing the tea, steeping it in the pot, and pouring it into tiny, ornately painted cups. She then took two tiny cups of tea out onto the back porch and offered one to her husband while they sat together to read the news and watch the birds.

In the above example, making of tea became imbued with new meaning. For the client, it was symbolic of what she still could do. She still had enough endurance and mobility to stand and make a cup of tea, and to manipulate all the components. The tea set served to connect her to her sister, who had died of breast cancer a few years earlier. The time on the porch with her husband was peaceful, a time to simply "be" and escape from the rigors of her treatment and thoughts of her prognosis.

Culturally significant and personally significant forms of ritual are both embedded in occupation. The form and meaning of rituals may be different than the everyday counterpart. As such, rituals contribute in a significant way to one's sense of self and sense of belonging in society. Understanding the significance of rituals assists the occupational therapy professional in identifying the most meaningful interventions to enhance health and well-being across the life course.

23.5 Roles

The Occupational Therapy Practice Framework – 4th Edition (American Occupational Therapy Association, 2020) defines roles as "behaviors that are shaped and defined by society, culture, context, as well as by the individuals, group or populations that embody or inhabit those roles" (p. 12). Roles are important to human doing because people engage in occupations in relation to their roles. As such, roles contribute to one's occupational identity. Multiple role theories exist, and while those theories may be informed by perspectives ranging from symbolic interactionism to organizational or cognitive social psychology, they are all concerned with how humans become socialized to assume certain roles and, along with those roles, the associated norms and expectations of behavior. Within the context of role theory, roles are seen as a necessary part of communal life as role conformity fosters social integration and maintenance of the social order (Jackson, 1998).

Despite the importance of roles to our behaviors, life choices, and occupational identities, as with habits, many of us become enculturated into roles and associated behavioral norms and expectations before we even become aware of it. A variety of structures, institutions, and traditions work in tandem to shape and reinforce what we come to see as "normal" and "appropriate". In many cases, our ideas about normative or expected behaviors, occupations, and roles are based on factors such as gender, age, racial background, religious orientation, or socioeconomic position. The same institutions, structures, and traditions that shape ideas about roles also serve to reproduce the social order, including norms and expectations. One such example is how religious institutions shape ideas about gender roles. Common understandings of Christian religious texts emphasize a woman's role as submissive, subservient, and focused on children and the household. Such ideas about gender norms are further reproduced when religious traditions disallow women to hold positions of authority as religious leaders.

Social reproduction is a concept which has origins in the work of Karl Marx (see Marx & Levitsky, 1965), but which has been a topic of interest to scholars in the social sciences for decades. Social reproduction refers to how social structures and systems are reproduced through a variety of mechanisms. Examples of social structures include families, religious groups, laws, and economic policies, whereas social systems refer to the systems (e.g., educational system, political system, and economic systems) in which structures are embedded. Together, structures and systems determine societal norms, and those norms are inextricably tied to roles. From the perspective of social reproduction, families might reproduce societally normative and expected gender roles by encouraging a little girl to play pretend in a toy kitchen while encouraging a little boy to play outside with a football. Obviously, such norms and expectations are eventually challenged and change with time, but they are enacted through social reproduction regardless, and within the performance of occupations (i.e., play). Roles and norms apply to all aspects of human doing, from what we do, to how we do it, to the outward symbols of role identification such as speech, attire, and so on.

It is important for the occupational therapy professional to understand the origin and evolution of roles because many of the challenges that clients face stem from how individuals balance, embody, resist, and adapt (or not) to expected societal roles and norms. For example, role imbalance is a known contributor to poor health and absenteeism in Western societies. Role balance refers to one's perception of the balance among their differing life roles (Marks, 2009) and is dynamic because a variety of factors impact one's perception of balance at any given time. For example, Evans et al. (2014) posit several key dynamics in their Model of Juggling Occupations that influence perceptions of role balance, including *between-role balance* (the degree to which one's occupational choices result in satisfying roles); *between-role enrichment* (e.g., the degree to which positive experiences within one role buffer negative experiences within another, or vice versa); and *between-role conflict* (e.g., stress that arises due to time demands or behavioral requirements of key roles).

Drawing on the Model of Juggling Occupations (Evans et al., 2014) a client could perceive positive role balance if they were having consistently positive experiences at work, despite challenging circumstances associated with a parenting role (between-role enrichment). However, a change in work schedule could tip the balance and lead to negative perceptions of balance overall due to increased role conflict (e.g., needing to spend more time in a worker role, which detracts from a parenting role). Further complicating the matter, the number and types of roles one embodies is inherently tied to a range of occupations they are expected to engage in, the totality of which may or may not be realistic. For example, in many Western cultures, there is high value placed on productivity and business, which can contribute to role overload.

Regardless of role balance or imbalance, some individuals may also experience distress because the roles they choose to fulfill, or the way they enact roles, runs counter to the normative expectations of the dominant group. For example, in the United States parenting roles have traditionally been closely tied to gender roles. As such, a traditional viewpoint could be that a normative parental unit includes a man and a woman, each with gender-normative roles in the parenting relationship. It might be expected that a mother cooks, arranges the family's schedule, and attends parent–teacher conferences, while the father faces less societal pressure to manage domestic life. In this context, a trans-female, lesbian couple may choose to adopt a child and may parent the child effectively, but encounter oppression, violence, or bigotry because others in society view their form of role enactment as outside of accepted norms of behavior.

Using another example, in 2016 Colin Kaepernik, an American professional football player in the National Football League, chose to kneel during the American national anthem, when it was customary to stand at attention as a show of nationalism. The gesture was made to protest police brutality and racial inequality in the United States. As part of the discourse that ensued, some segments of the population proposed that professional athletes should not engage in openly political acts. In essence, the argument suggested a professional athlete had role boundaries that excluded public displays of political activism.

Some of our most divisive social issues and significant social movements in contemporary society have at their root the issue of normative expectations and beliefs about roles. Societies change over time as individuals and groups resist and reinterpret roles. Roles contribute to a person's occupational identity and, as such, those who resist conventional role assignments or reinterpret what occupations are associated with their roles may face significant social stigma, which, in turn, could adversely affect emotional health and role satisfaction. It is important for the occupational therapy professional to understand how a client is constructing their identity through their occupations to support them in balancing and enacting roles in a way that promotes health and well-being. Since roles are a product of social processes, practitioners should also be mindful of their role as advocates for those who do not conform (either through choice or circumstance) to conventional roles.

23.6 Conclusion

In this chapter, we discussed how habits, routines, rituals, and roles create structure, give meaning to everyday life, and support human occupation. Habits are both a product of occupation and a building block of future occupational performance. Our habits of thought and action are interconnected with how we use our time. Habits of thought about what acceptable time use is influences one's routines. How stable or unstable one routine is, and how daily activities are distributed through time and space, influence the types of environments we are exposed to and, by extension, what habits develop. The relationship between habits and routines is, therefore, transactional and iterative. Habits and routines are intimately connected to roles and rituals. For example, rituals provide a reprieve from the mundane daily or weekly routine when we take everyday activities and enact them with special care. Habits, routines, and rituals are shaped by our roles and associated normative expectations about what roles one should take on and the occupations associated with those roles.

Each of those components of performance patterns is inextricably shaped by environing conditions, including social structures and systems. Taken together, those understandings allow the occupational therapy professional to identify root causes of occupational dysfunction and propose effective treatments. A deeper understanding of how social conditions shape the development of habits, routines, rituals, and roles, however, allows the practitioner to view the conditions that contribute to their development as an equally important target of intervention and professional advocacy.

23.7 Summary

- The patterning of everyday life influences occupational engagement, health, and well-being.
- Habits are formed in the context of occupational engagement and contribute to how occupations affect health and well-being.
- Habits develop in response to environmental conditions and cues, and help people to function within those environments.
- How we structure our routines contributes to health and well-being, yet not all people have the same level of control over how they structure their time.
- Routines and habits are connected as existing routines can support habit formation and changes to routines tend to disrupt one's habits.
- Rituals can be thought of as everyday activities that are elevated to the status of ritual because of the meaning attributed to them and how they are performed.
- Roles and how one fulfills one's roles are shaped by one's sociocultural context and expectations for normative behavior.

23.8 Review Questions

1. How are habits formed?
2. How do habits allow a client to function within a particular environment?

3. How does society influence the construction of an individual's routine?
4. How are rituals different from everyday occupations?
5. How do roles contribute to occupational identity?

References

American Occupational Therapy Association. (2020). Occupational therapy practice framework: Domain and process (4th ed.). *American Journal of Occupational Therapy, 74*(Suppl. 2), 7412410010p1–7412410010p87. https://doi.org/10.5014/ajot.2020.74S2001

Boyd, B. A., McCarty, C. H., & Sethi, C. (2014). Families of children with autism: A synthesis of family routines literature. *Journal of Occupational Science, 21*(3), 322–333. https://doi.org/10.1080/14427591.2014.908816

Christiansen, C. H., & Matuska, K. M. (2006). Lifestyle balance: A review of concepts and research. *Journal of Occupational Science, 13*(1), 49–61. https://doi.org/10.1080/14427591.2006.9686570

Dewey, J. (1957). *Human nature and conduct: An introduction to social psychology*. The Modern Library. (Original work published in 1922.)

Erlandsson, L. K., & Eklund, M. (2006). Levels of complexity in patterns of daily occupations: Relationship to women's well-being. *Journal of Occupational Science, 13*(1), 27–36. https://doi.org/10.1080/14427591.2006.9686568

Evans, K. L., Millsteed, J., Richmond, J. E., Falkmer, M., Falkmer, T., & Girdler, S. J. (2014). The complexity of role balance: support for the Model of Juggling Occupations. *Scandinavian Journal of Occupational Therapy, 21*(5), 334–347. https://doi.org/10.3109/11038128.2014.902988

Fiese, B. H. (2006). *Family routines and rituals*. Yale University Press.

Fishbein, A. B., Knutson, K. L., & Zee, P. C. (2021). Circadian disruption and human health. *Journal of Clinical Investigation, 131*(19), e148286. https://doi.org/10.1172/JCI148286

Fritz, H. (2014). The influence of routines on engagement in diabetes self-management. *Scandinavian Journal of Occupational Therapy, 21*(3), 232–240. https://doi.org/10.3109/11038128.2013.868033

Fritz, H., & Cutchin, M. P. (2016). Integrating the science of habit: Opportunities for occupational therapy. *OTJR: Occupation, Participation and Health, 36*(2), 92–98. https://doi.org/10.1177/1539449216643307

Gardner, B. (2015). A review and analysis of the use of 'habit' in understanding, predicting and influencing health-related behaviour. *Health Psychology Review, 9*(3), 277–295. https://doi.org/10.1080/17437199.2013.876238

Garrison, J. W. (2002). Habits as social tools in context. *OTJR: Occupation, Participation and Health, 22*(1_suppl), 11S–17S. https://doi.org/10.1177/15394492020220S103

Gawronski, B., & Creighton, L. (2013). Dual process theories. In D. E. Carlston (Ed.), *The Oxford handbook of social cognition* (pp. 282–311). Oxford University Press. https://doi.org/10.1093/oxfordhb/9780199730018.013.0014

Håkansson, C., & Ahlborg, G. (2018). Occupational imbalance and the role of perceived stress in predicting stress-related disorders. *Scandinavian Journal of Occupational Therapy, 25*(4), 278–287. https://doi.org/10.1080/11038128.2017.1298666

Jackson, J. (1998). Contemporary criticisms of role theory. *Journal of Occupational Science, 5*(2), 49–55. https://doi.org/10.1080/14427591.1998.9686433

Kielhofner, G. (1980). A Model of Human Occupation, part 2. Ontogenesis from the perspective of temporal adaptation. *American Journal of Occupational Therapy, 34*(10), 657–663. https://doi.org/10.5014/ajot.34.10.657

Lally, P., & Gardner, B. (2013). Promoting habit formation. *Health Psychology Review, 7*(Suppl. 1), S137–S158. https://doi.org/10.1080/17437199.2011.603640

Lally, P., Jaarsveld, C., Potts, H., & Wardle, J. (2010). How are habits formed: Modelling habit formation in the real world. *European Journal of Social Psychology, 40*(6), 998–1009. https://doi.org/10.1002/ejsp.674

Marks, S. (2009). Multiple roles and life balance: An intellectual journey. In K. Matuska & C. Christiansen (Eds.), *Life balance: Multidisciplinary theories and research* (pp. 43–58). SLACK.

Marshall, C. A., Roy, L., Becker, A., Nguyen, M., Barbic, S., Tjörnstrand, C., Gewurtz, R., & Wickett, S. (2020). Boredom and homelessness: A scoping review. *Journal of Occupational Science, 27*(1), 107–124. https://doi.org/10.1080/14427591.2019.1595095

Marx, K., & Levitsky, S. L. (1965). *Das Kapital: A critique of political economy*. H. Regnery.

Moore, A. (1996). Feasting as occupation: The emergence of ritual from everyday activities. *Journal of Occupational Science, 3*(1), 5–15. https://doi.org/10.1080/14427591.1996.9686403

Pace, J. C., & Mobley, T. S. (2016). Rituals at end-of-life. *Nursing Clinics, 51*(3), 471–487. https://doi.org/10.1016/j.cnur.2016.05.004

Sheeran, P., Aarts, H., Custers, R., Rivis, A., Webb, T. L., & Cooke, R. (2005). The goal-dependent automaticity of drinking habits. *British Journal of Social Psychology, 44*(1), 47–63. https://doi.org/10.1348/014466604X23446

Shordike, A., & Pierce, D. (2005). Cooking up Christmas in Kentucky: Occupation and tradition in the stream of time. *Journal of Occupational Science, 12*(3), 140–148. https://doi.org/10.1080/14427591.2005.9686557

Silva, A., Silva, A., Duarte, J., & da Costa, J. T. (2020). Shift-work: A review of the health consequences. *International Journal of Occupational and Environmental Safety, 4*(2), 48–79. https://doi.org/10.24840/2184-0954_004.002_0005

Smith-Gabai, H., & Ludwig, F. (2011). Observing the Jewish Sabbath: A meaningful restorative ritual for modern times. *Journal of Occupational Science, 18*(4), 347–355. https://doi.org/10.1080/14427591.2011.595891

Verplanken, B., & Wood, W. (2006). Interventions to break and create consumer habits. *American Marketing Association, 25*, 90–103. https://doi.org/10.1509/jppm.25.1.90

Wagman, P., Håkansson, C., & Björklund, A. (2012). Occupational balance as used in occupational therapy: A concept analysis. *Scandinavian Journal of Occupational Therapy, 19*(4), 322–327. https://doi.org/10.3109/11038128.2011.596219

Webb, T. L., & Sheeran, P. (2008). Mechanisms of implementation intention effects: The role of goal intentions, self-efficacy, and accessibility of plan components. *British Journal of Social Psychology, 47*(3), 373–395. https://doi.org/10.1348/014466607X267010

Wood, W., & Neal, D. T. (2007). A new look at habits and the habit-goal interface. *Psychological Review, 114*(4), 843–863. https://doi.org/10.1037/0033-295X.114.4.843

World Health Organization. (2001). *International classification of functioning, disability and health*. https://www.who.int/standards/classifications/international-classification-of-functioning-disability-and-health

CHAPTER 24

Evolving and Pluralistic

Understanding the Environment in Occupational Therapy

Tammy Aplin, Ana Paula Serrata-Malfitano, and Tim Barlott

Abstract
This chapter provides an overview of the evolving and pluralistic nature of the environment in occupational therapy. A historical perspective is used to examine the profession's changing understanding of the environment. A range of theories and models influencing the profession's conceptualizations is presented, including person-environment fit; ecological theories; the International Classification of Functioning, Disability and Health; social determinants and determination of health; rights-based approaches; community and territory; and Indigenous knowledge. The chapter concludes by examining how occupational therapy models view the environment from a transactive, interactional, or non-Western viewpoint. Overall, the chapter points to the significance of taking a contextually based approach to practice.

Authors' Positionality Statement
We represent a group of occupational therapists who have worked with clients, families, and communities as well as being educators and researchers. Our histories and experiences are from Australia, Brazil, and Canada, and we recognize that our positionality from these contexts influences the chapter presented, through different theories, vocabularies, and histories. Ana (Portuguese-speaking), Tim, and Tammy (English-speaking) are cis-gendered, white, and economically privileged. Ana and Tammy are the first in their families to be university educated. Tim lives in Amiskwacîwâskahikan (also known as Edmonton, Canada), which is part of Treaty 6 and the traditional and ancestral territory of the Nehiyawak (Cree), Dene, Blackfoot, Saulteaux, Nakota Sioux, a diversity First Nations, and also the home to the Métis people. Tammy lives and works in Brisbane, Queensland, Australia, on the unceded lands of the Turrbal and Jagera people. Ana lives in São Carlos, in the Brazilian countryside, where unfortunately there are no known historical registers about the First Nations' communities who used to live in this region. We acknowledge that our social locations have afforded us opportunities

to thrive in life, and our work seeks to be critical of social forces in crafting a more affirming world for and with marginalized people.

In the process of drafting this chapter, we have made a concerted effort to include evidence-based, scholarly, inclusive, culturally sensitive, gender-affirmative material in an attempt to embrace a diverse range of perspectives. However, we acknowledge that the contents of this chapter are not exhaustive, completely bias-free, or representative of every cultural, racial, gender, economic, political, or social reality. We hope that this text can foster critical, inclusive, respectful, and progressive debate among current and future occupational therapists, nationally and internationally.

> **Objectives**
> This chapter will provide readers with:
>
> - A historical context of occupational therapy's understanding of the environment.
> - An overview of how the environment is understood from a range of occupational therapy and guiding models and frameworks.
> - A broad understanding of the environment from a range of worldviews.
> - An understanding of the key elements of the environment as described in the OTPF-4.

> **Key terms**
> - environment
> - context
> - ecology
> - human rights
> - community
> - territory
> - decolonization
> - social determinants and determination of health
> - Indigenous knowledge

24.1 Introduction

Since the inception of occupational therapy, the environment has been a core construct informing our knowledge and practice. The profession's understanding of the environment is influenced and situated within our historical and cultural context and continues to evolve. This chapter presents a range of perspectives on the environment to provide an overview and initiate discussion on the pluralistic nature of the environment in occupational therapy. In using the term "pluralistic", we mean that the environment can be understood in many ways and that these can co-exist at the same time. The chapter begins by presenting the historical context of occupational therapy and the implications of this history on the profession's epistemology relating to the environment. Epistemology refers to the theory of knowledge or how we know and understand concepts and theories (Hooper, 2006), and in this chapter, we will examine how our ways of knowing evolved and continue to develop in different ways, informed by different theoretical backgrounds. Following this historical discussion key models and theories outside of occupational therapy theory are presented to provide a broad understanding of the many perspectives of the environment that have shaped, and continue to shape, our epistemology or understanding of the environment. Following this, key occupational therapy models are discussed in relation to how they conceptualize the environment as transactional, interactional, or outside the predominant theoretical discussions in occupational therapy from Anglo-Saxon or Western worldviews.

In this chapter, we refer to Western worldviews as those that stem from Western European culture rather than specific nations, although this would describe the dominant culture in nations such as the United States, Australia, the United Kingdom, and many nations in the European Union (Khan et al., 2022). We have intentionally used Western to acknowledge the dominance that the West has over other nations and cultures, including through processes of colonization, economic exploitation, and affiliation to liberal views of society. When we refer to non-Western concepts and models in this chapter, we mean to include Eastern perspectives; knowledge produced outside of the dominant Anglo-Saxon worldview, e.g., in colonized countries; Indigenous knowledge; and collective and socially oriented approaches to occupational therapy, such as social occupational therapy.

The terms "context" and "environment" are used interchangeably in this chapter to reflect the broad way in which they are used across a range of perspectives, models, and theories in occupational therapy and other literature informing our understanding of the environment. This chapter does not seek to represent all viewpoints given the diverse nature of occupational therapy's epistemology and provision across nations. It is intended to provide a brief overview and understanding of the pluralistic and changing nature of the environment in occupational therapy, one that will continue to develop and evolve over time.

24.2 History of the Environment in Occupational Therapy: Notes from the North

Since its beginnings, occupational therapy has acknowledged the role of the environment in health and well-being. The profession's foundations (in the United States) from the moral treatment and arts and crafts movements were a response to the environmental conditions of the time; for example, the inhumane conditions in mental asylums and poor living conditions due to industrialization (Andersen & Reed, 2017; Christiansen & Haertl, 2019). It is important we understand our history, as how the environment is conceptualized in occupational therapy is situated within our historical context. This historical context varies in different parts of the world, as do each country's political, economic, cultural, and social characteristics.

In the early 1900s, occupational therapy emerged in the United States where curative occupations such as weaving and pottery were used in working with people with mental and physical illness to restore health and well-being within settlement houses, asylums, and hospitals (Christiansen & Haertl, 2019). In 1917, this was formalized with the establishment in New York of the Society for the Promotion of Occupational Therapy

(Christiansen & Haertl, 2019). The First World War was a significant and influential event during this period and progressed the profession's development in Global North countries, where reconstruction aides, serving civilian women, were trained in orthopedic interventions and arts and crafts to facilitate the rehabilitation of military service personnel (Christiansen & Haertl, 2019).

Another important influence was the profession's quest for legitimacy in response to the scientific focus of medicine, under which occupational therapists most often worked (Andersen & Reed, 2017). During the 1920s and 1930s, occupational therapy drew closer to medicine, and the medicalization of the profession continued in the period leading up to the outbreak of the Second World War, especially within the warring countries (Christiansen & Haertl, 2019). Numbers of occupational therapists increased as did the sharpening of focus on rehabilitation using scientific techniques (Christiansen & Haertl, 2019).

In the mid-20th century, the profession, influenced by positivist theoretical understandings in science, becomes reductionistic in its practice by, for example, focussing on how activities can increase motor function, with occupation becoming less of a focus. In the 1950s, occupational therapy began to grow outside the United States, with educational programs commencing in the United Kingdom, India, Canada, Israel, Germany, Norway, Denmark, Sweden, South Africa, New Zealand, and Australia (World Federation of Occupational Therapists, 2022). Reflecting the new economic and political world order and globalization processes, the profession continued to expand throughout the latter half of the 20th century as occupational therapists from Europe and the United States established new courses in places such as Latin America. Through the 1960s and 1970s, numerous countries joined the World Federation of Occupational Therapists (WFOT), including Japan, Venezuela, Switzerland, Spain, Portugal, Philippines, Netherlands, Kenya, Italy, Ireland, Iceland, France, Finland, Columbia, Belgium, Austria, and Argentina. Today, the WFOT has 105 nation members (WFOT, 2022).

As the profession expanded globally, each country's epistemology, history, and practice of occupational therapy has been influenced by its own historical context and sociocultural environment. It is important, however, to reflect on the origins of the profession – emerging from the United States, it first expanded to other Western nations such as Denmark, Sweden, Ireland, New Zealand, Canada, Australia, and the United Kingdom. The values and belief systems of these Western worldviews therefore formed the foundations of the profession, and as occupational therapy expanded to other countries it followed the colonization model of economic and social global organization. As the profession reached wider cultures throughout the mid- and latter 20th century, the need for culturally specific theories emerged to counter the tension between Western-developed occupational therapy and the different cultures in which it was being taught and practiced (Kondo, 2004).

For example, in Japan, the United States' values of individualism and independence that predicated much of the theoretical basis of occupational therapy when it was first being taught in Japan was difficult to understand or endorse as it did not align with the Japanese cultural context of interdependence, social positioning, and concepts such as "gimu" (obligation) and "sekinin" (responsibility) (Kondo, 2004, 2018). The Kawa Model (Iwama, 2006), which is discussed below, was developed in response to these tensions. Similarly, in Latin American nations such as Brazil and Chile, the Global North profession's values, based on the positivistic perspective, did not fit these countries worldviews and values. As such, new epistemologies underpinned by more collective worldviews emerged to influence practice, for example, social occupational therapy (Lopes & Malfitano, 2021).

From the early 2000s and beyond, the need for practice to be responsive to the unique ways of knowing, doing, and being of the populations served began to emerge in a range of contexts (Nelson, 2007). It was during this time that the profession began to examine its colonial history and reproduction of the economic order and work toward decolonizing the profession (Taff & Putnam, 2022) by acknowledging Western privileged perspectives in occupational therapy discourse, education, and practice (Rudman et al., 2021). In countries such as Australia, New Zealand, and Canada, Indigenous occupational therapists are driving the change to decolonize practice and increase the profession's cultural capability (Emery-Whittington, 2021; Emery-Whittington & Te Maro, 2018; Gibson, 2020; Gibson et al., 2015; Phenix & Valavaara, 2019). This developing criticality of the profession's tenets, values, and beliefs, and learning from Indigenous cultures will continue to evolve the profession's epistemology and, therefore, understanding of the environment.

In Latin America, critical debates have emerged surrounding occupational therapy practices in the social sphere, including communities and territories; human rights; knowledge and knowledge production; the concept of critical analysis and reflection; gender and feminism; and the Global South (Díaz-Leiva & Malfitano, 2023). These debates have served to advance epistemologies of the profession in the region, changing the notion of environment and adding further theoretical perspectives, concepts, and vocabularies.

While the profession continues to evolve, it is important to understand that the Global North has predominantly shaped the profession and its scholarship; inside, however, there are resistance movements. The profession in its early history was focussed on restorative approaches, and only shifted to a rehabilitation focus following the two world wars. With this change our sense of occupation changed – originally viewed as a restorative tool, occupation and everyday life began to be seen as a productive tool to rehabilitate productive members of society. During the mid-20th century, there was also a focus on medicine and medically focussed interventions, resulting in a move toward physical therapies, away from the profession's roots of mental health, engagement in daily occupations, and the connection between environment and well-being.

The focus on legitimizing occupational therapy with science meant that different approaches from the scientific or medically focussed viewpoint were de-valued. As a result, the profession has been largely influenced by English-speaking Western scholars. For those from the Global South, Indigenous peoples, or those outside academia, this created numerous barriers to having their perspectives heard and providing opportunities to influence the profession (Malfitano, 2022). Only recently has there been push back with the emergence of a greater diversity of voices from the Global South and Indigenous communities that serve to influence the profession. The following sections describe some of the key theories and models which have influenced our understanding of the environment over time.

24.3 Models and Theories that Have Influenced Occupational Therapy's Understanding of Environment

Occupational therapy is grounded in an understanding of the interconnected nature of person, environment, and occupation/everyday life. Early models in occupational therapy such as the Occupational Performance Model (Pedretti, 1981) and Model of Human Occupation (Kielhofner, 1985) included the environment as a core construct. Over the profession's history, there have been a number of key theories and models that have influenced the profession's understanding of the environment, and new influences continue to emerge. While early influencers were the behavior-environment models and theories that focussed more on individuals, more recently a broader range of cultures and perspectives have influenced the profession with collective models and concepts changing the way we conceptualize the environment. This section looks first at the early influences on the profession which include person-environment fit and ecological viewpoints. It then moves on to consider more recent influences such as the World Health Organization's (WHO) International Classification of Functioning, Disability and Health (ICF), social determinants and social determination of health, rights-based approaches and ends with contemporary influences, including community, territory, and social occupational therapy, along with Indigenous knowledge.

24.3.1 Person-environment Fit

An early guiding principle in our understanding of the environment is the concept of person-environment fit which was first discussed by Lawton and Nahemow in *Ecological Theory of Aging* (1973). Person-environment fit is presented in the press-competence model, in which a person's competences or abilities interact with the environment resulting in their behavior and affect. Competence is described as including one's biological health, sensory and perceptual skills, motor skills, cognitive function, and psychological strength (Lawton, 1982). The environment includes a wide variety of physical and social factors, including cultural, socioeconomic, and intuitional, as well as social norms and values (Lawton, 1982; Shalinsky, 1986).

The model explains that the environment can be both supportive and disruptive to individuals, exerting differing levels of press depending on their personal characteristics. For example, for an older adult with osteoarthritis who has painful joints and balance problems, a home environment with stairs between levels may be difficult to use and limit their daily activities. While for another older adult the same stairs may be seen as an opportunity for exercise. The model is useful when thinking about how we can change the environment to better support the person's behavior and affect, or what they do and how they feel. For example, modifying a bathroom to make it easier and safer to bathe for someone who fatigued easily.

Person-environment fit has most often been used to understand the influence of the physical environment; yet, it is also helpful in considering broader aspects of the environment such as the socioeconomic environment. For example, for an older adult who owns their home and has an ongoing stable income, the everyday costs of life do not cause stress and they can enjoy a reasonable lifestyle. In contrast, for an adult living on a limited income and with ongoing housing costs, the everyday expenses of life are stressful and they may have to forgo basic necessities such as adequate food, housing, and health and social care. As a result, their physical and mental health will be impacted.

24.3.2 Ecological Systems Theory

Bronfenbrenner's Ecological Systems Theory focusses on child development and is another model widely used in occupational therapy to examine the influence of the environment on the person. In Bronfenbrenner's (1977) theory, child development is influenced by four environmental layers: micro, meso, exo, and macro level systems.

The microsystem describes the close or immediate surroundings of the individual such as home, school, health services, and peer groups (Bronfenbrenner & Morris, 2006). The mesosystem describes the inter-relationships between microsystems, e.g., the connections between home and a local club or health service. The exosystem describes settings in which the individual is not situated but is influenced by, e.g., a parent's workplace can influence a child's life and development (Tudge et al., 2009). The macrosystem describes the broader systems within society such as laws, customs, and policies, and includes cultures and social structures (Bronfenbrenner & Morris, 2006; Tudge et al., 2009).

Bronfenbrenner's system also considers micro, meso, and macro time, known as the chronosystem. The chronosystem refers to the historical context in which one has developed and lived, and how this influences life (Tudge et al., 2009). Bronfenbrenner's work paved the way for future ecological models in occupational therapy, including the Ecological Systems Model of Occupational Therapy (Howe & Briggs, 1982) and the Ecology of Human Performance (EHP; Dunn et al., 1994).

24.3.3 WHO's International Classification of Functioning, Disability, and Health

The ICF, released in 2001, has had a significant influence on occupational therapy practice and the profession's conceptualization of the environment. The ICF classifies health and health-related domains and includes a list of environmental and personal factors which interact with an individual's body functions and structures, health condition that may result in activity restrictions and participation limitations (Schneidert et al., 2003). It is a biopsychosocial model of disability which integrates medical and social models of disability (WHO, 2002). The ICF includes five environmental chapters: (1) products and technology; (2) natural environment and human-made changes to the environment; (3) support and relationships; (4) attitudes; and (5) services, systems, and policies (WHO, 2002). One of the purposes of the ICF was to establish a common language between people with disability, professionals, researchers, and policy makers (WHO, 2002). Its reach and influence are now widespread in occupational therapy, as reflected in the Occupational Therapy Practice Framework – Fourth Edition (OTPF-4) in which the environmental factors mirror the ICF's five categories (American Occupational Therapy Association, 2020). These are described in more detail in Table 24.1.

24.3.4 Social Determinants and Social Determination of Health

The ICF also includes personal factors, although they are not defined, and alongside environmental factors they comprise the contextual factors of the ICF. As contextual factors they can influence a person's health and participation in life, and can be considered social determinants of health (Froehlich-Grobe et al., 2020). The WHO defines social determinants of health as the non-medical factors that influence health, and include the "conditions in which people are born, grow, work, live, and age, and the wider set of forces and systems shaping the conditions of daily life" (WHO, 2022, para 1). These conditions, forces, and systems include education, unemployment and job security, food security, housing, access to health services, overarching economic policies and systems, development agendas, social norms, social policies, and political systems (WHO, 2022).

Social determinants of health are frequently associated with the unequal conditions of life and struggles for justice. For occupational therapy, these social determinants of health conceptualize the environmental factors which influence the health and life chances of the clients, groups, and populations we work with. By providing a broad range of environmental factors to consider in relation to a person's health or well-being, it differs from other occupational therapy models which may not clearly delineate or consider as wide an array of factors.

While the social determinants of health are a useful communication tool and framework for understanding non-medical factors that influence health, scholars from Latin America contest this perspective. Harvey et al. (2022) argue that social determinants of health oversimplify the social processes and forces generating unhealthy social conditions. They contend that the notion of social determinants of health, in its understanding of social conditions as discreet factors which influence health, does not reflect the multidimensional, complex, and interrelated processes that characterize social reality. The authors suggest that instead of social determinants, we consider social *determination* of health as the central concern (Harvey et al., 2022).

Social determination recognizes that health is produced throughout the life course by structural forces related to social life and inequalities present in our environment; in contrast, however, to the social determinants of health it does not seek to provide causal relationships between social factors and health (Harvey et al., 2022). Instead, the relationship between health and the multidimensional environment is viewed holistically (Spiegel et al., 2015). This difference in language is important because language matters in how we approach our practice and research (Spiegel et al., 2015). Social determination allows us as professionals and researchers to consider the social factors beyond simple risk factors or causal agents for health, providing an understanding of the complexity of the social processes and interconnections within the environment that influence our health. This perspective brings to occupational therapists the necessity of understanding the social determination of life, and that we need to consider this in our research and practice. We should always be cognizant that the environment is composed of unequal social determination, and this should form part of our professional lens and inform our reasoning for action.

24.3.5 Rights-based Approaches

The incorporation of occupational justice and related concepts as discussed in Chapter 10 was an important shift in occupational therapy theory and practice. Underpinned by human rights documents such as the Universal Declaration of Human Rights (UDHR), occupational rights include the right to education, the right to participate in the cultural life of the community, and the right to a standard of living adequate for health and well-being, including food, clothing, housing, medical care, and social services (United Nations General Assembly, 1948). As social rights were not clearly delineated in the UDHR, the International Covenant on Economic, Social and Cultural Rights (United Nations General Assembly, 1966) was created to highlight the significance of social rights. These include the right to involvement in social participation, working for a sufficient wage, and living free from discrimination.

A rights-based approach to practice has broadened occupational therapists' conceptualization of the environment and moves beyond simplistic understandings of the societal context. For example, it is not limited to an individual's immediate environment but thinks more deeply and broadly to consider factors such as government programs, funding, culture, and other systems and structures that influence the lives of individuals, groups, and populations (Crawford, 2017). In considering the broad array of factors, an intersectional perspective of rights is necessary for occupational therapists to understand and enact change at the political level. When we think about rights intersecting, such as the right to education and the right to live free of discrimination, we can see how the intersecting nature of the environment shapes people's lives, with some groups having more or less access to these rights (Balanta-Cobo et al., 2022).

Governments commit to human rights responsibilities by signing human rights documents such as the UDHR and the Convention on the Rights of Persons with Disabilities (United Nations General Assembly, 2007). Taking a rights-based approach to occupational therapy practice can therefore provide leverage by invoking governments' legal obligations when working toward social change such as enhanced funding, developing programs, or advocating for access to a service (Crawford, 2017). Rights-based approaches, social determinants of health, the ICF, Bronfenbrenner's ecological theory, and person-environment fit are for the most part Western-developed concepts which have influenced the profession's understanding of the environment. The chapter now turns to theories and knowledge outside of the Global North which are currently growing the profession's concept of environment.

24.3.6 Community, Territory, and Social Occupational Therapy

In Latin America, occupational therapy has been influenced by its historical context and sociocultural environment, which has resulted in two important concepts related to occupational therapy practice: community and territory. Community is a concept that has been present in professional practice in many Latin American countries since the 1970s, and is related to popular organization and access to services. Territory as a concept emerged in Latin America in the 1990s as a result of social and economic experiences related to social policies (Bianchi & Malfitano, 2022). The historical and socioeconomic contexts of these nations include colonization, military dictatorships, limited health services, and extreme social inequalities (Bianchi & Malfitano, 2022). This context has led to a politically active occupational therapy profession and practice outside of what would be considered traditional settings, where territorial and community action is taken by occupational therapists (Lopes & Malfitano, 2021).

Territory and community are based on the understanding that there is an inseparability between individuals and the groups and social history that constitute them, with social history, including current socioeconomic, political, and cultural conditions (Bianchi & Malfitano, 2022). Territory is a concept that was first developed by geographer Milton Santos, who suggested that territory should be seen as used (Santos, 2017).

A *territory* is therefore a geographic space that includes its historical, social, and material aspects as well as how its people use it in their everyday lives (Bianchi & Malfitano, 2022; Melgaço & Prouse, 2017; Santos, 2017).

For example, consider the neighborhood in which you live as a territory – there is a history of how it was developed and evolved, who has lived there, and the sociocultural factors such as migration and economic and housing policies that contributed to this, all of which shapes the place it is today. The streetscape, dwellings, buildings, and greenspaces all constitute its material aspects. Also consider how the space is used, or all the occupations that occur within this space, including work, school, play, socializing, and cultural occupations/everyday life. All these factors combine to make a territory and are inseparable from each other in understanding the territory.

Community is defined as a social group which constantly evolves and is connected by a sense of social identity, belonging, and common interests and needs (Bianchi & Malfitano, 2022). A community can be within a territory, e.g., a community within a neighborhood, and communities can also cross territories, e.g., a professional community, or a community of people with shared interests such as a social cause or enjoyed occupation.

Territory and community action by occupational therapists are those actions which work with and at the level of territory and community. This might include working with people in their communities or territories to identify and describe social inequalities or issues that need to change, as well as the actions of working toward this change. This would include community development work, such as working with a group of older women who are at risk of homelessness to develop a housing strategy in their community. These territory and community actions are reflective of occupational therapy in Latin American countries which have a more collective or community level focus than Western occupational therapy.

Malfitano et al. (2014) describe this territorial action approach in the context of social occupational therapy. Social occupational therapy advocates for the possibility of acting outside the funded health system and acts against social exclusion and injustice, focussing on social issues and change in the real context of where people live (Malfitano et al., 2014). While not always named social occupational therapy, this approach to practice has been occurring in Latin American nations since the 1970s and 1980s. It can be viewed as a demonstration of resistance to the individualization of social problems in capitalist, Western societies, and therapists' rejection of the biomedical model's predominant influence in the profession at the time (Lopes & Malfitano, 2021).

24.3.7 Indigenous Knowledge and Perspectives on the Environment and Occupational Therapy

Indigenous perspectives on occupation, environment, health, and well-being have long been ignored in occupational therapy and the provision of health care, to the detriment of Indigenous peoples (Fijal & Beagan, 2019; Ward, 2015). Indigenous knowledge and perspectives are diverse and unique and, in this chapter, we acknowledge that we cannot represent the diversity of perspectives and knowledge that crosses different groups of Indigenous peoples across nations and within countries such as Australia, where there are over 250 Aboriginal and Torres Strait Islander language groups (Australian Institute of Aboriginal and Torres Strait Islander Studies, 2020). We also acknowledge that, as non-Indigenous authors writing within a Western-developed textbook, we cannot adequately explore or understand Indigenous perspectives of the environment and how this relates to occupational therapy. It is important, however, to discuss the work that is being done by Indigenous authors.

Recent works by Indigenous authors and others have called for the profession to decolonize its knowledge and practice (Emery-Whittington & Te Maro, 2018; Gibson, 2020; Rudman et al., 2021). Decolonizing our knowledge and practice requires a deep and critical consideration of the historical and sociocultural context in which we live and work, the legacy of colonization, and the power and social imbalances that linger in its wake. This epistemology requires the profession to consider the environment or context far more deeply than it has previously done, and it likely signals the beginnings of a paradigm shift in the profession, with our core models, theories, and practice being challenged – and evolving in response.

Decolonizing actions are occurring at the micro and macro level in occupational therapy. For example, Occupational Therapy New Zealand – Whakora Ngangahau Aotearoa has a treaty model in place with two equal first delegates, one with Tāngata Whenua (the First peoples of Aotearoa) and the other with Tāngata Tiriti (all others who have come to Aotearoa). Changes such as this indicate that while there is more work to be done, there has been a shift in occupational therapy knowledge and practice, and significantly in the context of this chapter a shift in how the environment is considered. In considering the environment more deeply than before, we have started to look inward and consider how we as individuals and as a profession are part of the context that influences the groups and individuals we work with.

These changes have only been achieved by listening to and promoting Indigenous authors, and in giving them opportunities to lead their voices have brought a critical and differing view of the environment to occupational therapy. For example, the Integrated Canadian Model of Occupational Performance and Engagement (ICMOP-E) incorporates Canadian Indigenous worldviews on the environment, in which the environment and person are not seen as discrete entities; rather the person is simultaneously their environment (Fijal & Beagan, 2019). The authors describe how for Canadian Indigenous peoples the concept of land is central to community and individuals' health. Person and land are inseparable and as such the health of the community and individuals is the health of the land and all living things. Therefore, access to land and being able to conduct land-based activities is a critical contributor to individuals' health and well-being, which is why reconnecting with land is important to Indigenous people's health (Fijal & Beagan, 2019).

Inseparability in the health of an individual, community, and land is also central for Aboriginal and Torres Strait Islander peoples in Australia (Gibson, 2020; Trzepacz et al., 2014). Similarly, Emery-Whittington (2021) discusses the Māori perspective that whenua (land) and wai (waters) are sacred gifts to be looked after for the benefit of all, describing how Māori are of the land and that success is seen through occupations of kaitiaki (guardians and protectors) of Earth Mother.

Occupations of kaitiaki reflect Emery-Whittington's concept of decolonizing occupations which demonstrate resistance to Westernized notions of occupation and the colonization of Indigenous peoples' doing and being. She describes how decolonizing occupations involve "deliberate reconnection of purpose with spiritual, reverent aspects of collective being and doing" which include connecting with and guardianship of Earth Mother (Emery-Whittington, 2021, p. 158).

Gibson's concept of cultural occupations is similar to decolonizing occupations and reflects the significance of Country to Aboriginal and Torres Strait Islander peoples. Cultural occupations are those "driven by cultural connection" to family, kin, community, culture, mind, emotion, and the spiritual and physical (Gibson, 2020, p. 14). These concepts of decolonizing and cultural occupations indicate a much closer connection between environment and occupation than has previously been considered in occupational therapy's understanding of the environment, and highlights the significance of elevating and appreciating Indigenous perspectives in decolonizing our practice.

24.4 Occupational Therapy Models and the Environment

The concepts and theories discussed above have influenced occupational therapy models, which have changed over time as new needs are identified. In this chapter, we present a range of models to understand how the environment has been conceptualized, rather than present a comprehensive overview of all models in occupational therapy.

Models of occupational therapy were developed in the 1990s and those that are in common use in practice today, such as the Person, Environment, Occupation (PEO) model (Law et al., 1996), take an ecological approach to understanding person and environment, in which one cannot be understood without the other. These models were either implicitly or explicitly influenced by ecological theories like Bronfenbrenner's Ecological Systems Theory and John Dewey's concept of "transactionalism" (see Chapter 16). Dewey suggested that people and environment are inseparable and co-constitute one another in an ongoing dynamic process. As such, these models view person, environment, and occupation as transactive, where they cannot be considered separately (Turpin & Iwama, 2011).

In the early 2000s, there was a move away from this ecological understanding of the environment. Models such as the Person-Environment-Occupation-Participation (PEOP) (Baum & Christiansen, 2005) and Canadian Model of Occupational Performance and Engagement (CMOP-E) (Townsend & Polatajko, 2007) conceptualize the environment and person as separate but interactional, with occupation the bridge that connects person and environment (Turpin & Iwama, 2011). More recently, however, the Canadian Model of Occupational Participation (CanMOP) (Egan & Restall, 2022) has transitioned back to a more transactional focus.

24.4.1 Transactional Models

The PEO model (Law et al., 1996) has a strong focus on the relationship between the person and their environment, influenced by concepts such as Ecological Systems Theory. In this model, occupational performance is seen to be the dynamic interwoven product of person, environment, and occupation (Law et al., 1996). The environment is described broadly and includes cultural, socioeconomic, institutional, physical, and social elements. Importantly, the model emphasizes that these environmental domains are considered from the perspective of the person, household, neighborhood, or community (Law et al., 1996). The model also incorporates temporal aspects acknowledging that people, our contexts, and occupations change over time.

Another model which utilizes a transactive approach is EHP (Dunn et al., 1994). This model again discusses the person, occupation, and environment as being interdependent and inseparable. The environment is described broadly to include physical, temporal, social, and cultural elements (Dunn et al, 1994). The focus is on the environment, the lens through which all human performance should be viewed, and the context in which people act and are influenced and shaped by those actions (Turpin & Iwama, 2011).

The CanMOP (see Chapter 5) places renewed emphasis on the environment and, in particular, the role of social determinants/determination in occupational participation (Egan & Restall, 2022). The CanMOP invites analysis on how an individual's or group's life course (e.g., histories, relationships, and trajectories) and context (e.g., micro, meso, and macro) shapes occupational participation, where occupational participation is defined as "having access to, initiating, and sustaining valued occupations within meaningful relationships and context" (Egan & Restall, 2022, p. 76). This new model shows that scholarship and theory in occupational therapy are increasingly drawing on ecological and rights-based approaches to contextualize how occupations are shaped by person-environment transactions.

24.4.2 Interactional Models

Models including the PEOP (Baum & Christiansen, 2005), CMOP-E (Townsend & Polatajko, 2007), and OTPF-4 (AOTA, 2020) take a more interactive approach to understanding the environment. The PEOP model was developed to focus on improvement of performance and meaningful participation for individuals, organizations, and populations (Baum & Christiansen, 2005). It conceptualizes the environment as being separate from the person, whereas the occupational performance component unites the person and environment. The environment is seen to place demands on or provide affordances to occupational performance and participation, and includes social support, social and economic systems, culture and values, the built environment and technology, as well as the natural environment (Baum & Christiansen, 2005).

Similarly, the CMOP-E conceptualizes the environment as separate to the person, with occupation acting as the bridge between the person and environment. Individuals are seen to live within an environmental context which includes cultural, institutional, physical and social elements, and affords occupational opportunities (Townsend & Polatajko, 2007). As described above, the updated Canadian model positions itself as more transactional, embracing ecological and rights-based approaches.

The OTPF-4, developed by the American Occupational Therapy Association (AOTA) (2020), describes occupational therapy practice for the US context. It includes two main aspects, *Domain* and *Process*. The *Domain* outlines the profession's purview, or the key areas of knowledge and expertise, while *Process* describes the actions occupational therapists take when providing services. *Context* is defined by the OTPF-4 as a broad construct, being the environmental and personal factors specific to each client that influence engagement and participation in occupations (AOTA, 2020). This description and use of the ICF environmental factors in the OTPF-4 reflects an interactional understanding of the environment, in which environmental factors are seen to be barriers to, or facilitators of, performance and participation (AOTA, 2020). Table 24.1 presents the environmental factors as described by the OTPF-4; it is important to note, however, that this is just one way to conceptualize the environment.

The PEO, EHP, PEOP, CMOP-E, OTPF-4, and other models created during similar time periods have most often focussed on individuals, and reflect the Western worldview and the profession's early history. The Kawa and ICMOP-E models described below

Table 24.1 Example of an Interactional Approach to Understanding the Environment – OTPF-4 Environmental Factors

Environmental factor	Components described in OTPF-4
Attitudes	The beliefs and practices held by individuals, groups, and broader societal groups. These include customs, practices, ideologies, values, norms, cultural beliefs, and religious beliefs held by others.
Services, systems, and policies	The systems, policies, rules, regulations, conventions, and standards established by governments or other authorities at local, regional, national, and international levels. These include benefits, structured programs, and regulations for operations provided by institutions in various sectors of society that are designed to meet the needs of persons, groups, and populations.
Support and relationships	This includes all the people in our lives who support us and with whom we have relationships: immediate and extended family; friends; acquaintances; neighbors and community members; people in authority; people in subordinate positions; people providing support; and domesticated animals such as pets or therapy dogs.
Products and technology	All natural and human-made products or systems of products, equipment, and technology that we use, produce, manufacture, or gather. This includes food, drugs, household items, assistive technology, vehicles and other mobility transportation, communication systems and products, education processes and methods, workplaces and work systems, cultural, recreational, and sporting places and systems, religious places' systems and products, indoor and outdoor human-made environments (e.g., buildings, houses, gardens, and parks), money, property and other assets for economic exchange, and virtual environments.
Natural environment and human-made changes to the environment	Includes physical geography, population, plants and animals, the climate, natural events, human-caused events, light, and time or temporal aspects such as natural or regularly occurring rhythms.

Source: AOTA (2020).

Note. The OTPF-4 provides an overview of environmental factors. These are, however, described in quite neutral or positive terms, which may limit our understanding of the consequences and intersectionality of environmental factors, such as oppressive, racist, or inequitable services systems and policies.

have been developed from non-Western perspectives, and indicate a return to more ecological-oriented models that blur the conceptual boundaries between the person and environment. These models also ask us to critically consider Western-developed models by highlighting their focus on the individual and conceptualization and understanding of occupation through the lens of individuals (Turpin & Iwama, 2011). The Kawa and ICMOP-E models present differing viewpoints and seek to provide models of practice that can be used in a greater range of contexts.

24.4.3 Kawa Model

The *Kawa Model* originates from Japan and, as the first model developed from a non-Western viewpoint, it represents an important shift in occupational therapy thinking. The Kawa (meaning river in Japanese) was developed by Iwama (2006) in response to a need for a contextually relevant model in Japan. It uses a metaphor of a river, incorporating the elements of water, rocks, driftwood, river floor, and walls. The environment's role in the life-flow of an individual, family, or organization forms the river walls and river floor (kawa no sku-heki and kawa no zoko). These are described as the physical and social environment and are perhaps the most important influence on life-flow for individuals in a collectivist social context (Iwama, 2006).

The Kawa Model focusses more on the social environment and provides examples of family members, pets, friends, workmates, and others who form the close social circle of individuals, families, and organizations. The importance of environment or context in shaping life-flow can be easily understood from the river metaphor: the course of the river and strength of flow is dependent on the combination of geography, driftwood, and rocks. Using this metaphor, one can see how one's life river course is influenced by the context at every life step from birth to death, as it flows toward the sea. Turpin and Iwama (2011) caution, however, that the model can easily be interpreted as individualistic when viewed through a Western lens, and therefore emphasize that it must be understood as an integrated whole.

24.4.4 Integrated Canadian Model of Occupational Performance and Engagement (ICMOP-E)

Another recent model is the ICMOP-E, developed by Fijal and Beagan (2019). This model integrates Indigenous perspectives on health and wellness with the CMOP-E, and presents a different conceptualization of the environment. In the CMOP-E's worldview, health and well-being are viewed not just as a person's well-being – the interconnected nature of community and land mean that their health is also the person's health (Fijal & Beagan, 2019). Previous models have tended to filter how a model could be used, e.g., the PEO model could be used to understand an individual or community, whereas the ICMOP-E does not distinguish individuals from their community or lands – they can only be understood as a whole. The ICMOP-E signals the beginning of new knowledge in occupational therapy and, hopefully, the start of a new era of occupational therapy models and approaches to practice which are culturally and contextually based.

24.5 Conclusion

This chapter has shown that occupational therapy's understanding of the environment is pluralistic and ever-changing. It has provided a historical perspective of the environment in occupational therapy, including an overview of a range of concepts that have influenced our understandings and a review of models. Overall, the chapter highlights the value of taking a flexible and contextually based approach to considering the environment and our approach to practice. A contextually based approach to practice asks us to consider the territories in which we are working, where we must consider the historical, political, economic, and social factors relevant and important to the people we work with. It also requires deep reflection on our own understanding of person, environment, and occupation/everyday life and how this may be different to those we are working with.

24.6 Summary

- Occupational therapy's understanding of the environment is influenced and situated within a historical and sociocultural context, and continues to evolve.
- A range of models and theories have influenced our understanding of the environment and its relationship to person and occupation.
- Recently, non-Western models and theories have begun to influence occupational therapy's perspective of the environment, bringing more collective and holistic understandings to the complex concept of the environment, as well as challenging the profession to decolonize its practice and reflect on the taken-for-granted Western influence that permeates our scholarship.
- More recent models and theories have focussed on the transactional nature of person and environment, as well as the intersectionality of environmental factors.

24.7 Review Questions

1. Describe the components of the Kawa Model and its relationship to our understanding of the environment.
2. What are the key features of a Westernized view of the environment?
3. What is meant by person-environmental fit?
4. Explain what is meant by the terms "cultural occupations" and "decolonizing occupations"?
5. What are four features of the Global North's view of the environment?
6. What are the features of the ICMOP-E?

References

American Occupational Therapy Association. (2020). Occupational Therapy Practice Framework: Domain and process (4th ed.). *American Journal of Occupational Therapy, 74*(Suppl. 2), 7412410010p1–7412410010p87. http://doi.org/10.5014/ajot.2020.74S2001

Andersen, L. T., & Reed, K. L. (2017). *The history of occupational therapy: The first century.* Slack.

Australian Institute of Aboriginal and Torres Strait Islander Studies. (2020). *Indigenous Australians: Aboriginal and Torres Strait Islander people.* https://aiatsis.gov.au/explore/indigenous-australians-aboriginal-and-torres-strait-islander-people

Balanta-Cobo, P., Fransen-Jaïbi, H., Gonzalez, M., Henny, E., Malfitano, A. P. S., & Pollard, N. (2022). Human and social rights and occupational therapy: The need for an intersectional perspective. *Brazilian Journal of Occupational Therapy, 30*, e30202203. https://doi.org/10.1590/2526-8910.ctoED302022032

Baum, C., & Christiansen, C. (2005). Person-Environment-Occupation-Performance: A occupation-based framework for practice. In C. H. Christiansen, C. M. Baum, & J. Bass-Haugen (Eds.), *Occupational therapy: Performance, participation and well-being* (3rd ed., pp. 243–259). Slack.

Bianchi, P. C., & Malfitano, A. P. S. (2022). Occupational therapy in Latin America: Conceptual discussions on territory and community. *Scandinavian Journal of Occupational Therapy, 29*(3), 210–228. http://doi.org/10.1080/11038128.2020.1842492

Bronfenbrenner, U. (1977). Toward an experimental ecology of human development. *American Psychologist, 32*(7), 513–531. https://doi.org/10.1037/0003-066X.32.7.513

Bronfenbrenner, U., & Morris, P. A. (2006). The bioecological model of human development. In W. Damon & R. M. Lerner (Eds.), *Handbook of child psychology, volume 1: Theoretical models of human development* (6th ed., pp. 794–828). Wiley & Sons.

Christiansen, C. H., & Haertl, K. L. (2019). A contextual history of occupational therapy. In B. Schell & G. Gillen (Eds.), *Willard & Spackman's occupational therapy* (13th ed., pp. 11–42). Lippincott Williams & Wilkins.

Crawford, E. (2017). Continuing the dialogue: A rights-approach in occupational therapy. *Australian Occupational Therapy Journal, 64*(6), 505–509. https://doi.org/10.1111/1440-1630.12416

Díaz-Leiva, M. M., & Malfitano, A. P. S. (2023). Controversies and debates around occupational therapy: An analysis of bibliographic productions in South America (2010–2018). *Brazilian Journal of Occupational Therapy, 31*, e3344. https://doi.org/10.1590/2526-8910.ctoAO256433442

Dunn, W., Brown, C., & McGuigan, A. (1994). The ecology of human performance: A framework for considering the effect of context. *American Journal of Occupational Therapy, 48*(7), 595–607. http://doi.org/10.5014/ajot.48.7.595

Egan, M., & Restall, G. (Eds.). (2022). *Promoting occupational participation: Collaborative, relationship-focused occupational therapy*. Canadian Association of Occupational Therapists.

Emery-Whittington, I., & Te Maro, B. (2018). Decolonising occupation: Causing social change to help our ancestors rest and our descendants thrive. *New Zealand Journal of Occupational Therapy, 65*(1), 12–19. https://search.informit.org/doi/10.3316/informit.779745338782955

Emery-Whittington, I. G. (2021). Occupational justice – colonial business as usual? Indigenous observations from Aotearoa New Zealand. *Canadian Journal of Occupational Therapy, 88*(2), 153–162. http://doi.org/10.1177/00084174211005891

Fijal, D., & Beagan, B. L. (2019). Indigenous perspectives on health: Integration with a Canadian model of practice. *Canadian Journal of Occupational Therapy, 86*(3), 220–231. http://doi.org/10.1177/0008417419832284

Froehlich-Grobe, K., Douglas, M., Ochoa, C., & Betts, A. (2020). Social determinants of health and disability. In D. J. Lollar, W. Horner-Johnson, & K. Froehlich-Grobe (Eds.), *Public health perspectives on disability: Science, social justice, ethics and beyond* (2nd ed., pp. 53–89). Springer. https://doi.org/10.1007/978-1-0716-0888-3

Gibson, C. (2020). When the river runs dry: Leadership, decolonisation and healing in occupational therapy. *New Zealand Journal of Occupational Therapy, 67*(1), 11–20. https://link.gale.com/apps/doc/A628283412/AONE?u=anon~d697c535&sid=googleScholar&xid=8ef19ee4

Gibson, C., Butler, C., Henaway, C., Dudgeon, P., & Curtin, M. (2015). Indigenous peoples and human rights: Some considerations for the occupational therapy profession in Australia. *Australian Occupational Therapy Journal, 62*(3), 214–218. http://doi.org/10.1111/1440-1630.12185

Harvey, M., Piñones-Rivera, C., & Holmes, S. M. (2022). Thinking with and against the social determinants of health: The Latin American social medicine (collective health) critique from Jaime Breilh. *International Journal of Health Services, 52*(4), 433–441. http://doi:10.1177/00207314221122657

Hooper, B. (2006). Epistemological transformation in occupational therapy: Educational implications and challenges. *OTJR: Occupation, Participation and Health, 26*(1), 15–24. https://doi.org/10.1177/153944920602600103

Howe, M. C., & Briggs, A. K. (1982). Ecological systems model for occupational therapy. *American Journal of Occupational Therapy, 36*(5), 322–327. http://doi.org/10.5014/ajot.36.5.322

Iwama, M. (2006). *The Kawa Model: Culturally relevant occupational therapy*. Churchill Livingstone-Elsevier Press.

Khan, T., Abimbola, S., Kyobutungi, C., & Pai, M. (2022). How we classify countries and people – and why it matters. *BMJ Global Health, 7*(6), e009704. https://doi.org/10.1136/bmjgh-2022-009704

Kielhofner, G. (1985). *A Model of Human Occupation: Theory and application*. Williams and Wilkins.

Kondo, T. (2004). Cultural tensions in occupational therapy practice: Consideration from a Japanese vantage point. *American Journal of Occupational Therapy, 58*(2), 174–184. http://doi.org/10.5014/ajot.58.2.174

Kondo, T. (2018). History and current practice of occupational therapy in Japan. *Annals of International Occupational Therapy, 2*(1), 43–52. https://doi.org/10.3928/24761222-2018 1116-01

Law, M., Cooper, B., Strong, S., Stewart, D., Rigby, P., & Letts, L. (1996). The Person-Environment-Occupation Model: A transactive approach to occupational performance. *Canadian Journal of Occupational Therapy, 63*(1), 9–23. https://doi.org/10.1177/000841749606300103

Lawton, M. P. (1982). Competence, environmental press, and the adaptation of older people. In M. P. Lawton, P. G. Windley, & T. O. Byerts (Eds.), *Aging and the environment* (pp. 33–59). Springer.

Lawton, M. P., & Nahemow, L. (1973). Ecology and the aging process. In C. Eisdorfer & M. P. Lawton (Eds.), *The psychology of adult development and aging* (pp. 619–674). American Psychological Association.

Lopes, R. E., & Malfitano, A. P. S. (2021). *Social occupational therapy: Theoretical and practical designs*. Elsevier.

Malfitano, A. P. S. (2022). An anthropophagic proposition in occupational therapy knowledge: Driving our actions towards social life. *World Federation of Occupational Therapists Bulletin, 78*(2), 70–82. https://doi:10.1080/14473828.2022.2135065

Malfitano, A. P. S., Lopes, R. E., Magalhães, L., & Townsend, E. A. (2014). Social occupational therapy: Conversations about a Brazilian experience. *Canadian Journal of Occupational Therapy, 81*(5), 298–307. https://doi:10.1177/0008417414536712

Melgaço, L., & Prouse, C. (2017). Milton Santos and the centrality of the periphery. In L. Melgaço & C. Prouse (Eds.), *Pioneers in arts, humanities, science, engineering, practice: Volume 11: Milton Santos: A pioneer in critical geography from the Global South* (pp. 1–24). Springer. http://doi:10.1007/978-3-319-53826-6_1

Nelson, A. (2007). Seeing white: A critical exploration of occupational therapy with Indigenous Australian people. *Occupational Therapy International, 14*(4), 237–255. http://doi:10.1002/oti.236

Pedretti, L. W. (1981). *Occupational therapy practice skills for physical dysfunction*. Mosby.

Phenix, A., & Valavaara, K. (2019). Occupational therapy responses to the Truth and Reconciliation Commission. *Occupational Therapy Now, 21*(4), 3. https://caot.ca/document/6761/July_OTNow_2019_test.pdf

Rudman, M. T., Flavell, H., Harris, C., & Wright, M. (2021). How prepared is Australian occupational therapy to decolonise its practice? *Australian Occupational Therapy Journal, 68*(4), 287–297. https://doi.org/10.1111/1440-1630.12725

Santos, M. (2017). The return of the territory. In L. Melgaço & C. Prouse (Eds.), *Pioneers in arts, humanities, science, engineering, practice: Volume 11: Milton Santos: A pioneer in critical geography from the Global South* (pp. 25–31). Springer. https://doi.org/10.1007/978-3-319-53826-6_2

Schneidert, M., Hurst, R., Miller, J., & Üstün, B. (2003). The role of environment in the International Classification of Functioning, Disability and Health (ICF). *Disability and Rehabilitation, 25*(11–12), 588–595. https://doi.org/10.1080/0963828031000137090

Shalinsky, W. (1986). Disabled persons and their environment. *Environments, 17*(1), 1–8.

Spiegel, J. M., Breilh, J., & Yassi, A. (2015). Why language matters: Insights and challenges in applying a social determination of health approach in a North-South collaborative research program. *Globalization and Health, 11*, Article 9. https://doi:10.1186/s12992-015-0091-2

Taff, S. D., & Putnam, L. (2022). Northern philosophies and professional Neocolonialism in occupational therapy: A historical review and critique. *Brazilian Journal of Occupational Therapy, 30*, e2986. https://doi.org/10.1590/2526-8910.ctoAO22642986

Townsend, E. A., & Polatajko, H. J. (2007). *Enabling occupation II: Advancing an occupational therapy vision for health, well-being and justice through occupation.* CAOT Publications.

Trzepacz, D., Guerin, B., & Thomas, J. (2014). Indigenous country as a context for mental and physical health: Yarning with the Nukunu Community. *Australian Community Psychologist, 26*(2), 38–53. https://psychology.org.au/aps/media/acp/trzepacz-acp-26-2-dec-2014.pdf

Tudge, J. R. H., Mokrova, I., Hatfield, B. E., & Karnik, R. B. (2009). Uses and misuses of Bronfenbrenner's bioecological theory of human development. *Journal of Family Theory & Review, 1*(4), 198–210. https://doi.org/10.1111/j.1756-2589.2009.00026.x

Turpin, M., & Iwama, M. K. (2011). *Using occupational therapy models in practice.* Churchill Livingstone.

United Nations General Assembly. (1948). *Universal Declaration of Human Rights.* United Nations. https://www.un.org/en/about-us/universal-declaration-of-human-rights

United Nations General Assembly. (1966). *International Covenant on Economic, Social and Cultural Rights.* United Nations. https://www.ohchr.org/en/instruments-mechanisms/instruments/international-covenant-economic-social-and-cultural-rights

United Nations General Assembly. (2007). *Convention on the Rights of Persons with Disabilities.* United Nations. https://www.un.org/development/desa/disabilities/convention-on-the-rights-of-persons-with-disabilities/optional-protocol-to-the-convention-on-the-rights-of-persons-with-disabilities.html

Ward, R. (2015). Health and wellbeing. In K. Price (Ed.), *Knowledge of life: Aboriginal and Torres Strait Islander Australia* (pp. 141–151). Cambridge University Press.

World Federation of Occupational Therapists. (2022). *List of member organisations.* WFOT. https://wfot.org/membership/member-organisations/list-of-wfot-member-organisations

World Health Organization. (2002). *Towards a common language for functioning, disability and health: ICF.* WHO. https://cdn.who.int/media/docs/default-source/classification/icf/icf-beginnersguide.pdf?sfvrsn=eead63d3_4&download=true

World Health Organization. (2022). *Social determinants of health.* WHO. https://www.who.int/health-topics/social-determinants-of-health#tab=tab_1

SECTION FOUR

Human Occupation across the Lifespan and Life Course

CHAPTER 25

Human Occupations of Infants, Toddlers, and Preschoolers

Rondalyn V. Whitney

Abstract
This chapter uses a theory-based approach to discuss the occupational patterns of children during critical periods of development spanning birth to the time they enter preschool. Primary theories that guide practice and support therapists in developing a clinical hypothesis to guide intervention are presented, helping readers recognize the function-dysfunction criteria during development. Milestones are broadly categorized into social-emotional, language, cognitive, adaptive behavior, and motor skills. An occupational profile follows one child and their family, demonstrating embedded play in family routines, significant practices for early child development, and promoting participation in meaningful and purposeful pursuits.

Author's Positionality Statement
When I was 3, my mother kept losing the washcloths only to discover I was folding and delivering them to our elderly neighbors when she wasn't looking. I have no idea why I did that but I can tell you my first job as an occupational therapist was delivering washcloths to elderly patients on the skilled nursing unit for their morning ADLs: I suppose I was meant to be an occupational therapist from early in life. I didn't hear about the profession until after I'd received my Bachelor of Arts in Medical Psychology but once I did discover occupational therapy, I felt I'd found a profession big enough to hold all my curiosity and passion. I am deeply grateful that I landed here where Ora Ruggles says to "reach for the heart as well as the hands; that the heart does the healing". That resonates with me. Most of my clinical work has focused on pediatric mental health and empowering social engagement for children. The primary variable of interest in my scholarship is mother-child co-regulation, maternal stress, and how to co-create a sense of coherence in families through occupation. My two most important occupational roles in my life are that of mother and writer, and my favorite part of the Occupational Therapy Practice Framework – 4th Edition is *Performance Patterns: The habits, routines, roles and rituals as they contribute to health and wellness.*

RONDALYN V. WHITNEY

> **Objectives**
> This chapter will allow the reader to:
>
> - Describe patterns in adaptive and occupational engagement in children aged birth to preschool.
> - Use current evidence and theory to create occupation-based interventions.
> - Explore the elements of the common theories that guide clinical reasoning in occupational therapy interventions for early childhood development.
> - Understand the function-dysfunction continuum relevant to early childhood development.
> - Use case examples illustrating occupational profiles to frame clinical reasoning and serve as a problem-solving tool in practice.
> - Understand the data-driven decision-making process.

> **Key terms**
>
> - **function-dysfunction continuum**
> - **occupational profile**
> - **adaptive behavior**
> - **occupational engagement**
> - **play**
> - **infant, toddler, and preschooler**

25.1 Introduction

Between the journey of life and death, human beings grow and develop in sequential patterns. These patterns can be conceptualized longitudinally as *stages* or hierarchies of prerequisite skills that build upon one another. While the beginnings of each stage are frequently debated, in general, the developmental arc includes infancy, early childhood, middle childhood, adolescence, early adulthood, middle adulthood, and old age. This chapter discusses the critical development, transitional arcs, and contextual influences that support or impede occupational engagement during the early stages of growth and development for infants, toddlers, and preschoolers. Occupations are central to a child's developmental competency, occur in contexts, and are influenced by the interplay among performance patterns, skills, and client factors (AOTA, 2020). A case study focusing primarily on the performance patterns of early childhood (the habits, routines, roles, and rituals) is presented to demonstrate how interactions between the child, the environment, and occupational engagement promote growth across the developmental arc of the age span, birth to five. For the purposes of this chapter, the Centers for Disease Control and Prevention (CDC) is used to outline the developmental stages of early childhood: *infant, toddler,* and *preschooler* (CDC, n.d.).

25.2 Stages of Early Childhood

Most people tacitly know what an infant is and recognize a toddler as distinct from a preschooler. However, the boundaries between these stages can be liminal; children can simultaneously occupy a position on both sides of the boundary. Still, there are *general* agreements of both the time (ages) when children move from one stage to the next and developmental milestones (acquired skills) predicted within the three stages. Parents and caregivers need to understand developmental milestones and recognize the organization of the nervous system, that is, to understand that a child takes in information through the sensory system (Whitney, 2018; Whitney & Luebben, 2016). Daily routines are organizing for children, and they feel safe to explore and develop in their environment. Therapists use their understanding of theory and developmental expectations to create clinical hypotheses, develop intervention plans, and support development during critical periods. When we "see" typical development, we look for a range of behaviors across motor, language, and social interactions (see Table 25.1), and, when atypical development is observed, the therapist provides environmental support, support to the child themselves, and informed selection of sensory-rich occupations that promote development through play.

25.3 Infant

>Having children is like living in a frat house – nobody sleeps, everything's broken and there's a lot of throwing up.
>
>*Ray Romano (n.d.)*

Infancy is the stage between birth and the end of the first year (0–12 months) (CDC, n.d.), during which a child develops along a predictive continuum, meeting social-emotional milestones (playing peek-a-boo), language/communication (waving bye-bye, understanding "no"), cognitive skills (looking for a Cheerio hidden under a cup), and motor abilities (sitting without support, using fingers to rake food toward themselves). In addition to motor development, infants gain a sense of trust during the first year when caregivers are responsive to their needs. Thus, the caregiver-child relationship and the co-occupations of parenting become the primary focus of therapeutic intervention, parent education, and the development of healthy family routines. Play routines include encouraging interaction with the caregiver, mimicking expressions and sounds, and body awareness (like encouraging the infant playfully taking socks off their newly discovered feet) (see Figure 25.1).

25.4 Toddler

>A child is a curly, dimpled lunatic.
>
>*Ralph Waldo Emerson*

The threshold between *infant* and *toddler* is enigmatic; babies stop being babies both "overnight" and "over time". Still, after the first year of life children begin to move on their own volition, follow the direction of a caregiver who points to and names an object, begin to follow directions, and assert their autonomy. *NO!* becomes the defining word of toddlerhood. By two years of age, most children can read and respond to facial expressions of others, communicate using two-word sentences, open and close

Table 25.1 Observing Normal Development

	In infants we look at	In toddlers we look at	In preschoolers we look at	These build toward the development of early elementary
Gross motor	Creeping, crawling, walking, running, movement patterns, reflexes	Running, hopping, jumping, climbing, posture, equilibrium, reactions	Catching, shifting, hanging, sitting and attending, smooth pursuit, calibrations (cuddling pets, tool use, crayons)	Calibration of movement (force, speed, and directional control)
Fine motor	Raking small bits of food from the tray, holding, grasping, self-feeding	Use of two hands, release, refined grasps, stacking, twisting, opening	Tracing lines, coloring, lacing, placing, threading, imitation of shapes (drawing), careful work	Copying shapes, coloring in lines, writing in spaces, playing with letters and shapes, mature grasps (mature motor patterns in the hands, e.g., tripod/chuck, lateral key, and pincer)
Language	Zerbers (making silly sounds with the mouth), pops, coos, sounds (moo, baa, grunt)	Mimicry, back and forth, labeling, wanting to talk, earnest "babbles", frustration	Being understandable, participating in conversations, "chatting" and telling stories	"Reading", telling stories, songs, answering when asked
Self-care	Cries, holds out arms/legs to help with dressing (1 year)	Pulls off socks, helps by pushing arms through sleeves (2 years), pulls pants down, finds arms in t-shirt	Puts on t-shirt and shoes, socks, basic fasteners, unties/removes shoes, removes pants (3 years) Puts on shoes/socks, dresses with few errors, e.g., front/back of garment (4 years)	Independent in opening zip lock bags, backpacks, potty care, helps with setting the table and other simple chores, bath/teeth/dressing/eating all independent
Social	Turn-taking/reciprocal interactions with caregiver, smiling when seeing a familiar face	Following the intention of caregiver's pointing (e.g., "Look, a plant!")	Innate drive to find solutions, self-efficacy ("I can do it!")	Working with peers in small groups, self-regulation, frustration tolerance
Temperament/ Psychological	ME! The world is about ME!!!!	Self-mastery –Ta da!	Self-mastery – "Look what I can do?"	Win/lose I'm the best!
Curiosity/Play	Playfulness	Parallel play, playfulness	Associative play (one other), constructive play, fantasy plan, playfulness	Cooperative play (others), playfulness

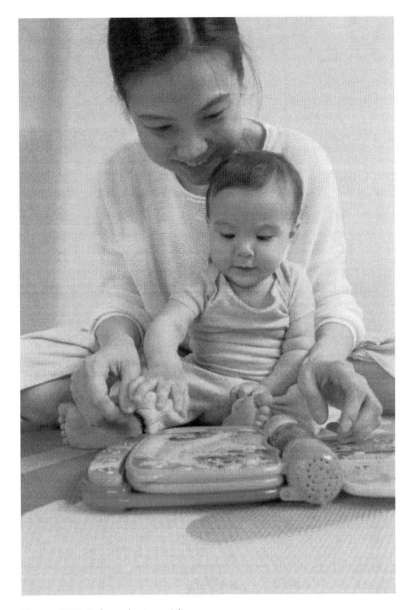

Figure 25.1 Infant playing with toy.

Source: Photo by Meruyert Gonullu, image used under license from pexels.com.

containers, and run and kick a ball. Six months later (18 months), their vocabulary soars to about 50 words (CDC, n.d.). They can follow a simple routine and two-step directions, play beside another child, turn pages of a book, and take off an open jacket.

Parents and caregivers need to understand developmental milestones, and recognize that typically developing toddlers are emotional. If a child is not meeting developmental milestones or had then lost a skill, parents and caregivers are in-situ observers who can raise critical concerns. Therapists use their understanding of theory and developmental

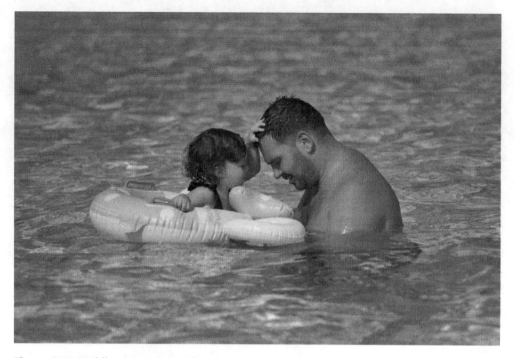

Figure 25.2 Toddler swimming with parent.
Source: Photo by Ali Danaci, image used under license from pexels.com.

expectations to create a clinical hypothesis, develop intervention plans, and support development during critical periods. For example, play routines, including turn-taking games, hide and seek, simple word games (what does the cow say?), dress-up play, and games to promote emotional regulation (e.g., blowing bubbles, quiet times to explore, and play in homemade tents) (see Figure 25.2).

25.5 Preschoolers

Play is the highest form of research.

Albert Einstein

Preschool is defined as being between the ages of three- and five-year-old, and this period of development is a time of exploration outside the family. The child's world opens up to new experiences, routines, and greater challenges. Developmental milestones during this period include using scissors, playing with others, and learning about boundaries (and challenging limits set on their exuberance). Beginning preschool is a significant transition, both for the child and for the family. The threshold between *toddler* and *preschooler* is more defined as the child leaves the family context and enters a community context. Play routines during this period include playing with another child, taking turns with a toy or a simple game, including the child in family chores, making gifts for others using scissors and glue, and gross motor play such as building forts out of tree branches or raking, then jumping in leaf piles in the back yard (see

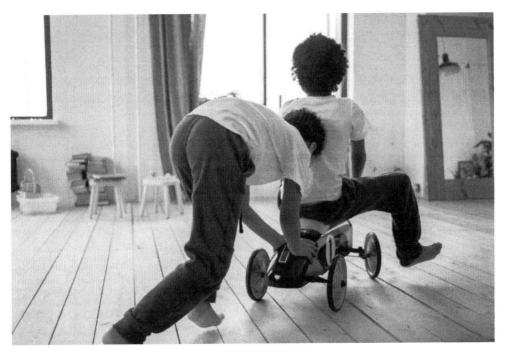

Figure 25.3 Child pretending to drive a sports car while being pushed by sibling.
Source: Photo by Monstera, image used under license from pexels.com.

Figure 25.3). Play schemes should include tool use (write name, paint/draw), eye-hand coordination games, opportunities for socializing, and self-regulation (Whitney & Gibbs, 2020).

25.6 Intervention

Intervention should be grounded in theory and focused on the child's functional performance and occupational needs rather than a diagnosis. Occupations are organized into broad categories (e.g., activities of daily living (ADL), instrumental activities of daily living, education, play and leisure, rest and sleep, and social participation) (AOTA, 2020; Whitney & Luebben, 2016) that serve as the framework for outcomes of intervention. Skill acquisition occurs through practice, and children practice through play (Knox, 2008). Occupational therapy practitioners use play to entice children to participate in interventions. For infants, toddlers, and preschoolers, play is often used as a means for meeting occupational goals. Occupation is used as an intervention (having a teddy bear tea party) and outcome (social participation during snack time at preschool).

Performance patterns, the acquired habits, routines, roles, and rituals can either support or hinder the performance of occupations during early development. Routines, in particular, establish structure in daily life and promote healthy development (see Table 25.2). In early childhood (birth to five), shared routines (those that involve two or more people) are understood to occur in a dance between parent and child. These co-occupations are nested within routines. For example, a toddler might engage in the occupation of meal prep (tearing lettuce and putting it into a bowl) as part of the family's preparation of dinner (child's daily routine). The parent's daily routine (co-occupation)

Table 25.2 Using Routines for Development

	Milestones	Family routines	Play schemes	Examples of play
Infant (9 months)	Social: Pat-a-cake, smile, follow when Mom points to a far object Language: wave bye-bye, mama/dada Cognitive: look for a toy hidden under a cushion Motor: Cruises (walks holding on to furniture), eats a bit of food using thumb/pointer finger	During daily walks, point and name trees, birds, etc. Encourage Matthew to follow your gaze (reciprocal gaze). Wave bye-bye to pets in the neighborhood, name pets (bye bye doggie!). Encourage hand use during meal prep (give Matthew food items in cups to dump into a bowl, push chocolate chips into dough, etc.) and dressing (let Matthew pull off his socks)	Establish sleep routine: Hide naughty teddy bear before bedtime (name your facial expressions and emotions – You found teddy, I'm so happy!). Use singing/reading as part of calming routines. Add sensation to bath time – squeeze toys, bubbles, fuzzy towels	Mom is making dinner. Matthew is in his high-chair beside the counter. He has several cups filled with cereal, puffs, and small bits of cheese, a large bowl, and a wooden spoon. He dumps, stirs, and nibbles while he and Mom "chat"
Toddler (2 years)	Social: Notices / responds to other's feelings Language: Points to body parts when you ask them to, two-word sentences, uses gestures (nods yes) Cognitive: plays with two or more toys, i.e., a stuffed toy on a wagon	While reading, look for facial expressions (look, that bird is so happy! Where's your happy face?) When dressing, ask Matthew to point to his body parts and help you (Matthew, where is your elbow? Put your elbow in this sleeve)	Evening routines include milk and cookies with Teddy, Teddy and Matt brushing teeth, Teddy and Matt have a story and a song, and then all boys are tucked into bed!	Bedtime: Walk like a bear with Teddy, brush teeth (brush Teddy's teeth), tuck in Teddy, tuck in Matt, read and sing the good night song to Teddy!

(Continued)

HUMAN OCCUPATIONS OF INFANTS, TODDLERS, AND PRESCHOOLERS

Table 25.2 (Continued)

	Milestones	Family routines	Play schemes	Examples of play
	Motor: Walks, kicks a ball, eats with a spoon, holds an item in one hand while using the other	During meal prep, Matthew helps open containers to retrieve grapes, cherry tomatoes, etc.	(Sometimes Teddy is naughty, and Matt has to help him be a good friend)	
Preschooler (4 years)	**Social:** Pretend play, avoids danger (like heights on the playground) **Language:** 4+ word sentences, can say one thing that happened in their day, answer simple questions **Cognitive:** Draws a person with 3+ body parts **Motor:** Pours, unbuttons some buttons, holds crayon between thumb and fingers	Pretends to be the firefighter and puts out pretend fire using a rope. Tells Mom how to play, "You hold the hose" Uses a crayon to draw what he saw on his daily walk He can take off his jacket by himself Has a daily chore: Waters the plants outside, sets utensils on the table, matches socks from the laundry basket	After-school routine: Make a snack, read 10 minutes with Mom (quiet time), outdoor play, chores	Matthew and Mom spend time each day side-by-side reading. They complete chores around the house in a playful routine before making and enjoying dinner together. He likes to make bread sticks for dinner, using the canned dough to form M&Ms (for Mom and Matt)

can be seen as they set out the lettuce, place the bowl on the counter for the child to use, and cut tomatoes beside the child to contribute to the salad being made. The routine provides a daily "dose" of practice for essential skill development (e.g., bilateral hand use, discrimination of sensation, and awareness of body position in space).

Children learn through *doing*, by engaging in the day-to-day routines of their families and peers (see Table 25.2). Learning is the acquisition of knowledge, skills, and occupations through shared routines nested in co-occupations (Lawlor & Mattingly, 2019). Thus, the goal of intervention within the lens of occupational therapy is to provide opportunities for children that allow occupational performance to be successful, to create routines through which the demands of the task, the skills of the child, and the features of the environment are congruent (AOTA, 2020). Learning within routines leads to permanent change in behavior and performance (see Table 25.2). For example, a two-year-old engaged in the daily routine of tearing lettuce during meal preparation gains a sense of belonging within a family who has meals together as part of a family routine. While all children benefit from sustained, routine-based practice, children with developmental delays especially benefit from the consistent dose (daily intervention) of the routine.

25.7 Case Study

Matthew is a 4.6-year-old with a history of developmental delays (see Table 25.3). He has been seen by an occupational therapist as part of the Birth to Three program (beginning at 2 months) until three years of age, at which time he transitioned to SunnyDays Preschool. He received services consistently there and he will transition to pre-kindergarten in the fall.

Table 25.3 Occupational Profile of Case

Name: Matthew
Age: 4y 6m
Medical Conditions: Level 1 Autism Spectrum Disorder and Mild Intellectual Impairment.

Client Report	The reason the client is seeking service and concerns related to engagement in occupations	Why is the client seeking service, and what are the client's current concerns relative to engaging in occupations and daily life activities? (This may include the client's general health status.)
		Reason: Evaluation for Occupational Therapy (OT) services through special education in preparation for the transition to pre-kindergarten in the fall.
		Concern areas: History of delays in ADL and expressive communication, functional motor skills, social participation, and behavioral regulation
		Parent concerns: Matthew can become overwhelmed at times and may not listen to instructions. He does not play with kids in his neighborhood, and his play at SunnyDays has been primarily parallel. He is more socially comfortable with adults.

(Continued)

Table 25.3 (Continued)

	Occupations in which the client is successful (p. S5)	In what occupations does the client feel successful, and what barriers affect success? Matthew has many skills. He knows his letters of the alphabet and can count to 100. He enjoys reading time, and books are calming for him. Matthew is right-handed and uses an appropriate hand pattern in school tasks. He does well with routines and works well in 1:1 situations.
	Personal interests and values (p. S7)	What are the client's values and interests? Matthew enjoys playing outdoors and helps neighbors with outdoor chores, like raking leaves, picking berries, and watering plants. Matthew is very active and is uncomfortable sitting for long periods. He seems to have little interest in most structured group or classroom activities. He loves to cook and is easily engaged in activities he finds familiar.
	Occupational history (i.e., life experiences)	What is the client's occupational history (i.e., life experiences)? Matthew was born following a full-term pregnancy. He lives with both parents and an older sister. Matthew was inconsistently compliant with adults at school and at home, with particular problems with mealtimes and bedtimes but has benefitted from routines to support these areas of occupation. Matthew can become distressed in new situations and around new people. He tantrums and can be quite disruptive when confronted with the unexpected.
	Performance patterns (routines, roles, habits, and rituals) (p. S8)	What are the client's patterns of engagement in occupations, and how have they changed over time? What are the client's daily life roles? (Patterns can support or hinder occupational performance.) *Motor Skills*: Matthew has mastered the basic motor milestones and walks and runs on even and uneven surfaces. He is able to get in and out of both the car and the school bus. Matthew has established hand dominance and has no significant problems producing legible written work at grade level. Matthew demonstrates awareness of household routines and self-care activities but completes these tasks following a pre-ordered plan.

(Continued)

Table 25.3 (Continued)

		Process Skills: Matthew has a short attention span and is easily frustrated. He is very sensitive to sounds and touch within the classroom setting. With novel tasks, Matthew needs frequent prompting to complete assignments. He understands the use of everyday items and knows the names of many things. He benefits from being pre-warned when a change in routine is anticipated, helping him make a plan (ideate the task), and being reminded to take a break if he feels overwhelmed.	
		Social Interaction Skills: Matthew can repeat basic safety and social rules but does not always remember to comply with these. Matthew expresses affection and a wide variety of emotions, with fair emotional modulation. He inconsistently conforms to social norms and has emerging skills to modify his behavior in accordance with social context.	
Environment	What aspects of the client's environments or contexts do they see as: Supports to occupational engagement and barriers to occupational engagement?		
	Physical (p. S28) (e.g., buildings, furniture, and pets)	Matthew has full physical access to all areas of his home and his classroom.	Matthew has poor safety awareness and needs supervision when routines are disrupted.
	Social (p. S28) (e.g., spouse, friends, and caregivers)	Matthew's family and teachers are supportive.	Matthew has no close friends and engages in few after-school activities.
Context	Cultural (p. S28) (e.g., customs and beliefs)	Matthew's family is from a suburban community in the Midwestern United States.	
	Personal (p. S28) (e.g., age, gender, SES, and education)	Matthew is part of a loving, supportive family with strong community connections.	Matthew comes from a family of low average SES. As a result, the family has limited resources for special toys or devices.
	Temporal (p. S28) (e.g., stage of life, time, and year)	Matthew likes routines and understands time and schedules.	Matthew has trouble with transitions, especially when they are unexpected.

(Continued)

Table 25.3 (Continued)

	Virtual (p. S28) (e.g., chat, email, and remote monitoring)	
Client Goals	Client's priorities and desired targeted outcomes (p. S34)	Consider: occupational performance – improvement and enhancement, prevention, participation, role competence, health and wellness, quality of life, well-being, and occupational justice. Matthew's parents want him to be successful at school and as independent as possible. He has benefited from the routines-based interventions, and the family is astute in using routines to support his development. As he transitions to pre-K next year, Matthew will benefit from developing a wider range of skills to support frustration tolerance, self-regulation, and social play.

25.8 Theories

Theories are scientifically acceptable general principles used broadly to describe, explain and predict behavior and relationships between concepts and events. Theories guide intervention and provide clinical hypotheses. A frame of reference is often defined as a set of assumptions or concepts derived from a theory, and like the frame of a house guides the focus of each room, a frame of reference guides routine practice.

25.9 Theory Analysis

Theory frames intervention, guides practice, and allows for the prediction of what will occur under a given circumstance. Theory is used to organize observations that translate into clinical practice and therapists use theory to identify problems and generate solutions in practice. While moving from theory to practice can be challenging, theory allows the clinician to predict the relationship between intervention and subsequent outcomes. In general, theory allows for the understanding of which observations are indicators of function (typical development) and dysfunction (e.g., developmental lags or delays) (Hinojosa et al., 2017).

Postulates are statements that describe the relationship between two or more concepts. Occupational therapists commonly use eight types of theoretical postulates: temporal, spatial, quantitative, qualitative, correlative, causal, hierarchical, and hypothesis. Postulates state the relationship between concepts. Within the theoretical base, all concepts are related in some way; the relationship between important concepts is made clear by postulates which serve as the linking mechanism between concepts.

Postulates often relate to more than one category. For example, the postulate "Students in Asia spend more time in school than students in the United States" is both quantitative and spatial. Postulates in the frame of reference "Making contact with persons of the opposite sex as an adolescent" are as follows: Postulate: Flirting is usually a socially appropriate way of making contact with someone of the opposite sex; Postulate: Making eye contact and smiling at the same time is an acceptable way of flirting (Hinojosa et al., 2017).

The next part in a frame of reference is referred to as the function-dysfunction continua and this section clearly identifies those areas of function with which the frame of reference is concerned and focuses on. As you read through the theoretical base, you should be able to identify the specific areas of performance important to the child's development of skills and abilities. These are the areas that the therapist evaluates to determine whether the child's development is *functional* or *dysfunctional*. Concepts and their definitions from the theoretical base identify what therapists who use this frame of reference consider to be functional. Likewise, concepts and definitions identify what represents dysfunction. Each function-dysfunction continuum covers one area of performance important to the particular frame of reference. A frame of reference generally has several function-dysfunction continua, which are labeled as such because human performance rarely can be classified as good or bad and abled or disabled. The situation usually is not so clear-cut. Function is at one end of the spectrum and dysfunction is at the other end, and human performance may fall at any point along this scale: Function to Dysfunction. The functional end of the continuum represents what the therapist expects the child to be able to do, whereas the dysfunctional end of the continuum represents disability. The following are some of the core theories most often used to build frames of references for use by occupational therapy practitioners who work with the pediatric population.

25.10 Psychodynamic and Theories of Motivation

Freud and the neo-Freudians focused on motivation, on what drives people to act as they do. Erik Erikson's theory, which addresses primarily psychosocial development, includes the Freudian understanding of the dynamic influences of psychological structures. In addition, Erikson's theory expanded Freud's earlier work by incorporating sociocultural influences on development. Erikson describes human development as a series of conflicts or crises to be resolved, and these crises can be resolved positively or negatively, thereby determining future function (Cronin & Mandich, 2015).

Abraham H. Maslow (1987) also focused on human motivation, developing his *hierarchy of needs* which is usually represented by a pyramid, as shown in Figure 25.4. Physiological needs are at the base of the pyramid, followed by safety, and progressing up the pyramid, love and belonging, esteem, and self-actualization. Maslow theorized that a person acts according to the priority of needs at any given time. Love and belonging reflect the need for intimacy and close interpersonal relationships; esteem is the need to be thought of well; and self-actualization is the realization or fulfillment of one's potentialities (Cronin & Mandich, 2015).

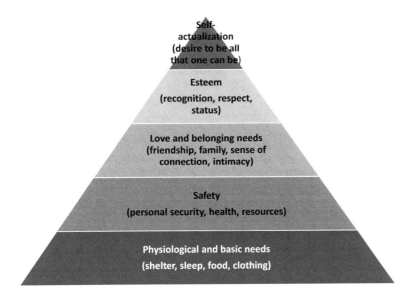

Figure 25.4 Maslow's hierarchy of needs (Maslow, 1987).
Source: Image created by chapter author, Rondalyn V. Whitney.

25.11 Attachment

John Bowlby believed that an intimate and continuous relationship with the mother was necessary for the young child to develop emotional attachments. In collaboration with Mary Ainsworth, three categories of attachment were described: secure, avoidant, and ambivalent. Infants are classified based on the child's response to being reunited with the mother after separation. Securely attached children use the mother as a "home base", referencing her when she is present; avoidant children do not seek proximity to the mother and avoid her when she returns; and ambivalent children have decreased exploratory behavior in the mother's presence. These children are considered ambivalent because they are distressed when the mother leaves and when she returns (Cronin & Mandich, 2015).

25.12 Cognitive Development

Jean Piaget developed a theory of cognitive development that postulated two functional invariants: organization and adaptation. Organization is the tendency to integrate parts into a whole and adaptation is a basic biologic need to permit functioning in a given environment. From adaptation, Piaget further identified the processes of assimilation and accommodation. Assimilation is the process of changing elements of the environment so they can be incorporated into the organism's structure. The function of adaptation is to modify observations and experiences to fit the child's cognitive structures which in Piaget's theory are known as *schema*. These refer to a class of similar sequences of action or mental representations that are related. The process by which assimilation and accommodation are balanced is known as *equilibration* which occurs when neither assimilation nor accommodation is dominant (Cronin & Mandich, 2015).

Piaget named four stages of cognitive development in which thought processes are qualitatively different from previous stages. The first stage is the sensorimotor stage, which can be divided into six substages and runs from birth to two years of age. Substage 1 is *reflexive* and lasts from approximately birth to one month. During this stage the infant performs little volitional activity and most activity is reactive to stimuli, e.g., the infant displays sucking and kicking patterns. Substage 2 involves *primary circular reactions* where the infant can repeat interesting actions volitionally, e.g., the infant will begin to swipe or bat at objects repetitively. In Substage 3, *secondary circular reactions*, the infant begins to act intentionally to make events that are interesting last longer. Secondary circular reactions roughly coincide with four to eight months of age. During Substage 4, *coordination of secondary circular reactions* which occurs from approximately 8–12 months, the infant begins to use objects instrumentally to accomplish a goal.

In Substage 4 of the sensorimotor stage, the infant develops the concept of *object permanence,* in which the infant knows that something continues to exist even when it is out of sight. One of the exercises infants will do to "test" this hypothesis is to drop things off the highchair tray, visually following the object to the floor. When the parent obligingly returns the object to the tray, the infant drops it again, and it is through this type of exploratory play the infant "learns" that objects exist even when out of sight.

The second year of life comprises Piagetian Substages 5 and 6, which last 12–18 and 18–24 months, respectively. In Substage 5, *tertiary circular reactions* occur as the infant experiments with actions and determines consequences. In this stage, the child can solve problems by trial and error, e.g., pulling a blanket to obtain a toy that is out of reach. In Substage 6, *invention of new means through mental combinations,* the child can mentally, without overt experimentation, devise means of manipulating the environment. The stages that follow the sensorimotor stage are preoperational (2–7 years), concrete operations (7–12 years), and formal operations (12 years and up) (Cronin & Mandich, 2015).

25.13 Social Constructivism

The theorist Lev Vygotsky differed from Piaget by emphasizing sociocultural influences on cognitive development, arguing that to understand cognitive development, we must evaluate what is significant in the cultural milieu in which the child is living. Vygotsky (1978) used the term "zone of proximal development" (ZPD) to refer to the child's readiness to comprehend a fact or perform a task. In the ZPD, a child will need minimal support from others to complete the task successfully; this support from others is known as *scaffolding* (Cronin & Mandich, 2015). See Figure 25.5.

25.14 Principles of Development

Arnold Gesell's study of human maturation was guided by three postulates: (1) behavior has a characteristic pattern; (2) the nature of that pattern reflects the underlying maturation of neural structure; and (3) the emergence of the pattern is tied to the genetically driven maturational process. Gesell's formulated *laws of developmental direction* (Cronin & Mandich, 2015) summarized the trends of developmental milestone acquisition as follows:

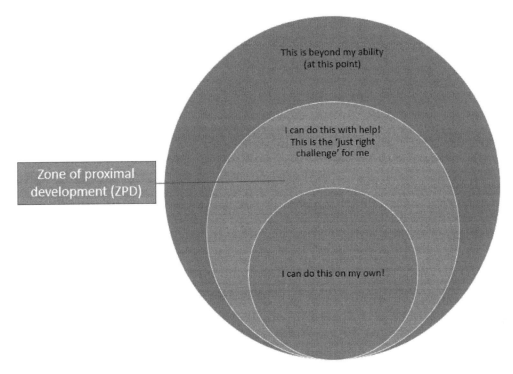

Figure 25.5 Zone of proximal development (Vyotsky, 1078).
Source: Image created by chapter author, Rondalyn V. Whitney.

1. *Development proceeds in a cephalocaudal direction.* As a result, the infant gains control progressively of the head, shoulders, spine, and, ultimately, the lower legs.
2. *Development proceeds proximally to distal.* As a result, the infant gains control of the shoulder and hip before control of the hand and foot.
3. *Development proceeds from medial to lateral.* Medial to lateral development is similar to proximal to distal development, e.g., grasp development moves from the ulnar (medial) side of the hand to the radial (lateral) side.
4. *Development proceeds up against gravity.* First, the infant progresses from completely prone to prone on elbows, then supported by hands, all four limbs, and, finally, standing and walking.

25.15 Behaviorism

This theoretical perspective, known as behaviorism, covers all domains of behavior and has its origins in the classical conditioning experiments conducted by Ivan Pavlov. Pavlov documented how hungry dogs could be conditioned to salivate to the sound of a bell by pairing it with the presentation of food. Salivation was the conditioned response (CR); the sound of the bell, the conditioned stimulus (CS); and the presentation of the meat, the unconditioned stimulus (UCS).

John Watson proposed that behavioral psychology is objective and seeks to predict and control behavior. Watson saw the stimulus-response relationship as the essential one between organism and environment. B. F. Skinner built on Watson's work with his theory of operant conditioning, adding the concept of reinforcement in which the type and rate of responses are directly related to the outcome the individual desires (Cronin & Mandich, 2015).

25.16 Ecological Systems

Learning occurs not only in the brain as the body and environment are always interacting and influencing one another. Intervention, then, considers not only impairments in development, physical, and social systems but also constraints in the environment and with the task. For example, children who spend significant time in constraints (e.g., car seats and strollers) will have fewer opportunities to walk, crawl, and run. Children who never have the opportunity to play with tools (scissors, markers, paint, etc.) will be less prepared for the preschool learning environment than peers exposed to these activities. The child, the environment, and the task (the occupation) overlap individually and work synergistically to promote development (Bronfenbrenner, 1978, 1992).

25.17 Play

Play is self-directed, intrinsically motivated, internally controlled, and freely chosen (Skard & Bundy, 2008). Once activities become directive, they are not play. Routines that are playful offer a child the opportunity to explore their world sensorially. For example, tearing lettuce for the salad, four-year-old Brianna creates a game of tossing the leaves into the bowl, taking turns with Mom, who tosses the cherry tomatoes into the bowl. Children understand their world through the senses (see, hear, smell, taste, feel, move) and children's actions and habits are based on what they learned from their senses. Children who play learn to coordinate their bodies (arms, hands, and fingers); they learn cause and effect; and they experiment and learn to try something new. Later, they can move their bodies more deliberately, take turns, and share in organized play. When learning to play, children will gain mastery of their body, learn to act upon their environment, and build their frustration tolerance and problem-solving capabilities.

While consideration of all categories of play is beyond the scope of this chapter, Brown's work helpfully organizes play broadly (Brown, 2022). The first play-state, *attunement play*, can be seen when a caregiver and infant engage in reciprocal sing-song interchanges. Repeated attunement experiences create neural pathways in the brain that become foundations for trust and motivate future playfulness. Infants begin playing with their bodies early, grabbing their feet, pulling off their socks, enjoying their fingers. *Body and movement play* begins in the womb and lays down the pathway for early muscle control. *Object play*, being curious about objects (e.g., spoons, socks, and sister's earrings), form the intrinsic motivation to explore, manipulate, and understand objects. Later, this play evolves to opening containers, solving a puzzle, and building a block tower. *Imaginative play* can be seen around the time a child becomes a toddler when children begin to tell stories without the need for a beginning, middle, or end, and instead enjoy the narrative for its own sake, using real and make-believe (Eberle, 2014).

Play schemes, where stuffed animals become connected train cars and boxes transform into magical portals, provide a rich environment for magical play. A cleared-out cupboard in the kitchen with flashlights and toilet paper tools can be a source of infinite amusement. Human beings are social beings and *social play* begins with a game of peek-a-boo. It evolves from parallel play to joint engagement, games with rules, and eventually satisfying friendships (Eberle, 2014).

25.18 Conclusion
The time between birth and the fifth year is a chaotic, exciting, and exuberant period of growth for human beings. During this time, an environment that invites, promotes, and facilitates playful engagement with caregivers, friends, objects, and imagination affords a child a precious time to develop. When barriers are presented, intervention focuses on removing barriers to playful exploration through daily routines. Theorists provide the framework for therapists to predict growth patterns and enrich opportunities for development.

25.19 Summary
- Play is self-directed; otherwise, the task becomes work.
- Theory guides practice and supports therapists in developing a clinical hypothesis to guide intervention.
- Milestones are critical to recognizing function and dysfunction during development.
- Milestones can be broadly categorized into social-emotional, language, cognitive adaptive behavior, and motor skills.
- Children learn through the senses; play that provides sensory-rich experiences promotes optimal learning.
- Embedding play into family routines is critical for early child development.

25.20 Review Questions
1. What are the best practice principles of occupational therapy that promote participation?
2. What are important concepts of family centered care?
3. How do foundational theories inform occupational therapy intervention approaches?
4. What is the influence of motivation and self-efficacy on learning?
5. How do play routines change during early development (infant, toddler, and preschool age)?

References
American Occupational Therapy Association. (2020). Occupational Therapy Practice Framework: Domain and process (4th ed.). *American Journal of Occupational Therapy*, 74(Suppl. 2), 7412410010p1–7412410010p87. https://doi.org/10.5014/ajot.2020.74S2001

Bronfenbrenner, U. (1978). *The ecology of human development*. Harvard University Press.

Bronfenbrenner, U. (1992). Ecological systems theory. In R. Vasta (Ed.), *Six theories of child development: Revised formulations and current issues* (pp. 187–249). Jessical Kingsley Publishers.

Brown, S. (2022). What is Play? National Institute for Play. https://www.nifplay.org/what-is-play/types-of-play/

Centers for Disease Control and Prevention (CDC). (n.d.). Milestones checklist. https://www.cdc.gov/ncbddd/actearly/pdf/FULL-LIST-CDC_LTSAE-Checklists2021_Eng_FNL2_508.pdf

Cronin, A., & Mandich, M. (2015). Human development and performance across the lifespan (2nd ed.). Cengage.

Eberle, S. G. (2014). The elements of play: Toward a philosophy and a definition of play. *American Journal of Play, 6*(2), 214–233. https://eric.ed.gov/?id=EJ1023799

Einstein, A. (1962). As quoted by N. V. Scarfe "play is education". *Childhood Education, 39*(3), 120. Association for Childhood Education International.

Emerson, R. W. (n.d.). Goodreads quotable quotes. https://www.goodreads.com/quotes/84615-a-child-is-a-curly-dimpled-lunatic

Hinojosa, J., Kramer, P., & Howe, T. (2017). Structure of the frame of reference: Moving from theory to practice. In J. Hinojosa, P. Kramer, & T. Howe (Eds.), *Frames of reference for pediatric occupational therapy* (4th ed., pp. 3–19). Wolters Kluwer.

Knox, S. (2008). Development and current use of the revised Knox Preschool Play Scale. In L. D. Parham & L. S. Fazio (Eds.), *Play in occupational therapy for children* (2nd ed., pp. 55–70). Mosby.

Lawlor, M., & Mattingly, C. (2019). Family perspectives on occupation, health, and disability. In B. A. Boyt-Schelle & G. Gillen (Eds.), *Williard and Spackman's occupational therapy* (13th ed., pp. 196–211). Wolters Kluwer.

Maslow, A. H. (1987). *Motivation and personality* (3rd ed.). Pearson Education.

Romano, R. (n.d.). Goodreads Quotable Quotes. https://www.goodreads.com/quotes/63411-having-children-is-like-living-in-a-frat-house--

Skard, G., & Bundy, A. C. (2008). Test of Playfulness. In L. D. Parham, & L. S. Fazio, (Eds.), *Play in occupational therapy for children* (2nd ed., pp. 71–93). Mosby Elsevier.

Vygotsky, L. S. (1978). *Mind and society: The development of higher psychological processes.* Harvard University Press.

Whitney, R. (2018). Sensory integration and sensory processing frames of reference. In A. Cronin & G. Graebe (Eds.), *Clinical reasoning in occupational therapy* (pp. 123–141). AOTA Press.

Whitney, R., & Gibbs, V. (2020). *Using sensory strategies to improve family life.* Prufrock Press.

Whitney, R., & Luebben, A. (2016). Interpretation and documentation. In J. Hinojosa & P. Kramer (Eds.), *Evaluation in occupational therapy: Obtaining and interpreting data* (pp. 188–203). AOTA Press.

CHAPTER 26

Human Occupations of School-aged Children

Evguenia S. Popova, Jane C. O'Brien, Mong-Lin Yu, Jarrett Wolske, Adam DePrimo, and Ted Brown

Abstract
This chapter discusses the occupations of school-aged children and the influence of social determinants of health and well-being on occupational participation. The chapter examines contextual influences on occupational development and explores how habits, roles, routines, and rituals create performance patterns that impact occupational participation. Case examples illustrate occupational therapy's role in examining school-aged children's occupations.

Objectives
This chapter will allow the reader to:

- Describe the development of occupations in school-aged children (5–14 years old).
- Examine occupational therapy's role in assessing school-aged children's occupations.
- Describe social determinants of health and well-being for school-aged children.
- Examine how the environment and cultural contexts influence school-aged children's occupations.
- Describe how habits, roles, routines, and rituals create performance patterns for school-aged children.
- Examine how well-being (e.g., physical, mental, and social) contributes to and is influenced by school-aged children's occupational participation.

> **Key terms**
> - Bronfenbrenner's Ecological Theory
> - environment and contexts
> - occupational competency
> - occupational identity
> - occupational participation
> - self-determination
> - school-aged culture
> - social determinants of health and well-being

Authors' Positionality Statement

The authors of this chapter include occupational therapists with experience working with school-aged children and their families. They have earned doctoral degrees, taught in academia, and completed research that examined influences on occupational participation. The material presented may represent socio-political orientations of occupational engagement relevant to their experiences in Australia, Canada, Taiwan, Russia, and the US. The authors aimed to explore evidence-based and demographically diverse perspectives on the occupations of school-aged children. However, the content is not exhaustive nor representative of every cultural and social reality. Readers are urged to critically assess the authors and their positionality as they explore the complexity of the occupations of school-aged children.

26.1 Introduction

School age (5–14 years old) is a critical phase in which children begin formal learning and education either at home or in a school environment. School-aged children develop core life skills, meaningful occupations, and strategies to support their transition into adulthood. Occupations and activity participation for school-aged children evolve with the child's development and are influenced by the child's home, school, and community environments.

This chapter offers descriptions of the occupational characteristics and assessments specific to each of the nine categories of human occupations delineated in the Occupational Therapy Practice Framework – 4th Edition (OTPF-4) (AOTA, 2020). The chapter specifically focuses on the occupations of school-aged children, the social determinants of health and well-being, and environmental influences across contexts. The components that form the structure of a child's performance patterns, including roles, habits, routines, and rituals, are also discussed. In examining social determinants of health and well-being, we consider how occupations and occupational participation of school-aged children can be influenced by the child's and the family's economic stability, as well as access to education, health care, and resources in their social and community contexts (Office of Disease Prevention and Health Promotion, n.d.). Box 26.1 highlights examples of the influence of social determinants on health and well-being.

Box 26.1 Social Determinants of Health and Well-being

Social determinants of health and well-being refer to societal, physical, and economic factors that impact children's occupational choices, opportunities, and outcomes related to health and well-being (WHO, 2022). Common barriers experienced by marginalized families include accessibility, affordability, acceptability, utilization, and quality and continuity of care (Spencer et al., 2019). For example, Dutta et al. (2020) found that the risks of anemia and absenteeism due to sickness were greater for school-aged children from less advantaged castes than those from the most advantaged castes in rural India. Similarly, Ahmed et al. (2022) found social inequities in access to health care for women and children in Pakistan, resulting in poorer health outcomes.

Policies that strengthen access to inclusive health care, family economics, family friendly work, and high-quality early childcare and education promote occupational choices and participation (Ahmed et al., 2022; Klevens et al., 2021). Occupational therapy practitioners play a critical role in service access and can engage in community-level advocacy and program development to provide opportunities for school-aged children that support their health and well-being.

26.2 Occupations of School-aged Children

School-aged children experience critical transitions from early childhood to middle childhood and adolescence. Occupations in this life stage occur within the contexts of home, school, and community, and can be characterized into nine categories (AOTA, 2020):

- activities of daily living (ADLs)
- instrumental activities of daily living (IADLs)
- health management
- rest and sleep
- education
- work and volunteerism
- play
- leisure
- social participation.

A child's environment (e.g., physical, social, virtual, and political) and culture (e.g., beliefs, values, rituals, and patterns) influence occupational choices and how occupations are performed. For example, despite core similarities in play occupations, school-aged children's play varies across cultures. Different social contexts and social expectations may influence how much time children spend in child-led (vs. adult-led) play activities, and Western concepts of a "play date" that are common in the US and Canada may not be familiar to immigrant families and families who live outside of North America. Examples of occupations within each of the nine categories are presented in Table 26.1, and an in-depth discussion of each category is presented later in this chapter.

Table 26.1 Occupations of School-aged Children

OTPF-4 definition and examples (AOTA, 2020)	Illustration of occupational participation
Activities of Daily Living (ADLs): Activities oriented toward taking care of one's own body and completed on a routine basis, including: - Eating and feeding - Dressing - Hygiene and grooming - Bathing and showering - Toileting and toilet hygiene - Functional mobility - Personal device care - Sexual activity	Kylie is a five-year-old girl who loves to swim. Kylie's parents hope to enroll her in a community swim class. However, Kylie experiences frequent accidents because she cannot tell her parents that she needs to go to the bathroom. At home, Kylie indicates when she needs to use the toilet by pointing to the bathroom door. However, in the community, she does not yet communicate her needs. To help Kylie be more independent and participate in community activities, Kylie's parents are exploring ways to reinforce their bathroom routine outside the home.
Instrumental Activities of Daily Living (IADLs): Activities to support daily life within the home and community, including: - Care of pets - Care of others - Driving and community mobility - Financial management - Home establishment and management - Meal preparation and cleanup - Religious and spiritual activities and expression - Safety and emergency maintenance - Shopping	Marx is an 11-year-old boy who is enrolled in fifth grade. Marx got a dog for his birthday. Although Marx loves to play with the dog and take it on walks, he often forgets to feed, groom, and train the dog. With help from his parents, Marx created a digital to-do list on his phone to ensure his pet's needs were met. The visual organizer is clear and helps Marx follow the daily routine, and he can independently record the completion of each task throughout the day.
Health Management: Activities related to developing, managing, and maintaining health and wellness routines, including: - Social and emotional health promotion and maintenance - Symptom and condition management - Medication management - Physical activity - Nutrition management	Jovan is a nine-year-old boy who is enrolled in fourth grade. Jovan carries his asthma inhaler in a small pack, easily accessible throughout the day. He learned how often he could use the inhaler during the day and knows internal cues of needing to use it.
Rest and sleep: Activities related to obtaining restorative rest and sleep, including: - Rest - Sleep preparation and participation	Isis is 14 years old, is enrolled in ninth grade, and uses they/them pronouns. Before bed, they like to take a warm bath, have a hot drink, and read. They shut off all electronics at 9:00 pm and typically fall asleep by 9:30. This routine helps Isis feel awake, rested, and ready for school by 7:00 am.

(Continued)

Table 26.1 (Continued)

Education: Activities needed for learning and participating in the educational environment, including: • Formal educational participation • Information educational participation and exploration	Alessandro is 12 years old and is about to transition from sixth to seventh grade. Alessandro's school team meets with Alessandro and his family to develop a transition plan for the next school year. The team assesses Alessandro's academic progress and preferences for extracurricular activities. The team also assesses Alessandro's technology use and discusses ways to improve his independence in using the computer.
Work and Volunteerism: Labor or exertion related to the development, production, delivery, or management of objects or services, including: • Volunteer exploration and participation • Work exploration and acquisition • Work participation and performance	Peyton is 13 years old and is passionate about horses. Peyton's mother hopes to help Peyton develop more work, social, and community navigation skills. The family helps Peyton volunteer at the horse barn, where she previously received hippotherapy to learn pre-vocational work and social skills while pursuing her interests and passion.
Play: Activities that are intrinsically motivated, internally controlled, and freely chosen may include suspension of reality, including: • Play exploration and participation	Damian is an eight-year-old boy with a dual diagnosis of autism and ADHD. He lives in a multi-generational apartment with his parents and grandmother. Damian's parents are concerned that he does not express any interest in social play with peers outside of school. Damian's occupational therapist met with Damian and his family to assess and problem-solve ways to encourage opportunities for Damian to participate in play with peers at home and in the community.
Leisure: Non-obligatory activity that is intrinsically motivated and engaged in during discretionary time, including: • Leisure exploration and participation	Grace is a seven-year-old girl with a recent diagnosis that has resulted in progressive vision loss. Low vision has impacted Grace's ability to participate in her interests, including reading, video games, and baking. The occupational therapist and Grace collaborated on developing goals to increase her leisure participation through environmental modifications and assistive technology.
Social Participation: Activities that involve social interaction with others, including: • Interactions with family, friends, and peers • Social participation in the community	Theo is a six-year-old child who enjoys spending time with his friends and family. During the week, Theo looks forward to going to school to be with his teacher, aide, and friends in the playground. On the weekends, he visits his grandparents and attends the local Orthodox liturgies with his parents and siblings.

26.3 Influence of Environment and Cultural Context

A child's environment and cultural context can influence the occupation and the expectations of the child's occupational performance. Ecological system theorists, such as Bronfenbrenner (2005), view child development as a complex process involving five interrelated systems that influence children's choice of occupation and performance: *microsystem* (child's immediate environment), *mesosystem* (interaction between the microsystem and the exosystem), *exosystem* (social influences on the child), *macrosystem* (ideological influences on the child), and *chronosystem* (time influences on the child). The interaction between these systems is illustrated in Figure 26.1.

Occupational therapy practitioners must consider the influence of each system on both the child and the occupation, and recognize how these influences can impact the child's participation across home, school, community, cultural, and virtual environments. The interaction between these systems influences the child and the child's occupations. For example, as a child participates in school, their motivation and performance in learning are influenced by their teacher and others in their community. In this example, a fifth-grade teacher (*microsystem*) may introduce the child and their classmates to climate change. To do this, the teacher develops a class project in which the students work together to create a documentary on the influence of climate change on animals in their country. The students work together to visit a local zoo and interview subject matter experts (*exosystem*) on this topic. The teacher facilitates the interaction between the students and the zookeepers (*mesosystem*) and helps the students develop questions for the interview. She also helps the students research the topic of climate change and engages the class in a debate on policies (*macrosystem*) to address climate

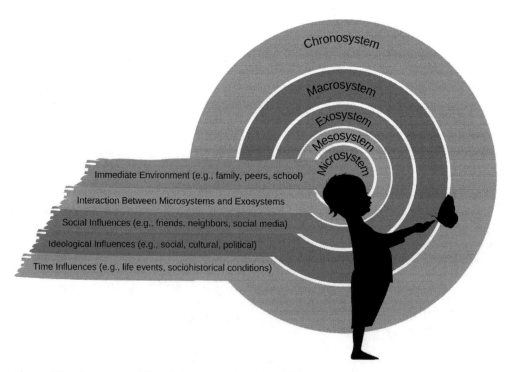

Figure 26.1 Depiction of Bronfenbrenner's Ecological Theory.

change in their city. At the end of the project, the teacher hosts a viewing party and the students share how this experience changed their views on climate change over time (*chronosystem*).

26.3.1 Home Environment

Home is the place where children live with their parents and/or caregivers. The home environment impacts children's development, physical health, and emotional and mental well-being. It can also provide children with a sense of belonging and security. Within the home environment, many factors such as physical space and objects, cultural norms, family structure and routines, family values, family members' roles, parents' time availability, socioeconomic resources, parents' relationship, and parent-child relationships influence children's occupations. For example, children living in an urban apartment building may be more likely to participate in indoor activities such as watching television, reading, playing video games, or baking, compared to children living in a suburban house with a backyard or nearby parklands. Single-parent or dual-earning families may have less time available for parent-child co-occupations, but that does not mean they do not value or have quality parent-child time. Parents' discipline, family routines, and the amount of time and attention parents devote to monitoring and supporting children's occupations contribute to participation in constructive activities such as reading, socializing with friends, and sports (Inoa, 2017).

26.3.2 School Environment

Schools are settings where children receive educational instruction. Schools may be buildings or outside spaces. Children come together at school to engage in education which often includes reading, math, language, and science tailored to challenge students at their level. The culture and policies influence the curriculum of the school and the information provided to students within the classroom may impact their attitudes and worldview. For example, books and learning materials representing cultural and social diversity, humility, and understanding have been shown to promote positive coping strategies, resilience, belongingness, and inclusiveness within the school context (Di Maggio et al., 2022; Williams et al., 2021). As children learn about different cultures and social diversity, they develop an understanding of others, and research suggests that classmates' attitudes toward peers with disabilities are associated with the representation of peers with disabilities that focuses on their strengths (Di Maggio et al., 2022).

While some children feel welcomed in the school environment, others may be fearful that they will not be accepted and experience social exclusion (Laninga-Wijnen et al., 2021). Despite the importance of representation, there remains a need to support positive illustrations of disability culture in children's books, related media, and educational materials. For example, Golos et al. (2012) found that children's literature depicting d/Deaf characters did not consistently illustrate d/Deaf characters from a cultural perspective, and instead was more likely to focus on disability from the perspective of needing intervention to best "fit" into the hearing world.

This research highlights opportunities for occupational therapists to advocate for increased inclusion and celebration of disability culture. An example of how occupational therapists have advocated for increased diversity, equity, and inclusion can be seen through curricula like Every Moment Counts, developed by Bazyk et al. (2018) in the US. This initiative has supported schools in incorporating programming to promote students' mental health, resilience, and well-being, including recognizing and distinguishing emotions and ways to respond to bullying.

26.3.3 Community Environment

Community refers to the local environment where the child resides and spends their time outside of home and school. School-aged children's participation in the community is impacted by safety, facilities, funding, accessibility, and social policy (Marino et al., 2018; Visser & Aalst, 2021). For example, home confinement during the COVID-19 pandemic led to compromised daily family routines, family members' mental health, physical activity participation, and eating behaviors (Ammar et al., 2020).

A child's independence in the community varies depending on the child's and family's preferences, routines, and expectations. For example, two children residing in the same city may have different levels of community participation due to environmental influences. One child residing in a rural part of town may be allowed to visit friends next door, walk to the neighborhood store by themselves, or walk to and from school. However, parents of another child residing in the urban neighborhood may be hesitant to allow their child to leave home without adult supervision due to safety concerns.

Limited facilities and resources, such as playgrounds, parks, sports facilities, and community groups, available in the immediate community may reduce participation in the community or require that children spend more time traveling to access the facilities. Likewise, health and social care funding significantly influence occupational participation for children with disabilities. Additionally, community mobility is a major aspect of the childhood experience and is heavily influenced by the community environment. As children gain safety awareness they begin to explore the community independently from their parents. Children engage in less independent outdoor play if parents are concerned about neighborhood safety and accessibility (Visser & Aalst, 2021).

26.3.4 Cultural Environment

Culture broadly influences the direct and indirect environments where children explore and participate in occupations, and expectations and occupations for children vary among cultures (Guthold et al., 2020; Li & Xie, 2020; Pinquart & Ebeling, 2019). For example, children from East Asian families influenced by Confucianism may be expected to excel academically and are more likely to spend increased time in sedentary academic activities. Commonly, children in East Asia start learning mathematics, reading, written expression, music, or a foreign language at preschool age. They are also expected to complete homework and participate in tutoring outside school hours to achieve rigorous academic expectations and progress in the educational system during school years. As preschoolers, children in Australia commonly engage in play and social activities and attend extracurricular events that often focus on expanding children's interests in sports, music, and the arts. While parents from East Asian cultures may see themselves in teaching, directing, and disciplinary roles and choose to support children in academic tasks, parents from Australia may spend more time playing or engaging in leisure activities with their children.

Families within the same culture may also hold different attitudes toward their children's occupational participation. For example, some families may view their child's education as a way to secure a better economic and social future. As a result, children may feel pressure to pursue career options based on their perceived status and prestige (e.g., law, medicine, dentistry, and engineering) rather than on their interests. Understanding the expectations and beliefs of families about educational expectations, occupational roles, and engagement levels with their children empowers family centered occupational therapy.

Due to the complexity of cultural nuances and the vastness of different cultures, occupational therapy practitioners must be cognizant of intersectionality between cultures, and practice cultural humility to understand the occupations of school-aged children. Box 26.2 illustrates the intersectionality between language and disability cultures.

Box 26.2 Supporting Language Learners with Disabilities

As demographics shift globally, occupational therapy practitioners must be aware of the intersectionality between immigrant and disability experiences of language learners. In the US, educators are becoming increasingly aware of the influences of the "language-or-disability" filter, where educators may only examine the student's experience from language or disability perspectives while missing the impact of systemic influences on English language learners with disabilities (Kangas, 2021). As a result, practitioners may overlook the needs of children with disabilities if a language barrier exists that impacts their educational needs. To support language learners with disabilities, occupational therapy practitioners and educators must be cognizant of culturally responsive education practices (Orosco & O'Connor, 2013) and seek training in bilingual and special education teaching practices (Wang & Woolf, 2015). For example, occupational therapy practitioners and teachers can work together to incorporate students' cultures and lived experiences in the classroom by integrating diverse customs, perspectives, and narratives into the curriculum.

26.3.5 Virtual Environment

The internet has become an indispensable resource in everyday life. Children may spend time online for play, leisure, social participation, education, and exploration of future work interests (Daoud et al., 2020; Park & Kwon, 2018). Additionally, school-aged children are increasingly found to use the internet as a means of social participation, identity exploration, and engagement in cyberculture (Kennedy & Lynch, 2016). Tablet and online applications are commonly introduced to children in elementary school to promote teaching, learning, physical activity, testing, and evaluation. Online games and social media platforms are popular entertainment and socialization tools among children and adolescents. Beyond serving as a social tool to connect with friends and families, social media is critical in promoting children's culture. School curriculum, parents' attitudes, financial resources, and internet access may influence children's accessibility to the online environment.

Parents and educators may worry about cyber safety and bullying, the quality of online resources, and online screen time regarding children's health and safety. For example, parents and caregivers may express concern that extensive use of social media will place their children at risk for personal safety, privacy concerns, access to inappropriate material, and mental health risks (specifically related to cyberbullying and access to explicit materials). Research also suggests that school-aged children report negative effects of internet overuse (Kennedy & Lynch, 2016).

To promote participation in virtual environments, occupational therapy practitioners can support initiatives to promote internet safety and protective factors. The benefits of social connectedness within online communities are increasingly recognized in research (Dyer, 2018), and increased social connectedness is a protective factor and primary coping strategy for youth experiencing bullying (Monks et al., 2012). Youth who are more socially connected have a stronger capacity to actively cope with cyberbullying, including increased help-seeking behaviors and positive mental health (Hamm et al., 2015).

Occupations that encourage social connection, such as participation in video games, have been recognized for their therapeutic potential in promoting mental health, positive behaviors, and social participation in children and youth (Cahill et al., 2020). Additionally, virtual spaces are increasingly examined for their therapeutic potential. For example, the game Re-Mission (Kato et al., 2008) was designed to support the health promotion of children undergoing cancer treatment. Within the game, the player can control nanobots to attack cancer cells, overcome infections, and manage symptoms (e.g., nausea and constipation), and the game has been shown to increase adherence to treatment, self-efficacy, and cancer-related knowledge in the treatment group (Kato et al., 2008).

26.4 Performance Patterns

Performance patterns include the child's *roles* (set of behaviors expected and shaped by society and culture), *habits* (specific and automatic behaviors), *routines* (observable patterns of behavior), and *rituals* (symbolic actions with spiritual, cultural, or social meaning), and support the child's occupational choices, participation, and identity (AOTA, 2020; Taylor, 2017). *Roles* are socially defined, context-dependent, and culturally influenced. They exert an organizing influence on performance by indicating which occupations a child is expected to perform relative to given life roles. Through role participation, a school-aged child develops the necessary skills and patterns of performance to participate in daily occupations. While expectations vary, a school-aged child's roles may include being a student, friend, sibling, hobbyist, volunteer, sports team member, and worker.

The degree that *habits* support or hinder occupational participation depends on the child's self-efficacy and consistency in contexts and environments. For example, in some cultures, such as the US, a child may be in the habit of making their bed when they get up in the morning, brushing their teeth after having breakfast, cleaning up after meals, and completing homework before bedtime. As the child completes these daily habits, they may receive praise or encouragement from their parents and develop positive feelings reinforcing those habits and patterns. However, an adolescent who participates in the worker role part-time may struggle to balance the demands of their academic, familial, social, and work expectations. This can lead to ineffective study habits, feelings of anxiety, and poor-quality sleep routines.

While habits are tendencies that can support or hinder consistent occupational participation, *routines* are the pairing of multiple occupations performed over a definite period. For example, a school-aged child's morning routine may include expectations of grooming, bathing, eating, and packing for school before the bus arrives. Researchers have examined the intersection of habits, routines, and time use, sometimes called temporal adaptation, in school-aged children (Mullan, 2019). Watson et al. (2020) found that engaging in light physical activity is related to better numeracy and literacy skills in school-aged children. In contrast to the automaticity of habits, routines and rituals allow for moments of pause and reflection.

School-aged children also carry out *rituals* as co-occupations with their families and loved ones. These rituals may include Sunday dinners, participating in liturgies, assisting parents or grandparents with celebratory activities, and preparing for holidays. Rituals may include classroom or school activities (e.g., morning announcements with reflection, singing after recess, or at the end of the workday organizing your desk for the following day).

Figure 26.2 illustrates the connection between the concepts that influence performance patterns. As school-aged children develop their performance patterns, they develop a sense of occupational identity. For example, a nine-year-old child who excels in art class may begin to view themselves as a good artist or art student. If their artistic talents are reinforced and recognized, they may seek opportunities to work on creative projects at home and in the community. They may find new art-related hobbies and spend time with peers who share this interest. As they engage in creative projects (e.g., occupational participation), they develop supportive performance patterns and it becomes who they are (e.g., occupational identity), which leads to a positive sense of self (i.e., occupational competency). These experiences can influence the child as they grow to base their decisions on their artistic occupational identity and purposefully choose to engage in occupations that lead to further study and an art career.

The following case vignette (Amar; Box 26.3) illustrates how environmental changes (i.e., impact) affect a child's roles, habits, routines, and rituals that influence occupational participation, identity, and competence. The case highlights the importance of viewing the interactions between multiple factors (e.g., personal, social, cultural, economic, environmental, and contextual) before making assumptions and planning programming.

26.4.1 Developmental Expectations for Occupational Participation in School-aged Children

As school-aged children grow and develop, they participate in more complex and diverse activities independently, with peers, or with adult assistance (or supervision). While age expectations, tasks, and performance patterns vary within cultures and families, parents begin to shift responsibility for daily tasks to their children as they start school, with the majority of children taking on full responsibility by 15 years of age (Kao et al., 2021). Even with increasing levels of independence and responsibility, children and adolescents participate in daily occupations and organized family events with their relatives. Occupational therapy practitioners analyze the occupational expectations for each child and family to accurately address the child's and family's

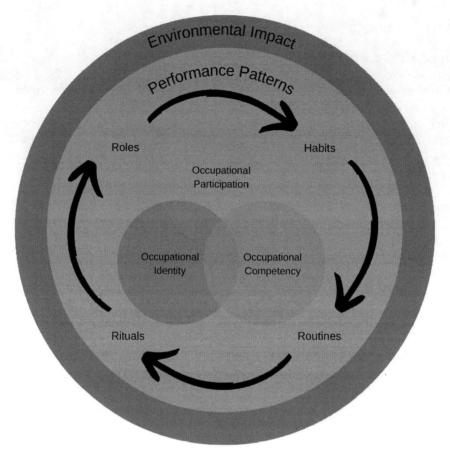

Figure 26.2 Factors influencing school-aged children's performance patterns.

Box 26.3 Case Vignette Amar

Amar is a ten-year-old student who recently enrolled in a new school district due to a cross-country move. Amar's parents immigrated from the Punjab region of India, and Amar grew up in a bilingual household of Punjabi and English. His previous school and community contexts supported his cultural identity as Southeast Asian, and Amar had friends who practiced the same faith as him, Sikhism.

At his new school, Amar struggles with finding academic success. When Amar first started the new school, the school administration attempted to place him into an English as a Second Language (ESL) program, despite Amar and his family being fully bilingual. The experience of his parents advocating for him made Amar weary of the new school. Since that event, Amar has completed assignments late and with poor quality. His parents are concerned about his low grades and general disengagement. Amar reports that he does not have any close friends at the new school and that he misses his old school and community. He also misses spending time with his cousins and having Sunday meals with his grandparents. He is nervous and worries that something bad may happen to his grandparents because he is not with them.

The move significantly disrupted Amar's valued social roles as a family member and friend, and impacted his performance patterns, occupational identity, and competency as a student. Amar missed being close to his family and friends and found it hard to make new friends at school. Being far from his family and friends made it challenging for Amar to maintain his previous routines of studying and playing with friends after school. Instead, Amar found himself doing homework alone and staying up late playing video games to stay in touch with his friends from home.

While online gaming helped Amar stay connected with friends, it made it challenging for him to get enough sleep and feel rested in school. As the school year progressed, Amar's teachers became more concerned that Amar frequently falls asleep in class. They were also concerned that instead of playing with peers at recess, Amar spent time alone doing homework at the library.

The teachers met with Amar's parents to discuss how to best support Amar's connection with same-aged peers at school and in the community. Amar's parents shared that Amar had a strong interest in gaming, which has been a way for him to stay connected with his friends from home. The teachers recommended that the family explore opportunities for Amar to get involved in afterschool clubs, including the robotics club, to build and expand upon his interest in gaming.

goals. Table 26.2 provides examples of the developmental progression of selected IADLs within the context of the United States.

As children enter kindergarten at five years old, their fine and gross motor skills support mastery of various occupations and activities, including play, sports, art, and music. This leads to a sense of occupational competence and identity further supported by cognitive and social-emotional capacities. By six years old, children engage in multi-step projects and activities, such as drawing a self-portrait. At the same time, social play expands in complexity and between seven and nine years old, children show increased interest in structured play activities with peers. Children between eight and nine years old begin to understand that a single problem can have multiple solutions, setting the stage for play that incorporates rules, giving instruction, and storytelling. By nine or ten years old, children participate in structured games and can also narrate detailed stories about their experiences and the experiences of others.

Middle childhood and adolescence increase awareness and understanding of personal identity and social relationships. Children reflect on their unique selves, gender identity, and sexual orientation through this process. The transition to adolescence also introduces new nuances to social relationships as children transform their relationships with their family, friends, and peers, and explore possibilities of romantic relationships. Through self-discovery, children may renegotiate their connections with others and explore different social groups. For example, a parent may find that their child is less interested in spending time with family and is more focused on spending time with their friends on week nights and weekends. Children may also explore new interests related to hobbies, volunteerism, and work. In addition to exploring new social roles,

Table 26.2 Developmental Progression of Independence during IADL within Home Context

Kindergarten-2 Grade (5–8 years old)	3–5 Grade (8–11 years old)	6–8 Grade (11–14 years old)
Taking care of clothes		
Assisting with laundry by loading and unloading the washer and dryer. Folding, hanging, and sorting clothes.	Selecting and putting on an outfit while getting ready for school or preparing a school uniform to wear.	Doing simple mending by sewing a button. Doing simple sewing, such as making a dress for a doll.
Preparing food		
Assisting with meal prep by stirring and mixing. Make simple cold dishes, such as a salad or sandwich.	Making simple hot dishes, such as scrambled eggs or waffles.	Preparing simple meals, such as tacos and guacamole. Preparing complex hot meals, such as baking a chocolate cake.
Taking care of a pet		
Feeding the dog and teaching it simple commands.	Walking the dog around the block accompanied by an adult or caregiver.	Taking the dog to a dog park. Working as a dog walker or sitter.
Yard work		
Watering the plants and raking leaves.	Planting flowers.	Tending to a garden and mowing the lawn.
Taking care of others		
Feeding a younger sibling. Helping a younger sibling get dressed.	Reading to a younger sibling.	Watching younger siblings. Working as a babysitter.
Taking care of technology		
Using a tablet or iPad for online learning, games, or leisure. Taking care of the iPad by ensuring it is safely stored and charged.	Using a personal computer, including managing the contents saved on the computer, and installing new software (e.g., games) with parents' or older siblings' assistance.	Updating personal computers, including independently installing or upgrading software and hardware with parents' or older siblings' assistance.

children become increasingly independent at home, school, and community. For example, at home children may acquire new responsibilities by completing increasingly complex chores such as cleaning, gardening, taking care of pets, or supervising siblings and younger family members.

Adolescents engage in school activities and become involved in leadership and service through clubs and other student or service organizations. Outside of school, adolescents may begin to explore opportunities for paid employment and earn money through activities like babysitting, yard work, and dog walking. This expanded capacity and motivation for independence fosters a desire to participate in activities with minimal adult supervision, including participation in social events with peers, such as parties, movies, shopping, or trips around the community. Motivation for independence and expanded interests also require youth to become skilled in community mobility, money management, and time management. An overview of developmental expectations for occupational participation by age and grade level is presented in Table 26.3.

26.5 Research Specific to Occupational Participation in School-aged Children

Engagement and participation in occupations is an essential contributor to the health and well-being of school-aged children. Yet, disparities in occupational engagement between children with and without developmental disabilities remain prevalent. For example, children with and without an autism diagnosis who experience motor challenges are more likely to experience difficulty participating in daily occupations such as

Table 26.3 Developmental Expectations for Occupational Participation of School-aged Children

Kindergarten–2 Grade (5–8 years old)

ADL and IADL

- Completes basic self-care (e.g., dressing, toileting, and bathing)
- Completes simple errands and chores (e.g., cleaning up while following 2–3 step instructions)
- Maintains simple money management (e.g., lunch money and allowance)

Rest/sleep and health management

- Taking care of minor health care needs

Play

- Games with rules: board games, computer games, competitive, and cooperative games
- Dramatic play: role play stories with themes, emphasis on reality, and reconstruction of the real world
- Social play: participates in group activities and organized play in groups and teams

Education

- Keeps track of and brings homework home
- Keeps track of time and completes work independently for up to 20 minutes

Work and volunteerism

- Developing a plan to reach a goal
- Begins exploration of different worker role identities

Social participation

- Follows social expectations for school and community activities with adult supervision (e.g., raising a hand before speaking in class)

(Continued)

Table 26.3 (Continued)

3–5 Grade (8–11 years old)

ADL and IADL
- Completes simple errands with increased time delay and distance from an adult
- Completes multi-step chores for 15–30 minutes
- Saves money and plans how to earn money

Rest/sleep and health management
- Follows instructions while participating in health management and medical treatment activities

Play and leisure
- Games with rules: computer games, card games, board games, and games that require problem-solving and abstract thinking
- Sports: participates in cooperative and competitive organized sports with other children with an emphasis on winning
- Social play: begins to play with a consistent group of friends, peer play predominates at home and school, and play includes storytelling and humor (e.g., telling jokes)

Education
- Keeps track of and completes homework for up to 60 minutes
- Plans and completes simple projects (e.g., art project and book report)

Work and volunteerism
- Begins exploration of community engagement through volunteering

Social participation
- Uses internet safely
- Follows social expectations for school and community activities with minimal adult supervision (e.g., able to follow directions while an adult is away from the room)
- Visiting relatives, attending holiday celebrations, and taking family holidays

6–8 Grade (11–14 years old)

ADL and IADL
- Completes multi-step errands and responsibilities for up to 60–90 minutes
- Increased independence in community mobility (biking, public transportation, may begin to explore driving)

Rest/sleep and health management
- Establishes and manages bedtime routine
- Sleeps 8–10 hours

Play and leisure
- Plans and uses leisure time to pursue recreational activities

Education
- Follows a complex school and extracurricular schedule with minimal reminders
- Plans and organizes school, work, and leisure opportunities
- Begins to manage projects and schoolwork effectively, including following deadlines and effectively responding to feedback from others

(Continued)

Table 26.3 (Continued)

Work and volunteerism

- Begins to explore vocational interests
- Begins to identify and work toward long-term goals (e.g., plans for work, college, and independent living)
- Begins to participate in unpaid volunteer and paid employment opportunities (e.g., babysitting and yard work)

Social participation

- Establish a sense of emerging identity and seeks to belong to a peer group
- Follows social expectations for in-school and community activities without adult supervision (e.g., able to follow directions without any adults present)
- Manages relationships (e.g., friendship and romantic) with others

---

dressing, bathing, health management, cleaning up and organization, meal preparation and cleanup, education, and safety (Travers et al., 2022).

As outlined in Table 26.3, age strongly predicts participation across home, school, and community settings. For example, younger children may be more likely to participate in household activities that rely on parent-child co-occupations instead of community activities (Little et al., 2014). Meanwhile, older children may be more likely to participate in outdoor and faith-based activities (Little et al., 2014). The shift of responsibility from parents to children (with and without disabilities) for completing everyday occupations is associated with the child's age, cognition, and birth order (i.e., older children assume greater responsibility). However, across the different age groups, children and youth with developmental disabilities (e.g., general developmental delay, intellectual disability, or physical disabilities) take on less responsibility than their peers without a disability.

Beyond personal factors (e.g., cognitive, physical, and social-emotional), context plays a critical role in how children participate in everyday occupations. As children participate in occupations across home, school, and community contexts they are influenced by the physical and social environments around them. For example, maternal college education was positively associated with the frequency of participation in social activities in the neighborhood (Little et al., 2014). Parents of young children with developmental disabilities perceive the daycare or preschool environment as less supportive of their child's participation (Benjamin et al., 2017). Environmental resources and support have been reported as an especially relevant barrier to occupational participation in community settings (Marino et al., 2018).

26.5.1 Activities of Daily Living (ADLs)

ADLs encompass occupations that help children take care of their bodies, including eating, toileting, bathing, dressing, and functional mobility (AOTA, 2020). School-aged children can manage most ADLs with minimal to no support from parents, caregivers, or teachers. The family context is a critical contributor to the child's participation in ADLs. For example, Levin and Currie (2010) found that family and home environments can be crucial in oral health routines. Families from higher socioeconomic backgrounds were significantly more likely to have greater odds of toothbrushing twice daily or more. Additionally, occupational therapy practitioners must be aware of cultural considerations in ADLs. For example, hair care within the Black community includes emphasis on protective hairstyles, differences in the frequency of hair washing, and routines specific to post-washing care products (Roseborough & McMichael, 2009).

As children near adolescence, they begin to demonstrate an increased desire for privacy and need for independence. Additionally, as school-aged children approach puberty, they gain increased interest in the ADL of sexual activity. With the transition to adolescence, occupational therapy practitioners play a critical role in supporting families and youth in addressing puberty-related changes. Specifically, they must be equipped to address emotional regulation, personal hygiene needs, and self-care associated with menstruation, masturbation, and safety (Larson et al., 2021). Practitioners must be mindful of cultural differences in personal hygiene and self-care preferences within this role. For example, families from Asian countries may prefer sanitary pads over tampons (or other menstrual products) (Grose & Grabe, 2014).

26.5.2 Instrumental Activities of Daily Living (IADLs)

IADLs encompass occupations that support everyday participation in the home and community, including home management, meal preparation, religious and spiritual expression, taking care of others (including family members and pets), community mobility, financial management, shopping, and maintaining safety (AOTA, 2020). IADLs require planning, organization, problem-solving, and physical, cognitive, and social-emotional skills. Since IADLs are more complex than ADLs, parents and teachers may provide instruction and supervision as children develop the ability to complete the IADL.

IADL participation is an important contributor to occupational participation across home, school, and community contexts. For example, religious and spiritual expression is an IADL associated with improved school adaptation (Carol & Schulz, 2018), and individuals with autism and Down syndrome diagnoses may report increased spirituality (Büssing et al., 2017; Liu et al., 2014). Occupational therapy practitioners must be mindful of individuals' interests and preferences in engaging in religious and spiritual activities, and can support community-based organizations to ensure equitable and accessible spaces for the worship of children and youth with disabilities.

A growing area of research highlights the importance of the IADLs of driving and community mobility, and community access for school-aged children and youth. Plummer et al. (2021) found that parents of children with an autism diagnosis were significantly less likely to participate in activities outside of the home if the child was reported to attempt to elope or display aggressive or self-injurious behaviors while driving. As children and youth with autism transition to adolescence, they may require specialized driving instruction to ensure community access due to mental flexibility, distractibility, difficulties understanding social cues, and motor coordination (Myers et al., 2021). In addition to supporting driving instruction, occupational therapy practitioners can support family education in understanding their children's strengths. For example, adolescents with autism have been found to exhibit increased adherence to road rules, decreased risk-taking, and attention to detail while driving (Myers et al., 2021).

26.5.3 Health Management

Health management encompasses occupations that support children in developing, managing, and sustaining their health, including participation in activities that promote physical, social, and emotional health, such as symptom management, nutrition management, communication with health care providers, and care for personal devices (AOTA, 2020). For example, children diagnosed with diabetes need to manage their blood sugar, monitor their caloric intake, be aware of their physical activity levels, and ensure they have adequate supplies of insulin (as well as manage their medical equipment, such as insulin pumps) (Rankin et al., 2018). Likewise, school-aged children with asthma must learn to manage their symptoms and respond when an asthma episode occurs (He et al., 2019). As children manage chronic conditions, they may also experience increased anxiety and stress (McClure et al., 2018).

A growing area of research in pediatrics explores the impact of concussions on children and youth. Moen et al. (2022) found that children and youth experience a wide variety of symptoms post-concussion, including variability and lability in mood and negative impact on occupational engagement. Furthermore, children and youth report the impact on them (or their families) of insufficient knowledge of medical management post-concussion (Moen et al., 2022).

26.5.4 Rest and Sleep

Rest and sleep support participation in other occupations, including relaxation and routines that contribute to the preparation of and participation in sleep (AOTA, 2020). The recommended amounts of sleep per 24-hour day are 10–13 hours for children 3–5 years old; 9–12 hours for children 6–12 years old; and 8–10 hours for children 13–18 years old (Paruthi et al., 2016). The most common sleep problems include difficulty initiating sleep, disturbed sleep, poor sleep quality, and poor sleep habits or hygiene. Insufficient or inadequate sleep patterns affect mental health, learning, school participation, and quality of life.

Regular, balanced engagement in daily occupation at home, school, and community and bedtime routines influence the quality and quantity of sleep. When daily routines of active engagement are disrupted or not achieved, children may need additional support to maintain habits of rest and sleep routine. Research suggests a significant relationship between differences in sensory processing and sleep behaviors, including findings that sensory under responsivity and sensory seeking may predict different arousal levels (Shochat et al., 2009).

26.5.5 Education

Education encompasses occupations that support learning and participation in formal and informal educational environments, including academic activities, recess, extracurricular activities (e.g., sports and clubs), and prevocational activities (AOTA, 2020). While educational expectations depend on the child's age and context, many academic institutions aim to prepare school-aged children for daily living, work, and community life.

Educational expectations are scaffolded, so children take on more roles and activities over time. Children learn and use enhanced social, communicative, and executive functioning skills as they advance to middle school. They may rely on technology and assistive technologies to support independence in academic participation in and outside of class (Rodrigues & Seruya, 2018). As children enter middle school, they seek to develop their own occupational identity; they may enjoy spending time separate from their families (while still being supported by their families). They prepare for high school by developing social and academic routines, curiosity for learning, and following through with responsibilities. They may become involved in work and volunteer roles in the community.

26.5.6 Work and Volunteerism

Work and volunteerism include occupations that support paid or unpaid pursuits leading to the production or delivery of some object or service, including work exploration, seeking, and participation (AOTA, 2020). Many occupations and activities of school-aged children prepare them for work and volunteering. For instance, social participation teaches school-aged children the skills necessary for effective collaboration in partnerships and teams at future work or volunteer sites. Social participation and the communication skills developed from it are essential for successfully undertaking work and volunteer tasks (Eismann et al., 2017).

School-aged children engage in work exploration (e.g., caring for pets, babysitting, and lawn care) that may prepare them for future work experiences. They may volunteer to complete activities associated with work, such as caring for family members, raising money, and completing service projects. They may complete community work, such as engaging in simple chores (e.g., dishwashing, mowing lawns, raking leaves, picking up trash, and delivering groceries) to give back to their community. They may engage in school service opportunities (e.g., food drive and community service) that promote belongingness and work skills. As children enter high school (around 14 years of age), they begin to focus on post-secondary transitions (i.e., college, work, and volunteering after high school) (Rosner et al., 2020).

26.5.7 Play

Play refers to occupations that are intrinsically motivated, freely chosen, and suspended from reality, including activities that involve play exploration and participation (AOTA, 2020). Play is fun, a spontaneous activity that is:

- Imaginative and spontaneous
- Flexible, non-linear, and iterative
- Free of externally imposed rules and involves active engagement, and
- Emphasizes the process rather than the outcome (Lynch & Moore, 2016).

School-aged children enjoy various play opportunities, especially outdoor play and active play that offer varied sensory experiences and motor play that encourages running, climbing, and jumping (Fahy et al., 2020).

Children develop cognitive, social, language, emotional, and physical skills as they engage in play. They also develop flexibility, negotiation, problem-solving skills, and an attitude or approach toward play (termed playfulness). Play is a vital co-occupation for parents and children. In children with autism, parental playfulness was a predictor of parental self-efficacy (Román-Oyola et al., 2017). However, parents may not consistently focus on play for the sake of play. For example, in the US and Europe, parents of children diagnosed with cerebral palsy view play in terms of the need to promote "typical play," burden of play, the need to expand play, and play as a motivation or reward for the child's participation in therapy (Graham et al., 2015).

Children with disabilities may experience limited access to play opportunities, play equipment, and equitable spaces that promote play and social interactions with others. For example, children with physical disabilities perceive their participation in play differently than their peers, reporting increased engagement in play by observing others, feeling extreme emotions during play, and imagining themselves without a disability as part of the play (Graham et al., 2019). Children with sensory processing challenges engage in less complex play, spend less time playing, and show an increased preference for sensory-based activities that satisfy a sensory need (Roberts et al., 2018; Watts et al., 2014). Additionally, children diagnosed with autism demonstrate challenges with imitative praxis, ideation, and participation in age-appropriate play and leisure activities (Bodison, 2015).

Play objects allow children to learn about themselves and the world around them. Consistently, representation of human diversity (e.g., race, ethnicity, gender, and disability) supports access, inclusion, and representation in play, and toy makers have shifted their designs to incorporate a more inclusive offering (e.g., #toylikeme campaign). In a study examining parents' perspectives on toys representing physical disabilities, Jones et al. (2020) found that (1) there was no direct association between the openness of parents to talking about disability and perceived willingness to play with the toys, and (2) increased parental openness to disability predicted the child's perceived willingness to play with the toys indirectly. This relationship was mediated by the parents' perception of whether their child wanted to be friends with other children with disabilities (Jones et al., 2020).

26.5.8 Leisure

Leisure consists of occupations that are non-obligatory and intrinsically motivated and includes activities that promote exploration and participation (AOTA, 2020). In school-aged children, play and leisure can look similar and be distinguished by the level of spontaneity and suspension from reality. Common leisure activities in school-aged children include sports, music, reading, cooking, games, watching TV, shopping, and outings with family or friends.

Engagement in leisure promotes children's health, well-being, and skill development (Fernandez et al., 2018). A child's age influences their leisure participation, skill level, and interests, as well as their parents' or caregivers' support, attitude, availability, and financial capacity (Fernandez et al., 2018). Leisure is an important aspect of occupational identity in school-aged children, and leisure pursuits expand in their complexity as children grow and develop. Participation in social leisure activities, such as extracurricular clubs and activities, can help children expand their friend networks, while individual leisure activities can promote the exploration of future work occupations.

26.5.9 Social Participation

Social participation refers to occupations that involve interactions with others, including family, friends, peers, and other people in the community (AOTA, 2020). School-aged children engage in social participation as part of their typical routine. They learn to get along, control their thinking and emotions, and develop and maintain relationships with others (Pascoe & Brennan, 2017). Children interact with others on and in the playground, cafeteria, classroom, and during transportation to and from school. They use social skills to develop relationships and communicate their needs with peers, friends, family, and community members. Challenges in self-awareness, executive functioning, and sensory processing can affect how children evaluate their behaviors and adjust them to match the social context (Challita et al., 2019).

Peer interactions are critical in supporting social participation and communication skills in children with developmental disabilities (Cahill & Beisbier, 2020). Participation in occupations that facilitate peer interactions (e.g., sports, video games, and camps) reinforces social participation and positively impacts mental health and behavior (Cahill & Beisbier, 2020). Research suggests that students' attitudes toward peers with disabilities are more likely to be positive if they have a friend with a disability and receive information about disabilities from their parents or media (Vignes et al., 2009).

26.6 Assessment of Occupational Participation in School-aged Children

Occupational therapy practitioners use a variety of assessments to evaluate school-aged children's strengths and challenges influencing occupational participation and performance. Assessments may be categorized as performance-based and self-report. Performance-based assessments examine how children engage in desired occupations and they may include observations of the child engaging in the occupation (such as feeding, dressing, play, and schoolwork), questionnaires, checklists, or criterion-referenced tests (requiring children to complete specific items). Self-report measures promote client-centered collaboration and gather information on children's subjective experiences or perceptions of their performance. School-aged children can reflect on the meaning of their everyday activities and their subjective experience is correlated with their objective participation (Rosenberg et al., 2019). Furthermore, children's preference is a significant predictor of participation in activities outside of school across multiple domains (e.g., recreation, physical, skill-based, and self-improvement) (Shields et al., 2018).

Occupational therapy practitioners may choose a combination of assessments to understand fully the child's occupational performance and participation. For example, while evaluating an adolescent's independence shopping in the community, the practitioner may use an observational assessment (e.g., Short Child Occupational Profile (SCOPE)) to evaluate the influence of the child's motivation, habits, skills, and environment on their participation. Through these observations the therapist may notice that while the adolescent participates in the shopping task, they demonstrate increased purposeful interactions with community members and a sense of pride by being able to complete the shopping tasks independently. The therapist may also observe the physical, cognitive, and social-emotional demands placed on the adolescent depending on the store layout and shopping list familiarity. Furthermore, they may observe how the store's physical layout, availability of social support, and social norms related to the shopping experience may further facilitate or restrict participation. The practitioner may also choose to pair their clinical observation with the client's self-report (e.g., Child Occupational Self Assessment [COSA]) to learn more about the adolescent's perceived competence and value of different occupations.

Occupational therapy assessments should be administered based on the instructions and guidelines provided in the associated manual. Additionally, occupational therapy practitioners should be aware of the constructs measured by the assessment. For example, bottom-up assessments may be appropriate to examine the child's body structure and function or skills, such as grip strength, range of motion, sensory processing, gross and fine motor skills, self-determination, anxiety, depression, or pain. In other instances, a top-down evaluation may be appropriate to support the therapists' understanding of the child's interests, routines, and performance during everyday occupations. Examples of top-down, occupation-centered assessments that can inform the evaluation of occupations for school-aged children are presented in Table 26.4.

Table 26.4 Occupation-centered Assessments for School-aged Children

Activities of Daily Living (ADLs)

Functional Independence Measure for Children (WeeFIM)

- **Ages:** 6 months to 7 years
- **Description:** Observational evaluation or proxy/health professional report to assess and grade a person's functional status based on their required level of assistance. FIM™ consists of 18 items grouped into two subscales – motor and cognition
- **Cost:** $4100 USD in/outpatient; $2200 USD inpatient only
- **Reference:** Granger, C. V., & McCabe, M. A. (1990). *Functional Independence Measure for Children (WeeFIM)*. Uniform Data System for Medical Rehabilitation

Pediatric Evaluation of Disability Inventory (PEDI)

- **Ages:** 6 months to 7 years
- **Description:** Observational or report standardized on a normative sample, allowing calculation of standard and scaled performance scores. Examines functional skills, caregiver assistance, and modifications across three domains:
  - Self-care
  - Mobility
  - Social function
- **Cost:** $123.40 USD
- **Reference:** Haley, S. M., Coster, Q. J., Ludlow, L. H., Haltiwanger, J., & Andrellos, P. (1992). *Pediatric Evaluation of Disability Inventory (PEDI): Development, standardization, and administration manual.* Boston University

(Continued)

Table 26.4 (Continued)

Vineland Adaptive Behavior Scales – 3rd edition (VABS-3)

- **Ages:** 0+ years
- **Description:** Measures the adaptive behavior of children with intellectual and developmental disabilities; autism spectrum disorders (ASDs); ADHD; post-traumatic brain injury; and hearing impairment
- **Cost:** $250–$500 USD
- **Reference:** Sparrow, S. S., Cicchetti, D. V., & Saulnier, C. A. (2016). *Vineland Adaptive Behavior Scales* (3rd ed.). Pearson Assessments

Instrumental Activities of Daily Living (IADLs)

Child Helping Out: Responsibilities, Expectations, and Supports (CHORES)

- **Ages:** 6–14 years
- **Description:** The assessment gathers parents' perspectives on children's performance and assistance needed while participating in household tasks. Includes two subscales:
  - Self-care household tasks
  - Family care household tasks
- **Cost:** N/A
- **Reference:** Dunn, L., Magalhaes, L. C., & Mancini, M. C. (2014). The internal structure of the Children Helping Out: Responsibilities, Expectations, and Supports (CHORES) measure. *American Journal of Occupational Therapy, 68,* 286–295. https://doi.org/10.5014/ajot.2014.010454

Children Participation Questionnaire (CPQ) & Children Participation Questionnaire–School (CPQ-S)

- **Ages:** 4–6 years
- **Description:** Parent proxy report
  - Participation diversity
  - Participation intensity
  - Independence
  - Child enjoyment
  - Parent satisfaction
- **Cost:** Free
- **Reference:** Rosenberg, L., Jarus, T., & Bart, O. (2010). Development and initial validation of the Children Participation Questionnaire (CPQ). *Disability and Rehabilitation, 32*(20), 1633–1644. https://doi.org/10.3109/09638281003611086

Roll Evaluation of Activities of Life (REAL)

- **Ages:** 2–18 years
- **Description:** Caregiver proxy report; reports standard scores, percentile ranks, and standard error of measure
  - ADL
  - IADL
- **Cost:** $215.20 USD
- **Reference:** Roll, K., & Roll, W. (2013). *The REAL™*. NCS Pearson.

Health Management

ARC Self-Determination Scale (ARC)

- **Ages:** 6+ years

(*Continued*)

Table 26.4 (Continued)

- **Description:** Norm-referenced self-report scale consisting of 72 items that measure 4 attributes related to self-determination: autonomy, self-regulation, psychological empowerment, and self-realization. It can be used to identify students' strengths and challenges related to self-determination
- **Cost:** Free
- **Reference:** Wehmeyer, M. (1995). *The ARC's Self-Determination Scale: Procedural guidelines.* Zarrow Center for Learning Enrichment, University of Oklahoma

Pediatric Quality of Life Inventory (PedsQL)

- **Ages:** Child self-report for ages 5–18 and parent proxy-report for ages 2–18
- **Description:** Norm-referenced scale that measures health-related quality of life (HRQOL) in healthy children and adolescents; designed for use with community, school, and clinical pediatric populations. Includes the following subscales:
  - Physical functioning (8 items)
  - Emotional functioning (5 items)
  - Social functioning (5 items)
  - School functioning (5 items)
- **Cost:** Licensing cost varies
- **Reference:** Varni, J. W., Seid, M., & Kurtin, P. S. (2001). PedsQL 4.0: Reliability and validity of the Pediatric Quality of Life Inventory version 4.0 generic core scales in healthy and patient populations. *Medical Care, 39*(8), 800–812. https://doi.org/10.1097/00005650-200108000-00006

Self-Control and Self-Management Scale (SCMS)

- **Ages:** 9+ years
- **Description:** Norm-referenced self-report scale; consists of 16 items and 3 factors: Self-monitoring, Self-evaluating and Self-reinforcing
- **Cost:** Free
- **References:** Herr, S., Herc, H., Navarre, K., & Mezo, P. (2019). *Evaluating the validity of the Self-Control and Self-Management Scale in a child and adolescent sample.* Midwestern Psychological Association & University of Toledo; Mezo, P. G., & Short, M. M. (2012). Construct validity and confirmatory factor analysis of the Self-Control and Self-Management Scale. *Canadian Journal of Behavioural Science, 44*(1), 1–8. https://doi.org/10.1037/a0024414

Rest and Sleep

Bedtime Routines Questionnaire (BRQ)

- **Ages:** 2–8 years
- **Description:** Parent-reported questionnaire; consists of 31 items yielding 3 subscales: Routine consistency, Reactivity to changes in routines, and Adaptive and maladaptive activities
- **Cost:** Free
- **Reference:** Henderson, J. A., & Jordan, S. S. (2010). Development and preliminary evaluation of the Bedtime Routines Questionnaire. *Journal of Psychopathology and Behavioral Assessment, 32,* 271–280. https://doi.org/10.1007/s10862-009-9143-3

(Continued)

Table 26.4 (Continued)

Children's Report of Sleep Patterns (CRSP)

- Ages: 8–12 years
- Description: The child self-report questionnaire consists of 62 items and includes 3 subscales: Sleep patterns, Sleep hygiene, and Sleep disturbance
- Cost: Free
- Reference: Meltzer, L. J., Avis, K. T., Biggs, S., Reynolds, A., Crabtree, V. M., & Bevans, K. B. (2013). The Children's Report of Sleep Patterns –Sleepiness Scale: A self-report measure for school-aged children. *Sleep Medicine, 9*(3), 235–245. https://doi.org/10.5664/jcsm.2486

Children's Sleep Habit Questionnaire (CSHQ)

- Ages: 4–10 years
- Description: Parent-reported questionnaire; consists of 45 items and includes 8 subscales: Bedtime resistance, Sleep onset delay, Sleep duration, Sleep anxiety, Night waking, Parasomnias, Sleep-disordered breathing, and Daytime sleepiness
- Cost: Free
- Reference: Owens, J. A., Spirito, A., & McGuinn, M. (2000). The Children's Sleep Habits Questionnaire (CSHQ): Psychometric properties of a survey instrument for school-aged children. *Sleep, 23*(8), 1–9. https://doi-org.ezproxy.lib.monash.edu.au/10.1093/sleep/23.8.1d

Education

School Assessment of Motor and Process Skills (School AMPS)

- Ages: 3–15 years
- Description: Observational and standardized assessment that assesses a student's performance in school-based tasks. There are 24 tasks in the assessment, including coloring, drawing, pasting, and cutting
- Cost: $65.00 USD
- Reference: Fisher, A. G., Bryze, K., Hume, V., & Griswold, L. A. (2007). *School AMPS: School version of the assessment of motor and process skills* (2nd ed.). Three Star Press

School Function Assessment (SFA)

- Ages: 5–13 years
- Description: Criterion-referenced assessment includes three sections: Participation, Task performance, and Activity performance
- Cost: $268.00 USD
- Reference: Coster, W., Deeney, T., Haltiwanger, J., & Haley, S. (1998). *School Function Assessment user's manual*. Psychological Corporation/Therapy Skill Builders

School Setting Interview (SSI)

- Ages: 10–18 years
- Description: Non-standardized ecological assessment that includes 16 items of a questionnaire regarding the student's participation in school and the impact of their disability
- Cost: $40.00 USD
- Reference: Hemmingsson, H., Egilson, S., Hoffman, O., & Kielhofner, G. (2005). *The School Setting Interview (SSI) version 3.0*. University of Illinois at Chicago

(*Continued*)

Table 26.4 (Continued)

Work and Volunteerism

CareerScope v10 (CareerScope)
- **Ages:** 11+ years
- **Description:** The CareerScope v10 is a self-administered aptitude and interest assessment that assists with the transition planning process
- **Cost:** $12.00 USD per administration
- **Reference:** Vocational Research Institute. (2010). *O*Net products at work*. O*Net Resource Center. http://www.onetcenter.org/paw/entry/8

Transition Planning Inventory – Updated Version (TPI-UV)
- **Ages:** 14–21 years
- **Description:** This inventory solicits feedback from multiple parties involved in the high school to the post-secondary transition process, including students, parents, and staff, via open-ended questions and rating scales. The inventory contains nine forms in total.
- **Cost:** $363.00 USD
- **Reference:** Patton, J. R., & Clark, G. M. (2014). *Transition Planning Inventory*. Pro-Ed.

Volunteer Functions Inventory (VFI)
- **Ages:** N/A
- **Description:** Clients respond to 30 questions on a Likert scale from 1 to 7 to assess volunteer motivation. The inventory consists of six subscales:
  - Protective measures
  - Values
  - Career
  - Social
  - Understanding
  - Enhancement
- **Cost:** Free
- **Reference:** Clary, E. G., Snyder, M., Ridge, R. D., Copeland, J., Stukas, A. A., Haugen, J., & Meine, P. (1998). Understanding and assessing the motivations of volunteers: A functional approach. *Journal of Personality and Social Psychology, 74*(6), 1516–1530. https://doi.org/10.1037//0022-3514.74.6.1516

Play

Test of Playfulness (ToP)
- **Ages:** 6 months to 18 years
- **Description:** Comprises 29 items scored following observation of the individual's free play in both indoor and outdoor settings. It measures a child's approach or attitude toward play by examining:
  - Intrinsic motivation
  - Internal control
  - Freedom from constraints
  - Framing (giving and reading social cues)

(Continued)

Table 26.4 (Continued)

- Cost: $36.53 USD
- References: Bundy, A. (2014). *Test of Playfulness manual*. Colorado State University; Skard, G., & Bundy, A. (2008). The Test of Playfulness (ToP). In L. D. Parham & L. S. Fazio (Eds.). *Play in occupational therapy for children* (2nd ed., pp. 71–93). Elsevier.

My Child's Play (MCP)

- Ages: 3–9 years
- Description: Parent-reported questionnaire consisting of 50 items to measure parents' perception of children's play performance related to:
  - Executive functions (20 items)
  - Interpersonal relationships and social participation (11 items)
  - Play choice and preference (14 items)
  - Play opportunities in the environment (5 items)
- Cost: Free
- Reference: Schneider, E., & Rosenblum, S. (2014). Development, reliability, and validity of the My Child's Play (MCP) questionnaire. *American Journal of Occupational Therapy*, 68, 277–285. https://doi.org/10.5014/ajot.2014.009159

Children's Play Scale (CPS)

- Ages: 5–11 years
- Description: Parent-reported questionnaire measuring children's time spent in play in seven spaces:
  - at home or in others' homes
  - outside at home or others' homes
  - at a playground
  - in green space (not at home or others' homes)
  - in the street or public space close to home
  - outdoor near water
  - indoor play centers and pools

Generates four time-use variables: (1) total hours spent playing; (2) total hours playing outdoors; (3) total hours spent playing in nature; and (4) total hours spent playing in adventurous places

- Cost: Free
- Reference: Dodd, H. F., Nesbit, R. J., & Maratchi, L. R. (2021). Development and evaluation of a new measure of children's play: The Children's Play Scale (CPS). *BMC Public Health*, 21, 878. https://doi.org/10.1186/s12889-021-10812-x

Leisure

Children's Assessment of Participation and Enjoyment / Preferences for Activities of Children (CAPE/PAC)

- Ages: 6–21 years
- Description: Self-reported measure estimates children's participation outside of school; consists of 55 items. CAPE provides five aspects of participation: diversity (number of activities participated), intensity (frequency of participation), enjoyment, and with whom and where participation occurs. PAC measures preferences for participation and groups test items into five categories: Recreational activities, Physical activities, Social activities, Skill-based activities, and Self-improvement activities

(Continued)

Table 26.4 (Continued)

- Cost: $165.80 USD
- Reference: King, G., Law, M., King, S., Hurley, P., Rosenbaum, P., Hanna, S., & Young, N. (2004). *Children's Assessment of Participation and Enjoyment and Preferences for Activities of Children*. Psychological Corporation.

Children's Leisure Assessment Scale (CLASS)

- Ages: 10–18 years
- Description: Self-report questionnaire; contains 40 leisure activities and one open item "Other activity"; assesses four leisure factors (instrumental indoor activities; outdoor activities; self-enrichment activities; games & sports activities) across five dimensions of leisure participation: Variety, Frequency, Sociability, Preference, and Desired activities
- Cost: Free
- References: Rosenblum, S., Sachs, D., & Schreuer, N. (2010). Reliability and validity of the Children's Leisure Assessment Scale. *American Journal of Occupational Therapy*, 24(4), 633–641. https://doi.org/10.5014/ajot.2010.08173; Schreuer, N., Sachs, D., & Rosenblum, S. (2014). Participation in leisure activities: Differences between children with and without physical disabilities. *Research in Developmental Disabilities*, 35(1), 223–233. https://doi.org/10.1016/j.ridd.2013.10.001

Pediatric Activity Card Sort (PACS)

- Ages: 6–12 years
- Description: Self-report test; consists of 75 cards with pictures of typical childhood activities and occupations in 4 categories: Personal care, School/productivity, Hobbies/social activities, and Sports
- Cost: $165.95 CAD
- Reference: Mandich, A., Polatajko, H. J., Miller, L., & Baum, C. (2004). *Pediatric Activity Card Sort: PACS*. Canadian Association of Occupational Therapists

Social Participation

Evaluation of Social Interaction (ESI)

- Ages: 2.5+ years
- Description: The interview and observer report include 27 skills related to verbal and non-verbal behaviors that support social interaction
- Cost: $75 USD
- Reference: Fisher, A. G., & Griswold, L. A. (2010). *Evaluation of Social Interaction* (2nd ed.). Three Star Press.

Participation Objective, Participation Subjective (POPS)

- Ages: N/A
- Description: Self-report consists of 26 items sorted into 5 categories: Domestic life; Major life activities; Transportation; Interpersonal interaction and relationships; and Community, recreation, and civic life. Generates two scores:
  – Participation objectives
  – Participation subjective
- Cost: Free
- Reference: Brown, M., Dijkers, M., Gordon, W., Asbman, T., Charatz, H., & Cheng, Z. (2004). Participation Objective, Participation Subjective: A measure of participation combining outsider and insider perspectives. *Journal of Head Trauma Rehabilitation*, 19(6), 459–481. https://doi.org/10.1097/00001199-200411000-00004

(Continued)

Table 26.4 (Continued)

Social Profile (SP)
- **Ages:** 18 months to 11 years (child version); 12+ years (adult version)
- **Description:** Observational assessment completed by therapists, teachers, or group leaders; measures the level of cooperation and performance within a group, sorted into three sections:
  - Activity participation
  - Social integration
  - Group memberships and roles
- **Cost:** $157.96 USD
- **Reference:** Donohue, M. V. (2005). Social Profile: Assessment of validity and reliability with preschool children. *Canadian Journal of Occupational Therapy, 72*(3), 164–175. https://doi.org/10.1177/000841740507200304

26.7 Occupational Participation and Well-being

Occupational participation is critical to the well-being of children and youth. As children engage in daily occupations, they develop across physical, cognitive, and social-emotional domains. In fact, school-aged children have been shown to describe well-being in terms of their perceived participation in valued occupations, including play and social participation (Moore & Lynch, 2018). Occupational therapy practitioners play a critical role in promoting physical, social, and emotional well-being by enhancing support and addressing barriers that impact occupational participation across home, school, and community settings. Practitioners use knowledge of children's internal assets (e.g., personality traits, prosocial skills, attitudes, and beliefs) and external assets (e.g., support from home, school, and community) to help them cope with adversity and participate in occupations (Holmes et al., 2015). In doing so, occupational therapists empower resilience (e.g., children's capacity to cope and develop competence in the face of adversity) and self-determination in school-aged children (Sui et al., 2022).

As children make their own choices, they develop their self-determination and their occupational identity. Self-determination contributes to well-being and includes children's perceptions of (1) autonomy (e.g., belief that you have a choice), (2) competence (e.g., belief that you are effective), and (3) relatedness (e.g., belief that you belong). Children who exhibit self-determination feel free to make choices (e.g., I want to write a story about my visit to the zoo), believe they can perform (e.g., I am good at making up stories), and feel they belong (e.g., I am excited to read my story in class). Conversely, children with low self-determination may feel they do not have choice or control over what they do, feel they cannot perform as required, and feel excluded from groups, preventing them from engaging in school occupations. Self-determination influences how children participate in everyday occupations and is influenced by the child's home, school, and community environments. Box 26.4 illustrates the influences of a global pandemic (COVID-19) on children's occupational participation, well-being, and self-determination.

Box 26.4 Impact of COVID-19 on Occupational Participation of School-aged Children

The COVID-19 pandemic affected all facets of everyday life at global and local societal levels. To try and limit exposure and transmission, states, local governments, and municipalities enacted safeguards, such as closing down schools and places of employment; requiring individuals and families to quarantine for several weeks after receiving positive diagnoses; and enacting social distancing efforts in combination with the use of personal protective equipment during essential travel into the community.

The new precautions significantly changed school-aged children's everyday roles, routines, and habits. Schools and educational institutions scrambled to provide access to virtual attendance and families suddenly found themselves spending their routines across all life roles (e.g., work, school, leisure, and play) in the same space. Social circles became smaller as children spent most of their time at home with family and transitioned to online learning.

These changes shaped children's self-determination by altering their relationships with others, ability to make choices, and feelings of success and competency in their everyday occupations. As children and youth experienced social isolation and loneliness for extended periods, they faced mental health challenges, including depression and anxiety (Loades et al., 2020). As a result of the pandemic, children experienced decreased prosocial behaviors (i.e., positive, helpful, and socially acceptable conduct) and increased behavioral challenges associated with a lower frequency of participation in school and community activities (Chien, 2022).

26.8 Conclusion

School-aged children engage in academic, social, and physical occupations and activities in the home, school, and community. They spend their days within their communities (at school or home), meeting other children and adults, developing habits and routines to promote learning, and communicating their needs. They must complete physical tasks and develop new relationships, negotiate, and problem-solve. As they develop skills, they participate in more complex occupations, such as education, socialization, and leisure (sports or clubs) that require following rules, making decisions, caring for themselves, and organizing, planning, and completing tasks (such as schoolwork, social games, and competitions). They develop friendships, follow the rules (such as family, school, and community rules), face challenges, and strive to belong.

The child's family, community, culture, and society influence occupational participation. Occupational therapy practitioners examine those factors (both internal and external) that facilitate or hinder the child's participation in desired activities within their community. They provide support to promote resilience and self-determination for health and well-being. Using knowledge of the developmental progression of occupations, they work with children and families to facilitate occupational participation. They assess the child's occupational performance through various assessments and consider cultural and contextual factors, age, grade expectations, and the child's strengths and challenges.

26.9 Summary
- School-aged children's occupational choices, opportunities, and outcomes are influenced by social determinants of health (such as race, access to health care, education, financial well-being, and community mobility).
- Culture influences the direct (e.g., physical, societal opportunities, facilities, accessibility, institutions, and economic) and indirect (e.g., values, beliefs, expectations, and attitudes) environments where children explore and participate in occupations.
- Performance patterns encompass (i) roles that exert an organizing influence on performance by indicating which occupations a child is expected to perform relative to given life roles; (ii) habits that support or hinder occupational participation; (iii) routines which are the pairing of multiple occupations performed over a period; and (iv) rituals that allow for moments of pause and reflection.
- The main occupations of school-aged children include ADLs, IADLs, health management, rest and sleep, education, work and volunteerism, play, leisure, and social participation.
- Mental health challenges interfere with school-aged children's occupational participation, affecting their health and well-being. Children who exhibit positive self-determination believe they can make choices, do things, and connect with others. Children with low self-determination, anxiety, depression, trauma, or other mental health issues have difficulty engaging in occupations and may miss opportunities.

26.10 Review Questions
1. What social determinants of health and well-being influence school-aged children?
2. How do environmental and cultural contexts influence school-aged children's occupations?
3. How do habits, roles, routines, and rituals create performance patterns for school-aged children?
4. What are the main occupations of school-aged children? What are the contributors to children's participation in ADLs, IADLs, health management, rest and sleep, education, work and volunteerism, play, leisure, and social participation?
5. How does occupational participation influence well-being in school-aged children?

References
Ahmed, K. A., Grundy, J., Hashmat, L., Ahmed, I., Farrukh, S., Bersonda, D., Shah, M. A., Yunus, S., & Banskota, H. K. (2022). An analysis of the gender and social determinants of health in urban poor areas of the most populated cities of Pakistan. *International Journal for Equity in Health, 21*, 52. https://doi.org/10.1186/s12939-022-01657-w

American Occupational Therapy Association. (2020). Occupational Therapy Practice Framework: Domain and process – Fourth edition. *American Journal of Occupational Therapy, 74*(Supplement_2), 7412410010p1–7412410010p87. https://doi.org/10.5014/ajot.2020.74S2001

Ammar, A., Mueller, P., Trabelsi, K., Chtourou, H., Boukhris, O., Masmoudi, L., Bouaziz, B., Brach, M., Schmicker, M., Bentlage, E., How, D., Ahmed, M., Aloui, A., Hammouda, O., Paineiras-Domingos, L. L., Braakman-Jansen, A., Wrede, C., Bastoni, S., Pernambuco, C. S., ... Hoeckelmann, A. (2020). Psychological consequences of COVID-19 home confinement:

The ECLB-COVID19 multicenter study. *PLOS ONE, 15*(11), e0240204. https://doi.org/10.1371/journal.pone.0240204

Bazyk, S., Demirjian, L., Horvath, F., & Doxsey, L. (2018). The Comfortable Cafeteria program for promoting student participation and enjoyment: An outcome study. *American Journal of Occupational Therapy, 72*, 7203205050. https://doi.org/10.5014/ajot.2018.025379

Benjamin, T. E., Lucas-Thompson, R. G., Little, L. M., Davies, P. L., & Khetani, M. A. (2017). Participation in early childhood educational environments for young children with and without developmental disabilities and delays: A mixed methods study. *Physical & Occupational Therapy in Pediatrics, 37*(1), 87–107. https://doi.org/10.3109/01942638.2015.1130007

Bodison, S. C. (2015). Developmental dyspraxia and the play skills of children with autism. *American Journal of Occupational Therapy, 69*(5), 6905185060p1–6905185060p6. https://doi.org/10.5014/ajot.2015.017954

Bronfenbrenner, U. (2005). Ecological systems theory (1992). In U. Bronfenbrenner (Ed.), *Making human beings human: Bioecological perspectives on human development* (pp. 106–173). https://psycnet.apa.org/record/2004-22011-010

Büssing, A., Broghammer-Escher, S., Baumann, K., & Surzykiewicz, J. (2017). Aspects of spirituality and life satisfaction in persons with Down syndrome. *Journal of Disability & Religion, 21*(1), 14–29. https://doi.org/10.1080/23312521.2016.1270179

Cahill, S. M., & Beisbier, S. (2020). Occupational therapy practice guidelines for children and youth ages 5–21 years. *American Journal of Occupational Therapy, 74*(4), 7404397010p1–7404397010p48. https://doi.org/10.5014/ajot.2020.744001

Cahill, S. M., Egan, B. E., & Seber, J. (2020). Activity- and occupation-based interventions to support mental health, positive behavior, and social participation for children and youth: A systematic review. *American Journal of Occupational Therapy, 74*, 7402180020. https://doi.org/10.5014/ajot.2020.038687

Carol, S., & Schulz, B. (2018). Religiosity as a bridge or barrier to immigrant children's educational achievement? *Research in Social Stratification and Mobility, 55*, 75–88. https://doi.org/10.1016/j.rssm.2018.04.001

Challita, J., Chapparo, C., Hinitt, J., & Heard, R. (2019). Patterns of cognitive strategy are common in children with reduced social competence derived from parent perceptions. *Australian Occupational Therapy Journal, 66*, 500–510. https://doi.org/10.1111/1440-1630.12574

Chien, C.-W. (2022). Brief Report: Effects of the change in activity participation during the COVID-19 pandemic on children's mental health. *American Journal of Occupational Therapy, 76*, 7602345010. https://doi.org/10.5014/ajot.2022.047118

Daoud, R., Starkey, L., Eppel, E., Vo, T. D., & Sylvester, A. (2020). The educational value of internet use in the home for school children: A systematic review of literature. *Journal of Research on Technology in Education, 53*(4), 353–374. https://doi.org/10.1080/15391523.2020.1783402

Di Maggio, I., Ginevra, M. C., Santilli, S., & Nota, L. (2022). Elementary school students' attitudes towards peers with disabilities: The role of personal and contextual factors. *Journal of Intellectual & Developmental Disability, 47*(1), 3–11. https://doi.org/10.3109/13668250.2021.1920091

Dutta, A., Mohapatra, M. K., Rath, M., Rout, S. K., Kadam, S., Nallala, S., Balagopalan, K., & Tiwari, D. (2020). Effect of caste on ehealth, independent of economic disparity: Evidence from school children of two rural districts of India. *Sociology of Health & Illness, 42*(6), 1259–1276. https://doi.org/10.1111/1467-9566.13105

Dyer, T. (2018). The effects of social media on children. *Dalhousie Journal of Interdisciplinary Management, 14*. https://doi.org/10.5931/djim.v14i0.7855

Eismann, M. M., Weisshaar, R., Capretta, C., Cleary, D. S., Kirby, A. V., & Persch, A. C. (2017). Centennial topics: Characteristics of students receiving occupational therapy services in transition and factors related to postsecondary success. *American Journal of Occupational Therapy, 71*, 7103100010. https://doi.org/10.5014/ajot.2017.024927

Fahy, S., Delicâte, N., & Lynch, H. (2020). Now, being, occupational: Outdoor play and children with autism. *Journal of Occupational Science, 28*(1), 114–132. https://doi.org/10.1080/14427591.2020.1816207

Fernandez, Y., Ziviani, J., Cuskelly, M., Colquhoun, R., & Jones, F. (2018). Participation in community leisure programs: Experiences and perspectives of children with developmental difficulties and their parents. *Leisure Sciences, 40*(3), 110–130. https://doi.org/10.1080/01490400.2017.1408509

Golos, D. B., Moses, A. M., & Wolbers, K. A. (2012). Culture or disability? Examining deaf characters in children's book illustrations. *Early Childhood Education Journal, 40*(4), 239–249. https://doi.org/10.1007/s10643-012-0506-0

Graham, N., Mandy, A., Clarke, C., & Morriss-Roberts, C. (2019). Play experiences of children with a high level of physical disability. *American Journal of Occupational Therapy, 73*(6), 7306205010p1–7306205010p10. https://doi.org/10.5014/ajot.2019.032516

Graham, N. E., Truman, J., & Holgate, H. (2015). Parents' understanding of play for children with cerebral palsy. *American Journal of Occupational Therapy, 69*(3), 6903220050p1–6903220050p9. https://doi.org/10.5014/ajot.2015.015263Grose, R. G., & Grabe, S. (2014). Sociocultural attitudes surrounding menstruation and alternative menstrual products: The explanatory role of self-objectification. *Health Care for Women International, 35*(6), 677–694. https://doi.org/10.1080/07399332.2014.888721

Guthold, R., Stevens, G. A., Riley, L. M., & Bull, F. C. (2020). Global trends in insufficient physical activity among adolescents: A pooled analysis of 298 population-based surveys with 1.6 million participants. *The Lancet Child & Adolescent Health, 4*(1), 23–35. https://doi.org/10.1016/s2352-4642(19)30323-2

Hamm, M. P., Newton, A. S., Chisholm, A., Shulhan, J., Milne, A., Sundar, P., Ennis, H., Scott, S. D., & Hartling, L. (2015). Prevalence and effect of cyberbullying on children and young people. *JAMA Pediatrics, 169*(8), 770. https://doi.org/10.1001/jamapediatrics.2015.0944

He, Y., Stephenson, M., Gu, Y., Hu, X., Zhang, M., & Jin, J. (2019). Asthma self-management in children: A best practice implementation project. *JBI Database of Systematic Reviews and Implementation Reports, 17*(5), 985–1002. https://doi.org/10.11124/JBISRIR-2017-003775

Holmes, M., Yoon, S., Voith, L., Kobulsky, J., & Steigerwald, S. (2015). Resilience in physically abused children: Protective factors for aggression. *Behavioral Sciences, 5*(2), 176–189. https://doi.org/10.3390/bs5020176

Inoa, R. (2017). Parental involvement among middle-income Latino parents living in a middle-class community. *Hispanic Journal of Behavioral Sciences, 39*(3), 316–335. https://doi.org/10.1177/0739986317714200

Jones, S., Ali, L., Bhuyan, M., Dalnoki, L., Kaliff, A., Muir, W., Uusitalo, K., & Uytman, C. (2020). Parents' responses to toys representing physical impairment. *Equality, Diversity and Inclusion: An International Journal, 39*(8), 949–966. https://doi.org/10.1108/edi-08-2019-0213

Kangas, S. E. (2021). "Is it language or disability?": An ableist and monolingual filter for English learners with disabilities. *TESOL Quarterly, 55*(3), 673–683. https://doi.org/10.1002/tesq.3029

Kao, Y.-C., Coster, W., Cohn, E. S., & Orsmond, G. I. (2021). Preparation for adulthood: Shifting responsibility for management of daily tasks from parents to their children. *American Journal of Occupational Therapy, 75*(2), 7502205050. https://doi.org/10.5014/ajot.2020.041723

Kato, P. M., Cole, S. W., Bradlyn, A. S., & Pollock, B. H. (2008). A video game improves behavioral outcomes in adolescents and young adults with cancer: A randomized trial. *Pediatrics, 122*(2), e305–e317. https://doi.org/10.1542/peds.2007-3134

Kennedy, J., & Lynch, H. (2016). A shift from offline to online: Adolescence, the internet and social participation. *Journal of Occupational Science, 23*(2), 156–167. https://doi.org/10.1080/14427591.2015.1117523

Klevens, J., Treves-Kagan, S., Metzler, M., Merrick, M., Reidy, M. C., Herbst, J. H., & Ports, K. (2021). Association of public explanations of why children struggle and support for policy solutions using a national sample. *Analyses of Social Issues and Public Policy, 22*(1), 268–285. https://doi.org/10.1111/asap.12285

Laninga-Wijnen, L., van den Berg, Y. H. M., Mainhard, T., & Cillessen, A. H. N. (2021). The role of aggressive peer norms in elementary school children's perceptions of classroom peer climate and school adjustment. *Journal of Youth and Adolescence, 50*, 1582–1600. https://doi.org/10.1007/s10964-021-01432-0

Larson, S. K., Nielsen, S., Hemberger, K., & Klug, M. G. (2021). Addressing puberty challenges for adolescents with autism spectrum disorder: A survey of occupational therapy practice trends. *American Journal of Occupational Therapy, 75*, 7503180020. https://doi.org/10.5014/ajot.2021.040105

Levin, K. A., & Currie, C. (2010). Adolescent toothbrushing and the home environment: Sociodemographic factors, family relationships and mealtime routines and disorganization. *Community Dental Oral Epidemiology, 38*, 10–18. https://doi.org/10.111/j.1600-0528.2009.00509.x

Li, W., & Xie, Y. (2020). The influence of family background on educational expectations: A comparative study. *Chinese Sociological Review, 52*(3), 269–294. https://doi.org/10.1080/21620555.2020.1738917

Little, L. M., Sideris, J., Ausderau, K., & Baranek, G. T. (2014). Activity participation among children with autism spectrum disorder. *American Journal of Occupational Therapy, 68*, 177–185. https://doi.org/10.5014/ajot.2014.009894

Liu, E. X., Carter, E. W., Boehm, T. L., Annandale, N. H., & Taylor, C. E. (2014). In their own words: The place of faith in the lives of young people with autism and intellectual disability. *Intellectual and Developmental Disabilities, 52*(5), 388–404. https://doi.org/10.1352/1934-9556-52.5.388

Loades, M. E., Chatburn, E., Higson-Sweeney, N., Reynolds, S., Shafran, R., Brigden, A., Linney, C., McManus, M. N., Borwick, C., & Crawley, E. (2020). Rapid systematic review: The impact of social isolation and loneliness on the mental health of children and adolescents in the context of COVID-19. *Journal of the American Academy of Child & Adolescent Psychiatry, 59*(11), 1218–1239.e3. https://doi.org/10.1016/j.jaac.2020.05.009

Lynch, H., & Moore, A. (2016). Play as an occupation in occupational therapy (Editorial). *British Journal of Occupational Therapy, 79*(9), 519–520. https://doi.org/10.1177/0308022616664540

Marino, E. D., Tremblay, S., Khetani, M. A., & Anaby, D. (2018). The effect of child, family and environmental factors on the participation of young children with disabilities. *Disability & Health Journal, 11*, 36–42. https://doi.org/10.1016/j.dhjo.2017.05.005

McClure, N., Seibert, M., Johnson, T., Kannenberg, L., Brown, T., & Lutenbacher, M. (2018). Improving asthma management in the elementary school setting: An education and self-management pilot project. *Journal of Pediatric Nursing, 42*, 16–20. https://doi.org/10.1016/j.pedn.2018.06.001

Moen, E., McLean, A., Boyd, L. A., Schmidt, J., & Zwicker, J. G. (2022). Experiences of children and youth with concussion: A qualitative study. *American Journal of Occupational Therapy, 76*, 7604205040. https://doi.org/10.5014/ajot.2022.047597

Monks, C. P., Robinson, S., & Worlidge, P. (2012). The emergence of cyberbullying: A survey of primary school pupils' perceptions and experiences. *School Psychology International, 33*(5), 477–491. https://doi.org/10.1177/0143034312445242

Moore, A., & Lynch, H. (2018). Understanding a child's conceptualisation of well-being through an exploration of happiness: The centrality of play, people and place. *Journal of Occupational Science, 25*(1), 124–141. https://doi.org/10.1080/14427591.2017.1377105

Mullan, K. (2019). A child's day: Trends in time use in the UK from 1975 to 2015. *British Journal of Sociology, 70*(3), 997–1024. https://doi.org/10.1111/1468-4446.12369

Myers, R. K., Carey, M. E., Bonsu, J. M., Yerys, B. E., Mollen, C. J., & Curry, A. E. (2021). Behind the wheel: Specialized driving instructors' experiences and strategies for teaching autistic adolescents to drive. *American Journal of Occupational Therapy, 75*, 7503180110. https://doi.org/10.5014/ajot.2021.043406

Office of Disease Prevention and Health Promotion. (n.d.). Social determinants of health. *Healthy People 2030*. US Department of Health and Human Services. https://health.gov/healthypeople/objectives-and-data/social-determinants-health

Orosco, M. J., & O'Connor, R. (2013). Culturally responsive instruction for English language learners with learning disabilities. *Journal of Learning Disabilities, 47*(6), 515–531. https://doi.org/10.1177/0022219413476553

Park, E., & Kwon, M. (2018). Health-related internet use by children and adolescents: Systematic review. *Journal of Medical Internet Research, 20*(4), e120. https://doi.org/10.2196/jmir.7731

Paruthi, S., Brooks, L. J., D'Ambrosio, C., Hall, W. A., Kotagal, S., Lloyd, R. M., Malow, B. A., Maski, K., Nichols, C., Quan, S. F., Rosen, C. L., Troester, M., & Wise, M. S. (2016). Consensus statement of the American Academy of Sleep Medicine on the recommended amount of sleep for healthy children: Methodology and discussion. *Journal of Clinical Sleep Medicine, 12*(11), 1549–1561. https://doi.org/10.5664/jcsm.6288

Pascoe, S., & Brennan, D. (2017). *Lifting our game: Report of the review to achieve educational excellence in Australian schools through early childhood interventions*. https://www.education.vic.gov.au/Documents/about/research/LiftingOurGame.PDF

Pinquart, M., & Ebeling, M. (2019). Parental educational expectations and academic achievement in children and adolescents: A meta-analysis. *Educational Psychology Review, 32*(2), 463–480. https://doi.org/10.1007/s10648-019-09506-z

Plummer, T., Bryan, M., Dullaghan, K., Harris, A., Isenberg, M., Marquez, J., Rolling, L., & Triggs, A. (2021). Parent experiences and perceptions of safety when transporting children with autism spectrum disorder. *American Journal of Occupational Therapy, 75*(5), 7505205010. https://doi.org/10.5014/ajot.2021.041749

Rankin, D., Harden, J., Barnard, K., Bath, L., Noyes, K., Stephen, J., & Lawton, J. (2018). Barriers and facilitators to taking on diabetes self-management tasks in pre-adolescent children with type 1 diabetes: A qualitative study. *BMC Endocrine Disorders, 18*, Article number: 71. https://doi.org/10.1186/s12902-018-0302-y

Roberts, T., Stagnitti, K., Brown, T., & Bhopti, A. (2018). Relationship between sensory processing and pretend play in typically developing children. *American Journal of Occupational Therapy, 72*(1), 7201195050p1–7201195050p8. https://doi.org/10.5014/ajot.2018.027623

Rodrigues, S. M., & Seruya, F. M. (2018). Current practice patterns and perceived needs of occupational therapy practitioners in middle schools. *Journal of Occupational Therapy, Schools, & Early Intervention, 12*(1), 144–155. https://doi.org/10.1080/19411243.2018.1512066

Román-Oyola, R., Reynolds, S., Soto-Feliciano, I., Cabrera-Mercader, L., & Vega-Santana, J. (2017). Child's sensory profile and adult playfulness as predictors of parental self-efficacy. *American Journal of Occupational Therapy, 71*(2), 7102220010p1–7102220010p8. https://doi.org/10.5014/ajot.2017.021097

Roseborough, I. E., & McMichael, A. J. (2009). Hair care practices in African American patients. *Seminars in Cutaneous Medicine and Surgery, 28*(2), 103–108. https://doi.org/10.1016/j.sder.2009.04.007

Rosenberg, L., Pade, M., Reizis, H., & Bar, M. A. (2019). Associations between meaning of everyday activities and participation among children. *American Journal of Occupational Therapy, 73*, 7306205030. https://doi.org/10.5014/ajot.2019.032508

Rosner, T., Grasso, A., Scott-Cole, L., Villalobos, A., & Mulcahey, M. (2020). Scoping review of school-to-work transition for youth with intellectual disabilities: A practice gap. *American Journal of Occupational Therapy, 74*(2), 7402205020p1–7402205020p23. https://doi.org/10.5014/ajot.2019.035220

Shields, N., Adair, B., Wilson, P., Froude, E., & Imms, C. (2018). Characteristics influencing diversity of participation of children in activities outside school. *American Journal of Occupational Therapy, 72*, 7204205010. https://doi.org/10.5014/ajot.2018.026914

Shochat, T., Tzischinsky, O., & Engel-Yeger, B. (2009). Sensory hypersensitivity as a contributing factor in the relation between sleep and behavioral disorders in normal schoolchildren. *Behavioral Sleep Medicine, 7*(1), 53–62. https://doi.org/10.1080/15402000802577777

Skard, G., & Bundy, A. (2008). The Test of Playfulness (ToP). In L. D. Parham & L. S. Fazio (Eds.), *Play in occupational therapy for children* (2nd ed., pp. 71–93). Elsevier.

Spencer, N., Raman, S., O'Hare, B., & Tamburlini, G. (2019). Addressing inequities in child health and development: Towards social justice. *BMJ Paediatrics Open, 3*(1), e000503. https://doi.org/10.1136/bmjpo-2019-000503

Sui, X., Massar, K., Reddy, P. S., & Ruiter, R. A. C. (2022). Developmental assets in South African adolescents exposed to violence: A qualitative study on resilience. *Journal of Child & Adolescent Trauma, 15*, 1–13. https://doi.org/10.1007/s40653-021-00343-3

Taylor, R. R. (2017). *Kielhofner's Model of Human Occupation: Theory and application* (5th ed.). F. A. Davis.

Travers, B. G., Lee, L., Klans, N., Engeldinger, A., Taylor, D., Ausderau, K., Skaletski, E. C., & Brown, J. (2022). Associations among daily living skills, motor, and sensory difficulties in autistic and nonautistic children. *American Journal of Occupational Therapy, 76*, 7602205020. https://doi.org/10.5014/ajot.2022.045955

Vignes, C., Godeau, E., Sentenac, M., Coley, N., Navarro, F., Grandjean, H., & Arnaud, C. (2009). Determinants of students' attitudes towards peers with disabilities. *Developmental Medicine & Child Neurology, 51*(6), 473–479. https://doi.org/10.1111/j.1469-8749.2009.03283.x

Visser, K., & Aalst, I. (2021). Neighbourhood factors in children's outdoor play: A systematic literature review. *Tijdschrift Voor Economische En Sociale Geografie, 113*(1), 80–95. https://doi.org/10.1111/tesg.12505

Wang, P., & Woolf, S. B. (2015). Trends and issues in bilingual special education teacher preparation: A literature review. *Journal of Multilingual Education Research, 6*(4). https://research.library.fordham.edu/jmer/vol6/iss1/4

Watson, A., Dumuid, D., & Olds, T. (2020). Associations between 24-hour time use and academic achievement in Australian primary school-aged children. *Health Education & Behavior, 47*(6), 905–913. https://doi.org/10.1177/1090198120952041

Watts, T., Stagnitti, K., & Brown, T. (2014). Relationship between play and sensory processing: A systematic review. *American Journal of Occupational Therapy, 68*(2), e37–e46. https://doi.org/10.5014/ajot.2014.009787

Williams, N. J., Frederick, L., Ching, A., Mandell, D., Kang-Yi, C., & Locke, J. (2021). Embedding school cultures and climates that promote evidence-based practice implementation for youth with autism: A qualitative study. *Autism, 25*(4), 982–994. https://doi.org/10.1177/1362361320974509

World Health Organization. (2022). *Social determinants of health.* https://www.who.int/health-topics/social-determinants-of-health#tab=tab_1

CHAPTER 27

Human Occupations of Adolescence and Youth

Sandra L. Rogers

Abstract
The breadth of occupations that is available to adolescents and youth rapidly expands as biological (e.g., physical, physiological, and cognitive) maturation unfolds. This chapter will highlight the numerous options that adolescents can access as they mature, and will highlight some of the joys, barriers, and challenges they may experience because of this rapid expansion of motor, cognitive, social, sexual, and emotional skills. While the experience of every adolescent is unique, there are some continuities in the progression of adolescent development that allows us to understand and thus pair our interventions in occupational therapy appropriately.

Author's Positionality Statement
As a young person, I always remembered being drawn to health care; in high school, I volunteered as a candy-striper in a hospital and worked as a nursing assistant in an older adult care facility. I found my way to occupational therapy when I met the Certified Occupational Therapy Assistant who worked in the care facility where I worked and she shared her love of fostering independence. With my job as a certified nursing assistant, I was able to pay my way through college; it gave me a deep appreciation for dedication and hard work which I continue to value in my work as an occupational therapist. Admittedly, while I was eager to be independent in high school, I was fearful about going to college as I did not think of myself as smart and was worried that college was beyond my capabilities. My striving for independence also placed me in some very risky positions and without parents to guide me, I did find a lot of trouble – as many teenagers do. The idea that one caring person can make a difference resonated with me, as a high school teacher encouraged and helped me to choose an occupational therapy program that was within my reach at a local public university, and gave me the courage to pursue my dream. Much later in life I discovered that I had a congenital hearing impairment, that went undiagnosed until I was in my 30s, and so even as

a child I learned from books and grew into a voracious reader. I also grew to enjoy leisure pursuits in just about any activity that involves the water – kayaking, sailing, paddleboarding, and windsurfing. In occupational therapy, I have found a rich and diverse career that allows me to be independent and to facilitate that same independence, or partial independence, in others.

> **Objectives**
> This chapter will:
>
> - Highlight the connection between adolescent development, including the formation of physical, cognitive, emotional, social, and emotional skills, to the formation of occupational options.
> - Connect adolescent and youth development to the context in which it unfolds, and as it relates to the transition to school, work, and social life, in readiness for the occupations of adulthood.
> - Explain how environmental contexts of socioeconomic conditions, gender identity exploration, and risk-taking behavior might be experienced, and how those behaviors impact the acquisition of occupation and occupational choices.
> - Discriminate typical sexual development and activities of daily life from problematic activities and outcomes.

> **Key terms**
> - occupations of adolescents
> - development in adolescents
> - gender and sexuality development

27.1 Introduction

In adolescence, the rapid expansion of physical, cognitive, physiological, emotional, and social development allows for the exploration and engagement into a wide array of occupations. This expansion of both developmental and physiological growth also presents numerous challenges for adolescents and youth. This is primarily due to the unfolding of development in an uneven sequence. The consequences are that youth engagement in some occupations does not match their developmental skills, making them susceptible to harm. This chapter will highlight the numerous options that adolescents can access as they mature, and also highlight some of the joys, barriers, and challenges they may experience because of this rapid expansion of motor, cognitive, social, sexual, and emotional skills. While the experience of every adolescent is unique and asynchronous, there are some continuities in the progression of adolescent development that allows us to understand and thus pair our interventions in occupational therapy appropriately. Identifying developmental areas of the dyssynchronous development is important; for example, individuals may acquire the physical capacity for sexual intimacy long before they possess the emotional capacity to engage in long-term relationships. These mismatches between physical capacity and emotional skill can sometimes contribute to challenging situations for youth and pose health, emotional, and social risks with which a youth is not prepared to cope.

27.2 Defining Adolescence

Defining precise stages of adolescence is difficult given the breadth of individual differences in a youth's body and the enormous variation in the environments they experience as they become adults. Most resources consider the ages between 12 and 19 to represent adolescence; however, variation includes younger adolescents, starting at age 10, and older youth up to 21 years of age. This age categorization is oftentimes too simplistic to capture the differences from the initiation of adolescence to late adolescence. Children reach adolescence at a wide variety of ages, with some children entering emerging adolescence at 10 years of age, while others do not begin until they are 14 or 15 years of age. Consequently, it is common practice to identify ages in terms of developmental stage vs. simply identifying an age range. It is often more helpful to discuss youth development in two or three stages, capturing emerging adolescence and middle-to-late adolescence. Other researchers choose to include additional stages, with a developmental epic into young adulthood (18–22 years). For this chapter, we will consider those in adolescence in two stages: 12–15 years of age as young-to-middle adolescence and 15–18 years of age as middle-to-late adolescence.

While youth are often still closely attached to their family, they are also developing strong relationships outside of the family that support their social and emotional development. Youth develop the capacity for abstract thought and construction of personal ethics and spirituality. They can begin to grapple with complex societal issues that do not have definitive solutions and require examination of multiple issues at the same time. They are generally very healthy as most youth have been exposed to many childhood illnesses which have allowed their immune systems to recognize a variety of pathogens and respond robustly. Additionally, youth add musculoskeletal strength to allow engagement in competitive sports, improved fine motor precision to allow use of tools more accurately, and heightened mental focus to achieve personal goals (see Figure 27.1). In multidisciplinary activities, like the arts, youth are combining mastery of both physical and mental art forms (e.g., dance, music, and drama). For many, it is a time of scaffolding important physical, cognitive, emotional, and social skills that support their transition to successful adulthood.

27.3 Stages of Development in Adolescence
27.3.1 Typical Developmental Trajectories
- Cognitive
- Physical
- Social
- Emotional
- Activities of daily living (ADLs)
- Ethics/morality
- Sexuality/gender identity

SANDRA L. ROGERS

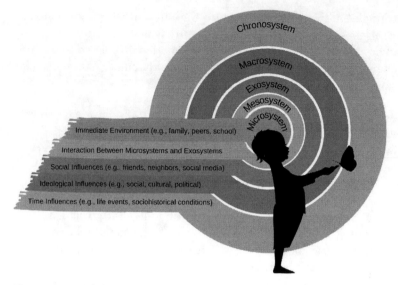

Figure 27.1 Adolescents gain musculoskeletal strength that allow engagement in competitive sports, improved fine motor precision for tool use, and heightened mental focus to achieve personal goals.

Source: Photo by frstudio, pexels.com; photos on Pexels are free to use and attribution to photographer is provided.

27.3.2 Categories of Development
- Physical changes/brain development
- Social rituals and sexuality
- Cognitive changes
- Moral reasoning
- Emotional changes
- Motor skill changes
- Communication skills

27.3.3 Young-to-Middle Adolescence (Ages 12–15)
Adolescence is defined by changes that affect a youth's physical, mental, emotional, sexual, and social characteristics. Development of hormones that drive those changes occurs at a range of ages; however, there is often little continuity between social readiness and physical changes. These hormonal changes are often most obvious in physical and secondary sex characteristics for adolescents. Most commonly, we identify the beginning of adolescence with the emergence of rapid growth and development of secondary sex characteristics. This growth encompasses an increase in musculoskeletal, neurological, and hormonal characteristics.

Specifically, these body changes include bone growth; increases in muscle to body weight measures and body weight proportions; hair growth under the arms and near the genitals; breast development, distribution of body fat, and menstruation in females; enlargement of the testes, growth of the penis, first ejaculation of seminal fluid (e.g., spermarche), appearance of facial hair, and a deepening of voices in males. Development in females usually starts a year or two earlier than in males, and it can be normal for some changes to start as early as age 10 for females and age 11 for males. Many females may start their period at around age 12, on average 2–3 years after the onset of breast development. These body changes can inspire curiosity and/or anxiety in youth, particularly if youth do not know what to expect of their bodily changes or understand how widely these changes vary for any given individual. Some youth may also question their gender identity at this time, and the onset of puberty can be a difficult time for transgender persons. Growth spurts occur in bones when perceptible changes in height take place rapidly. Many adolescents are often deeply affected by these changes and how the changes are seen by others, having moved from a more egocentric perspective to greater self- and social consciousness.

Early on in emerging adolescence, youth tend to have more concrete or definitive thinking. For example, youth at this stage tend to think in terms of absolute right or wrong, and good or bad, without considering subtle and diverse perspectives or looking at a multiplicity of issues. Socially and emotionally, many youths find this an exciting yet daunting time. As youth expand their social connections beyond their family to members of the same sex, opposite sex, different ethnic, religious, and social groups, and other adults, like teachers or coaches, they are exposed to a wide range of ideas and possibilities of choices in life. Youth are often beginning this stage in a more egocentric state – a term used to describe their focus on themselves. When they consider another's perspective, they tend to overextend the belief that someone is thinking about them.

As a result, youth also become self-conscious about their appearance and the appearance of others, as they feel they are being judged. Due to many bodily changes, youth feel an increased need for privacy. They begin to explore ways of being independent from their family both socially and emotionally and begin to form friendships and share private thoughts with their friends instead of family members (see Figure 27.2). In this process, they may push boundaries and may react strongly if parents or guardians reinforce limits.

Other important considerations are changes occurring in a youth's brain. While young children experience a massive growth, with 90%–95% of brain size developed by age 6, the brain requires tremendous remodeling to enable higher level analysis, planning, and decision making. This remodeling occurs as neuronal pruning (e.g., unused neuronal connections are eliminated and others are strengthened) allowing for more efficient use of brain resources. This brain development, triggered by hormonal changes, begins in the occipital cortex and moves to the prefrontal cortex – consequently decision making, planning, impulse control, and problem solving occur later in the unfolding of adolescence. It is hypothesized that early stage adolescents rely more heavily on their amygdala, because it develops earlier than the prefrontal cortex, to make decisions and solve problems. Emotions, impulses, aggression, and instinctive behavior are less restricted or inhibited by the prefrontal lobe. Adolescents do seem to vacillate between mature behaviors and illogical ones. Risky behavior and experimentation with sex, drugs, and alcohol may also be linked to this development. Emotional development is also linked to the amygdala and, subsequently, youth seem moodier than they did in elementary school and often lose the self-confidence they had as their younger selves. They are also at risk for mental health issues, depression, eating disorders, and substance use.

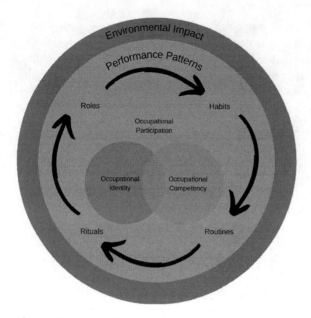

Figure 27.2 In adolescence, youth begin to explore ways of being independent from their family both socially and emotionally and begin to form friendships and share private thoughts with their friends instead of family members.

Source: Photo by Kat Wilcox, pexels.com; photos on Pexels are free to use and attribution to photographer is provided.

27.3.4 Middle-to-Late Adolescence (Ages 15–19)

Physical changes from puberty continue during middle adolescence. These changes will begin to effect males who will experience physical growth in height and weight, and have begun developing more secondary sex characteristics. All youth may experience changes to their voice, skin, and hair, development of body fat, and musculoskeletal changes that may propel them to try competitive sports. While physical changes may be nearly complete for females at this stage, they may just be starting for males.

The brain continues its maturation, particularly in the frontal lobes – a process that extends until a person is well into their 20s. This disparity between physical development and cognitive, mental, and social development can potentially create challenges for youth. While the brain continues to mature, primarily by improving neuronal connectivity and myelination, there are still many differences in how a typically developing middle adolescent thinks compared to an adult. The frontal lobes play a big role in coordinating complex decision making, impulse control, and being able to consider multiple options and consequences. However, middle-to-late adolescents are now more able to think abstractly and consider multiple and competing issues from more perspectives, but they still may lack the ability to apply it in the moment.

Youth at this stage begin to experience a crystallization of their self-concept. Self-concept is posited by researchers to represent multiple components, including self-image, self-esteem, and a representation of an ideal self. It also includes the concepts of self-efficacy and self-awareness. The dawning of self-image leads at this stage to concern about their appearance, and the influence of peer pressure may peak at this age. This over-projection of self-image lends itself to youth over estimating the amount of attention others pay to them and they can become acutely embarrassed and feel as if they are being watched and judged by others in their social group.

At this later stage of development, many adolescents become interested in romantic and sexual relationships. They may question and explore their sexual identity, which may be stressful if they do not have support from peers, family, or community. Friendships and romantic relationships toward the end of this stage become more stable. Many families experience increasing arguments with youth in middle adolescence as they struggle for more independence, gradually becoming further emotionally and physically separated from their family. They may opt to spend less time with family and more time with friends. Teens entering early adulthood also have a stronger sense of their own individuality now and can identify their own values. They may become more focused on future planning and base decisions on their hopes and ideals. Adolescents prepare for more independence and responsibility, many teenagers start working, and many will be leaving home soon after high school to pursue work or continue their education (see Table 27.1).

Table 27.1 Changes During Adolescent Development

Typical stages of adolescent development	*Emerging-early adolescence*	*Middle-late adolescence*
Cognitive, ethical, and moral development	Concrete thinking and moral reasoning are rule bound	Concrete thinking is replaced with the ability to think more abstractly, which allows consideration of more subtle differences in morality
Physical development	Obvious growth period, including height and body proportions	Growth slows and equilibrates; thus, youth achieve height and body proportions they will have as adults
Gender and sexuality development	Secondary sexual characteristics emerge as do more specific feelings and thoughts about gender	Exploring sexuality, sexual intimacy, and gender identity is a hallmark of older adolescents
Social development	Closely tied to family, but development of close friend relationships is established	Expansion of social networks and friendships to potentially more diverse social groups in a variety of realms
Development of self and self-identity	Self-identity is relational and focuses on more superficial characteristics	Development of a stronger sense of self and self-efficacy, self-esteem, and self-identity

27.4 Health and Adolescence

Adolescents, overall, are among the healthiest people in the Western world with low rates of disease and mortality (Centers for Disease Control and Prevention, 2020). In 2019, there were nearly 42 million children (41.8 million) and adolescents ages 10–19, representing roughly 13% of Americans. In the past ten years, the adolescent population has grown by more than 7%, with the largest gains seen among young adults ages 20–24. Additionally, while not specific to the adolescent population, about 51% of the population were counted as female, 49% were male, and an estimate of the transgender population concluded that for 1 in 250 adults, their gender identity does not match their sex assigned to them at birth. Adolescents in the Western world are a wonderfully diverse group of young people, reflecting society's increasing diversity as racial and ethnic minority groups continue to expand (U.S. Census Bureau, 2020).

The overall health of the adolescent population is reflected by the percentage of adolescents aged 12–17 years who are in fair or poor health, which stood at 3.2% in 2020. The percentage of adolescents aged 12–17 years who missed 11 or more days of school in the 2019–2020 school year because of illness or injury was 4.1% (Centers for Disease Control and Prevention, 2020). The National Vital Statistics Database System indicates that mortality is also very low, with the number of deaths for adolescents aged 15–19 years tallied at 12,278, indicating a death rate of 58.6 per 100,000 in 2021 (National Center for Health Statistics, 2021a). This is the only age group where the leading causes of death – accidental death, homicide, and suicide – are largely preventable (National Center for Health Statistics, 2021a).

While adolescents may be healthier, in general, than other age groups the data also suggest that health status depends largely on socioeconomic standing, positive and safe home and community environments, and access to high-quality public education and health care. Additionally, many Black or Hispanic youths and/or those who live in high-density urban settings are often overrepresented in many categories of disease and mortality. These include violence, mental distress, mental illness, poor dental health, asthma, allergies, and attention-deficit-hyperactivity-disorder (ADHD); a parent who is incarcerated; and living with someone who has a drug or alcohol problem/disorder. Society has propagated many of these issues through systemic racism, a situation that promulgates the disparities between White, Black, and Hispanic youth populations.

The major categories of health challenges in adolescence differ from other age groups in important ways, and in ways which may affect their life trajectories. The primary health challenges for adolescents in Western countries are obesity, sexually risky behaviors, teen pregnancy, early experimentation and continued substance use of alcohol and tobacco, and mental illness. Table 27.2 illustrates the ways in which adolescents aged 12–19 are affected by health challenges (all data are from the National Center for Health Statistics, 2021b).

27.5 Development in Adolescence

27.5.1 Developmental Theorists/Theories of Adolescent Development

While there are many developmental theories focusing on the acquisition of developmental skills early in life, less attention has been paid to adolescent development. The exceptions are the theorists Maslow and Piaget whose theories explicitly include this stage of development.

Table 27.2 Health Conditions, Prevalence, and Occupational Risk in Adolescence

Health condition	Prevalence and health risks in the United States	Risks to occupational engagement
Obesity, nutrition, and physical activity	The percentage of adolescents aged 12–19 years who are obese stands at 21.2%. Youth who are obese tend to remain overweight throughout adulthood.	Potentially limits a youth's participation in a full range of social and physical activities, and exposes youth to long-term health consequences (e.g., diabetes).
Sexual risky behaviors and teen pregnancy	Fewer teens aged 15–19 are having children than ever before; the birth rate for teenagers aged 15–19 has fallen almost continuously since 1991, reaching historic lows for the nation every year since 2009, and despite declines in all racial and ethnic groups, teen birth rates continue to vary considerably by race and ethnicity. Importantly, the US teen birth rate remains higher than in other industrialized countries, and childbearing by teenagers continues to be a matter of public concern. This represents recent and long-term trends and disparities in teen childbearing by race and Hispanic origin (Hamilton et al., 2021).	Youth who become parents as teenagers are more likely to live at or below the poverty line, raise children as single parents, and experience limitations in exploring job and educational opportunities.
Substance abuse, and use of alcohol and tobacco	In 2019, the percentage of adolescents aged 12–17 years who reported smoking cigarettes in the past month was 2.3%; those who reported using alcohol was 9.4% (National Center for Health Statistics, 2021c).	Early use of alcohol and tobacco are associated with higher risk of developing substance dependence later in life (Handren et al., 2016; von Diemen et al., 2008).
Mental health conditions	Access to health care that supports mental health services is rare. The percentage of adolescents aged 12–17 years that have access to health care is 96.4%. The percentage of adolescents aged 12–17 years without health insurance is 4.6% (National Center for Health Statistics, 2022).	

(Continued)

Table 27.2 (Continued)

Poverty	Of the 37.2 million people living in poverty, 11.6–13 million are children, thus 16%–18% of all children in the US are living in poverty. Stated another way, this equates to approximately 1 out of 6.5 children. Child poverty occurs when a child lives in a household where the combined annual earnings of all adults fall below a federally set income threshold. This threshold varies by family size and composition. In 2018, a family of two adults and two children were officially living in poverty if their household earnings fell below $25,465 annually.	Poverty elevates a child's risk of experiencing behavioral, social, emotional, and health challenges. Poverty also reduces skill-building opportunities and academic outcomes, undercutting a youth's capacity to learn, graduate high school, and more. In one study, affluence, neighborhood safety, and family resources during adolescence accounted for 4.5% of the differences in health 15–20 years later (Troxel & Hastings, 2014).

Abraham Maslow (1908–1970) was a humanistic psychologist who viewed people as naturally healthy individuals who seek opportunities for self-fulfillment and personal growth (Maslow, 1970). Maslow suggested that we are all driven by an inner need to fulfill our potential and achieve a sense of self-actualization (Milevsky, 2014). While Maslow acknowledged that we are all driven toward growth by an inner need, we are only motivated to pursue activities that fulfill our specific needs. Maslow proposed a hierarchy of needs that was common to all people. This now widely taught model starts with the need for food and safety at the base, progresses through social contact and self-esteem, and finishes with self-actualization as the pinnacle (see Figure 27.3). As a powerful conceptual tool for helping people deal with life difficulties, Maslow's work spurred the development of clinical psychology and with it the notion that one has inner needs that one can control. Understanding people's need to grow and develop is crucial in enabling parents, health care providers, and educators to support adolescents as they work through their emotional and social needs during this time of change.

Jean Piaget (1896–1980) was primarily interested in how children learn and acquire knowledge about their environment, and how those differences and limitations in thinking evolve and effect the way children and adolescents interact with concepts, objects, and people. His observations and interviews with children allowed him to develop a profoundly influential theory that continues to resonate in cognitive assessment, intervention, and education (Crain, 2005). Most relevant to adolescents is the idea that the basis of learning occurs in early childhood and is the foundation upon which the ability to generalize and scaffold complexity and abstract concepts lies, without which movement into adulthood and total independence is difficult.

Adolescents transition to the stage that Piaget named "formal operations" around the age of 12. Formal operations include the ability of a youth to begin to think

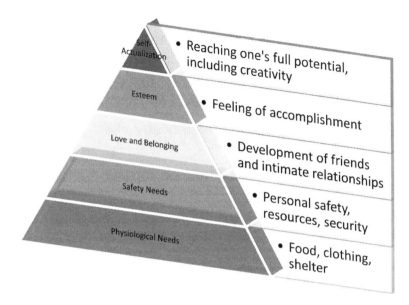

Figure 27.3 Maslow's hierarchy of needs.
Source: Maslow, 1970; reproduced with permission.

abstractly and reason about hypothetical problems. In this stage, adolescents are more able to think about moral, philosophical, ethical, social, and political issues that require theoretical and abstract reasoning; and initiate the ability to apply deductive logic or reasoning from a general principle to specific information. A youth who uses formal operations is more organized in their approach to a problem and therefore makes fewer errors in thinking. They can generalize principles and make connections between areas of life; for example, they can see precision in an abstract work of art or appreciate the contrasts in dissonance in music, whereas a younger child will not make these connections. Understanding that these processes unfold gradually throughout adolescence allows educators, parents/caregivers, and health care providers insight into behavior, and facilitates support for youth in this time of pivotal change.

27.6 Occupations in Adolescents

27.6.1 Occupational Range for Adolescence: Basic and Instrumental Activities of Daily Living (IADLs)

Neurotypically developing children gain their independence in grooming, bathing/showering, hand washing, oral-facial hygiene, toileting, dressing, eating, and functional mobility by seven years of age. Therefore, adolescents' development in ADLs is focused on acquisition of IADLs. These activities, highlighted in Table 27.3, reflect the gradual attainment of the cognitive, social, and physical skills needed to complete more complex activities (Beisbier & Laverdure, 2020; Cahill & Beisbier, 2020; Janssen, Elzinga et al., 2021; Janssen, Verkuil et al., 2021; Lamash et al., 2022; Twenge & Park, 2019).

Most cultures have rites that recognize the passage from childhood to adulthood, some of which are celebrated by ceremonies. These rites of passage are usually based

Table 27.3 Highlighted Occupations for Youth in Young-Middle and Middle-Late Adolescence

Task (AOTA, 2020)	Young-middle adolescence (12–15)	Middle-late adolescents (15–19+)
ADL		
Bathing, showering, toileting, dressing, eating, functional mobility, personal hygiene, grooming	Independent	Independent
Sexual activity	May engage in self-stimulation. Typically, youth will explore kissing and hugging at this age.	Youth become more engaged in romantic and sexual relationships, and they will potentially explore gender expression. For those beginning engagement in the broad possibilities of sexual expression, experiences with self or others will vary widely depending on individuals, culture, and interest (e.g., hugging, kissing, foreplay, masturbation, oral sex, and intercourse).
IADLs		
Care of others	Able to babysit children over 2 years of age safely. Can assist parent in daily care for younger siblings.	Able to babysit all children, including infants for shorter periods. Able to care for siblings' basic needs.
Care of pets	Able to care for a pet with support and supervision. Will need a lot of assistance with purchasing food, establishing and management of a care routine, and managing health (e.g., veterinarian care) and behaviors.	Able to care for a pet with occasional support and can arrange or teach how to care for a pet with others.
Communication management	Able to send, receive, and use a variety of systems and equipment, including phones, computers, and telecommunication, but will need help with interpretation of information and management of appropriate use of devices.	Able to send, receive, and use a wider variety of systems and equipment, including phones, computers, telecommunication, communication boards, and personal digital assistants, and will only occasionally require help with interpretation of information.

(Continued)

Table 27.3 (Continued)

		Able to manage a calendar to keep track of assignments in school and activities at home or for extracurricular activities. Able to anticipate needs for a weekly schedule (e.g., rehearsing a schedule, ensuring clothing is clean, communicating with family to make sure that they have transportation to events).
Community mobility	Able to navigate immediate environment (e.g., neighborhood and community). Able to use bike to go short distances (e.g., neighborhood school and store). Can use public transportation on anticipated routes and can begin to recognize usual driving route.	With exposure/practice, able to move around in the community using public or private transportation, such as driving, walking, bicycling, or accessing and riding in buses, taxi cabs, or other transportation systems.
Financial management	Learning to understand money management. Needs assistance with banking and financial transactions. Beginning to understand basic fiscal concepts (e.g., value of products and saving money). Able to set short-term goals.	Independent in managing cash and daily money use, along with money earned from any work. However, banking (e.g., checking or savings accounts) and finances, including keeping track of bank accounts and paying bills, will require support. Able to start setting longer-term goals for money use.
Health management and maintenance	Relies on parent caregiver to manage and maintain routine for medical appointments and medication management. Establishing own routines for physical activity and eating. May be exposed to and utilize activities like meditation and yoga at school or with family and friends.	Has developed more set health management habits, including managing and maintaining routines for engaging in health and wellness promotion, such as physical fitness, nutrition, decreasing health risk behaviors, and responsibility for medication routines.

(*Continued*)

Table 27.3 (Continued)

Home establishment and management	At this age youth can engage in a variety of personal and household management. This includes making their own bed, cleaning their own room (e.g., dusting, vacuuming, and picking up things), picking up around the house, putting things away, light housecleaning, folding clothing, and learning how to use appliances.	Youth are now able to engage in a wider range of activities for home management. This includes shopping in stores for clothing and groceries, helping with home repairs that are non-technical in nature (e.g., changing light bulbs or repairing a loose screw). They can also begin doing their own laundry, including use of a washing machine and dryer, and folding and putting away clothing. They may also be assisting with outdoor maintenance (if dwelling is a home), including picking up sports equipment, lawn maintenance (e.g., mowing, weeding, and planting).
Meal preparation and clean-up	Preparing simple foods requiring no mixing or cooking, including sandwiches, cold cereal, etc. Mixing and cooking simple foods, e.g., frying eggs, make pancakes, and heating foods in microwave. Preparing a simple complete meal, e.g., pasta. They are also able to help with meal set-up and clean-up, e.g., setting and clearing table and washing dishes, including using a dishwasher.	Able to plan, prepare, and serve well-balanced, nutritional meals and clean up food and utensils after meals. Youth at this age may begin to take responsibility for their own meals or will prepare meals for family or friends independently.
Religious observance	Youth generally participate in organized system of beliefs, practices, rituals, and symbols that are part of family traditions. Depending on family or culture, may opt to complete rites of passage that mark adulthood into a religious group.	Participating in an organized system of beliefs, practices, rituals, and symbols may be similar to or different from family or culture. Youth are tending to choose their own beliefs. Again, depending on family or culture, may opt to complete rites of passage that mark adulthood into a religious group.

(*Continued*)

Table 27.3 (Continued)

Safety and emergency management	Able to know and perform preventive procedures to maintain a safe environment; recognize sudden, unexpected, hazardous situations; and initiate emergency action to reduce threats to health and safety. Decisions may be more reactive and less informed and based on life experience.	Able to know and perform preventive procedures to maintain a safe environment; recognize sudden, unexpected, hazardous situations; and initiate emergency action to reduce threats to health and safety more independently. Able to make decisions regarding safety and emergency situations in a more informed, rational, logical, and mature manner.
Shopping	Youth can assist with making shopping lists for preferred food items, shop with family/carer to select clothing items, and typically rely on family resources to pay for any food or clothing. Able to help with the physical tasks of shopping and putting items away.	Youth can prepare shopping lists (grocery and other), selecting, purchasing, and transporting items. They continue to need assistance with payment, and completing money transactions.
Education	Youth can participate in a wide range of academic coursework (e.g., reading, writing, math, science, and arts), non-academic (e.g., recess, lunchroom, and hallway), online/technological and basic exploration of pre-vocational learning opportunities, and extracurricular activities (e.g., sports, science, and debate). In most cultures and in countries with higher incomes, youth in this age group are involved as students full-time.	By age 18 youth are progressing to completion of mandatory education in many cultures. Youth will make decisions about advanced academic coursework and continue their studies, e.g., academic coursework in college. Most youth will begin consideration of jobs they might do as adults, e.g., pre-vocational learning. In some cultures, or countries, youth may be transferring skills to more adult-like work and less education.
Rest and sleep	Youth who are between 12 and 14 may require 9–12 hours of sleep and with a desire to start sleeping later and arising later emerging. Youth are intrigued by concepts of "staying up all night." Sleep health, however, is increasingly seen as crucial to learning, concentration, and mental health in youth.	Youth at this age require 8–10 hours of sleep. Preferences for sleep times are established and while youth can seemingly engage in their daily activities energetically with less than 8 hours of sleep, research indicates that this takes a toll on concentration, academic readiness, and overall mental health.

(*Continued*)

Table 27.3 (Continued)

	Youth require support to develop healthy sleep habits and routines.	Youth may need to be encouraged to develop habits for relaxation prior to bed and engaging in routines that will help facilitate sleep, e.g., reading, listening to music, and meditation.
Work/volunteering	Youth may be exposed to helping others through engagement in clubs (e.g., girl scouts) and do volunteer work with other youth and adults. Youth may express interest in various jobs, including those of their own family or friends. May work doing babysitting, yard work, household chores, or house sitting.	Many youths have part-time jobs that require them to complete application materials, interviews, and training. Some youth do training (e.g., life guarding) to attain jobs for seasonal work. Typically, work required is routine or scripted, but requires development of communication skills, being consistent, completing required jobs independently, using time effectively, and developing interactional skills with fellow employees. Volunteer work is more directed to causes that youth care about and find interesting. Volunteering may be done in conjunction with family.
Leisure exploration and participation	Engagement in a variety of leisure activities is associated with youth health development. Youth may engage in a wide array of physical activities, creative activities (e.g., dance, music, art, and theater), video gaming, and social (e.g., meeting friends) or more solitary pursuits (e.g., reading). Youth may pursue these activities sequentially, for example discovering that they enjoy team vs. individual sports. They may also pursue these interests simultaneously (e.g., playing basketball and learning the piano).	Youth are more likely to find a balance between leisure pursuits with the most meaning and are more confident about choosing among the activities they enjoy. Leisure pursuits may become related to part-time work, full-time work, or educational pursuits. For example, a youth who becomes exceptionally proficient at piano may begin teaching lessons to younger children or may pursue a degree in music.

(*Continued*)

Table 27.3 (Continued)

	Youth require adults to help to manage schedules, finances, manage objects needed, and help to manage balance of needs.	May still require financial support but are able to schedule activities, care for objects, manage need for participation, and balance interests.
Social participation	Social interactions and expanding one's peer group, while building friendships, is a key component to healthy adolescence. Friendships may still change but are becoming more solidified. Youth identify small groups, usually 3–5 friends, as close friends and spend a lot of time with those friends. Friendships are formed within different groups depending on school and extracurricular activities, and may be related to proximity and family interests.	Social interactions continue to expand and include a wider array of people. While building relationships with close friends, friend networks may continue to expand. Friendships are formed outside of proximity to school, leisure interests, or family ties (e.g., establishing a friendship with another counselor at a summer camp who lives in another state). Intimate relationships with one person may be established for longer periods. Youth spend more time with friends and pursuing joint interests, which are oftentimes preferred over family (Khetani & Coster, 2019).

on a particular society's, religion's, or even family's expectations, and rites of passage are quite different between Western and Eastern societies. Table 27.4 highlights those rites from a Western perspective and contrasts the relationship between rites and the development of occupations. These rites often coincide with sexual, physical, and social maturation. Additionally, some youth assert their independence by rejecting rites of passage, as they may not represent their newly developed values.

Many youths view the transition from childhood to adulthood as recognition that they are being accepted into society, family, and community with all the rights that adults have, and most are eager to attain this status. Table 27.5 highlights the overarching goals that are often associated with the benefits and challenges of reaching adulthood. Recently, researchers have documented the timing of transitions to the acquisition of skills for adulthood; this provides an important perspective on how responsibility slowly shifts over five years, in many cases, for typically developing youth. In youth who have disabilities, these shifts may take up to 15 years (Kao et al., 2021). Few researchers have investigated perceptions of how adolescents experience occupations as they transition from adulthood. Wilcock and Hocking (2015) assert that dimensions of being (having time to be), becoming (developing through engagement in occupations),

Table 27.4 Typical Western Society Rites of Passage

Rite of passage	Occupation	Symbolic purpose
Attainment of a Driver's License	Independent community mobility allowing pursuit of social, work, and leisure activities outside family,	Independence from family and establishment of independent routines.
Voting	Recognizing and taking social responsibility within a society.	Signifies adoption of the rights of citizenship.
Sexual intimacy	Dating and sexual intimacy signal a belief in readiness for longer-term relationships and commitment to one person.	Demonstrates personal choice in partners and responsibility for sexual intimacy.
Military service	Military service for periods of 4 years when youth reach the age of 18.	Signifies the adoption of citizenship in a country (some countries have mandatory service for men and women).
Acceptance into a religious or other organization (bar/bat mitzvahs, confirmation, baptism, Quinceanera)	Can be solemn, vibrant, and colorful, or both. These rites are typically a thoughtful acceptance of adult responsibilities within the religious community.	Provides special meaning (cognitive) to the adolescent through family and community support (religious programs).

Table 27.5 Developmental Goals of Adolescence

Goal to accomplish/prepare for in adolescence	Occupations that support this goal	Challenges
Prepare for financial independence and life as a productive citizen (work).	■ Education progression (high school diploma and post-secondary education) for more complex math and money. ■ Experience as a part-time worker or volunteer. ■ Engaging in extracurricular activities, e.g., sports, music, and clubs.	Occupational exploration that is broad and covers art, science, technology, music, and education for a wide variety of career options. Balancing demands of school, social exploration, work, and discovery of interests.

(Continued)

HUMAN OCCUPATIONS OF ADOLESCENCE AND YOUTH

Table 27.5 (Continued)

Achieve emotional independence from parents and other adults.	Engaging in positive relationships with peers around a shared value. Identifying with positive adult role models outside of family role, e.g., teachers, religious leader, or coach. Be encouraged to express opinions. Initiate friendly interactions in low stakes situations.	Social relationships with peers valued over family relationships. Poorly developed social connections can lead to mental health issues. Bullying.
Prepare for sustained intimate relationship(s) and/or family life.	Opportunities for healthy dating. Continued participation in family traditions by helping to prepare for holidays. Express gender and sexual identities through clothing and hair style.	Development of gender identity that is not acceptable to family may cause fractures of family relationships. Inexperience with dating/intimate social relationships or substance use may lead to risk-taking behavior.
Identify and incorporate behaviors consistent with social expectations and personal value systems.	Opportunities to reconcile different worldviews with family, peer, school, work, and community expectations and values. Identify and incorporate consistent behaviors that reflect social and personal values.	Views of the world that are vastly different than family values may cause tension. Rejection of spiritual or religious values may cause disruptions in family life and social structures.
Learn to use one's body effectively.	Engaging in fluent peer-to-peer conversation. Participation in group activities. Working collaboratively with others for a purpose. Opportunities to give directions or instructions to others.	Lack of self-confidence may result from inexperience with sports or social exposure, and sets up a negative cycle of drawing away from others.
Establish a gender identity.	Participating in a gender identity curriculum with peers at school. Meeting a wide range of people who represent a range of gender identities in positive roles. Discussion of gender identity with peers in a positive manner.	Gender identity is not supported by family. Views gender identity very narrowly and sees gender distinctions outside of binary genders as negative.

(*Continued*)

CHAPTER 27

Table 27.5 (Continued)

Establish new and more mature relations with peers.	Can identify 2–3 close friends but is able to separate and mix with others. Makes eye contact and faces others when speaking. Maintains comfortable and socially appropriate space between self and others. Makes a new friend.	Rarely leaving a "safe" close peer group to meet others may attenuate social opportunities. Viewed as immature or socially inadequate.
Develop a set of values and an ethical system as a guide to behavior.	Explores questions like where and how do I fit into my world. Opportunities to discuss complex social issues and disparities. Takes part in volunteering for causes that are consistent with values.	Sees hypocrisy in adults or has been exposed to an inconsistent set of values (adults abusing drugs). Contradictions in society are seen as flaws that are irrevocable.
Develop positive self-esteem.	Volunteers for tasks and activities. Recognizes strengths, interests, and abilities.	Develops low self-esteem or mental health issues, e.g., depression and substance abuse.

and belonging (doing things with others) are crucial to humans as occupational beings. A group of researchers who asked adolescents how they would categorize occupations found that they would include experiences of time passing, periods of enjoyment, challenges, deeper engagement, relaxation, need/necessity, and self-identification (Widmark & Fristedt, 2019).

27.6.2 Occupational Profile

Jason is a 14-year-old young male who lives with his mother, who is remarried, and his stepfather. He has a strong, mostly positive relationship with his family. Jason has an older brother who is 18 years old and will be leaving for an apprentice program in a nearby town. The family lives in a single-family home in a suburban setting. Jason has periodic contact with his biological father whom he regards as family but does not feel close with or positive about. Jason enjoys playing soccer and self-taught himself to play an acoustic guitar. Jason can identify two friends with whom he is close. He also has a wider group of people of both sexes who he says are more casual friends from his middle school and neighborhood. He is transitioning into high school and he expresses a lot of anxiety about fitting in; Jason is sensitive to comments by his family and friends about his clothing and hair style. He enjoys math and science but has signed up for drawing in high school as well. He would like to experiment with doing more in the arts but is reluctant to show anyone his work for fear of judgment. He does not have a clear occupational goal but may want to explore drafting. His family is religiously observant and they attend services regularly; he states that he does not believe in much of the teachings of his church and often protests about having to attend services. He knows he is much more attracted to his male friends romantically and sexually but he has not talked about this with anyone. Jason feels that he will not be accepted by his family and fears that his friends will reject him if they find out. He has decided to discuss these feelings with a school counselor with whom he has a positive relationship. He is both excited about his future and sad that he cannot express his wholeness to his family or friends. His family sees that he has become stubborn about attending church services, seems reluctant to talk with them, and seems more withdrawn socially. Maslow's hierarchy suggests that healthy development requires Jason to resolve these issues to achieve his goals in adulthood.

27.6.3 Case Study

David is a deaf 15-year-old male with a cleft lip and palate. He is in eighth grade and lives with his adoptive parents and a nine-year-old female sibling. David was adopted at age 11 from Vietnam, where he had been placed in an orphanage at nine years old following the death of his grandmother who was caring for him. Upon entrance to the orphanage, he had had no formal schooling and, in addition to his cleft lip and palate and craniofacial anomalies, he was erroneously identified as having an intellectual impairment and genetic disorder. These errors were corrected upon medical testing on arrival in the US. While his cleft lip and palate had been repaired as an infant, David also had craniofacial anomalies, including hypoplasia of his upper jaw, right ear, bilateral external auditory canals, and inner ear (e.g., oval window, round window, ossicles with dysplastic malleus, incus, and loss of a normal air gap between the malleus head and epitympanic wall). He was initially fitted with bone-assisted hearing aids which failed due to numerous infections, and only in the past year was David ultimately and successfully fitted with bilateral cochlear implants.

He is currently enrolled in a deaf and hard of hearing program that encourages the use of total communication (e.g., spoken English and American Sign Language). David was determined to have normal intellectual functioning, which was initially masked because of language barriers. Upon supportive education and access to speech language pathology and occupational therapy, he has been making steady progress in language acquisition and IADLs. Academically, he is at sixth- to seventh-grade level but in the past year has improved one full grade. He will be moving into ninth grade on an individualized education plan and making a transition to high school, with a deaf and hard of hearing program that is embedded in a hearing/regular high school.

David is very social and readily engages in conversation with peers who hear and those who are deaf/hard of hearing. His teachers say he is well-liked by classmates and he identifies one close friend. David enjoys his teachers and completes his homework, stating that math is his favorite subject. He loves video games, playing soccer, basketball, and engaging in karate. He also attends computer coding workshops periodically. He says that he is not particularly good at anything and verbalizes his faults more than his skills (e.g., he states he hates his skin because of acne). David has reported to his family that he was bullied at the school he attended in Vietnam and was name called (e.g., dumb) and teased by the other children.

In many ways David is a typical teenager; however, he does have emotional regulation challenges. He has intense outbursts when he is frustrated, primarily at home with his parents. He tends to hit things and has punched holes in walls and doors on several occasions. Seemingly innocuous events appear to trigger these outbursts. When he is sad or disappointed (e.g., loses a soccer game or cannot master a video game) he catastrophizes and withdraws. David can reconcile his emotions and talk to his family following these outbursts. He states that he feels ashamed of his outbursts but claims that he cannot "control" his mind. He becomes particularly upset when he perceives that he is being teased or bullied by other students in school.

David's goals are to make more friends, improve his soccer skills, and learn to drive. His parents share his goals to help him expand his social network and find a sport which he enjoys and can be successful at; however, they feel that he is too immature to drive. His parents also want him to learn more appropriate outlets for his frustration and to see himself more positively. In addition, they are very concerned that he catches up to his grade level academically to enable him to eventually pursue a career. His teachers have recommended that a counselor be added to his services at school to help him develop coping strategies when he feels that he is being bullied or experiences disappointment. David's family will encourage use of these strategies at home, will consistently check in with him about any bullying, and will request support when needed. He and his parents will pursue family counseling, see a dermatologist to manage his acne, and reinforce a good hygiene routine. He will be encouraged to invite friends over to his home or to engage in a social activity with peers at least twice a month. David will take driver education classes and allow the teachers to determine if he is mature and able to safely pursue driving (e.g., read signs and complete exam). He will continue with all his sports, gaming, and coding if he utilizes coping strategies and talks with family and his counselor about his feelings.

27.7 Conclusion

Adolescence is a time of change, full of opportunities as well as challenges; most obvious are physical changes and the development of secondary sex characteristics, as well as growing independence in basic and instrumental self-care. Numerous and more subtle changes are also taking place: an emotional and social movement away from family; development of abstract reasoning and complex inductive thought; increasing self-awareness and self-concept; and changing peer dynamics. All these changes occur in diverse environments that include opportunities to alter engagement in family life, peer relationships, community involvement, educational opportunities, and leisure exploration. Healthy adolescents, usually later in adolescence, achieve a balance between social interests, romantic relationships, and family commitments; make choices about education and work; and find satisfying leisure pursuits. While adolescence is, in general, a time of life where good health is experienced, some adolescents may experience poor health, particularly if they live in marginalized communities and lack access to good education, opportunities for physical activity, and consistent health care. The primary health challenges for youth are mental illness (e.g., depression and suicide risk), risk-taking behavior (e.g., unprotected sex, reckless driving, and substance use), handling conflict through violence (e.g., bullying and access to guns), and poor physical fitness due to diet and physical activity. The goal of adolescence is to emerge into adulthood with skills that can be scaffolded into positive engagement in society with productive contributions. Thus, IADLs become a focus of development. In emerging-early adolescence, youth require support and encouragement to take on new roles, while older adolescents may take a lead in orchestrating their education, leisure, and social life, and require little assistance. Most adolescents begin to explore work options and attain a part-time job, explore a variety of leisure options, and may move away from values expressed by family or their religious communities. These differences may cause strife and angst in families and cause youth to seek support from friends or adults outside of the family. Youth also experience a wide array of social challenges and may need support and help to navigate negative self-concepts, bullying, or gender diversity. Healthy development often requires a blend of allowing individual development with caring adult support which understands the challenges youth face and encourages their independence as they move through adolescence.

27.8 Summary

- For an adolescent, engagement in a variety of occupations often reflects the demands of the external environment and internal physiological development.
- Developmental trajectories diverge for adolescents and are highly dependent on individual characteristics; familial, cultural, and social expectations; and demands of the physical environment.
- Adolescence is characterized by:
  - Rapid growth and maturation
  - Refinement of skills
  - Increased self-determination
  - Development of a sense of identity and positive self-concept
  - Critical thinking and reasoning skills
  - Increased social development and sense of responsibility.
- Occupational therapists promote the following outcomes for adolescents, including adolescents with disabilities:
  - A sense of personal identity
  - Autonomy in daily life activities
  - Independent decision making
  - Life skills for adulthood
- All health care providers, educators, and family who have adolescents can benefit from understanding the developmental tasks and trajectories for youth as they move from childhood to adulthood.
- Adolescents, despite perceptions, are often healthier than other age groups; however, they experience mortalities from largely preventable conditions, including suicide and violence – a sad statistic which society has yet to grapple with.
- Adolescents are particularly vulnerable to health conditions that oftentimes arise during this age (e.g., mental health issues, substance use, and obesity) and which have the potential to affect them throughout life.

27.9 Review Questions
1. What unique perspectives do some adolescents have about occupations?
2. What are the most likely causes of mortality in adolescents?
3. What health conditions most affect adolescents?
4. How can educators, health care providers, and families support adolescents as they move through this developmental stage?
5. How long does it take neurotypical youth to move from dependence to relative independence in ADLs?
6. Which areas of occupation are most affected as youth move through adolescence?
7. Who are the two theorists discussed in this chapter and how do their theories help practitioners to support adolescents?
8. What are the broad occupational goals and challenges for adolescents to transition to adulthood?
9. What are rites of passage for adolescents? What is thought to be the purpose of these rites?

References

American Occupational Therapy Association. (2020). Occupational Therapy Practice Framework: Domain and Process (4th ed.). *American Journal of Occupational Therapy, 74*(Suppl. 2), 7412410010p1 -7412410010p87. https://doi.org/10.5014/ajot.2020.74S2001

Beisbier, S., & Laverdure, P. (2020). Occupation- and activity-based interventions to improve performance of instrumental activities of daily living and rest and sleep for children and youth ages 5–21: A systematic review. *American Journal of Occupational Therapy, 74*(2), 7402180040p1–7402180040p32. https://doi.org/10.5014/ajot.2020.039636

Cahill, S. M., & Beisbier, S. (2020). Occupational therapy practice guidelines for children and youth ages 5–21 years. *American Journal of Occupational Therapy, 74*(4), 7404397010p1–7404397010p48. https://doi.org/10.5014/ajot.2020.744001

Centers for Disease Control and Prevention. (2020). *Interactive Summary Health Statistics for Children – 2019–2020*. Centers for Disease Control and Prevention. https://wwwn.cdc.gov/NHISDataQueryTool/SHS_child/index.html

Crain, W. (2005). *Theories of development concepts and applications* (5th ed.). Pearson.

Hamilton, B., Rossen, L., Lu, L., & Chong, Y. (2021). *U.S. and state trends on teen births, 1990–2019*. National Center for Health Statistics.

Handren, L., Donaldson, C., Crano, W., Handren, L. M., Donaldson, C. D., & Crano, W. D. (2016). Adolescent alcohol use: Protective and predictive parent, peer, and self-related factors. *Prevention Science, 17*(7), 862–871. https://doi.org/10.1007/s11121-016-0695-7

Janssen, L. H. C., Elzinga, B. M., Verkuil, B., Hillegers, M. H. J., & Keijsers, L. (2021). The link between parental support and adolescent negative mood in daily life: Between-person heterogeneity in within-person processes. *Journal of Youth & Adolescence, 50*(2), 271–285. https://doi.org/10.1007/s10964-020-01323-w

Janssen, L. H. C., Verkuil, B., van Houtum, L. A. E. M., Wever, M. C. M., & Elzinga, B. M. (2021). Perceptions of parenting in daily life: Adolescent-parent differences and associations with adolescent affect. *Journal of Youth & Adolescence, 50*(12), 2427–2443. https://doi.org/10.1007/s10964-021-01489-x

Kao, Y.-C., Coster, W., Cohn, E. S., & Orsmond, G. I. (2021). Preparation for adulthood: Shifting responsibility for management of daily tasks from parents to their children. *American Journal of Occupational Therapy, 75*(2), 7502205050p1–7502205050p11. https://doi.org/10.5014/ajot.2020.041723

Khetani, M. A., & Coster, W. (2019). Social participation. In B. A. B. S. G. Gillen (Ed.), *Willard and Spackman's occupational therapy* (13th ed., pp. 847–860). Wolters.

Lamash, L., Ricon, T., & Rosenblum, S. (2022). Time organization patterns of adolescents: Agreement between self-report and parent report. *Physical & Occupational Therapy in Pediatrics, 42*(3), 319–332. https://doi.org/10.1080/01942638.2021.1982839

Maslow, A. (1970). *Motivation and personality* (2nd ed.). Harper & Row.

Milevsky, A. (2014). *Understanding adolescents for helping professionals.* Springer.

National Center for Health Statistics. (2021a). *Health, United States, 2019: Table 20.* Centers for Disease Control and Prevention. https://www.cdc.gov/nchs/hus/contents2019.htm

National Center for Health Statistics. (2021b). *National vital statistics system, mortality 1999–2020 on CDC WONDER Online Database.* Centers for Disease Control and Prevention. http://wonder.cdc.gov/ucd-icd10.html

National Center for Health Statistics. (2021c). *Use of selected substances in the past month among people aged 12 years and over, by age, sex, and race and Hispanic origin: United States, selected years 2002–2019.* https://www.cdc.gov/nchs/data/hus/2020-2021/SubUse. pdf

National Center for Health Statistics (2022). *Percentage of ever having asthma for children under age 18 years, United States, 2019—2022.* National Health Interview Survey. https://wwwn.cdc.gov/NHISDataQueryTool/SHS_child/index.html

Troxel, N., & Hastings, P. (2014). Poverty during childhood and adolescence may predict long-term health. *Policy Brief - Center for Poverty Research, 2*(10). https://poverty.ucdavis.edu/sites/main/files/file-attachments/policy_brief_troxel-hastings_poverty_stress.pdf

Twenge, J. M., & Park, H. (2019). The decline in adult activities among U.S. adolescents, 1976–2016. *Child Development, 90*(2), 638–654. https://doi.org/10.1111/cdev.12930

U.S. Census Bureau. (2020). *2019 population estimates by age, sex, race and Hispanic origin, April 1, 2010 to July 1, 2019.* census.gov/newsroom/press-kits/2020/population-estimates-detailed.html

von Diemen, L., Bassani, D. G., Fuchs, S. C., Szobot, C. M., & Pechansky, F. (2008). Impulsivity, age of first alcohol use and substance use disorders among male adolescents: A population based case-control study. *Addiction, 103*(7), 1198–1205. https://doi.org/10.1111/j.1360-0443.2008.02223.x

Widmark, E., & Fristedt, S. (2019). Occupation according to adolescents: Daily occupations categorized based on adolescents' experiences. *Journal of Occupational Science, 26*(4), 470–483. https://doi.org/10.1080/14427591.2018.1546609

Wilcock, A. A., & Hocking, C. (2015). *An occupational perspective on health, third edition.* Slack Incorporated.

CHAPTER 28

Human Occupations of Early Adulthood

Louise Gustafsson

Abstract

Early adulthood (18–40 years) is a period of identity consolidation and transition toward the independence, responsibility, and autonomy typical of an adult. Two representative stages have been described to represent and expand this lifespan. First, emerging adulthood, spanning the ages of 18–29 years and, second, established adulthood from the ages of 30–45 years. The key developmental tasks of early adulthood are closely linked to changes in occupations and performance patterns and have been described as completing education, leaving home, commencing full-time work, forming an intimate relationship, and entering parenthood. The order and timing of the developmental tasks occur variably due to individual and cultural factors, societal influences, and personal preferences. Therefore, the trajectory and experience of early adulthood is a uniquely personal and context-specific pathway and age cannot be considered a clear indicator of when a person becomes an adult.

Author's Positionality Statement

I am a cis-gender, heterosexual, white female who was afforded a privileged education in Australia, on the unceded lands of the traditional custodians, the Turrbul and Jagera peoples. I am an ally for the LGTBQI+ community and have personal experience of supporting people who live with neurological and mental health conditions. I have traveled and worked across different areas of the world and may bring some of these experiences to my writing, but I do not assume that I can represent the diverse experiences of all peoples. Formative personal and professional experiences shaped my early understanding of bias, exclusion, and injustice, and I am on a continual path of learning to understand and dismantle the mechanisms that exclude and disadvantage First Nations peoples and other populations. Finally, although I am now in middle adulthood, I have experienced the career-and-care-crunch of established adulthood, am a parent of emerging adults, and work with young adults experiencing the vastly different trajectories of early adulthood.

> **Objectives**
> This chapter will allow the reader to:
>
> - Describe the developmental tasks of early adulthood from an occupational perspective.
> - Differentiate the performance patterns of emerging and established adulthood.
> - Articulate a global and diverse perspective of early adulthood.
> - Develop an occupational profile for people and groups in early adulthood.

> **Key terms**
>
> - emerging adulthood
> - established adulthood
> - intimacy versus isolation
> - career-and-care-crunch
> - autonomy
> - responsibility
> - education
> - employment
> - parenting
> - child rearing

28.1 Introduction

Early adulthood has traditionally been described as the period of life between the chronological ages of 18–40 (Arnett, 2000). It is the lifespan period in which individuals strive toward a clear sense of who they are and what their place is in the world. Engagement in an expanding repertoire of occupations within and outside of the home assists the young adult to explore possibilities, make choices, and establish personal preferences, values, beliefs, and goals. The early adulthood lifespan is portrayed as two stages: emerging adulthood (18–29 years) and established adulthood (30–45 years) (Arnett, 2000; Mehta et al., 2020). The developmental tasks of early adulthood are considered a series of transitions toward independence, responsibility, and autonomy. They include leaving the childhood home and caregivers, finishing education, commencing employment, forming intimate relationships with or without cohabitation, and becoming a parent. Erikson (1950) believed that early adulthood is a time of intimacy versus isolation, underscoring the importance of developing close, honest, and committed friendships and relationships with people outside of the family during this lifespan period. In this chapter, the reader will consider the developmental tasks of early adulthood from an occupational perspective, distinguish between the stages of emerging and established adulthood, and explore the diverse occupational profiles of early adulthood with a range of illustrative vignettes.

28.2 Developmental Tasks of Early Adulthood

In some cultures, there are rituals and ceremonies to acknowledge the period in the lifespan in which an individual enters adulthood. For example, on the second Monday of January in Japan, men and women who turned 20 in the previous year celebrate Seijin no Hi or their "Coming of Age Day". On this day, the young adults wear traditional clothing and attend formal ceremonies in the local city (or prefecture) offices before celebrating with family and friends. In the Philippines, women celebrate their transition from a girl to a woman with a Debut on their 18th birthday, a grand party with family and friends. In contrast, men in the Philippines celebrate their coming of age on their 21st birthday, with a less lavish affair. These are symbolic celebrations for what is otherwise a complex, gradual, and often poorly defined process.

At the simplest level, a person is considered to have achieved adulthood when they have established financial independence and taken responsibility for themselves (Arnett, 2003). The developmental tasks of early adulthood (see Table 28.1) have been described predominantly from the perspective of the developed world and have evolved from when first described by Havighurst (1972). For example, changing social and societal influences led to the introduction of developmental tasks related to substance use avoidance in the early 2000s (Roisman et al., 2004; Schulenberg et al., 2004). It is suggested that five major transitions occur during early adulthood, and they form the foundation of this chapter: people leave their childhood home and caregivers; finish their education; begin employment, find intimate relationships with or without cohabitation; and they may become a parent (Skogbrott Birkeland et al., 2013).

When considered from an occupational perspective, the developmental tasks of early adulthood represent transitions or changes to the roles of the young adult with corresponding adjustments to their routines and occupational profile. For instance, leaving the childhood home leads to increased or new participation in instrumental activities of daily living (IADLs) and health management. Increasing occupations of social

Table 28.1 Developmental Tasks of Early Adulthood

Havighurst (1972)	*Schulenberg et al. (2004)*	*Schulenberg and Schoon (2012)*
■ Achieving autonomy	■ Education	■ Completing education
■ Establishing identity	■ Work	■ Leaving home
■ Developing emotional stability	■ Financial autonomy	■ Commencing full-time work
■ Establishing a career	■ Romantic involvement	■ Forming a romantic relationship
■ Finding intimacy	■ Peer involvement	■ Entering parenthood
■ Becoming part of a group or community	■ Healthy lifestyle/substance abuse avoidance	
■ Establishing a residence and learning how to manage a household	■ Citizenship	
■ Becoming a parent and rearing children		
■ Making marital or relationship adjustments and learning to parent		

participation are important as the young adult consolidates their identity through increasing community involvement, development of new friendships, and establishment of intimate relationships. The links between developmental tasks of early adulthood and occupational profiles are explored in further detail later in this chapter.

There is no socially mandated order for the transition to adulthood, and indeed the timing and sequence of the developmental tasks is based on unique factors, contexts, and preferences (Institute of Medicine and National Research Council, 2015). The young adult may achieve independence and autonomy early in the early adulthood lifespan period while for others there is more incremental development across their 20s, and even into their 30s. Vignettes are included here to briefly introduce the reader to two differing occupational profiles within early adulthood. The two profiles are representative of how individual and cultural factors, societal contexts, and personal preferences can influence the trajectory to adulthood.

> Peter is 20 years old and has a permanent full-time position working in a clothing store. Peter experienced bias and exclusion during his high school years and chose to move away from his hometown after school. He received initial financial support from his parents but is now financially independent and living in a rental apartment with his intimate partner Toby. They share responsibility for all household-related IADLs and caring for their dog.

> Simon is 20 years old, living in his childhood home with his parents, and is currently single. He is completing tertiary education at the nearby university and is employed to work 15–20 hours a week at a local restaurant. Simon has taken responsibility for the management of some of his finances (e.g., paying for select expenses such as clothing, entertainment, and car expenses) but is otherwise reliant on his parents for all other financial support. Simon is learning to live with a newly diagnosed chronic health condition and take responsibility for the related health management occupations. He is not required to attend to any of the household-related IADLs, although he will occasionally prepare meals for himself and his parents.

In the first vignette, Peter is now financially independent and has taken charge of decisions, managed challenges, and solved problems independent of his childhood caregivers (parents). Peter is demonstrating the independence, responsibility, and autonomy of adulthood, including the establishment of an intimate relationship. In contrast, Simon has not fully achieved any of the developmental tasks of adulthood and is illustrative of an incremental transition to adulthood. He demonstrates many of the characteristics of the first stage of early adulthood, appropriately termed "emerging adulthood".

28.3 The Stages of Early Adulthood

Early adulthood is typically the period of life when the individual separates from their family or childhood caregivers from a personal, emotional, and financial perspective. As a person enters early adulthood, they are developing a clear sense of their individuality (personal and sexual), their values, and views of the future. It is difficult to identify the point of transition to adulthood based on a specific age. Imagine a typical 22-year-old: they may live with their childhood caregivers and have a job; they may attend university and live with a group of friends; they may have a job and live with their partner; and so on. In each of these scenarios there are different levels of responsibility or indicators of entry into adulthood demonstrated by the individual. Because of this adulthood is now defined around responsibilities and adoption of appropriate occupations rather than age. Two stages have been identified within early adulthood: the first stage applies to people aged 18–29 years and is termed "emerging adulthood"; the second applies to people aged 30–45 years and is called "established adulthood". Remember that these are suggested stages and ages, and the trajectory of individuals into the responsibilities and occupations of adulthood is highly variable.

28.3.1 Emerging Adulthood

Positioned between adolescence and established adulthood, emerging adulthood is described as the age of identity exploration, instability, self-focus, feeling in-between, and possibilities (Arnett, 2000). During this period, an individual explores life independent of childhood caregivers, possibilities for careers, and intimate relationships. Identity development occurs as people change jobs, residences, and relationships, often more frequently than in any other period in the lifespan. The emerging adult may remain financially dependent on their childhood caregivers as they complete formal education, explore different career options, and make decisions about their future directions. Generational changes have led to an increase in people engaging in further education into their twenties, often remaining at home with their childhood caregivers for longer and delaying transition to developmental tasks related to career, home, and relationships.

Although people in emerging adulthood may be adult size, their behavior is different to people in their thirties and their behavior can be considered immature (Hochberg & Konner, 2020). Brain development is continuing and although risk taking during emerging adulthood may appear different to that of an adolescent, it also differs to that of people in the latter stage of early adulthood (Hochberg & Konner, 2020). Postformal thought is considered a key cognitive development of this stage, supporting the emerging adult to move beyond a right and wrong perspective of the world. The development of postformal thought supports the individual to appreciate and synthesize ideas and feelings that may be at conflict into a new understanding (Sinnott, 2014). This complex form of adult cognition is considered essential for solving everyday problems such as those in the workplace and is beneficial for successful intrapersonal and interpersonal relationships (Sinnott, 2014). It has been proposed that only one-third of early adults will have reached this advanced level of thinking by the age of 30 (Labouvie-Vief, 2006), with possible consequences for successful transition to, and participation in, the occupations of early adulthood.

Individuals enter emerging adulthood with a trajectory that has been influenced by their personal capacities and the opportunities available to them. The trajectory of emerging adulthood can be negatively influenced by factors that can marginalize, including economic and social inequality. Equally, people who have experienced disadvantage due to race, ethnicity, sexuality, or disability may exhibit differing trajectories. Importantly, some people will prevail and successfully transition to established adulthood despite marginalization and disadvantage. Perhaps one of the best ways to

Marcus is 20 years old and lives with his partner Sofia (20 years old) and their 8 month old daughter in a one-bedroom apartment. Marcus is training to be a carpenter and works as a food delivery driver on the weekend so that he can support his family financially.

Kareem is 20 years old and lives in a house with two of his friends from high school. The three housemates share responsibility for all domestic activities. Kareem works in a business owned by his family and plans to develop his career within the business.

Noah is 21 years old and lives with his grandparents. He is responsible for all domestic activities within the home and has recently completed vocational training as a hairdresser. He and his girlfriend plan to move into an apartment next year.

Jose is 20 years old and lives with his parents and older brother. Jose receives financial support from his parents so that he can focus on his university education. He would like to get a part-time job but is worried about going against his parent's wishes.

Tao is 19 years old and has received a scholarship to attend university at a nearby town. He lives in student accomodation on the university campus and works in the student cafeteria to support himself financially. He is unable to meet with his football friends each week and is thinking of joining the university football team.

Figure 28.1 Emerging Adulthood Vignettes.

illustrate the diversity of emerging adulthood is through exploration of the lives and occupations of a group of friends who meet regularly with others to play football (see Figure 28.1). Members of the group have played football together from early in their teenage years. They are now all in their late teens and early twenties and although they have grown to have diverse lives, the shared occupation of football continues to draw them together on a regular basis. The groups of friends demonstrate how emerging adults can enter their twenties with different trajectories related to home, work, education, relationships, and caring responsibilities (children or family).

28.3.2 Established Adulthood (30–45 Years)

Transition into adulthood is taking longer and is more likely to be dictated by personal choices rather than societal expectations (Institute of Medicine and National Research Council, 2015). The term "established adulthood" has been recently proposed (Mehta et al., 2020) to describe a unique period in the lifespan often marked by the intersection of work and relationship or family responsibilities – called the "career-and-care-crunch" (p. 436). Individuals in this lifespan may be engaged in career development while simultaneously experiencing relationship satisfaction or breakdown, and making decisions about parenthood or negotiating parenting roles. Individuals in established adulthood have achieved the independence, responsibility, and autonomy of adulthood and yet continue to exhibit variable experiences and trajectories. For example, the end of a heterosexual relationship with children in the late twenties may lead to the formation of a LGBTQI+ step family as an individual claims a bi-sexual identity in their thirties.

HUMAN OCCUPATIONS OF EARLY ADULTHOOD

Yasmina (32 years old) has recently moved back to her home town after the end of a long-term relationship. Yasmina is finding it difficult to reconnect with her old school friends and is looking for community groups to extend her social connections. She rents her apartment and continues to work online in her previous job.

Helen and Karen (31 and 32 years old) met at school and have been in a relationship for 11 years. They have bought their own home and are busy building their careers while also prioritising leisure occupations of hiking and camping on the weekends.

Lucia (31 years old) and Mateo (31 years old) have recently separated. Lucia is studying to become a teacher and is working part-time in retail. Lucia and Mateo share custody of their children, aged 10 and 12 years old. The children's grandparents assist with childcare so that Lucia can achieve her career goals.

Carla (32 years old) is married to Raphael (33 years old). Carla is the stay-at-home parent for their 1 and 3 year old children. She has plans to return to paid employment when the children commence school. During this time she is re-engaging in previously enjoyed leisure occupations of painting and drawing.

Linh (32 years old) owns and manages a popular restaurant with her sister. Linh is married to John (34 years old) who works as a car salesman. Linh and John value working hard and saving money so that they can financially support and visit Linh's parents who live overseas. They are unsure if they would like to have children.

Figure 28.2 Established Adulthood Vignettes.

Or at a population level, the longstanding systemic and structural racism that has limited educational opportunities and career development for First Nations people within Western countries can result in poorer employment outcomes and trajectories in adulthood (Monem & McDonald, 2023).

Established adulthood is generally considered a time when the competing demands of family and work are at their peak, with the career-and-care-crunch experienced at a greater level by women and those from lower socioeconomic groups (Mehta et al., 2020). Because of competing demands, the individual may sacrifice something from their work or home domain or reduce participation in occupations considered discretionary such as those from the leisure and social participation categories. Vignettes are provided (see Figure 28.2) to further support the demonstration of the diversity of established adulthood. The women have been friends from school and are now in their early thirties. Their unique trajectories through emerging adulthood have led to markedly different experiences in established adulthood.

28.4 A Global Perspective of Early Adulthood

It is not feasible to fully examine the global experience of early adulthood within this chapter and many of the previous studies of this lifespan can be critiqued as a heteronormative, ethnocentric, and classist representation of the developed world. Indeed, there are large areas of the global population for which there is limited research regarding the developmental tasks and lifespan of early adulthood. However, global differences can be gleaned from key international reports, and these have been used in this chapter to introduce the reader to a global perspective related to education, employment, and relationships and parenthood. Reports have also been included to highlight that different populations experience disparities within a country.

28.4.1 Education

Emerging adulthood is a phenomenon of predominantly industrialized, Organisation for Economic Co-operation and Development (OECD) countries (Arnett, 2011). The higher rates of post-school education and subsequent delay of marriage and parenthood that are synonymous with emerging adulthood are observed to last longer within Europe, perhaps due to generous social support systems and low-cost education (Douglass, 2007). Compulsory military service within European countries can also delay entry to post-school education and lengthen these timelines. For example, only 5% of people completing a university education in Israel entered directly from secondary (school) education, which is in stark contrast to the 90% of people completing a university education in the United States who entered directly from school (United Nations, 2023).

There is some evidence that a rising number of people experience emerging adulthood in non-OECD countries; however, these numbers are currently low and are isolated to people from affluent backgrounds. Monitoring of achievement toward the Quality Education Sustainable Development Goal (United Nations, 2023) demonstrates that there are significantly different completion rates for secondary (school) education worldwide which limit access to post-school education. Recent statistics indicate that completion rates range from approximately 30% in Sub-Saharan Africa, to between 50% and 70% in Oceania, Asia, North Africa, Latin America, and the Caribbean, and between 80% and 90% for Europe, North America, Australia, and New Zealand.

Worldwide there is evidence which highlights that although emerging adulthood is an established phenomenon in some countries it should not be considered a universal experience for all peoples. Disadvantage and marginalization within OECD countries can also limit educational attainment and outcomes. Within Australia, the completion rates for secondary (school) education are significantly lower for Aboriginal and Torres Strait Islander Peoples (65.9%) compared to 90.4% of all non-Aboriginal and Torres Strait Islander Peoples (Australian Institute of Health and Welfare, 2021). This is in stark contrast to New Zealand where significant focus on improving cultural understanding and teaching approaches has resulted in 80.6% of Māori Peoples and 83% of Pacific Peoples achieving a level 1 (secondary school) qualification, compared to 85.8% for the overall population (Stats New Zealand, 2020). Consequently, there are increasing numbers of Māori and Pacific young adults engaging in education occupations post formal schooling, but these are yet to match the rates of the total population.

28.4.2 Employment

Global trends for employment highlight a bias in our understanding of the developmental tasks of early adulthood toward a Western, ethnocentric, and classist perspective. In 2022, between 25% and 32% of young people (15–24 years) from North and

Sub-Saharan Africa, Oceania, and Central, Southern, and Western Asia were not in education, employment, or training (United Nations, 2023). This is in contrast to the comparatively low 8%–11% of young people (15–24 years) who were not in education, employment, or training in Europe, North America, Australia, and New Zealand. Worldwide, over 50% of the population are engaged in informal employment (United Nations, 2023) which is when individuals are engaged in work occupations that are not subject to income tax, are without entitlement to employment benefits, or are not registered by the government.

Examples of the informal labor market are wide ranging and can include domestic work, street vendors, babysitting, home-based workers such as garment repairs or laundering, home repairs, or car cleaners. The nature of informal employment contrasts significantly with the employment and career development generally described within the early adulthood literature. There is a need for our understanding to expand and better represent the range of work occupations, and associated developmental tasks, from a global perspective.

28.4.3 Relationships and Parenthood

Timelines to marriage vary greatly between and within countries. Comparison of emerging adults within Europe and countries such as Japan and South Korea suggest similar, long timeframes to marriage and parenthood. However, cultural differences exist within this comparison, with the emerging adults from an Asian cultural background demonstrating a higher sense of collectivism and family obligations and paying more attention to parental advice and wishes regarding partners (Douglass, 2007). Worldwide, one in five young women are married before they even enter early adulthood with rates higher in Sub-Saharan Africa, Latin America, and the Caribbean (United Nations, 2023). Finally, racial differences are reported within developed countries such as America, in which 36% of African Americans are not married by the age of 25 or older compared to 16% of white European Americans (Wang & Parker, 2014).

Becoming a parent may be an identified developmental task of early adulthood but there are some worldwide trends regarding the age at which women commence the occupations of caring for and rearing a child. Women living in Chad, Niger, and Bangladesh are generally aged 18 years or younger at the birth of their first child, while women in countries, including Burma, Kazakhstan, Sri Lanka, and Belarus, have a mean age of 25 years. The oldest first-time mothers (30–31 years of age) are from countries, including South Korea, Switzerland, Japan, Ireland, Italy, and Singapore (Central Intelligence Agency, 2023).

28.5 The Occupations of Early Adulthood

The developmental tasks and occupations of early adulthood are predominantly described in the literature for individuals. However, the shared occupations of groups are also pertinent during the early adulthood lifespan. Table 28.2 outlines the occupational profile of early adulthood mostly from the perspective of an individual with some examples of the shared occupations of groups included. *Italics* are used to indicate the developmental tasks of early adulthood and identify the links to occupation.

Table 28.2 An Occupational Profile of Early Adulthood

Activities of Daily Living

The early adult attends to their self-care needs on a routine basis (bathing, showering, dressing, toileting, toilet and personal hygiene, grooming, feeding, eating, swallowing, and functional mobility). An individual may adopt new routines or activities as their *identity develops* such as changes to grooming because of the growth of a beard. The young adult may find themselves participating in the shared occupation of a morning cup of tea or eating during lunch with others in the workplace. This can be a period of significant exploration of sexual expression and sexual experiences with self and others. The exploration of intimacy and sexual activities may occur within and outside of *intimate relationships* during adolescence and emerging adulthood (Boislard et al., 2016). Considered risky behavior by previous generations, exploration of intimacy and sexual activities through casual sexual relationships and experiences, such as one-time sexual encounters (one-night stands) or as "friends with benefits", are now considered a normal developmental experience of the early adult lifespan. It is important to recognize that sexual abstinence may also occur in early adulthood because of individual, peer, and family related factors (Boislard et al., 2016).

IADLs

Moving out of the childhood home leads to increasing responsibility and independence as the young adult establishes the home, learns to manage the household, and participates in the shopping, meal preparation, and clean up. *Financial independence* is a key marker of entry into adulthood and requires the demonstration of independent skills for managing a budget to support themselves financially and engage in activities such as paying bills on time. The *exploration of identity* during emerging adulthood can lead to individuals exploring beliefs and routines for religious and spiritual expression that are different to those of their childhood caregivers. Alternatively, early adulthood may sustain previously held beliefs while developing their own routines for religious and spiritual expression. *Becoming a parent and rearing children* is an identified developmental task of early adulthood and the activities of caring for a child can predominate during emerging or established adulthood, or for some individuals not at all. Young adults may also provide care, assistance, or support on an unpaid basis to a family member or other person with disability, chronic health, or mental health conditions. For some young adults this will be a continuing role for childhood and adolescence while for others it may be a newly adopted role. Finally, increasing responsibility and participation in the care of animals or pets may occur. Examples of when groups of young adults may engage in shared IADLs includes traveling to and from a football game together or working together to clean up the yard and garden of a home.

Health Management

Emerging adulthood is a time of exploration and uncertainty, and the emerging adult may engage in risky levels of health-compromising activities such as smoking, alcohol and other *illicit substance use,* disordered eating, and unsafe sex, which can lead to illness later in life or may require immediate health management. It can be a time of increased vulnerability to mental health conditions due to the multiple changes in living environments, education or workplaces, friendships, relationships, etc. (Taber-Thomas & Perez-Edgar, 2015).

(Continued)

Table 28.2 (Continued)

Increasing access to health care for social and emotional health promotion and maintenance can occur as the young adult first experiences the first symptoms of a mental health disorder with evidence of rising rates of depression, anxiety, eating disorders, substance abuse, and suicidal behaviors in emerging adults in developed countries (Jurewicz, 2015). Environmental and lifestyle changes as the emerging adult *leaves their childhood home* have been associated with negative changes to their nutrition management with associated weight gain and physical health risks (Winpenny et al., 2018). Most studies report decreased engagement in physical activity as the individual transitions into early adulthood with an increase in sedentary activities that is often greater for men (Corder et al., 2015, 2019). A study of Australian women aged 18–23 identified that the developmental tasks of *co-habitating, getting married, and becoming a mother* are strongly associated with decreases in physical activity (Bell & Lee, 2005). Young adults may support each other to continue to engage in shared physical activity by forming walking or running groups. Established adulthood is generally a time of good physical functioning (Mehta et al., 2020) and there is often an increase in health-promoting occupations and reduction of the risky activities that were prominent during emerging adulthood.

Rest and Sleep

A recent worldwide study across 63 countries (Coutrot et al., 2022) found that the twenties and early thirties were the period of the lifespan when people experienced decreasing sleep participation with the lowest participation at age 33. The busyness of early adulthood with changing environments, increasing responsibilities, and the *career-and-care-crunch* may explain this trend. It highlights the importance of the activities of sleep preparation and sleep participation to minimize this trend and ensure adequate rest and sleep to support engagement in other occupations.

Education

People may *engage in education* to achieve a range of goals during early adulthood, including literacy and numeracy skill development; work readiness skill development; knowledge, skill, and competency development for a range of vocational and avocational roles; self-improvement in areas of health and psychological well-being; spiritual and intellectual growth and enrichment; social or cultural training; or to obtain tools for community, social, and political advocacy. As indicated previously, participation in formal education is increasingly a feature of the emerging adult cohort that can take many different forms such as: university-based education, apprenticeship (workplace-based training), adults returning to school, community-based continuing education, or online training. It is important that the emerging adult also achieves the developmental task of *leaving education* and embarks upon their career. However, the young adult may continue to engage in informal personal education, either individually or in groups, across a range of interest areas such as self-development and leisure.

Work

Engaging in paid *employment and establishing a career* are key developmental tasks of early adulthood. Participation in employment seeking and acquisition occupations will predominate at critical periods during early adulthood as the individual either takes decisive action toward a chosen job or career, or chooses to change their employment or career direction to align with their preferred interests and pursuits.

(Continued)

Table 28.2 (Continued)

Successful participation in job performance and maintenance is an area of critical knowledge and skill development for the young adult, for whom success in employment equates to greater financial independence and transition toward adulthood. An individual's experience of work occupations is influenced by socioeconomic, racial, gender, and other factors. For example, young adults with insecure housing can experience greater difficulty obtaining employment and may engage in the underground economy or may not be able to establish employment. Volunteer participation during early adulthood (*taking on civic responsibility*) is more prominent in those who volunteered during adolescence and are attending post-school education, and less prominent in those engaged in full-time work or with parenting responsibilities (Oesterle et al., 2004). Volunteerism is often a shared occupation completed by a group of people with shared interests and motivations.

Play

Play can take many forms during early adulthood such as when groups of friends come together to play board games, a parent plays a game of hide-and-seek with their child, workplaces introduce a ping pong table, or an individual plays an endless game of tug'o'war with their dog. Emerging adulthood can be an emotionally challenging time and play may be important to help relieve stress, promote positive emotions, build resilience, enhance productivity, and improve relationships and connections to others.

Leisure

The young adult may expand their participation in new leisure occupations as their social networks extend to people with different interests. Equally, early adulthood can be a time when leisure exploration or participation are at their lowest. Gustafsson et al. (2017) found that adults aged 18–40 years reported retention of only 60% of recreation and relaxation activities and 40% of high/low impact physical activities. Although some of the change may represent a natural adjustment across the lifespan, it is most likely that the loss of activities is representative of the transitions of early adulthood and career-and-care-crunch previously described. Individual leisure occupations may be easier to retain as they can be completed at a flexible time for the young adult, while group-based shared leisure occupations may be less amendable to the flexibility required of the career-and-care-crunch.

Social Participation

Forming intimate relationships is a key developmental task of early adulthood. Following the development of a sense of self during adolescence, an individual enters early adulthood ready to share themselves with others, developing longer term relationships and commitments outside of the childhood circle and family. Young adults expand their networks and social participation by *becoming part of a group or community* with shared interests through leisure activities, volunteering, or activism, or connecting with people in a similar life stage (e.g., parenting groups). The expanding social interactions support establishment of identity, friendship groups, and people with whom they develop intimate partner relationships. Havighurst (1972) previously described early adulthood as a time when people *select a mate* with a focus on marriage. Although this may remain true for some early adults, it is now considered a time when people also *find intimacy* with their close, long-term relationships. As an individual traverses their twenties they may meet and remain with one person or may experience a series of relationships with or without resolution toward one partner. This is a time when personal preference and identity are powerful guides and a time that can lead to lifelong friendships and partners or, if a person is unable to establish these relationships, it can lead to isolation and loneliness.

28.6 Conclusion

Early adulthood is a lifespan period of significant change and transition toward the independence, responsibility, and autonomy of an adult. New roles and routines are adopted as the individual steps through the developmental tasks of moving away from the home of their childhood caregivers; finishing their education; commencing employment; developing intimate relationships; and becoming a parent. Importantly, the trajectory of early adulthood is highly unique and although the stages of emerging and established adulthood may describe a more contemporary pathway, we cannot assume that it is a universal experience. The trajectory of early adulthood is closely linked to if, and when, role changes occur such as when an individual completes their education, leaves their childhood home, enters the workforce, develops new intimate or romantic relationships with friends and lifelong partners, or becomes a parent.

Equally, the trajectory is influenced by when the individual engages in the occupations of the new roles with the independence, responsibility, and autonomy of adulthood. There is no socially mandated order for the transition to adulthood and it is experienced differently due to multiple influencing factors, contexts, and preferences. It is therefore essential that we understand the young adult's narrative as an occupational being with a past, present, and future.

28.7 Summary

- Early adulthood is a lifespan period of significant change, exploration, and uncertainty.
- Traditionally described as one stage, it is now recognized that the ages of 18–29 represent emerging adulthood and the ages of 30–45 represent established adulthood.
- The occupational profile of the early adult changes as they transition through the developmental tasks of leaving the childhood home, finishing education, commencing employment, developing intimate relationships, and becoming a parent.
- Individuals enter early adulthood with a trajectory that has been influenced by their personal capacities, contexts, preferences, and the opportunities available to them.
- A person is considered to have achieved adulthood when they are financially independent and have taken full responsibility for themselves.
- Our current understanding of early adulthood has a bias toward a heteronormative, ethnocentric, and classist representation of the developed world, and cannot be considered representative of all populations.

28.8 Review Questions

1. Why is early adulthood now depicted as two stages? Name and describe them.
2. What are the developmental tasks of early adulthood?
3. Describe the developmental tasks from an occupational perspective.
4. Why is it stated that the trajectories of early adulthood are highly unique?
5. When is it considered that an individual has achieved adulthood?

References

Arnett, J. J. (2000). Emerging adulthood. A theory of development from the late teens through the twenties. *American Psychologist*, *55*(5), 469–480. https://doi.org/10.1037/0003-066X.55.5.469

Arnett, J. J. (2003). Conceptions of the transition to adulthood among emerging adults in American ethnic groups. *New Directions for Child and Adolescent Development, 100*, 63–75. https://doi.org/10.1002/cd.75

Arnett, J. J. (2011). Emerging adulthood(s): The cultural psychology of a new life stage. In L. A. Jensen (Ed.), *Bridging cultural and developmental approaches to psychology: New syntheses in theory, research, and policy* (pp. 255–275). Oxford University Press.

Australian Institute of Health and Welfare. (2021). *Indigenous education and skills.* https://www.aihw.gov.au/reports/australias-welfare/indigenous-education-and-skills

Bell, S., & Lee, C. (2005). Emerging adulthood and patterns of physical activity among young Australian women. *International Journal of Behavioral Medicine, 12*(4), 227–235. https://doi.org/10.1207/s15327558ijbm1204_3

Boislard, M. A., van de Bongardt, D., & Blais, M. (2016). Sexuality (and lack thereof) in adolescence and early adulthood: A review of the literature. *Behavioral Sciences, 6*(1), 8. https://doi.org/10.3390/bs6010008

Central Intelligence Agency. (2023). Mothers mean age at first birth (field listing). In *The World Factbook.* https://www.cia.gov/the-world-factbook/field/mothers-mean-age-at-first-birth/

Corder, K., Sharp, S. J., Atkin, A. J., Griffin, S. J., Jones, A. P., Ekelund, U., & van Sluijs, E. M. (2015). Change in objectively measured physical activity during the transition to adolescence. *British Journal of Sports Medicine, 49*, 730–736. https://doi.org/10.1136/bjsports-2013-093190

Corder, K., Winpenny, E., Love, R., Brown, H. E., White, M., & Sluijs, E. V. (2019). Change in physical activity from adolescence to early adulthood: A systematic review and meta-analysis of longitudinal cohort studies. *British Journal of Sports Medicine, 53*, 496–503. https://doi.org/10.1136/bjsports-2016-097330

Coutrot, A., Lazar, A. S., Richards, M., Manley, E., Wiener, J. M., Dalton, R. C., Hornberger, M., & Spiers, H. J. (2022). Reported sleep duration reveals segmentation of the adult life-course into three phases. *Nature Communications, 13*, 7697. https://doi.org/10.1038/s41467-022-34624-8

Douglass, C. B. (2007). From duty to desire: Emerging adulthood in Europe and its consequences. *Child Development Perspectives, 1*(2), 101–108. https://doi.org/10.1111/j.1750-8606.2007.00023.x

Erikson, E. H. (1950). *Childhood and society.* W. W. Norton & Company.

Gustafsson, L., Hung, I. H. M., & Liddle, J. (2017). Test-retest reliability and internal consistency of the Activity Card Sort–Australia (18–64). *OTJR: Occupational Therapy Journal of Research, 37*(1), 50–56. https://doi.org/10.1177/1539449216681277

Havighurst, R. J. (1972). *Developmental tasks and education.* David McKay.

Hochberg, Z. E., & Konner, M. (2020). Emerging adulthood: A pre-adult life-history stage. *Frontiers in Endocrinology, 10*, 918. https://doi.org/10.3389/fendo.2019.00918

Institute of Medicine and National Research Council. (2015). *Investing in the health and well-being of young adults.* The National Academies Press. https://doi.org/10.17226/18869.

Jurewicz, I. (2015). Mental health in young adults and adolescents: Supporting general physicians to provide holistic care. *Clinical Medicine, 15*(2), 151–154. https://doi.org/10.7861/clinmedicine.15-2-151

Labouvie-Vief, G. (2006). Emerging structures of adult thought. In J. J. Arnett & J. L. Tanner (Eds.), *Emerging adults in America: Coming of age in the 21st century* (pp. 59–84). American Psychological Association. https://doi.org/10.1037/11381-003

Mehta, C. M., Arnett, J. J., Palmer, C. G., & Nelson, L. J. (2020). Established adulthood: A new conception of ages 30 to 45. *American Psychologist, 75*(4), 431–444. https://doi.org/10.1037/amp0000600

Monem, R. M., & McDonald, H. (2023). Closing the First Nations employment gap will take 100 years. *The Conversation.* https://theconversation.com/closing-the-first-nations-employment-gap-will-take-100-years-205290

Oesterle, S., Kirkpatrick Johnson, M., & Mortimer, J. T. (2004). Volunteerism during the transition to adulthood: A life course perspective. *Social Forces, 82*(3), 1123–1149. https://doi.org/10.1353/sof.2004.0049

Roisman, G. I., Masten, A. S., Coatsworth, J. D., & Tellegen, A. (2004). Salient and emerging developmental tasks in the transition to adulthood. *Child Development, 75*(1), 123–133. https://doi.org/10.1111/j.1467-8624.2004.00658.x

Schulenberg, J. E., Bryant, A. L., & O'Malley, P. M. (2004). Taking hold of some kind of life: How developmental tasks relate to trajectories of well-being during the transition to adulthood. *Development and Psychopathology, 16*(4), 1119–1140. https://doi.org/10.1017/S0954579404040167

Schulenberg, J., & Schoon, I. (2012). The transition to adulthood across time and space: Overview of special section. *Longitudinal and Life Course Studies: International Journal, 3*(2), 164–172. https://doi.org/10.14301/llcs.v3i2.194

Sinnott, J. D. (2014). The development of complex thought in adulthood: Some theories and mechanisms that grow with interpersonal experience. *Adult Development: Cognitive Aspects of Thriving Close Relationships* (online ed.), Oxford Academic. https://doi.org/10.1093/acprof:oso/9780199892815.003.0002

Skogbrott Birkeland, M., Leversen, I., Torsheim, T., & Wold, B. (2013). Pathways to adulthood and their precursors and outcomes. *Scandinavian Journal of Psychology, 55*, 26–32. https://doi.org/10.1111/sjop.12087

Stats New Zealand. (2020). *Education outcomes improving for Māori and Pacific peoples.* https://www.stats.govt.nz/news/education-outcomes-improving-for-maori-and-pacific-peoples

Taber-Thomas, B., & Perez-Edgar, K. (2015). Emerging adulthood brain development. In J. J. Arnett (Ed.), *The Oxford handbook of emerging adulthood* (pp. 126–141). Oxford University Press.

United Nations. (2023). *The sustainable development goals report: Special edition.* https://unstats.un.org/sdgs/report/2023/

Wang, W., & Parker, K. (2014). *Record share of Americans have never married: As values, economics and gender patterns change.* Pew Research Center's Social & Demographic Trends project, September. https://www.pewresearch.org/social-trends/2014/09/24/record-share-of-americans-have-never-married/

Winpenny, E. M., van Sluijs, E. M. F., White, M., Klepp, K.-I., Wold, B., & Lien, N. (2018). Changes in diet through adolescence and early adulthood: Longitudinal trajectories and association with key life transitions. *International Journal of Behavioral Nutrition and Physical Activity, 15*, 86. https://doi.org/10.1186/s12966-018-0719-8

CHAPTER 29

Human Occupations of Middle Adulthood (Ages 40–65)

Rosanne DiZazzo-Miller, Louise Gustafsson, and Tomomi McAuliffe

Abstract
This chapter discusses the lifespan period commonly referred to as middle adulthood or midlife. This is the least defined of all the lifespan periods and spans from 40 to 65 years of age. The occupations and experiences of middle adulthood are commonly shaped by the decisions and developmental tasks of early adulthood, together with cultural and societal influences. It is a period often marked by stress and challenge from balancing multiple occupations with caring, work, and health management occupations often predominating. Midlife in general is a time when people experience new challenges from all different angles; it is not a time full of dread and crisis and the need to "act out" as portrayed by the media. Rather, the re-evaluations and changes that occur during middle adulthood are considered a normal developmental transition.

Authors' Positionality Statement
The authors of this chapter identify as cisgender females from White Australian, White American, and Japanese cultural backgrounds. We acknowledge that we have written the chapter from a position of privilege as all have received a postgraduate education and work as researchers and educators in the higher education sector in Australia and the US. We recognize that our collective experiences are not representative of the global community, and we cannot assume to speak on behalf of all populations and groups, many of whom have, and continue to, experience systemic disadvantage and bias.

Objectives
This chapter will allow the reader to:

- Describe the middle adulthood lifespan.
- Articulate and understand a global and diverse perspective of middle adulthood.

- Describe theories of middle adulthood from an occupational perspective.
- Articulate the occupations of middle adulthood.
- Develop an occupational profile for middle adulthood by applying the Occupational Therapy Practice Framework – 4th Edition (OTPF-4).

Key terms

- middle adulthood
- sandwich generation
- generativity
- stagnation
- midlife crisis
- caring role
- occupational balance

29.1 Introduction

Middle adulthood spans the chronological ages of 40–65 and is typically a period of age-related changes in physical, mental, cognitive, and sensory abilities, immune system, and reproductive functioning (Lachman, 2004). In response, this period can be marked by increased attention to health maintenance and promotion as individuals traverse the challenges of the previously considered "midlife crisis." This chapter will outline the current knowledge and description of the lifespan from 40 to 65 years of age, with illustrative examples of the variable trajectories of middle adulthood. From an occupational perspective, this period can include dynamic caring responsibilities for older and younger family members, negotiating and renegotiating roles and occupations at work, in relationships, in the household, and society. The impact of contexts together with the choices and decisions made during early adulthood on occupational engagement during this period is explored. Finally, the chapter will introduce the reader to the diverse occupational profiles of middle adulthood that can emerge based on the early adulthood trajectory and from a global perspective. A range of client scenarios are included to support this exploration.

29.2 Defining Middle Adulthood

Middle adulthood (or midlife) has traditionally been described as a period where people experience decreasing energy, changing physical appearance, and general unhappiness or crisis (Lachman, 2004). Recently, however, it has been described as the peak of life, a time of wisdom, achievement, and control, with a greater focus on stress rather than crisis (Lachman et al., 2015). There have been generational changes following the first descriptions of middle adulthood that have led to a melding of the developmental stages traditionally considered part of early adulthood into middle adulthood. Chronological age is now considered less predictive of life stage and subsequent occupations due to the variable influencing factors such as gender, sexuality, socioeconomic status, race, culture, relationship status, health status, and employment status. Thus, it has become increasingly difficult to definitively identify and define the age range, occupations, and occupational roles of middle adulthood. A contemporaneous definition for middle adulthood is one that identifies it as a developmental transition period between early adulthood and retirement (Polan & Taylor, 2010). This definition allows for the variability evident today in the roles, life events, and life experiences during the chronological ages of middle adulthood (Lachman et al., 2015).

29.3 Middle Adulthood in the 21st Century

Middle adulthood is the least understood of the lifespan, and the absence of information about the developmental tasks of middle-aged adults leads to misinformation (Infurna et al., 2020). As the precursor to older adulthood, the differing personal and cultural influences can mean that some embrace older age while others resist aging. Various theories exist regarding middle adulthood, with some conflicting views, such as the existence of the midlife crisis. Regardless, the challenges that seem to be consistent across the theories include balancing the care of both younger and older family members, dealing with the onset of health concerns, whether it be acute or chronic and encompass physical, mental, or cognitive challenges, and the health care costs associated with them. Balance among work and life becomes increasingly challenging when added to responsibility related to health management, rest and sleep, play, leisure, and social participation (AOTA, 2020). However, the middle-aged adult's response to these life changes relies heavily on personal, social, and cultural factors and even geographical location. The predominantly traditional and Western knowledge regarding middle adulthood creates challenges for the occupational therapist working within a global perspective. Culture and context play an enormous role in the varying attitudes and practices related to aging. Globally, it has become increasingly clear that even the attitude of aging varies around the world with Japan, South Korea, and China showing the most concern and the US, Indonesia, and Egypt showing the least (Pew Research Center, 2014). This is true regarding just about any topic related to aging and is a critical component to bear in mind when working with people in the middle adulthood lifespan period.

The contexts, experiences, and decisions of early adulthood greatly shape the trajectory throughout middle adulthood. Relationships, marriage, children, employment, and home location are just a few major life contexts that impact experiences later in life. For example, choosing a life partner with or without marriage leads to in-laws and may also lead to children. The transition to middle adulthood has become more complex in the 21st century as people, regardless of gender, sexuality, race, or nativity, may participate in education throughout their young adult lives and leave home at later ages, thus delaying life partnership or marriage and family planning until their thirties (Moore-Ramirez et al., 2017). Individuals are then faced with the future possibility of not only caregiving for parents but also children while they themselves are aging and dealing with the beginning of specific types of health screenings and health changes. It is clear that a person's life situation or stage will exert a more significant impact on the occupations of middle adulthood than chronological age.

It is universally agreed that middle adulthood lends to stress overload due to attempts to balance too many commitments and occupations (Brim et al., 2004). Alternatively, stress is experienced due to disadvantages and a lack of opportunities for occupational engagement. Gender differences have been identified with women found to experience more "crossover" stressors linked to balancing work and family simultaneously compared to men (Brim et al., 2004). People from the LGBTQI+ community can experience additional stressors from familial and sociocultural sources as they negotiate the relationships, family planning, and caregiving of middle adulthood (Moore-Ramirez et al., 2017). Socioeconomic differences are evidenced when people with lower education levels report the same number of stressors as those with higher education levels, but rate the stressors as more severe (Grzywacz et al., 2004). The population of First Nations Peoples who have experienced systemic bias and disadvantage transition into middle adulthood with greater health disparities, economic disadvantage, and stress (Commonwealth of Australia, 2020). People displaced due to persecution, war, or natural disasters experience stress due to the substantial challenges in attaining occupational balance in occupations beyond basic self-care (Altuntaş et al., 2021). Understanding intersectionality, that is how an individual's identity and contexts shape their individual experiences, is essential when working with people in their midlife (Milton & Qureshi, 2022).

Across the lifespan of middle adulthood, people with children may experience many adjustments to their caregiving roles. There is first the adjustment to life with young children, the re-adjustment to life after the adult children leave home, and re-adjustment if those adult children return home, with or without their own partners and families. A phenomenon of the 21st century, the "boomerang generation" are the adult children who return to live at home with parents, most often for economic reasons. This was acutely experienced during the recent COVID-19 pandemic when government restrictions disrupted everyday activities, such as employment and education, forcing adult children to move back to their parents' places due to financial hardship or the need for emotional support (Hall & Zygmunt, 2021).

29.4 Psychosocial Developmental Tasks of Middle Adulthood and Occupation

Middle adulthood is a period of contrasting psychosocial experiences, following the individualism established during early adulthood and shaped by unique personality traits. Lachman (2004) identified that the key developmental tasks of middle adulthood were taking on caring roles for parents/caregivers or partners; the death of parents or caregivers; and preparing for late adulthood. Two developmental theories associated with this period are Erikson's stage of generativity versus stagnation (Erikson, 1950) and Levinson's description of the midlife crisis (Levinson, 1978).

29.4.1 Client Scenario 1: Generativity versus Stagnation

Eva is a 42-year-old single mother who has lost her parents due to chronic health conditions. She has a 3-year-old daughter and is a sister and an aunt. She has a close and supportive group of friends who she refers to as her "chosen family." Eva is self-employed and owns and manages a busy café in the city center, working long days during the week. Her network of friends assists with the caring responsibilities for her daughter, allowing Eva to meet the responsibilities of the business. Eva has been reflecting on the demands of her job and would like to be more available to spend time with her daughter. She has also been reflecting on her wider contribution to society and has recently started to explore educational options for a new career in the teaching profession.

The fundamental conflict of middle adulthood is generativity versus stagnation (Erikson, 1950). During midlife, a person involves themselves in occupations that contribute to the development of others or generate products and outcomes that will benefit future generations while continuing their own productivity. Erikson describes generativity as a means for adults to promote the next generation and leave a positive legacy through nurturing, teaching, and leading (Erikson, 1950). Middle adulthood presents unique opportunities to lead multiple generations through multiple roles such as educator, mentor, coach, parent, grandparent, and even in their role as caregiver to aging parents. This can be extended to people who adopt roles as leaders or activists and engage in collective actions with an aim toward a better future (e.g., climate change activists and cyber security specialists). Stagnation, however, occurs in the absence of passing along this torch from one generation to the next. Erikson theorized that the absence of generativity results in stagnation and, therefore, emotional despair (Malone et al., 2016). It is well documented throughout the literature that emotional despair (e.g., depression) has a negative impact on occupational performance (Daremo et al., 2015). This can lead to deficits in late-life cognitive and emotional functioning, which can present a myriad of issues related to occupational performance specific to memory, executive functioning, depression, and overall psychosocial engagement (Malone et al., 2016).

29.4.2 Client Scenario 2: Midlife Crisis or Time of Transition

Alejandro (48 years old) has been the primary caregiver for twin children born by surrogacy to him and his partner José. The twins are now entering high school and require less support from Alejandro, who is feeling the loss of a valued caring and parenting role. Alejandro has not worked for the last 12 years, and the family have been supported financially by José. This situation has been a cause of stress for Alejandro, who would like to make changes now that the children are older. However, he is aware that his previous work colleagues have received multiple promotions during this time, and he does not want to return to a workplace where he would be working alongside people whom he considers junior to him. Alejandro is at a transition point involving significant reflection, re-evaluation, adaptation, and decisions toward the future.

The premise of Levinson's theory of development in adulthood and the midlife crisis (Levinson, 1978) centered on the belief that middle-aged adults re-evaluate their life, comparing their previous plans and aspirations with their current reality, and making abrupt changes in response. It was proposed that this was a normal part of development. However, it is increasingly recognized that a "crisis" is not normative, and people may experience psychological distress without it being identified as a crisis. Middle adulthood is undoubtedly a time of change and re-evaluation, as children become self-reliant, older relatives require additional assistance, choice of career and career paths may be re-evaluated, etc. However, a disconnect between identity and reality may only result in a psychological crisis for 10%–20% of people (Infurna et al., 2020). That is, individuals may experience career discontent, relationship breakdown, or develop health issues either as a psychological crisis or perceiving them as a challenging transition (Wethington, 2000). Personality traits and other factors specific to the individual may influence how this transition is experienced.

Table 29.1 Middle Adulthood Occupational Profile

OTPF-4 Occupations[a]	Middle adulthood occupational profile
ADLs - Bathing, showering - Toileting and toilet hygiene - Dressing - Eating and swallowing - Feeding - Functional mobility - Personal hygiene and grooming - Sexual activity	ADLs in middle adulthood hold a multifaceted role. Personally, individuals begin to experience changes in their bodies with varying hormone levels and normal aging processes that can influence how they engage in ADLs. In addition, individuals in middle adulthood may provide caring for their parents who are moving into older adulthood and may require their adult children to provide or organize care for basic ADLs. While caregiving is classified as an IADL, performing ADLs are the most challenging area of care as they tend to require more energy physically and emotionally, and caregiver education related to ADL training is limited (Edemekong et al., 2022). This limitation in training and need to now assist with ADLs for their adult parents presents added stress and potential injury.
IADLs - Care of others - Care of pets and animals - Child rearing - Communication management - Driving and community mobility - Financial management - Home establishment and management - Meal preparation and clean-up - Religious and spiritual expression - Safety and emergency maintenance - Shopping	Providing care is perhaps the most common occupation in middle adulthood. The magnitude of this occupation can place individuals in middle adulthood in stressful and anxiety-producing situations. Many individuals find themselves in the sandwich generation, where they are caring for both their aging parents and their adolescent children and children with disabilities (Parker & Patten, 2013). Equally, people may be required to provide care to a partner, relative, or friend who is experiencing health issues. Caring for a pet or animals can help relieve stress and while this, too, is an occupational task, more often than not the sheer benefits of caring for a pet can have a positive impact on an individual. Meal preparation, clean-up, and shopping are additional demanding occupations that require the individual to plan and conduct for themselves and/or others in their household. Middle adulthood may also present with changing dietary requirements that people must incorporate into their daily lives. Religion and spirituality may be either set or evolving. Caregivers in middle adulthood may find that their faith or spirituality helps them through their daily activities and responsibilities (Reis & Menezes, 2017). Finally, safety and emergency maintenance are occupations that people in middle adulthood must have in place for themselves and those to whom they provide care.

(Continued)

Table 29.1 (Continued)

OTPF-4 Occupations[a]	Middle adulthood occupational profile
Health management - Social and emotional health promotion and maintenance - Symptom and condition management - Communication with the health care system	The occupation of health management becomes a focus during middle adulthood, with changes in appearance and body systems a characteristic of this stage. Often at this phase in life, individuals are diagnosed with conditions such as cardiac and orthopedic problems due to aging (Hoffnung et al., 2018). Regular exercise and a healthy diet can minimize cardiovascular, respiratory, and musculoskeletal system changes. Midlife adults may continue or adopt new physical activity occupations such as solitary or group exercise programs or joining a sporting team. There is often an increase in activities related to communication with the health care system and symptoms and condition management – those in middle adulthood will visit their physician and commence annual examinations that may reveal additional health risks. As such, people in middle adulthood need to be better equipped to deal with the social and emotional challenges involved in their health status, as well as manage their health and navigate the medical system. However, midlife adults may experience difficulty orchestrating health management occupations while fitting in other occupations, such as IADLs, due to their roles as caregivers or workers.
Rest and sleep - Rest - Sleep participation	Sleep is a main area of neglect for people in middle adulthood and includes common issues such as difficulty falling asleep and staying asleep, and therefore not achieving adequate, restorative rest (Li et al., 2022). A lack of sleep is one of the most powerful predictors of health and well-being among older adults. Finding a healthy sleep routine is critical to overall health. Restorative rest and "finding time for oneself" is often difficult for people to prioritize during middle adulthood due to competing demands.
Education - Formal educational participation - Informal personal educational needs or exploring interests - Informal educational participation	Some people in middle adulthood find themselves in unfulfilling work situations and therefore seek either formal or informal methods of education to support career consolidation or a change in career. Informal educational participation in middle adulthood also provides an opportunity where people might finally feel as though they have time to explore and pursue their interests, and find meaning and purpose through alternate avenues. Informal education may also be pursued to support personal development.

(Continued)

Table 29.1 (Continued)

OTPF-4 Occupations[a]	Middle adulthood occupational profile
Work - Employment interests and pursuits - Employment seeking and acquisition - Job performance and maintenance - Retirement preparation and adjustment - Volunteer exploration - Volunteer participation	Many people in middle adulthood are at the peak of their careers during this period of time. Engagement in work occupations supports retention of cognitive abilities that may otherwise decline during middle adulthood such as the ability to "multi-task" and shift attention between two tasks, or ignore irrelevant information and the working memory. However, while still working, people in middle adulthood may also become more aware of ageism in the workplace and find themselves needing to advocate and negotiate for their positions (Bauer & Sousa-Poza, 2015). Middle adulthood can be a time of career consolidation or it may be a time when people seek alternative pathways toward retirement. There may be reductions in work hours to support the pursuit of other occupations such as leisure, caring, or health management occupations. Later in this stage, people in middle adulthood become more focused on retirement planning and volunteering pursuits. These pursuits can bring great meaning and purpose, and may help the transition from retirement by providing continued structure and sense of purpose.
Play - Play exploration - Play participation	Play for people in middle adulthood provides an escape from reality and allows the individual to explore humor and competitions that bring about meaning and pleasure.
Leisure - Leisure exploration - Leisure participation	Middle adulthood is a time when people may continue engagement in hobbies or interests, return to previous hobbies or interests, or explore new ones. For some people there is reduced engagement in leisure due to increasing and competing demands such as caring for others, their own health management, or work demands. For those who now have aging parents to care for, inability to engage in play and leisure can present a void in their lives, leading to perceived burden and decreased quality of life (Tessier et al., 2007).
Social participation - Community participation - Family participation - Friendships - Intimate partner relationships - Peer group participation - Peer group participation	Social participation is another occupation that contributes to the quality of life. Social participation for people in middle adulthood brings about not only friendships and participation among family and peer groups but also provides an avenue to communicate with others on similar life challenges and provide and receive support from others. Intimate relationships and friendships (including internet or workplace friendships) are important during middle adulthood.

(Continued)

Table 29.1 (Continued)

OTPF-4 Occupations[a]	Middle adulthood occupational profile
	Social participation may be negatively impacted by the challenges of caring for others; however, it is likely that people in middle adulthood can experience a resumption in social participation from a post-caregiver experience, either when their adult children leave home or their older adult parents no longer require care. It is through the reconstruction of their daily life that people find themselves with time to resume participation and reconnect with family and friends (Afonso & D'Espiney, 2022).

[a]Occupations are taken from American Occupational Therapy Association (2020).

29.5 The Occupational Profile of Middle Adulthood

The occupations of middle adulthood can be explored with the OTPF-4 (AOTA, 2020). Specifically, activities of daily living (ADLs), instrumental activities of daily living (IADLs), health management, rest and sleep, education, work, play, leisure, and social participation. An occupational profile provides information related to an individual's needs, challenges, and concerns regarding their occupational performance (AOTA, 2020). Middle adulthood is a period when striking occupational balance and finding control over situations with purpose and plan are important outcomes. The development of an occupational profile forms a foundation for the occupational therapist to understand each client's unique circumstance. Questions from an occupational profile may include why the client is seeking services, what barriers inhibit performance, their values and interests, patterns of engagement, and their priorities and desired outcomes for occupational performance, health, well-being, and quality of life. Table 29.1 outlines the occupational profile of middle adulthood.

29.6 Caregiving of Middle Adulthood

As previously discussed in this chapter, it is common for individuals in middle adulthood to carry multiple roles, and many of their roles come with significant responsibilities and require a high time commitment. One such role is being a caregiver for family members. The World Health Organization (WHO) (2023) reports that global life expectancy increased by 6.6 years between 2000 and 2019. As longevity increases, people may live with a disability or chronic illness. When an older family member develops a chronic illness or experiences a disability, their adult children, who are usually in their middle adulthood, can assume the family caregiver's role.

29.6.1 Client Scenario 3: Caring for Older Adult Parents

Sharon is a 52-year-old woman, living with her partner and her son who is preparing to go off to college. She works full-time and is experiencing life changes related to menopause. Sharon reports that she was recently finding time to re-engage in play and leisure occupations with her partner because her son was less dependent on her for care. Sharon has a close relationship with her mother Gayle who she recently accompanied to the doctor. Due to perceived stigma, Sharon and her mother had both delayed the appointment to see the physician to discuss Gayle's memory and behavioral changes. Gayle has subsequently received a diagnosis of early stage dementia. Sharon feels a deep sense of obligation to care for her mother, although she is concerned about the impact caregiving will have on her employment, play, leisure, and family life.

Although it is common for people in middle adulthood to transition into a caring role for their aging parents, there are cultural differences and expectations. For example, the principle of filial piety in Chinese culture places significant importance on adult children's moral duty and responsibility to provide for and support their aging parents (Andruske & O'Connor, 2020). The principle of familism in Latino culture assumes that the family has a duty toward loyalty and reciprocity of caregiving as a collective, which can extend beyond family (Andruske & O'Connor, 2020). In contrast, caregivers from Western cultures are individualistic and generally feel a lower obligation toward caring (Knight & Sayegh, 2010). Therefore, it is important to understand the unique context and expectations for caring which can either reduce or add to the stress experienced. Nevertheless, the challenges of managing multiple commitments and the resulting stress when transitioning to a new caring role can be high for people in middle adulthood (Savla et al., 2008).

Accommodating a new role while balancing multiple existing occupational roles can negatively impact a person's health and well-being (Bauer & Sousa-Poza, 2015). The integration of a new caring role into daily routines requires people to juggle existing commitments, limiting the time available for other activities (Savla et al., 2008). Some people change to a part-time work arrangement or leave their paid work entirely to create extra time for this new role, with women most often reducing their working hours (Bauer & Sousa-Poza, 2015). Without organizational support, providing care can negatively affect a person's work performance because they may have to arrive at work late or suddenly leave work due to care commitments (Bauer & Sousa-Poza, 2015).

29.6.2 Client Scenario 4: The Sandwich Generation

Huong is a 47-year-old woman with two children: Anh is 11 years old and Binh is 7 years old and has cerebral palsy. Before having children, Huong completed both a Master's degree and PhD. Huong's husband is now completing his Master's degree and lives away from home. Huong's mother has been hospitalized due to a fall. As her mother is not confident communicating in English, Huong visits her at the hospital daily to assist. Now Huong has to manage this extra task while juggling several medical and therapy appointments for Binh and Anh's school activities. While Huong feels physically and mentally exhausted being a sandwich caregiver, she feels obliged to support her mother as she is the eldest daughter of three.

In middle adulthood, people often provide simultaneous care for their parents and children, and they are referred to as the "sandwich generation" (Parker & Patten, 2013). The sandwich generation is reported to experience poorer health than other caregivers (Do et al., 2014). When care recipients require ADL and IADL assistance or have cognitive impairments, the levels of care strain increase and caregivers often feel the care demand is beyond their capacity (Rubin & White-Means, 2009). Interestingly, the sandwich generation is less likely to engage in health-promoting occupations than other caregivers or non-caregivers (Chassin et al., 2010). The reasons for this are multifaceted and complex; for example, lack of time and placing other people's needs first (Chassin et al., 2010). While the importance of health-promoting occupation, including self-care is acknowledged among the sandwich generation, it is difficult to prioritize as their focus is on providing support to their care recipients (Evans et al., 2017). The experience of providing care for parents and children may intensify if their children have a disability or chronic illness. Providing care for children with a developmental disability is a lifelong process, and these children's caregivers have been found to experience more stressors than other caregivers (Wong & Shobo, 2017).

29.7 Conclusion

In conclusion, middle adulthood presents with many opportunities and challenges for occupational performance. There are varying opinions on middle adulthood; whether it is a time of decreasing physical and mental health as opposed to a time where people feel as though they are in the peak of their life. Various factors contribute to each individual experience, such as gender, socioeconomic status, health, and employment. These factors can cause a great deal of stress, impacting health and occupational performance. Physical activity and diet can positively impact areas that typically show a decline in middle adulthood, such as cardiovascular and musculoskeletal health. At the point in time when cognition begins to decline, engagement in meaningful and purposeful occupational performance can help retain and even gain cognitive skills. Caregiving for adult children and older adult parents can impact psychosocial development and adjustment among people in middle adulthood. Various theories are presented that address generativity, stagnation, and midlife experiences. It is known that experiences and decisions early on impact later life and bring with them stressors that impact occupational performance. Analyzing the occupational profile of middle adulthood can help occupational therapists better identify and address needed areas of assessment and intervention.

29.8 Summary

- Occupations of middle adulthood are greatly impacted by earlier life situations, decisions, and circumstance.
- Personal characteristics and contexts such as gender, socioeconomic status, health, and employment impact individual challenges and barriers to occupational performance.
- Middle adulthood presents with both positive and negative experiences that include some feeling as though they are in the peak of their lives, while others may experience a decline in health, stamina, and overall well-being.
- Balancing various occupations while dealing with outcomes of caring for others, working, and health management can cause a high degree of stress.
- Theories such as those proposed by Erikson and Levinson provide developmental approaches to understanding and addressing generativity, stagnation, and midlife experiences.
- An occupational profile can outline and address occupational engagement that may be at risk for people in middle adulthood, including ADLs, IADLs, health management, rest and sleep, education, work, play, leisure, and social participation.

29.9 Review Questions

1. Describe how the occupations of middle adulthood are influenced by earlier life decisions and circumstances.
2. How can the development of an occupational profile assist with understanding occupational issues in middle adulthood?
3. Describe the links between Erikson's psychosocial development theory and the occupations of middle adulthood.
4. What is meant by the term "sandwich generation" and what is the potential impact for people in middle adulthood?

References

Afonso, C., & D'Espiney, L. (2022). Reconstruction of daily life: The lived experience of the family post-caregiver. *New Trends in Qualitative Research, 11*. https://doi.org/10.36367/ntqr.11.2022.e541

Altuntaş, O., Azizoğlu, V., & Davis, J. A. (2021). Exploring the occupational lives of Syrians under temporary protection in Turkey. *Australian Occupational Therapy Journal, 68*(5), 434–443. https://doi.org/10.1111/1440-1630.12756

American Occupational Therapy Association. (2020). Occupational therapy practice framework: Domain and process – Fourth edition. *American Journal of Occupational Therapy, 74*, 7412410010p1 -7412410010p87. https://doi.org/10.5014/ajot.2020.74S2001

Andruske, C. L., & O'Connor, D. (2020). Family care across diverse cultures: Re-envisioning using a transnational lens. *Journal of Aging Studies, 55*, 100892. https://doi.org/10.1016/j.jaging.2020.100892

Bauer, J. M., & Sousa-Poza, A. (2015). Impacts of informal caregiving on caregiver employment, health, and family. *Population Ageing, 8*, 113–145. https//doi.org/10.1007/s12062-015-9116-0

Brim, O., Ryff, C., & Kessler, R. (2004). *How healthy are we? A national study of wellbeing at midlife*. University of Chicago Press.

Chassin, L., Macy, J. T., Seo, D., Presson, C. C., & Sherman, S. J. (2010). The association between membership in the sandwich generation and health behaviours: A longitudinal study. *Journal of Applied Developmental Psychology, 31*, 38–46. https//doi.org/10.1016/j.appdev.2009.06.001

Commonwealth of Australia. (2020). *Closing the gap report*. https://ctgreport.niaa.gov.au/content/closing-gap-2020

Daremo, Å., Kjellberg, A., & Haglund, L. (2015). Occupational performance and affective symptoms for patients with depression disorder. *Advances in Psychiatry, 2015*, 1–6. https://doi.org/10.1155/2015/438149

Do, E. K., Cohen, S., & Brown, M. J. (2014). Socioeconomic and demographic factors modify the association between informal caregiving and health in the sandwich generation. *BMC Public Health, 14*, 362–369. https://doi.org/10.1186/1471-2458-14-362

Edemekong, P. F., Bomgaars, D. L., & Sukumaran, S. (2022). *Activities of daily living*. StatPearls Publishing. https://pubmed.ncbi.nlm.nih.gov/29261878/

Erikson, E. H. (1950). *Childhood and society*. Norton & Co.

Evans, K. L., Girdler, S. J., Falkmer, T., Richmond, J. E., Wagman, P., Millsteed, J., & Falkmer, M. (2017). Viewpoints of working sandwich generation women and occupational therapists on role balance strategies. *Scandinavian Journal of Occupational Therapy, 24*(5), 366–382. https//doi.org/10.1080/11038128.2016.1250814

Grzywacz, J. G., Almeida, D. M., Neupert, S. D., & Ettner, S. L. (2004). Socioeconomic status and health: A micro-level analysis of exposure and vulnerability to daily stressors. *Journal of Health and Social Behavior, 45*(1), 1–16. https://doi.org/10.1177/002214650404500101

Hall, S. S., & Zygmunt, E. (2021). "I hate it here": Mental health changes of college students living with parents during the COVID-19 quarantine. *Emerging Adulthood, 9*(5), 449–461. https//doi.org/10.1177/21676968211000494

Hoffnung, M., Hoffnung, R. J., Seifert, K. L., Hine, A., Pausé, C., Ward, L., Signal, T., Swabey, K., Yates, K., & Burton Smith, R. (2018). *Lifespan development* (4th Australasian ed.). Wiley.

Infurna, F. J., Gerstorf, D., & Lachman, M. E. (2020). Midlife in the 2020s: Opportunities and challenges. *American Psychologist, 75*(4), 470–485. https://doi.org/10.1037/amp0000591

Knight, B. G., & Sayegh, P. (2010). Cultural values and caregiving: The updated sociocultural stress and coping model. *Journals of Gerontology: Series B, 65*, 5–13. https://doi.org/10.1093/geronb/gbp096

Lachman, M. E. (2004). Development in midlife. *Annual Review of Psychology, 55*, 305–331. https://doi.org/10.1146/annurev.psych.55.090902.141521

Lachman, M. E., Teshale, S., & Agrigoroaei, S. (2015). Midlife as a pivotal period in the life course: Balancing growth and decline at the crossroads of youth and old age. *International Journal of Behavioral Development, 39*(1), 20–31. https://doi.org/10.1177/0165025414533223

Levinson, D. J. (1978). *The seasons of a man's life*. Knopf.

Li, Y., Sahakian, B. J., Kang, J., Langley, C., Zhang, W., Xie, C., Xiang, S., Yu, J., Cheng, W., & Feng, J. (2022). The brain structure and genetic mechanisms underlying the nonlinear association between sleep duration, cognition and mental health. *Nature Aging, 2*(5), 425–437. https://doi.org/10.1038/s43587-022-00210-2

Malone, J. C., Liu, S. R., Vaillant, G. E., Rentz, D. M., & Waldinger, R. J. (2016). Midlife Eriksonian psychosocial development: Setting the stage for late-life cognitive and emotional health. *Developmental Psychology, 52*(3), 496–508. https://doi.org/10.1037/a0039875

Milton, S., & Qureshi, K. (2022). Reclaiming the second phase of life? Intersectionality, empowerment and respectability in midlife romance. *Sociological Research Online, 27*(1), 27–42. https://doi.org/10.1177/1360780420974690

Moore-Ramirez, A., Kautzman-East, M., & Gincola, M. M. (2017). LGBTQI+ persons in adulthood. In M. M. Ginicola, C. Smith, & J. M. Filmore (Eds.), *Affirmative counseling with LGTBQI+ people* (pp. 49–60). American Counseling Association. https://doi.org/10.1002/9781119375517

Parker, K., & Patten, E. (2013). *The sandwich generation: Rising financial burdens for middle-aged Americans*. Pew Research Center. http://www.pewsocialtrends.org/2013/01/30/the-sandwich-generation/

Pew Research Center. (2014). *Attitudes about aging: A global perspective*. https://www.pewresearch.org/global/2014/01/30/attitudes-about-aging-a-global-perspective/

Polan, E., & Taylor, D. (2010). Middle adulthood. In E. Polan & D. Taylor (Eds.), *Journey across the life span: Human development and health promotion* (pp. 183–194). F. A. Davis Company.

Reis, L. A. dos, & Menezes, T. M. de O. (2017). Religiosity and spirituality as resilience strategies among long-living older adults in their daily lives. *Revista Brasileira de Enfermagem, 70*(4), 761–766. https://doi.org/10.1590/0034-7167-2016-0630

Rubin, R. M., & White-Means, S. I. (2009). Informal caregiving: Dilemmas of sandwiched caregivers. *Journal of Family Economic Issues, 30*, 252–267. https://doi.org/10.1007/s10834-009-9155-x

Savla, J., Almeida, D. M., Davey, A., & Zarit, S. H. (2008). Routine assistance to parents: Effects on daily mood and other stressors. *The Journals of Gerontology: Series B, 63*(3), S154–S161. https://doi.org/10.1093/geronb/63.3.s154

Tessier, S., Vuillemin, A., Bertrais, S., Boini, S., le Bihan, E., Oppert, J.-M., Hercberg, S., Guillemin, F., & Briançon, S. (2007). Association between leisure-time physical activity and health-related quality of life changes over time. *Preventive Medicine, 44*(3), 202–208. https://doi.org/10.1016/j.ypmed.2006.11.012

Wethington, E. (2000). Expecting stress: Americans and the "midlife crisis". *Motivation and Emotion, 24*, 85–103. https://doi.org/10.1023/A:1005611230993

Wong, J. D., & Shobo, Y. (2017). Types of family caregiving and daily experiences in midlife and late adulthood: The moderating influences of marital status and age. *Research on Aging, 39*(6), 719–740. https://doi.org/10.1177/0164027516681050

World Health Organization. (2023). *The Global Health Observatory*. World Health Organization. https://www.who.int

CHAPTER 30

Human Occupations of Late Adulthood

Emily J. Balog

Abstract
This chapter discusses age-related changes and conditions that affect older adults' participation in their chosen daily occupations. It also addresses opportunities for older adults to continue participating in occupations through the collaborative therapeutic relationship with occupational therapy practitioners. Occupational therapy practitioners are skilled in using theory to support interventions and this chapter describes the most salient theories to promote participation in occupations that are meaningful to older adults.

Author's Positionality Statement
I am a White, English-speaking, American, cisgender woman, occupational therapy health care educator working in a higher education institution with a PhD focusing on self-advocacy and occupational justice. I come from a blue-collar working-class background, am a first-generation college graduate, first-generation PhD graduate, and a Veteran of the United States Air Force where I swore to uphold the Constitution of the United States of America. I acknowledge that, as a White person, my work has and will continue to be influenced by this lens.

Objectives
This chapter will allow the reader to:

- Understand functional occupational performance changes related to the aging process.
- Define and describe chronic conditions associated with late adulthood.

- Understand the occupational participation challenges of older adults related to the aging process and acute/chronic illness.
- Describe the opportunities for older adults who seek occupational therapy services.
- Identify appropriate theories, models, and frameworks that can guide evidence-informed, occupation-based practice aimed at late adulthood.

Key terms
- aging process
- chronic disease
- agism
- cultural sensitivity
- social determinants of health

30.1 Introduction
30.1.1 Background
Worldwide older adults are the fastest growing population with an expected increase of 21.1% by 2050 (World Health Organization, 2015). In Western societies, the majority of older people are community-dwelling (European Commission, 2019; Garner et al., 2018; Jansson, 2020). There has been a shift from institutional care to community care with the majority of adults seeking care in the community through primary settings. Occupational therapists are underrepresented in primary care, yet desperately needed by communities to provide integrated, person-centered care (Bolt et al., 2019) to older adults.

30.1.2 Occupations of Older Adults
The human occupations of older adulthood are similar to adulthood in many ways, yet there are also unique differences in mental, physical, and social wellness in later adulthood that may present challenges to meaningful occupational participation. As occupational therapy practitioners we must understand the intersection of contexts, occupations, and the person as a means for optimal engagement. As we age there is at least some degree of cognitive, physical, sensory, and psychosocial changes that potentially impact the ability to perform meaningful and necessary occupations.

This chapter will describe the unique challenges and opportunities faced by late adulthood as a group and the ways in which occupational therapy practitioners can support engagement in occupation by addressing these challenges and leveraging opportunities.

30.2 Occupations of Late Adulthood
30.2.1 Challenges
There is no uniform standard for aging – it is as unique a process as individual humans. Many older adults face challenges throughout the aging process ranging from personal

factors (e.g., demographics), normal age-related changes, chronic/health conditions, and psychosocial implications. This section will describe these challenges to more clearly understand how these factors, changes, and conditions impact the ability of the older adult to participate in meaningful occupations in their physical, virtual, and social environments.

30.2.2 Personal Factors

Personal factors are commonly understood as demographics and include age, gender identity, race, ethnicity, and socioeconomic and educational status. These are generally unchanging and intrinsic to who a person is. While not typically considered positive or negative (American Occupational Therapy Association [AOTA], 2020), society and social determinants that create disparities related to these factors can influence the health and well-being of older adults.

30.2.2.1 Agism

Much like other marginalized populations, older adults face discrimination from general society that continues as they grow older. Agism "include[s] direct discrimination …" (e.g., older workers excluded from job market, elder abuse), "… but also encompasses less direct, more insidious, stereotyping" (e.g., conceptualizing older adults as a burden) that results in the stigmatizing of older adults (Walker, 2016, pp. 57–58). This type of stigmatization also causes younger adults to procrastinate preparing for their own aging and hinders the larger society from developing policy that benefits older community members. The impacts of agism (lack of respect and social exclusion) result in isolation due to decreased community engagement and social participation. Furthermore, aging stereotypes may lead to monolithic assumptions about the needs of older adults that adversely impact quality care. These social aspects, coupled with often confusing or inaccessible support from health services and inaccessibility in community spaces (buildings, transportation, housing), further marginalize older adults from fully achieving participation in desired occupations. The results of agism directly impact the health outcomes of older adults (Palmore, 2015).

30.2.2.2 Misogyny

Misogyny, or prejudice against women, is important to understand and recognize particularly in the "old old" (age 76 and over) as they tend to be mostly women (Walker, 2016). Prejudice against older women is largely due to the gender inequalities associated with women who work lower paying jobs in their lifetime and are less likely to have pensions. Having less cumulative wealth to support themselves in retirement years (Jansson, 2015), older adult women face greater disparities.

30.2.2.3 Racism

The hegemonic (i.e., influences of the dominant group) historical and political policies of many nations, particularly the United States, has led to the marginalization of people of color. These racist policies are known to impact the health, wellness, and quality of life for Black and Indigenous communities, and people of color. Gentrification, or the process of changing poor, urban communities by bringing in affluent groups and displacing persons within said community (Cho & Kim, 2016; Versey, 2018), can threaten the independence of older adults, especially those with chronic conditions and disabilities, and their ability to age in place as it reduces their access to needed goods and services (Rosenwohl-Mack et al., 2020; Wu & Tseng, 2018).

30.2.2.4 Low Educational Attainment

Education is correlated with socioeconomic status (SES). As such, those individuals who are less educated are more likely to have lower SES. Low SES places older adults at a greater disparity in terms of experiencing low health literacy, less access to care, and less opportunity to participate in meaningful occupation.

30.2.2.5 Intersectionality

Intersectionality is when an individual has two or more, or an intersection, of known disparity groups. Those who experience intersectionality are at exponential risk for negative effects. For example, the disparity between an older adult White man and an older adult Black woman are significant.

30.3 Client Factors

Older adults are faced with increasing chronic conditions and impacts on their occupations due to the aging and disease processes. Age- and disease-related changes in body function and structure and associated challenges can be described relative to performance skills and performance patterns that intersect with personal and environmental factors (AOTA, 2020). Communities have yet to evolve to the changing needs of this growing population to accommodate older adults as they experience age-related changes, including chronic conditions. The following section will describe both normal age-related changes and health conditions associated with various body systems.

30.3.1 Client Factors and Age-related Change

Body function and structure changes in late adulthood span the spectrum of functional change in mental, sensory, neuromusculoskeletal, organ systems, skin, and other anatomical structures. Some common body function changes associated with age include visual changes, fine motor coordination decline, balance impairment, diminished or changed sensation, decreased muscle strength, genitourinary changes, and emotional changes (such as depression) associated with isolation and loss.

30.3.1.1 Cognitive Changes

Older adults' cognitive processes do not decline uniformly across individuals. There are normal age-related declines in cognition that do occur; however, there are also cognitive processes that improve with age, and those areas with mixed or maintained processes. While more research is needed, it has been found that sensory processes (i.e., vision and hearing), alternating attention, divided attention, working memory, and executive functioning decline with age. Sustained attention, semantic memory, non-declarative memory, prospective memory, and intelligence show no difference, or possibly improvements for older adults. Mixed results have been found for selective attention, short-term memory, and everyday problem solving (Bonder & Dal Bello-Haas, 2018). As occupational therapy practitioners, we must keep abreast of recent research and understand normal age-related changes in cognition.

30.3.1.2 Sensory Changes

Age-related sensory loss is a normal part of aging. While limiting in daily life function, sensory loss is often able to be accommodated by the older adult. At times, health conditions can also adversely impact sensory function of older adults. With normal age-related loss, older adults may be at risk for skin integrity issues (bumping into furniture, trips, and falls) and social withdrawal and isolation due to sensory impairment. It is critical for occupational therapy practitioners to assess sensation and associated functional/occupational impairment during evaluation and intervention planning.

30.3.1.3 Musculoskeletal Changes

As one ages, it is expected that structure and functional changes will occur in the muscles, tendons, bones, cartilage, and nerves. As such, musculoskeletal changes can be a normal age-related change. Decline in strength, flexibility, and range of motion are common as one ages. However, these changes can also result in risks and functional impairments. Occupational therapists can intervene at various stages associated with age-related musculoskeletal changes.

30.3.1.4 Neuromuscular Changes

Posture, coordination, balance, and gait are all affected by the aging process; however, the variability in how neuromuscular and movement function presents varies greatly from person to person. Balance screenings and exercise programs designed to address deficits in neuromuscular and movement function are critical in remediation, restoration, and maintenance of neuromuscular function. Yet, occupational therapy practitioners must go beyond assessment and intervention related to movement and exercise alone and consider the functional implications of deficits in these areas (e.g., consider the dangers of falling in the shower due to balance difficulties). As such, occupational therapists often conduct a home safety assessment with the client and develop recommendations for fall prevention.

30.3.1.5 Cardiovascular and Cardiopulmonary Changes

As with other organ systems, older adults experience cardiopulmonary and cardiovascular age-related changes. These include calcification, narrowing, and wasting of structures in and of the lungs and heart. As a result, oxygenation and blood flow decline and affect the functional performance of older adults through a range of symptoms such as fatigue, dizziness, shortness of breath, lightheadedness/fainting, instability, and disorientation when engaging in exercise, mobility, and occupations. Occupational therapy practitioners must be skilled in assessing normal age-related cardiopulmonary and cardiovascular function.

30.3.2 Client Factors and Chronic Conditions

Chronic conditions are "conditions that last one year or more and require ongoing medical attention or limit activities of daily living or both" (Centers for Disease Control and Prevention, 2022, para. 1). Chronic diseases include conditions such as cancer, substance use, head injury, mobility impairment, visual impairment, diabetes, heart disease, and arthritis (Grover & Joshi, 2014). Chronic conditions have known causal mechanisms that affect specific client factors. For example, diabetes is known to impact sensory, skin, and body systems and these impacts can cause additional disability when resultant outcomes such as amputation or vision loss begin to impact performance. As with age-related changes, chronic conditions impact all areas of occupation. When coupled with age-related changes, activities of daily living (ADLs), instrumental activities of daily living (IADLs), and other occupational domains can be increasingly difficult to manage.

30.3.2.1 Cognitive and Mental Health Conditions

Disorders of cognition in aging include dementia, stroke, and Parkinson's disease. With the prevalence of dementia expected to affect 75 million older adults by 2050, the presence of cognitive disorders such as dementia have enormous personal and social consequences. Dementia puts older adults at risk for costly institutionalization and decreases the economic productivity of caretakers (World Health Organization, 2015). According to a global study, one-third of Alzheimer's dementia cases worldwide are attributed to modifiable risk factors, including depression (Norton et al., 2014). Mental health conditions that contribute to cognitive impairment include depression, anxiety, and substance use. About 2%–3% of the world's community-dwelling older adults have depressive symptoms and that number increases significantly to 10% among frail and institutionalized older adults worldwide. Anxiety disorders often coexist with depressive disorders and result in significant disability and decreased quality of life (World Health Organization, 2015). The physical environment contributes to outcomes for mental health. When the physical environment is free from excessive noise and is walkable and pleasant, mental health outcomes are improved (Annear et al., 2014). Both mild cognitive impairment and mental health conditions such as depression are linked to functional decline (Morley, 2015).

30.3.2.2 Sensory Conditions

Low vision and blindness from conditions such as cataracts, macular degeneration, glaucoma, diabetic retinopathy, and Parkinson's and Alzheimer's disease impact nearly every occupation. This includes the ability to read for pleasure as well as, for example, reading medication labels that would allow for independence in health management. Visual conditions impact an older adult's ability to drive, navigate the home and community environments, and participate in basic ADL and IADL tasks. Both visual and vestibular disorders, such as vertigo, threaten the safety of individuals through increased risk of falls which can lead to catastrophic downward spirals of disability and death. Auditory disorders such as deafness, tinnitus, and hearing loss are known to have social consequences and some older adults may reduce their interactions, putting them at risk for isolation. Diminished olfactory and gustation can decrease interest in food and result in anorexia in aging. The skin is the first layer of protection against diseases and skin disorders such as dermatitis and pressure ulcers permit an avenue to infection and illness. Furthermore, health conditions such as diabetes and peripheral neuropathy create decreased blood flow to appendages which can result in skin breakdown, gangrene, and amputation. Lastly, pain is undertreated in older adults and disorders such as fibromyalgia, gout, and low back pain are common causes of pain that benefit from pain management (Bonder & Dal Bello-Haas, 2018).

30.3.2.3 Musculoskeletal Conditions

Conditions such as arthritis and osteoporosis are prevalent in the older adult population and may result in fractures or surgical interventions such as a joint replacement. These conditions impact functional mobility and ADL participation in older adults (Bonder & Dal Bello-Haas, 2018). Older adults have indicated that mobility both in the home and in the community are critical for maintaining a sense of well-being and independence (Black et al., 2015; Li, 2020).

30.3.2.4 Neuromusculoskeletal Conditions

Conditions such as Parkinson's disease and amyotrophic lateral sclerosis (ALS) are progressive neurological conditions that impact strength, balance, and coordination, resulting in impairment in functional mobility, feeding, and nearly all areas of occupation. Individuals with these conditions are at significantly increased risk for falls.

30.3.2.5 Cardiovascular and Cardiopulmonary Conditions

Occupational therapy practitioners must understand health related conditions/pathology marked by lifestyle (e.g., smoking, obesity) that result in cardiovascular and cardiopulmonary conditions such as hypertension, stroke, bronchitis, emphysema, and asthma. Furthermore, an understanding of intrinsic health conditions and their impact on the cardiovascular/cardiopulmonary system – such as cancer, diabetes, COPD, COVID-19, and heart disease, as well as the implications of extrinsic factors (e.g., surgery, medication) – are also warranted (Bonder & Dal Bello-Haas, 2018; Cohen & Tavares, 2020). Exposure to environmental toxins and "social toxins" (i.e., agism) contribute to cardiovascular disease, and low-income communities are disproportionately affected by these toxins (World Health Organization, 2015).

30.3.3 Health Conditions and Functional Ability

When the aging and disease processes begin to interfere with function, a person may begin to see themselves as having a disability. According to the World Health Organization (WHO), disability measured through six domains (cognition, mobility, self-care, getting along, life activities, and participation) predicts a number of factors, including service needs, level of care, outcome of the condition, length of hospitalization, receipt of disability benefits, work performance, and social integration (Üstün et al., 2010). Additionally, knowledge of disability can improve public health and policy decisions beyond knowledge of a diagnosis because needs may be better identified, treatment and intervention may be better matched, outcomes and effectiveness can be measured, and priorities and resources can be better allocated (Üstün et al., 2010). Occupational therapists design interventions to address or prevent these disruptions in function and enhance a person's ability to engage in meaningful occupation. Because occupational therapy practitioners use a strengths-based approach, use of the term *functional ability* is preferred over *disability*. Functional ability can be thought of as an individual's level of functioning in a given activity and measured by observable and self-reported performance skills (AOTA, 2020).

30.3.3.1 Age-related Changes, Disease, and Performance Skills

Motor, process, and social skills are impacted by age-related changes and often lead to a cascade of issues such as falls and inability to complete important ADL/IADL tasks such as reading, driving, taking medications, and safely engaging in all tasks (e.g., decreased balance impacts safety in ADLs in the bathroom and IADLs in meal preparation and cleaning). Decreased sensory functions impact ADLs and IADLs, but also meaningful leisure and social activities such as reading, dialing the phone, and working with computers. When faced with the implications of age-related loss, chronic conditions, and illness and accidents, older adults may require focused interventions addressing ADLs, health management, and sleep and rest, which support day-to-day living at the most basic level.

30.4 Environmental Factors

One's home and personal context – including family dynamics and living situation – are important considerations for aging adults. Because of the changing structures of families, older adults are more likely to live alone and have limited traditional caregiving support from family (Dupuis-Blanchard et al., 2015; Gitlin et al., 2013; Lehning, 2012; Narushima & Kawabata, 2020). Thus, an emphasis on support services that include assistance for basic ADLs as well as IADLs has been identified as a care need for older adults living alone, and also for all community-dwelling older adults. Green et al. (2022) emphasize the importance of social determinants related to housing, specifically the need for and access to home safety renovations, as a cost-effective strategy for aging in place that would cost less than 2% of the Centers for Medicare and Medicaid budget. The authors argue that, in part, the issue lies in policy development, where policymakers rarely fund non-medical programs and miss the opportunity to relate these services as a benefit to health.

Environmental factors beyond a person's home living environment must also be considered. Community characteristics of outdoor spaces, buildings, and roads were shown to be, in part, predictors of civic and social participation in older adult participants in Castelló, Spain. Older adults who live alone have a greater reliance on community support and health services (Flores et al., 2019).

30.4.1 Transportation

The ability to move about one's community impacts the opportunity to access services and participate socially and civically (World Health Organization [WHO], 2007). The ability to navigate one's community is a critical variable to measure in terms of access and participation. Investments in improving road conditions instead of addressing public transportation will disproportionately affect older adults (World Health Organization, 2015). Transportation is discussed further as an IADL.

30.5 Occupations of Older Adults

Before, in tandem, or after addressing the most basic needs, practitioners can also address in and out-of-home occupations related to more advanced IADLs, leisure, and social and community participation. There is no prescribed order to addressing the occupations of late adulthood; however, providers will often only cover the most basic of needs, thereby limiting the scope of the profession. There is a need to demonstrate the value of occupational therapy services in addition to and beyond basic ADL restoration because achieving health and wellness and living a full life are not marked simply by self-care. Practitioners should ensure intervention and education on ADL/IADL tasks can be generalized to other occupational areas that may not be readily covered by payors. For example, skills used to improve safety and energy in grocery shopping can be generalized to social events in the community.

30.5.1 ADL

ADL is an area of occupation that includes the tasks and activities of caring for oneself. Older minority adults with disability and chronic conditions are at higher risk for isolation and depression; have less ability to perform ADLs, leisure, and work; are more likely to be frail, have falls, and be hospitalized; and have a higher mortality rate. These poor outcomes are exacerbated by unsupportive home and community environments (Gitlin et al., 2013). Findings from a hazard analysis on determinants of aging in place behaviors show that individuals with a functional impairment are at greater risk for institutionalization (Sabia, 2008).

30.5.2 IADL

IADL is an area of occupation that focuses on one's personal business, such as caring for pets, preparing a meal, cleaning, managing bills, home and property maintenance, driving/community mobility, and going grocery shopping. Older adults both with and without functional disability have identified that community mobility is a barrier to participation. Access to transportation is a mediating source for social participation in communities and the lack of affordable, reliable, accessible, and convenient transportation is a barrier to social participation (Levasseur et al., 2015; WHO, 2007). Individuals who are living alone and potentially isolated may be suited for special services focusing on support for outings, meals, and housework, particularly because of the emphasized importance older adults place on community supports (Flores et al., 2019).

30.5.3 Health Management
Health management are those activities that relate to improvement or maintenance of health and wellness of the older adult (AOTA, 2020). Self-advocacy for one's health is threatened by the health care system, health care policies, and even health care team members, which collectively are known to be ageist, dismissive, and exclusionary when older adults seek health services (Wyman et al., 2018). Experiencing normal age-related changes and/or chronic disease can significantly impact the ability of an older adult to manage their health. For example, difficulties with vision or impairments in fine motor control can make taking medications that manage one's health difficult or impossible.

30.5.4 Rest and Sleep
Sleep is a passive occupation that impacts daily waking occupations. Occupational therapy categorizes sleep into preparation (self and environment) and participation (AOTA, 2020). Poor sleep can affect older adults, including increasing the incidence of morbidity and mortality; decreasing daily occupational performance; increasing risk of accidents; impairing function and judgment; creating dysfunction in family life and use of health care; and lessening overall quality of life (Colten & Altevogt, 2006).

30.5.5 Education
Normal age-related changes impact the ways in which an older adult learns. Increased effort is required due to diminished processing and divided attention, and conditions such as low vision can also impact the ability of older people to gain education. Learning has economic, social, and health impacts for all ages.

30.5.6 Work
The Occupational Therapy Practice Framework – 4th Edition (OTPF-IV) (AOTA, 2020) defines work as labor that is either paid or unpaid. Lengthening employment is often sought after by policy makers (Walker, 2016), but for older adults, civic participation is more than employment. The literature highlights the desire and need for opportunities for structured volunteerism and ways to "give back" (Black et al., 2015; Flores et al., 2019).

30.5.7 Leisure
Leisure interests are those activities that are non-obligatory and intrinsically engaging (AOTA, 2020). It is increasingly recognized since the passing of the Americans with Disabilities Act that designing community spaces to allow for physical access is imperative for inclusivity; however, calls for research to examine how older adults and persons with disabilities engage in occupation in these spaces is critical (Watchorn et al.,

2021). Barriers to inclusivity as a result of agism and discrimination impact the will of older adults to participate in their communities (Black et al., 2015; Sorrell, 2021). Complex conditions are known to negatively impact leisure participation (Gitlin et al., 2013). Older adult women, and those with physical or mental health symptoms and low educational status, were less likely to engage in leisure activities (Paillard-Borg et al., 2009). Similar to the disability rights movement, older adults have identified social attitudes and policies as greater barriers to leisure pursuit than disability (Hammel et al., 2008).

30.5.8 Social Participation

Social participation centralized around engagement with the community, family, and/or peers supports wellness in older adults and promotes aging in place. A National Association of Area Agencies on Aging survey indicates that communities are underprepared to address aging in place at a community level (Black et al., 2015). Under-preparedness has immense social and economic consequences (Au et al., 2020), yet over-reliance on communities could relieve government officials from provision of programing and policy that would support aging in place (Menec et al., 2011). Diversity-friendly and accommodating spaces are critical to facilitate socialization, but practitioners must think beyond space and access and consider occupational participation. This is because access does not necessarily offer the ability to engage in meaningful and preferred occupations (Watchorn et al., 2021). Eliciting older adults to participate socially in meaningful ways that bring value and purpose to their lives is an important outreach consideration; however, the information streams to elicit participation are decentralized and often web-based. Information using technology and internet-based outreach has been identified as a barrier to older adults, exacerbated by the COVID-19 pandemic during which many older adults did not have access to, or knowledge of, technology use (Kotwal et al., 2021). As such, social isolation and associated mental health conditions have worsened for many older adults over the spanning pandemic years, and efforts to address health needs have been difficult to navigate (Kotwal et al., 2021). Social isolation is known to negatively contribute to cardiovascular, immune, and nervous system disorders of older adults; as much as the serious health implications of smoking half a pack of cigarettes a day (Cagney et al., 2013; WHO, 2015).

30.5.9 Performance Patterns

Performance patterns include habits, roles, routines, and rituals of older adults. Occupational therapy practitioners understand that the healthful balance and embedment of occupations over time into performance patterns support occupational performance. When a person experiences a disruption in any one of these domains, they may experience a decline in health, well-being, and participation (AOTA, 2020).

30.5.10 Opportunities

As occupational therapy practitioners, we must understand the ways in which personal factors and performance patterns impact occupational performance. Advocating for our clients and helping to promote agency in one's daily life, as well as dispel misnomers about aging to curb agism, misogyny, and racism, must become common practice. Learning about the history of our profession can assist with this feat. For example, the profession has been dominated by White, Western, middle-class, and heterosexual perspectives and, as such, our assessments, interventions, and outcomes are designed to reintegrate clients into a society where these perspectives are seen as the norm (Grenier, 2020). We can better design interventions and prepare clients for satisfactory participation in meaningful occupation when we fully understand the personal context and history of person groups (Lucas & Washington, 2020). Due to known inequalities among minority races and ethnicities, accounting for this demographic in later life is critical for identifying inequalities and developing plans to address them using occupational consciousness – defined as an awareness of the dynamics of hegemony and appropriate selection of assessments and interventions (Walker, 2016). Furthermore, involving older adult minorities in the planning process in communities can bolster trust and participation within the community (Balog, 2021). Understanding individual, group, and community perspectives from minority and marginalized groups helps us to promote occupational justice, or the promotion of equal opportunity to have the right to engage in diverse and meaningful occupations (Townsend & Wilcock, 2004).

30.5.11 Personal Factors

As with occupations spanning the lifespan, culture and individual meaning must be considered when discussing occupations. Occupational therapy practitioners are called to provide culturally responsive and customized services (AOTA, 2017), and recognizing that late adulthood is not marked by a monolithic experience demonstrates this cultural sensitivity. Practitioners must intersect culture and personal attributes that impact human occupation when designing interventions (e.g., occupations that older adults find meaningful and important through needs and desire). Furthermore, occupational therapy practitioners are skilled in assisting clients to establish performance patterns that support meaningful and purposeful occupations.

30.6 Client Factors: Values, Beliefs, Spirituality

Client factors of values, beliefs, and spirituality are considered part of the philosophy of our profession which sees individuals as occupational beings who are internally motivated by what is interesting, important, and satisfying. These client factors are widely recognized as a theoretical driver to analyze a person's motivations, sense of self, and one's place in the world (Duncan, 2020). Collectively, older adults have articulated shared values in remaining in their homes and communities, or aging in place (Binette & Vasold, 2018). These core factors of an individual are drivers for participation and engagement. For example, an older adult who values civics may be more likely to engage in the voting process.

30.6.1 The Importance of Participation in Meaningful Occupation

Participation in society focuses on the constructs of sense of belonging, the act of meaningfully doing and influencing, and ultimately the inclusion in available opportunities (Cogan & Carlson, 2018; Sverker et al., 2020; Üstün et al., 2010; World Health Organization, 2007). Purpose in life and *mattering* have been shown to be predictors of wellness and well-being. Mattering is defined as a sense that you are important and valued (Flett & Heisel, 2021; Sorrell, 2021). Participation in society includes a variety of types of participation, including social and civic activities such as person-centered planning. Older adults have identified that they desire to have a choice and a voice in their communities that is respected, valued, and sought after (Black et al., 2015; Rosenwohl-Mack et al., 2020). Including older adults and developing accommodations are ways that occupational therapy practitioners can mediate purposeful participation in meaningful occupations.

30.7 The Intervention Process with Older Adults

Occupational therapy practitioners can provide older adults with the ability to continue engaging in meaningful occupation despite illness, chronic conditions, and the aging process. It is useful to move through the evaluative process beginning with a strengths-based approach to understand and capitalize on an individual's personal assets and existing function. Through therapeutic use of self and collaboration with the older client, the pair can uncover the ways in which function has been impacted and the methods by which strengths can be leveraged through values and goals. This is the process of developing the occupational profile of the older adult client (AOTA, 2020). Once the evaluation process is completed, the selection of an occupation-based theory (or theories) coupled with frames of reference can be selected. Theories that can support empowered aging are discussed later in this chapter.

Working with an occupational therapy practitioner to address age-related challenges associated with all occupations both in and out of the home can help older adults with interventions that aim to create, promote, establish, restore, maintain, modify, and/or prevent depending on the need of the individual or group (AOTA, 2020). Occupational therapists have a unique set of medical and social skills that enable them to provide these services in both community and institutional settings; however, a focus toward the community may enable more prevention focused approaches that reduce the need for institutionalization.

30.7.1 Occupational Interventions of Late Adulthood

The occupational therapy practitioner can work with the client to create, promote, establish, restore, maintain, modify, and/or prevent within any occupational domain. Below is a description of some of the ways that occupational therapy practitioners can address these domains with older adults.

30.7.1.1 ADL and IADL

Nursing home placement is based on cognition and/or functional impairment and the lack of support for ADL/IADL tasks (Luppa et al., 2010). Occupational therapy practitioners are equipped to address these barriers through home and community-based interventions. The Community Aging in Place, Advancing Better Living for Elders (CAPABLE) study demonstrated improved functional performance in older adult participants with a patient-directed approach, in collaboration with an occupational therapist, registered nurse, and handy worker team. At a $1,300 average budget per household, 94% of the intervention group reported an improvement in their lives by participating in the study as compared to only 54% in the control group (Szanton et al., 2011). This study is not only a demonstration of how occupational therapy practitioners are well suited to address the needs of older adults in their homes, but also a demonstration of how interdisciplinary collaboration of stakeholders can address barriers to aging in place. Developing self-motivating behaviors can lead to self-efficacy or how confidently a person is able to take a course of action in response to a situation (Bandura, 1977) through achievement of increased knowledge and understanding, and adopting behaviors associated with habit formation (AOTA, 2020; Michie et al., 2011).

Ultimately, older adults who utilize homecare have reduced mortality, hospitalization, institutionalization, and improved quality of life all at a reduced cost to the healthcare system. Social factors and determinants make the difference between an older adult being home with assistance and institutionalized. Interventions that address and enhance ADL and IADL participation are shown to improve social participation and are protective factors for institutionalization (Mah et al., 2021; Papageorgiou et al., 2016).

30.7.1.2 Health Management

With the rising rates of chronic disease impacting health and quality of life among older adults, the management of chronic disease is critical for the promotion of occupational performance. There is strong evidence for improving occupational performance and quality of life for older adults by working with an occupational therapy practitioner on health management at both individual- and group-level interventions (Berger et al., 2018). Occupational therapy practitioners must be skilled in the identification of assessments that can identify specific difficulties related to client factors and develop interventions to support health management. For example, the selection of a medication management assessment might better identify whether a client is experiencing cognitive versus fine motor impairment that is contributing to difficulty managing their medications. Tailored approaches to meet individual health management needs are a hallmark of occupational therapy intervention and must always be considered when utilizing assessments and protocols. Figure 30.1 shows Navy veteran, Rosa, power-walking through her community to manage her health.

30.7.1.3 Rest and Sleep

Sleep and rest impact every waking occupation (Balog, 2021) and can be particularly impacted in older adults who require health interventions. Assessing for sleep-related issues during the evaluation process can allow for the development of person-centered goals and treatment plans that enable intrinsic motivation and can lead to enhanced client safety, function, and overall quality of life (Mitchell et al., 2018).

30.7.1.4 Education

As our world moves toward web-based platforms, learning how to use devices and programs, and an awareness of information literacy and health literacy are areas older adults can benefit from to stay connected socially and confidently learn about a breadth

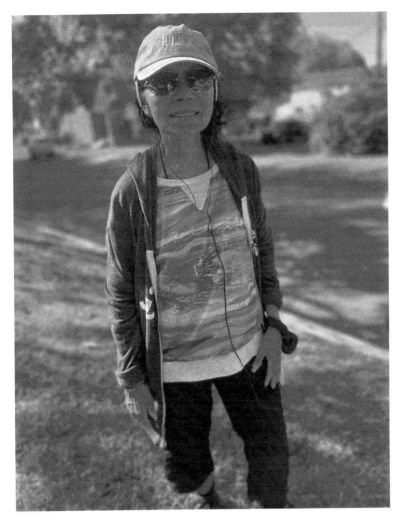

Figure 30.1 Navy veteran, Rosa, powerwalking through her community to manage her health.

Source: Photo by Emily Balog.

of topics. Health literacy allows for exertion of control in one's life and may mediate access to a larger pool of resources and social supports that facilitate participation in one's community (Miyashita et al., 2021). Providing supportive strategies for new learning and creating/adapting learning materials to ensure readability (i.e., grade level), comprehensibility (i.e., design quality and usefulness), and suitability (i.e., appropriateness) are ways that occupational therapists can support learning and health literacy in late adulthood (Fortuna et al., 2021).

30.7.1.5 Work

Because late adulthood is often marked by a period of non-paid work (retirement), it affords opportunities for civic engagement and volunteerism. Older adults have the opportunity to shape programs and activities within the community that can support aging in place and village mental models (e.g., "it takes a village to raise a child"). Advocacy work that empowers older adults to promote their own needs allows for investment in this work and true person-centeredness. Occupational therapy practitioners can work with clients to develop opportunities for older adults to meaningfully give back to society through volunteer efforts in the community. Such mentorship can help older adults to maintain independence and enhance community participation (Papageorgiou et al., 2016).

30.7.1.6 Leisure and Social Participation

Leisure participation is known to address areas of loneliness and boredom and promote health and wellness. Leisure participation is also closely linked with social participation as many leisure activities are co-occupations conducted in the community. Occupational therapy practitioners can utilize assessments to identify areas of interest (past, present, and future) for older adults and develop individual or group interventions and programs for engaging in meaningful leisure tasks (Smallfield & Molitor, 2018). Figure 30.2 depicts retired nurse, Jane, knitting on the beach as a way to keep her mind and hands occupied.

Communities can support leisure and social participation through age-friendly initiatives that prioritize universal design principles and inclusion within the community. Development of policies that can support communities in these critical domains is an avenue for occupational therapists to carve out roles in communities.

Information about community services, events, and activities must be clear and have reduced complexity of information. Simple messaging should be visually appealing and able to connect older adults to programs, services, and activities in their communities. For example, in Figure 30.3, Army Veteran, Frank, discusses plans for remembering fallen service members with a friend at his local Veterans' Club. Communications should have consistent messaging that can expand access and awareness of community information. These communications should be delivered through multiple sources or channels for information to be digested by older adults in the community as a spur for community participation (Black et al., 2015; De Wit et al., 2017; Miyashita et al., 2021; Rosenwohl-Mack et al., 2020). Designing not only the services and events, but also the means by which they are communicated to community-dwelling older adults is a skill within the field of occupational therapy.

30.7.2 Environmental and Community Intervention

The World Health Organization's (2007) Global Age-Friendly Cities Guide and checklist for communities can be leveraged to support community engagement. The checklist can serve as a self-assessment in beginning to understand where improvements can be made. Derived from the guide, the checklist provides eight domains where age-friendliness can be evaluated: outdoor spaces and buildings; transportation; housing (built environment); social participation; respect and social inclusion; civic participation and employment (social environment); communication and information; and community support and health services (service environment) (John & Gunter, 2016). This is an

HUMAN OCCUPATIONS OF LATE ADULTHOOD

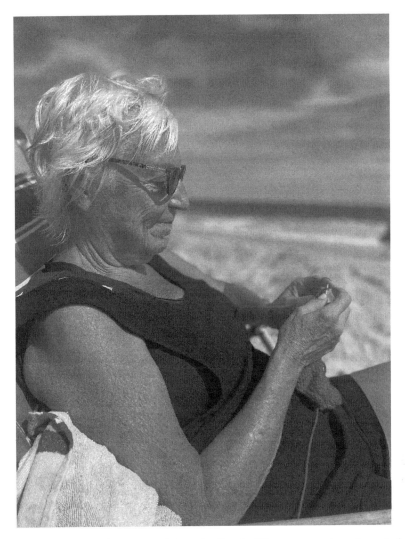

Figure 30.2 Jane knitting on Brigantine Beach, NJ, as a way to keep her mind and hands occupied.
Source: Photo by Emily Balog.

opportunity for occupational therapists to design interventions in the community by working with local governments, community organizations, and older adults in the community.

30.7.3 Performance Pattern Intervention

Qualitative studies and mixed-methods designs employed over the last decade have demonstrated the adaptive strategies of older adults when they are faced with challenges. Older adults assert agency through focusing on the strengths that do exist while also adapting their current routines. Agency is the capacity to make choices, to respond to threats, and maintain important life skills (Rosenwohl-Mack et al., 2020). Agency

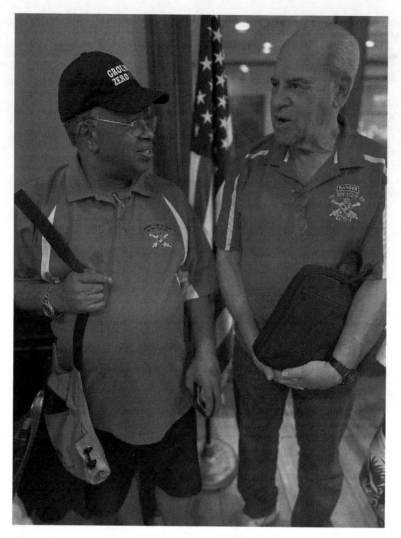

Figure 30.3 Army Veteran, Frank (left), discusses plans for remembering fallen service members with a friend from his Veterans' Club.

Source: Photo by Emily Balog.

also includes a choice in whether to age in place in their current residence or to move elsewhere, such as an institution. Empowered aging concepts encompass the idea of shared responsibility for participation for both the individual older adult and the community (Moulaert & Garon, 2016). Much like an occupational therapist grades up and down (modifies) activities to improve function or respond to difficulties, the idea of providing varied levels of opportunity should be considered during action planning and when designing opportunities for participation within the home and community.

30.8 Theories to Support Occupations of Late Adulthood

As we age there is at least some degree of cognitive, physical, sensory, and psychosocial changes that potentially impact the ability to perform meaningful and necessary occupations. In gerontology, these can be addressed through biological, psychological, and sociological theories (Bonder & Dal Bello-Haas, 2018). Achieving balance is a skill that occupational therapy practitioners can facilitate through several occupation-based models (e.g., MOHO and Kawa). One model, Sturmberg and Martin's (2013) somato-psycho-socio-semiotic model of health, encompasses these concepts as achieving a balance of health. When operationalized with occupation-based theory, health can be achieved by addressing/preventing problems in any of these constructs. When designing interventions for occupations at individual, group, and population levels, the needs of the client coupled with the selected theory can assist with the decision to restore, maintain, or modify performance patterns, client factors, and/or performance skills.

30.8.1 The Model of Human Occupation (MOHO)

The use of person-centered and volition focused theory can be utilized to promote and empower participation among older adults. The MOHO can be used throughout any age group and its utility with older adults can be particularly useful. This is because occupational identity is shaped over time reflecting cumulative life experiences. Older adults have lived long lives and as such are likely to have a deep understanding of their interests, roles, obligations, capacity for doing, and, for some, a familiar environment. Interruptions in performance capacity through normal age-related changes and/or health conditions affect an individual's volition and habits, interfere with life roles and identity, and change the way an individual interacts with the physical and social environment. Theoretical reasoning through the use of the MOHO can assist clinicians in a work-up of the occupational profile and development of the therapeutic process to maintain, restore, or modify occupational competence, performance, and participation (Duncan, 2020).

30.8.2 Ecological Theories

Ecological theories focus on the interaction between an individual and their environment. Three prominent ecological theories are described below and range from interactions at micro to macro levels, the fit of the individual within these varied contexts, and the ways in which performance can be addressed.

30.8.2.1 Ecological Systems Theory

Bronfenbrenner's (1986) Ecological Systems Theory considers (a) the *individual* and associated factors and abilities; (b) the *microsystem* of direct contacts such as family and church; (c) the *mesosystem* interconnecting the microsystem to the exosystem; (d) the *exosystem* which considers contexts such as neighbors and politics; and (e) the *macrosystem* reflecting the larger culture and attitudes.

30.8.2.2 Environmental Press Theory

Environmental Press Theory (Lawton & Nahemow, 1973) considers the individual characteristics of the older adult and the community characteristics in which one resides. Occupational therapy practitioners use the theory to consider the impacts of these characteristics on meaningful participation. This theory shows that individual function and environmental characteristics require alignment; for example, if an individual characteristic includes low functional mobility and the environment includes a high challenge, such as stairs, there will be high press or poor alignment. The opposite is also true and would result in boredom (high individual skill, low environmental challenge). The goal is to match the ability at the person level with an appropriate *just right challenge* (Rebeiro & Polgar, 1999) at the environmental level to achieve a zone of maximum comfort or fit. *Fit* of meaningful participation is often thought of on an individual level in the field of occupational therapy; however, the recent edition of the OTPF-IV (AOTA, 2020) extends this concept more explicitly to groups and populations.

30.8.2.3 Ecology of Human Performance

Ecology of Human Performance (EHP) can provide a focus for interventions at the person, context, or task level with a goal of enhancing occupational performance. The model uses five intervention approaches with a focus at each level: establish and restore (person), alter (context), adapt/modify (context or task), and prevent (primary intervention approach) (Cole & Tufano, 2020).

30.8.3 Kawa River Model and Occupational Justice

As the occupational therapy profession moves toward its community roots, theories that examine social determinants of health and analyze access and justice to occupations are critical lenses with which to support groups of older adults who most often live within communities. Social determinants of health are the conditions with which people live, work, play, and worship, whereby poor conditions compounding over time result in the manifestation of disease (Thornton et al., 2016).

The Kawa River Model (Iwama, 2006) uses river imagery to represent life flow and priorities (water), obstacles and challenges (rocks), assets and liabilities (driftwood), and environments (riverbed/walls). The role of the occupational therapy practitioner in collaboration with the client is to create space for an unimpeded flow. While the Kawa model has been traditionally applied to individuals, the model is especially helpful in understanding barriers to access and justice for older adults in the community.

Occupational Justice (Townsend & Wilcock, 2004) considers that people are occupational and social beings with the right to engage in meaningful occupations. Addressing societal constraints that limit access to participation in occupation is understood as a means to health, well-being, and survival, and empowers individuals and communities. Kawa and occupational justice provide powerful understanding of the complex public health phenomenon that baby boomers (post-WWII child boom era, born between 1946 and 1964) are embarking upon.

30.8.4 Knowledge to Action

Knowledge translation, implementation science, and team science (collectively called translational science) have emerged as a critical aspect of health care delivery. It takes an average of 17 years for research in health care to make its way into practice (Westfall et al., 2007). While not designed as an occupational therapy/science theory, the Knowledge to Action model is a useful tool for occupational therapy practitioners to embed evidence into practice and understand the impact of their interventions (Straus et al., 2013). When strategically combined with occupation-based theories, models, and frameworks, Knowledge to Action can ensure that clinicians adopt and implement occupation-based interventions that generate lasting outcomes for populations, groups, and individuals.

30.9 Conclusion

This chapter described the challenges related to the aging process, including stereotypes of personal factors (e.g., agism, misogyny) and age-related changes associated with client factors (e.g., musculoskeletal) that impact function. Common health conditions related to late adulthood were also discussed in terms of the older adult's performance skills, environmental factors, and the relationship to functional ability. Next, the occupations of late adulthood were described within the context of the OTPF – 4th Edition. The described occupations highlight the risks related to the aging process and health conditions. Opportunities for occupational therapy practitioners to collaborate with clients to address the challenges that affect meaningful and necessary occupations of late adulthood were described. Finally, theories that support therapeutic intervention for older adults were presented.

Occupational therapy practitioners must understand and address an individual's physical and mental health, the social and physical contexts they experience, and the ways in which older people ascribe meaning and purpose to their lives. It is this holistic and person-centered approach that allows for a culturally appropriate collaboration of therapeutic intervention that can lead to empowered aging and the best possible quality of life for clients.

30.10 Summary

- Occupational therapists have the capacity to address normal age-related changes as well as chronic conditions that restrict participation.
- Tailored, strengths-based interventions may lead to outcomes that improve function, address environmental barriers, enhance safety and participation, and, ultimately, improve quality of life.
- Evidence-based interventions that draw from occupation-based theory, the OTPF, and implementation/translational health science allow for occupational therapists to develop approaches related to the person, environment, and/or occupation from the micro through to the macro level, reinforcing the importance of a theoretical lens and offering opportunities for dissemination and scaling up.

30.11 Review Questions

1. Functional occupational performance changes related to the aging process occur in which body systems?
2. Older adults who experience illness or chronic disease may experience challenges in which areas?

3. Describe the opportunities for older adults who seek occupational therapy services. By participating in occupational therapy intervention, older adults may be able to do what?
4. Which theory most closely aligns with the occupational therapy intervention approaches *establish and restore, alter, adapt/modify, prevent*?

References

American Occupational Therapy Association. (2017). Vision 2025. *American Journal of Occupational Therapy, 71*(3), 7412410010p1 -7412410010p87. https://doi.org/10.5014/ajot.2017.713002

American Occupational Therapy Association. (2020). Occupational Therapy Practice Framework: Domain and process (4th ed.). *American Journal of Occupational Therapy, 74*(Supplement 2), 7412410010p1–7412410010p87. https://doi.org/10.5014/ajot.2020.74S2001

Annear, M., Keeling, S., Wilkinson, T. I. M., Cushman, G., Gidlow, B. O. B., & Hopkins, H. (2014). Environmental influences on healthy and active ageing: A systematic review. *Ageing & Society, 34*(4), 590–622. https://doi.org/10.1017/S0144686X1200116X

Au, A., Lai, D. W. L., Yip, H.-M., Chan, S., Lai, S., Chaudhury, H., Scharlach, A., & Leeson, G. (2020). Sense of community mediating between age-friendly characteristics and life satisfaction of community-dwelling older adults. *Frontiers in Psychology, 11*, 86. https://doi.org/10.3389/fpsyg.2020.00086

Balog, E. (2021). Sleep: Awakening to the opportunities for occupational therapy practitioners. *SIS Quarterly Practice Connections*, 15–17.

Bandura, A. (1997). *Self-efficacy: The exercise of control*. W H Freeman/Times Books/ Henry Holt & Co.

Berger, S., Escher, A., Mengle, E., & Sullivan, N. (2018). Effectiveness of health promotion, management, and maintenance interventions within the scope of occupational therapy for community-dwelling older adults: A systematic review. *American Journal of Occupational Therapy, 72*(4), 7204190010p1–7204190010p10. https://doi.org/10.5014/ajot.2018.030346

Binette, J., & Vasold, K. (2018). Home and community preferences: A National Survey of Adults Age 18-Plus. *AARP Research; Issues & Topics: Livable Communities.* https://doi.org/10.26419/res.00231.001

Black, K., Dobbs, D., & Young, T. L. (2015). Aging in community: Mobilizing a new paradigm of older adults as a core social resource. *Journal of Applied Gerontology, 34*(2), 219–243. https://doi.org/10.1177/0733464812463984

Bolt, M., Ikking, T., Baaijen, R., & Saenger, S. (2019). Occupational therapy and primary care. *Primary Health Care Research & Development, 20*, e27. https://doi.org/10.1017/s1463423618000452

Bonder, B. R., & Dal Bello-Haas, V. (2018). *Functional performance in older adults*. F. A. Davis.

Bronfenbrenner, U. (1986). Ecology of the family as a context for human development: Research perspectives. *Developmental Psychology, 22*(6), 723–742. https://doi.org/10.1037/0012-1649.22.6.723

Cagney, K. A., Browning, C. R., Jackson, A. L., & Soller, B. (2013). Networks, neighborhoods, and institutions: An integrated "activity space" approach for research on aging. In J. Waite & T. J. Plewes (Eds.), *New directions in the sociology of aging* (pp. 151–174). National Academies Press.

Centers for Disease Control and Prevention. (2022). *About chronic diseases*. https://www.cdc.gov/chronicdisease/about/index.htm

Cho, M., & Kim, J. (2016). Coupling urban regeneration with age-friendliness: Neighborhood regeneration in Jangsu Village, Seoul. *Cities, 58*, 107–114. https://doi.org/10.1016/j.cities.2016.05.019

Cogan, A. M., & Carlson, M. (2018). Deciphering participation: An interpretive synthesis of its meaning and application in rehabilitation. *Disability and Rehabilitation, 40*(22), 2692–2703. https://doi.org/10.1080/09638288.2017.1342282

Cohen, M. A., & Tavares, J. (2020). Who are the most at-risk older adults in the COVID-19 Era? It's not just those in nursing homes. *Journal of Aging & Social Policy, 32*(4–5), 380–386. https://doi.org/10.1080/08959420.2020.1764310

Cole, M. B., & Tufano, R. (2020). *Applied theories in occupational therapy: A practical approach* (2nd ed.). SLACK Inc.

Colten, H. R., & Altevogt, B. M. (2006). Extent and health consequences of chronic sleep loss and sleep disorders. In H. R. Colten & B. M. Altevogt (Eds.), *Sleep disorders and sleep deprivation: An unmet public health problem* (pp. 55–135). National Academies Press.

de Wit, L., Fenenga, C., Giammarchi, C., di Furia, L., Hutter, I., de Winter, A., & Meijering, L. (2017). Community-based initiatives improving critical health literacy: a systematic review and meta-synthesis of qualitative evidence. *BMC Public Health, 18*(1), 40. https://doi.org/10.1186/s12889-017-4570-7

Duncan, E. A. (2020). *Foundations for practice in occupational therapy*. Elsevier Health Sciences.

Dupuis-Blanchard, S., Gould, O. N., Gibbons, C., Simard, M., Éthier, S., & Villalon, L. (2015). Strategies for Aging in Place: The Experience of Language-Minority Seniors with Loss of Independence. *Global Qualitative Nursing Research, 2*, 2333393614565187. https://doi.org/10.1177/2333393614565187European Commission. (2019). *Ageing Europe. Looking at the lives of older people in the EU: 2019 edition. Statistical books*. Publications Office of the European Union.

Flett, G. L., & Heisel, M. J. (2021). Aging and feeling valued versus expendable during the COVID-19 pandemic and beyond: A review and commentary of why mattering is fundamental to the health and well-being of older adults. *International Journal of Mental Health and Addiction, 19*(6), 2443–2469. https://doi.org/10.1007/s11469-020-00339-4

Flores, R., Caballer, A., & Alarcón, A. (2019). Evaluation of an age-friendly city and its effect on life satisfaction: A two-stage study. *International Journal of Environmental Research and Public Health, 16*(24), 5073. https://doi.org/10.3390/ijerph16245073

Fortuna, J., Riddering, A., Shuster, L., & Lopez-Jeng, C. (2021). Assessment of modified patient education materials for people with age-related macular degeneration. *BMC Ophthamology, 20*, 391. https://doi.org/10.1186/s12886-020-01664-x

Garner, R., Tanuseputro, P., Manuel, D. G., & Sanmartin, C. (2018). Transitions to long-term and residential care among older Canadians. *Health Reports, 29*(5), 13–23. https://www150.statcan.gc.ca/n1/en/catalogue/82-003-X201800554966

Gitlin, L. N., Szanton, S. L., & Hodgson, N. A. (2013). It's complicated-but doable: The right supports can enable elders with complex conditions to successfully age in community. *Generations, 37*(4), 51–61. https://www.jstor.org/stable/26556011

Green, H., Fernandez, R., & MacPhail, C. (2022). Well-being and social determinants of health among Australian adults: A national cross-sectional study. *Health & Social Care in the Community, 30*(6), e4345–e4354. https://doi.org/10.1111/hsc.13827

Grenier, M.-L. (2020). Cultural competency and the reproduction of White supremacy in occupational therapy education. *Health Education Journal, 79*(6), 633–644. https://doi.org/10.1177/0017896920902515

Grover, A., & Joshi, A. (2014). An overview of chronic disease models: a systematic literature review. *Global Journal of Health Science, 7*(2), 210–227. https://doi.org/10.5539/gjhs.v7n2p210

Hammel, J., Magasi, S., Heinemann, A., Whiteneck, G., Bogner, J., & Rodriguez, E. (2008). What does participation mean? An insider perspective from people with disabilities. *Disability and Rehabilitation, 30*(19), 1445–1460. https://doi.org/10.1080/09638280701625534

Iwama, M. K. (2006). *The Kawa model: Culturally relevant occupational therapy*. Elsevier Health Sciences.

Jansson, B. S. (2015). *Social welfare policy and advocacy: Advancing social justice through 8 policy sectors*. SAGE Publications.

Jansson, I. (2020). Occupation and basic income through the lens of Arendt's vita activa. *Journal of Occupational Science*, 27(1), 125–137. https://doi.org/10.1080/14427591.2019.1646161

John, D. H., & Gunter, K. (2016). engAGE in community: Using mixed methods to mobilize older people to elucidate the age-friendly attributes of urban and rural places. *Journal of Applied Gerontology*, 35(10), 1095–1120. https://doi.org/10.1177/0733464814566679

Kotwal, A. A., Holt-Lunstad, J., Newmark, R. L., Cenzer, I., Smith, A. K., Covinsky, K. E., Escueta, D. P., Lee, J. M., & Perissinotto, C. M. (2021). Social isolation and loneliness among San Francisco Bay Area older adults during the COVID-19 Shelter-in-Place Orders. *Journal of the American Geriatrics Society*, 69(1), 20–29. https://doi.org/10.1111/jgs.16865

Lawton, M. P., & Nahemow, L. (1973). Ecology and the aging process. In C. Eisdorfer & M. P. Lawton (Eds.), *The psychology of adult development and aging* (pp. 619–674). American Psychological Association. https://doi.org/10.1037/10044-020

Lehning A. J. (2012). City governments and aging in place: community design, transportation and housing innovation adoption. *The Gerontologist*, 52(3), 345–356. https://doi.org/10.1093/geront/gnr089

Levasseur, M., Généreux, M., Bruneau, J. F., Vanasse, A., Chabot, É., Beaulac, C., & Bédard, M. M. (2015). Importance of proximity to resources, social support, transportation and neighborhood security for mobility and social participation in older adults: Results from a scoping study. *BMC Public Health*, 15, 503. https://doi.org/10.1186/s12889-015-1824-0

Li, S. (2020). Living environment, mobility, and wellbeing among seniors in the United States: A new interdisciplinary dialogue. *Journal of Planning Literature*, 35(3), 298–314. https://doi.org/10.1177/0885412220914993

Lucas, C., & Washington, S. (2020). Understanding systemic racism in the United States: Educating our students and ourselves. Continuing education article, CEA1020. American Occupational Therapy Association.

Luppa, M., Luck, T., Weyerer, S., König, H. H., Brähler, E., & Riedel-Heller, S. G. (2010). Prediction of institutionalization in the elderly. A systematic review. *Age and Ageing*, 39(1), 31–38. https://doi.org/10.1093/ageing/afp202

Mah, J. C., Stevens, S. J., Keefe, J. M., Rockwood, K., & Andrew, M. K. (2021). Social factors influencing utilization of home care in community-dwelling older adults: A scoping review. *BMC Geriatrics*, 21(1), 145. https://doi.org/10.1186/s12877-021-02069-1

Menec, V. H., Means, R., Keating, N., Parkhurst, G., & Eales, J. (2011). Conceptualizing age-friendly communities. *Canadian Journal on Aging*, 30(3), 479–493. https://doi.org/10.1017/S0714980811000237

Michie, S., van Stralen, M. M., & West, R. (2011). The behaviour change wheel: A new method for characterising and designing behaviour change interventions. *Implementation science: IS*, 6, 42. https://doi.org/10.1186/1748-5908-6-42

Mitchell, S. E., Laurens, V., Weigel, G. M., Hirschman, K. B., Scott, A. M., Nguyen, H. Q., Howard, J. M., Laird, L., Levine, C., & Davis, T. C. (2018). Care transitions from patient and caregiver perspectives. *The Annals of Family Medicine*, 16(3), 225–231. https://doi.org/10.1370/afm.2222

Miyashita, T., Tadaka, E., & Arimoto, A. (2021). Cross-sectional study of individual and environmental factors associated with life-space mobility among community-dwelling independent older people. *Environmental Health and Preventive Medicine*, 26(1), 9. https://doi.org/10.1186/s12199-021-00936-2

Morley, J. E. (2015). Aging successfully: The key to aging in place. *Journal of the American Medical Directors Association*, 16(12), 1005–1007. https://doi.org/10.1016/j.jamda.2015.09.011

Moulaert, T., & Garon, S. (2016). *Age-friendly cities and communities in international comparison: Political lessons, scientific avenues, and democratic issues*. Springer Link.

Narushima, M., & Kawabata, M. (2020). "Fiercely independent": Experiences of aging in the right place of older women living alone with physical limitations. *Journal of Aging Studies, 54*, 100875. https://doi.org/10.1016/j.jaging.2020.100875

Norton, S., Matthews, F. E., Barnes, D. E., Yaffe, K., & Brayne, C. (2014). Potential for primary prevention of Alzheimer's disease: An analysis of population-based data. *The Lancet Neurology, 13*(8), 788–794. https://doi.org/10.1016/S1474-4422(14)70136-X

Paillard-Borg, S., Wang, H.-X., Winblad, B., & Fratiglioni, L. (2009). Pattern of participation in leisure activities among older people in relation to their health conditions and contextual factors: A survey in a Swedish urban area. *Ageing and Society, 29*(5), 803–821. https://doi.org/10.1017/s0144686x08008337

Palmore, E. (2015). Ageism comes of age. *The Journals of Gerontology Series B: Psychological Sciences and Social Sciences, 70*(6), 873–875. https://doi.org/10.1093/geronb/gbv079

Papageorgiou, N., Marquis, R., Dare, J., & Batten, R. (2016). Occupational therapy and occupational participation in community dwelling older adults: A review of the evidence. *Physical & Occupational Therapy in Geriatrics, 34*(1), 21–42. https://doi.org/10.3109/02703181.2015.1109014

Rebeiro, K. L., & Polgar, J. M. (1999). Enabling occupational performance: optimal experiences in therapy. *Canadian Journal of Occupational Therapy, 66*(1), 14–22. https://doi.org/10.1177/000841749906600102

Rosenwohl-Mack, A., Schumacher, K., Fang, M. L., & Fukuoka, Y. (2020). A new conceptual model of experiences of aging in place in the United States: Results of a systematic review and meta-ethnography of qualitative studies. *International Journal of Nursing Studies, 103*, 103496. https://doi.org/10.1016/j.ijnurstu.2019.103496

Sabia, J. J. (2008). There's no place like home: A hazard model analysis of aging in place among older homeowners in the PSID. *Research on Aging, 30*(1), 3–35. https://doi.org/10.1177/0164027507307919

Smallfield, S., & Molitor, W. L. (2018). Occupational therapy interventions supporting social participation and leisure engagement for community-dwelling older adults: A systematic review. *American Journal of Occupational Therapy, 72*(4), 7204190020p1–7204190021p8. https://doi.org/10.5014/ajot.2018.030627

Sorrell J. M. (2021). Losing a generation: The impact of COVID-19 on older Americans. *Journal of Psychosocial Nursing and Mental Health Services, 59*(4), 9–12. https://doi.org/10.3928/02793695-20210315-03

Straus, S. E., Tetroe, J., & Graham, I. D. (2013). *Knowledge translation in health care: Moving from evidence to practice*. Wiley.

Sturmberg, J., & Martin, C. (2013). *Handbook of systems and complexity in health*. Springer.

Sverker, A., Thyberg, I., Valtersson, E., Björk, M., Hjalmarsson, S., & Östlund, G. (2020). Time to update the ICF by including socioemotional qualities of participation? The development of a "patient ladder of participation" based on interview data of people with early rheumatoid arthritis (the Swedish TIRA study). *Disability and Rehabilitation, 42*(9), 1212–1219. https://doi.org/10.1080/09638288.2018.1518494

Szanton, S. L., Thorpe, R. J., Boyd, C., Tanner, E. K., Leff, B., Agree, E., Xue, Q. L., Allen, J. K., Seplaki, C. L., Weiss, C. O., Guralnik, J. M., & Gitlin, L. N. (2011). Community aging in place, advancing better living for elders: a bio-behavioral-environmental intervention to improve function and health-related quality of life in disabled older adults. *Journal of the American Geriatrics Society, 59*(12), 2314–2320. https://doi.org/10.1111/j.1532-5415.2011.03698.x

Thornton, R. L., Glover, C. M., Cené, C. W., Glik, D. C., Henderson, J. A., & Williams, D. R. (2016). Evaluating strategies for reducing health disparities by addressing the social determinants of health. *Health Affairs, 35*(8), 1416–1423. https://doi.org/10.1377/hlthaff.2015.1357

Townsend, E., & Wilcock, A. (2004). Occupational justice and client-centred practice: A dialogue in progress. *Canadian Journal of Occupational Therapy, 71*(2), 75–87. https://doi.org/10.1177/000841740407100203

Üstün, T. B., Kostanjsek, N., Chatterji, S., & Rehm, J. (2010). *Measuring health and disability: Manual for WHO disability assessment schedule WHODAS 2.0*. World Health Organization.

Versey, H. S. (2018). A tale of two Harlems: Gentrification, social capital, and implications for aging in place. *Social Science & Medicine, 214*, 1–11. https://doi.org/10.1016/j.socscimed.2018.07.024

Walker, A. (2016). Population ageing from a global and theoretical perspective: European lessons on active ageing. In T. Moulaert & S. Garon (Eds.), *Age-friendly cities and communities in international comparison: Political lessons, scientific avenues and democratic issues* (pp. 47–64). Springer. https://doi.org/10.1007/978-3-319-24031-2_4

Watchorn, V., Hitch, D., Grant, C., Tucker, R., Aedy, K., Ang, S., & Frawley, P. (2021). An integrated literature review of the current discourse around universal design in the built environment – is occupation the missing link?. *Disability and Rehabilitation, 43*(1), 1–12. https://doi.org/10.1080/09638288.2019.1612471

Westfall, J. M., Mold, J., & Fagnan, L. (2007). Practice-based research: "Blue highways" on the NIH roadmap. *JAMA, 297*(4), 403. https://doi.org/10.1001/jama.297.4.403

World Health Organization. (2007). *Global age-friendly cities: A guide*. https://iris.who.int/handle/10665/43755

World Health Organization. (2015). *World report on ageing and health*. World Health Organization.

Wu, H. C., & Tseng, M. H. (2018). Evaluating disparities in elderly community care resources: Using a geographic accessibility and inequality index. *International Journal of Environmental Research and Public Health, 15*(7), 1353. https://doi.org/10.3390/ijerph15071353

Wyman, M. F., Shiovitz-Ezra, S., & Bengel, J. (2018). Ageism in the health care system: Providers, patients, and systems. In A. Ayalon & C. Tesch-Römer (Eds.), *Contemporary perspectives on ageism. International Perspectives on Aging*, volume 19. Springer. https://doi.org/10.1007/978-3-319-73820-8_13

CHAPTER 31

Future Considerations and Conclusion

Sharon Gutman and Ted Brown

Abstract
Humans are occupational beings and are shaped by the occupations to which they have access in a society. Access to occupational participation is commonly influenced by such social factors as race, ethnicity, socioeconomic and educational levels, gender, and gender orientation. Occupational participation is also influenced by occupations that are sanctioned and censured by the larger society in which humans live. This concluding chapter explores the social issues that impact occupational participation in Western society, including systemic racism, social intolerance, colonization, gender inequality, homophobia, agism, mental health stigmatization, and biased health care systems. It is anticipated that future occupational therapists will attempt to equalize disparities in health and social care delivery through bias-free strategies, inviting service recipients to be collaborators instead of passive receivers of care, providing services within the community to increase care accessibility, and addressing mental health challenges in all practice settings.

Authors' Positionality Statements: see Chapter 1, Section 1.9

Objectives
This chapter will allow the reader to:

- Understand that access to such commodities as effective public-school systems; safe neighborhoods; secure, livable-wage employment; bias-free, affordable health care; and technology, impacts one's occupational opportunities and participation.
- Understand that occupational access is also greatly influenced by one's race, ethnicity, educational level, socioeconomic status, ability status, age, gender, and gender orientation.

- Understand that humans are shaped by occupations that are sanctioned and censured by the larger society in which they live.
- Understand how social problems embedded in Western society erupted into mass consciousness during the global COVID-19 pandemic through increased awareness of systemic racism, social intolerance, cultural insensitivity, colonization, gender inequality, homophobia, mental health stigmatization, employment and income insecurity, and biased health care systems.
- Understand how future generations of occupational therapists will likely become more occupation-focused and community-based; routinely learn and use bias-free, culturally sensitive, inclusive strategies to equalize care for all recipients and their families; view service recipients as equal collaborators instead of passive receivers of care; and address mental health challenges in all practice areas.

Key terms
- systems of racism and agism
- stigmatization of mental illness
- racial, economic, and occupational injustice
- gender inequality and patriarchal oppression
- inaccessible and inequitable health and social care
- social intolerance and cultural insensitivity
- occupational access, opportunities, participation, and dissonance

31.1 Introduction

Humans are occupational beings and are shaped by the occupations that are available in their environments, cultures, societies, and families. The availability of occupations and the opportunities for occupational participation are also governed by whether people live in wealthy countries with access to capital assets and technology, or poorer developing nations with fewer needed resources. Occupational participation is additionally influenced by whether people are members of traditionally privileged groups having access to a greater array of occupational opportunities, particularly those requiring financial means, or members of marginalized, disadvantaged groups having far less access and even systemic restrictions to occupational opportunities. Occupational access is also greatly influenced by one's race, ethnicity, cultural background, educational level, ability status, age, socioeconomic status, gender, and gender orientation. Although Western capitalistic societies often promote the idea that anyone who works hard enough can become successful, historians and scholars have shown that societies embed overt and concealed restrictions on occupational access based on race, ethnicity, ability status, educational and socioeconomic level, gender, and gender orientation (Christian, 2019). In the West, dominant privileged groups have traditionally been white, male, well-educated, wealthy, able-bodied, and heterosexual. Today, this group

FUTURE CONSIDERATIONS AND CONCLUSION

continues to hold and control the highest amount of global wealth, political power, social privilege, and access to desired occupational opportunities (Moss et al., 2020).

Humans are also shaped by occupations that are both sanctioned and censured by the larger society in which they live. Such occupations are influenced by ethical values, belief systems, social norms and customs, political and educational systems, and the ethos which federal governments have established for their citizens. We grow up in a social culture that has already endorsed specific activities as appropriate or inappropriate for our age, gender, religious beliefs, ability-status, and socioeconomic level. When occupations endorsed by the larger society are not congruent with our own preferences, interests, or innate sense of self, we experience occupational dissonance. We may feel excluded from the larger society, feel devalued and demeaned, and eventually seek a community of similar others through which our collective voice generates greater political power. We may also engage in societally condemned activities – such as theft, drug use, violence toward others, or prostitution – if the environment in which we live does not support our basic needs for food, shelter, safety, education, income, and well-being. When the environment does not provide effective public schools; opportunities for secure, livable-wage employment; fair and bias-free protection from law enforcement agencies; and safe neighborhoods, few opportunities exist for advancement through education; steady and stable employment; home ownership; and the ability to create a safety net of financial savings. A lack of the most basic opportunities needed for daily living creates desperation. In such situations, people may turn to societally condemned, illicit, or illegal occupations for survival and as a means to cope with hopelessness.

This textbook dissected and examined human occupation through the various lenses of developmental and lifespan theories, cultural perspectives, gender ideologies, and critical race theory – acknowledging that all influence both the occupations to which we have access and to which we feel innately drawn or repelled. In a broad sense, human occupation and occupational participation have been considered through a lens of intersectionality with regard to race, socioeconomic status, gender, gender orientation, and presence of disability as a set of interconnected variables that shape and influence a person's occupational access and opportunities. The book also attempted to deconstruct and examine traditional Western perspectives of occupational participation from an international, global perspective. In doing so, human occupation and occupational participation were explored through the contemporary issues of decolonization, environmental sustainability, globalization, technology, disability rights, gender diversity and equality, and racial equity.

31.2 The Global COVID-19 Pandemic: Impact on Occupational Function and Participation

Perhaps more than any other singular world event in recent history, the worldwide pandemic brought us together as an international community. It also forced us to view each other as members of the global human family having the same experience of fear, anxiety, loss, illness, isolation, and restriction of daily life activities – instead of humans divided by social, economic, religious, cultural, and political borders with little in common. The COVID-19 pandemic brought about dysfunction in our occupational participation and patterns, forced severe activity limitations for prolonged periods, and eroded the social connections that maintained our well-being as socially connected creatures. However, while the pandemic generated novel experiences of dysfunction brought about by lockdowns and activity restrictions, it also heightened our awareness of societal problems surreptitiously and covertly embedded in Western society. The protracted periods of in-home confinement and sheltering in place left us with hours of time alone with our own thoughts, free from the distractions of typical daily life, as well as hours of time spent watching the drama of daily events unfold on 24-hour cable news and internet.

31.3 Racism: Diversity, Inequity, Exclusion, Injustice

In the United States, the murder of George Floyd in May 2020 while in police custody had become a national outrage, fueling protests across the country, and propelling momentum of the Black Lives Matter Movement (Boudreau et al., 2022). The murder of George Floyd, a Black man living in an impoverished area of Minneapolis, Minnesota, was the breaking point for and final affront to a Black community that had witnessed too many deaths of its community members over decades at the hands of police officers. Not since the Civil Rights Movement of the 1960s had the country been forced to look deeply at and confront its systems of racism and barriers to equality among Black and Brown communities (e.g., African American, West Indian, Jamaican, Hispanic, Latinx, and Mexican). Ineffective public-school systems; unsafe crime-ridden neighborhoods; lack of livable-wage, secure employment opportunities; deterrents to saving and transferring wealth to future generations; and mass incarceration of Black and Brown males became understood by the larger society as socially embedded systems that maintained the Western subjugation of Black and Brown communities over centuries (Delgado & Stefancic, 2017) (see Figure 31.1).

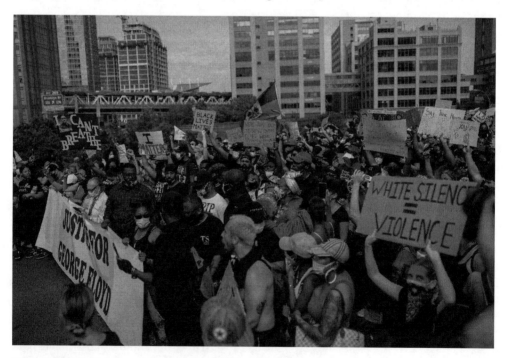

Figure 31.1 Protestors of systemic racism and the murder of George Floyd in police custody, New York City.

Source: Photo by Life Matters, pexels.com.

The adverse impact of colonization by dominant White, Western societies, however, was not isolated to Black and Brown cultures throughout the world. First Nation and indigenous peoples living for centuries in both global hemispheres were slaughtered; removed from tribal and ancestral lands; forced to live in segregated and unfertile regions; and stripped of civil rights and opportunities for income, health care, and education (Emery-Whittington, 2021). The decimation of First Nation peoples under the guise of White colonization was a genocide that continues to negatively affect the welfare of such groups today. In the United States, Canada, and Australia, it is estimated that 25%–30% of First Nation people live in poverty without access to secure, livable-wage employment or adequate health care and education (Allam, 2020; Canadian Centre for Policy Alternatives, 2022; Northwestern University Institute for Policy Research, 2020). Like Black and Brown communities worldwide, the COVID-19 pandemic disproportionately affected First Nation people who already lacked access to needed health care and were not included in the development of recovery policies, or consulted to address culturally appropriate recovery measures (United Nations, 2021a). First Nation communities that were already ravaged by White colonization have been further devastated by the global pandemic in ways that may be impossible to fully recover from.

31.4 Mental Health Stigmatization
The COVID-19 pandemic also challenged Western societies to confront the stigmatization of mental illness, the societal conditions that contribute to high levels of mental health concerns, including depression and substance use, and the lack of resources allotted to provide public health assistance. In Western society, the stigmatization of mental illness manifests through a significant economic disparity in health care coverage for physical versus mental health conditions, with physical conditions 5.2 times more likely to be covered than mental health conditions (King, 2019). Societal stigmatization also manifests as ridicule of people who need or seek care for mental health conditions, with the resultant effect of hindering people from attaining needed care or causing them to hide their care from others. During the pandemic, adults of all races reporting depression and/or anxiety rose 30%, from 11% in 2019 to 41% in 2021 (Panchal et al., 2021). Black and Brown adults were disproportionately affected by mental health concerns with 48% of Black and 46% of Brown adults reporting depression and/or anxiety in 2021. Similar to adults, adolescents of all races reporting feelings of depression or sadness increased 10% between 2009 and 2019, from 26.1% in 2009 to 36.7% in 2020. During the pandemic, the percentage of adolescents attempting to manage depression or sadness increased to 44.2%. The percentage of adolescents considering suicide increased from 13.8% in 2009 to 18.8% in 2019; at the height of the pandemic this figure rose to 20% (Jones et al., 2022).

While it is likely the pandemic worsened feelings of depression, sadness, and suicidal ideation in both adolescents and adults due to social isolation and financial concerns, it is equally as likely mental health conditions were underreported prior to the pandemic due to stigmatization. One positive outcome of the pandemic was the willingness of the larger society to acknowledge and accept mental health problems as legitimate and worthy of treatment. Public health announcements were routinely made encouraging people to seek assistance for feelings of depression and suicidality, and hotlines and virtual clinics were established to serve people desiring help (Tausch et al.,

2022). While this sanctioning of mental health concerns heightened public awareness, lessened stigmatization, and enhanced treatment accessibility, it also forced the larger society to examine societal attitudes and occupations that may erode mental health and well-being. During the pandemic, research examining social media usage revealed higher rates of depression and suicidality among youth of both genders (Jones et al., 2022), and clear links were made between female adolescents' use of social media and the prevalence of eating disorders (Gómez-Castillo et al., 2022). Depression and suicidality in adults were similarly linked to loss of employment, loss of home, and major traumatic life events such as victimization, domestic abuse, divorce, and death of a partner (Panchal et al., 2021).

31.5 Capitalism and Work

The pandemic, along with its requirements for lockdowns and sheltering in place, also forced millions of workers to begin working remotely from their homes. At least two primary occurrences resulted. One was that, although working remotely further reduced social connectedness, workers became aware that with the availability of technology, the need to be physically present at a worksite for eight hours a day, five days a week, was often unnecessary and even burdensome. Workers questioned the necessity for costly and lengthy daily work commutes, and the need to live within proximity to highly congested and expensive urban areas for employment. Environmentalists brought our attention to significantly reduced polluted atmospheres and the appearance of blue skies over urban metropolises for the first time in decades, resulting from the temporary discontinuance of human transportation (e.g., cars, buses, planes, and trains).

Western societies, particularly after the Industrial Revolution, had routinely promoted the Protestant work ethic as aspirational and desirable. Working remotely, and the flexibility it brought, now encouraged workers to begin questioning the occupational imbalance of working 40 or more hours a week over an adult lifespan. Those workers who were deemed essential and required to be physically present on site feared contracting the COVID-19 virus and risking their own and their family's lives. For various reasons which are still being examined, COVID-19 disproportionately affected disadvantaged, Black, and Brown communities (Golestaneh et al., 2020), and anger erupted over Western capitalistic societies that appeared to treat workers, particularly essential workers, as disposable commodities rather than as valued citizens. Likewise, the pandemic also negatively impacted a larger proportion of members of the disability community in comparison to the general public at large. Individuals with a physical, developmental, intellectual, or psychosocial disability had been historically disenfranchised and segregated from the workforce but are now actively making their collective voice heard to secure their right to livable-wage, stable employment in Western capitalistic societies. The COVID-19 pandemic brought social, racial, age, disability, gender, and cultural injustice and inequity to the forefront of our collective awareness.

A second major work-related occurrence resulting from the pandemic was the worldwide loss of employment affecting society's most marginalized. At the height of the pandemic, the United Nations (2021b) reported that over 200 million people worldwide had lost employment. Women, youth, older adults, people with a disability, and Black and Brown communities disproportionately sustained the highest economic losses from pandemic-related unemployment and many lost homes and became food insecure.

FUTURE CONSIDERATIONS AND CONCLUSION

The disparity between those living paycheck-to-paycheck whose daily survival became threatened by the pandemic's economic upheaval, and those who were financially protected by upper echelon corporate positions (and who were largely white, privileged males), became magnified as another societal problem of racial, economic, social, and occupational injustice. Anger further erupted over Western capitalism's greed, systemic racism, ableism, and gender inequality that have relegated the most vulnerable of our society to insecure, low-paying jobs over a lifetime.

With regard to gender, women faired far worse during the pandemic, both sustaining greater job losses and having to leave the workforce because of childcare and child education responsibilities (Carli, 2020). Those who were able to work remotely expressed concerns about the undue burden of having full-time employment and attempting to assist with their children's remote learning and home schooling (see Figure 31.2). Approximately 1.1 million female workers in the United States left the workforce during the pandemic to assume caregiver responsibilities (Gonzales, 2022). Women earn approximately 80 cents to every dollar earned by men, with Black and Brown women earning approximately 70 cents (Barroso & Brown, 2022). The occupational injustice of earning unequal pay for the same work as men while having to balance childcare further highlighted Western society's problems of gender inequality, racism, and occupational imbalance.

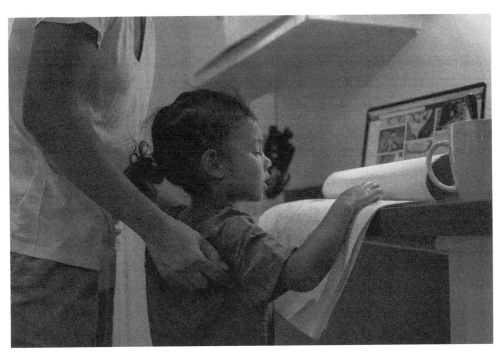

Figure 31.2 Women faired far worse during the pandemic, both sustaining greater job losses and having to leave the workforce because of childcare and child education responsibilities.

Source: Photo by Kamaji Ogino, pexels.com.

31.6 Technology and Occupation

For many, the protracted lockdowns and sheltering in place were experienced as isolating and served to diminish feelings of wellness and increase thoughts of hopelessness and powerlessness. For others, the prolonged periods of sequestering afforded a slower lifestyle pace, a chance to pause and reflect, and an enhanced awareness that Western society promotes occupational overload involving constant stimulation, cyber over-connectivity, information saturation, sensory sensitivity, and overactivity. We have become a society of multi-taskers and the proverbial city that never sleeps. With 24-hour cable television; internet connectivity; social media accessibility; and online shopping, banking, food ordering, and entertainment, we are infrequently left without activity in our waking hours. Rarely do we need to search long for something to occupy our attention – text messages, email, internet surfing, social media engagement, blogging, binge-viewing TV series, ordering food – the list is endless. But the list of activities is also superficial and may serve to erode our skills for the sustained attention needed to accomplish activities requiring higher level analytical, creative, critical thought processes. The impact of multi-tasking and split-tasking on higher order cognitive skills, often associated with high levels of screen-time use, may reduce efficiency and performance.

Technology has made our physical lives less stressful, but it has also intensified the pace of life and fragmented our social connections and support systems. Technology has enhanced our physical lives while paradoxically increasing anxiety about our ability to maintain occupational balance that supports well-being, formulates occupational roles through which we can meaningfully connect with others, and develops patterns of occupational participation that foster our resilience and perseverance. Technology usage has been shown to both promote and impede people's social determinants of health. As our industrialized technologies have polluted our oceans, lands, and skies, we must also ask if our technological occupations support environmental sustainability or the Western destruction of natural world resources embedded in the ideology that humans sit at the top of the evolutionary tree and no other life form in the natural world is as sacrosanct. Technologies that dissolve our connection to the natural world and pollute our lands and bodies may not in fact be signs of civilization's advancement, but rather indicative of Western ignorance and ethnocentrism.

31.7 Paradigm Shift in the Profession's Occupational Lens

Today, as a result of global events in previous years, Western society has become more aware of the need to acknowledge and support diversity, equity, and inclusion among all of its members. Voices of traditionally marginalized groups have become louder and have demanded not only recognition, but acknowledgment, of the trespasses, insensitivities, and injustices committed against such communities by a dominant white, heterosexual, male patriarchy. No longer is a world perspective characterized by white male dominance and privilege accepted without question. But change from patriarchal oppression is slow and stymied by solidly embedded racist, ableist, misogynistic, and homophobic attitudes, behaviors, beliefs, norms, and practices.

Women are still fighting for equality all over the world, including the United States, where laws protecting women's reproductive rights have been progressively eroded and laws supporting equal pay have been continuously blocked by conservative male politicians (Tanne, 2022). After 50 years of federal reproductive rights protection, and the

FUTURE CONSIDERATIONS AND CONCLUSION

civil right of women to make self-determining decisions about their own bodies, the United States Supreme Court overturned Roe v. Wade in June 2022 and gave the determination of abortion legality back to individual states (Totenberg, 2022). Within less than a month of this decision, 20 of the 50 US states illegalized abortion and another 11 states set in motion legislation designed to ban it. Such control over women, and their occupational choices regarding sexual activity, birth control use, family planning, and economic pressure to either leave the workforce or obtain multiple jobs to support children because of unequal pay disparities, will have enormous impact on women's occupational participation for generations. Most impacted by the restriction of reproductive rights are women of color who cannot afford travel to states with protected abortion rights (see Figure 31.3).

The MeToo Movement, which gained validation globally, brought awareness to the widespread sexual assault and exploitation of women worldwide. It is estimated that

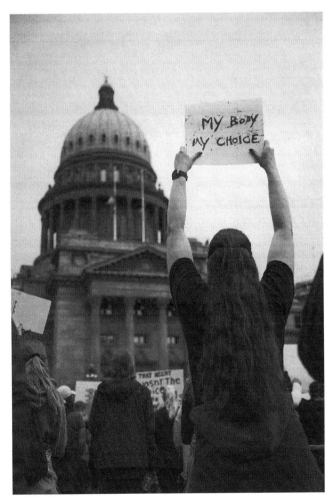

Figure 31.3 Protesters fighting for women's reproductive rights.

Source: Photo by Brett Sayles, pexels.com.

just under half a million women and girls continue to be assaulted each year in the United States (Morgan & Thompson, 2020). Although the Black Lives Matter Movement gained international recognition and commendation, Black and Brown communities continue to hold the highest rates of poverty in the world (Baker et al., 2021; Katayama & Wadhwa, 2019). Members of the disability community similarly continue to experience high rates of unemployment, varying levels of inclusivity from education and health care systems, and well entrenched ableist attitudes. While gender-diverse communities have gained greater acceptance with legal protections against housing and employment discrimination and the right to same-sex marriage in Western society, the white, heterosexual, conservative, male patriarchy holding political power are positioning the courts to reverse such decisions (Reinah, 2021). As a global society, people are striving for guidance to deal with the embedded problems that have erupted into conscious awareness.

The profession of occupational therapy, too, is struggling to deal with the societal problems and inequalities that have burgeoned into mass consciousness in recent years and called for systemic change in health and social care settings. It must be acknowledged that researchers have documented existing bias in the form of inaccessible and inequitable care among marginalized and disadvantaged groups (Lavizzo-Mourey et al., 2021). Occupational therapists are also challenged to provide care that is relevant and meaningful to service recipients and their families who do not fit within a dominant white, heteronormative culture. A paradigm shift is occurring in the profession's occupational lens that parallels society at large.

The generation of occupational therapists graduating in the ensuing years will not analyze occupation through a singular Western perspective but will understand occupational participation through a much broader frame of reference. Future occupational therapists will have an awareness of society's global problems and how those challenges impact the assumption of, and engagement in, occupational roles and performance. Poverty, inequality, the destruction of the world's natural resources, and the unequal division of resources and wealth among socioeconomic classes and countries will impact the way that therapists assess the supports and barriers of service recipients' occupational participation. Occupational therapy practitioners will routinely unearth and examine their own unconscious biases during their educational training and learn strategies to better provide bias-free care to all service recipients. Practitioners will also understand that the highest standard of care involves helping clients and their families to examine and adopt desired occupations that are most facilitative of their emotional health and self-actualization, rather than occupations that are societally sanctioned but violate a client's self-identity and self-determinism.

Occupational therapy practitioners will also be aware of the concept of intersectionality which refers to the "simultaneous experience of social categories such as race, gender, socioeconomic status, and sexual orientation and the ways in which these categories interact to create systems of oppression, domination, and discrimination" (Proctor et al., 2017, para 1). Intersectionality reflects the multi-faceted, cumulative lived experiences of marginalized individuals, families, and groups within society, and maintains that holding more than one of these identities can cause the experiences of oppression and discrimination to be additive. Intersectionality reminds occupational therapy practitioners to be cognizant of, and sensitive to, the potential intersection of service recipients' multiple identities and lived experiences, and the cumulative, intensified impact it can foster.

Future occupational therapists will also abandon the engrained Western overvaluing of individualism and independence, and will instead understand the importance of interdependence, commonality, dignity, and mutual respect in the establishment of social connection and well-being. The Western paradigm of the health care provider as an authority figure and the client as a passive recipient of care will be abandoned to achieve a more equalized and collaborative health care model. Service recipients and their families will be viewed as collaborators having life experience that cannot be replicated by health care providers with differing sociocultural backgrounds and life experiences.

Occupational therapy practitioners will also have an increased awareness of mental health issues and the need to address emotional and behavioral challenges in all care settings, including physical rehabilitation, the school system, and elder care. The profession will return to its strong roots in mental health intervention but armed with a 21st-century understanding of the societal triggers that propagate anxiety, depression, and substance use. Mental health intervention will become trauma-informed and therapists will tailor care in concert with the impact of trauma on a service recipient's emotional regulation and behavior. Trauma from war, natural disaster, assault, abuse, lifelong discrimination, imprisonment, institutionalization, oppression, and forced colonization will be analyzed with regard to their impact on occupational function. Occupational therapy practitioners will help service recipients assess both how trauma has impacted occupational participation and how occupational patterns, habits, and routines can be reconstructed and remodeled to facilitate recovery.

Similarly, occupational therapy practitioners will have an increased understanding of the impact of technology and how access to medical, assistive, computer, and communication technology can enhance quality of life. Conversely, addiction to technology in the form of videogaming, social media overuse, digital workaholism, and online shopping, gambling, and pornography can break down family relationships and cause severe occupational imbalances that interfere with daily life function. Future practitioners will help clients understand which technologies enhance emotional and physical health, which erode it, and how occupational balance can be regained through changes in occupational patterns, habits, and routines.

It is also likely that future occupational therapy practitioners will return to the profession's roots and become fully occupation-focused and community-based. Assessment and intervention will be carried out primarily in the community where people participate in their typical daily occupations, rather than in artificial clinical settings reliant upon simulated occupations. There will still be the need for occupational therapists to provide acute care in a formal hospital setting, but the majority of occupational therapy services will be provided in schools, worksites, homes, and the communities in which people carry out their daily self-care, work, education, play, leisure, and social occupations.

31.8 Conclusion

As we contemplate the profession's journey into the next decades, our path may parallel the vision of the early founders who envisaged occupational therapists helping people in their communities to newly learn or regain desired daily life activities despite physical injury, disability, disease, social disadvantage, mental health challenge, poverty, or intellectual disability. We have the potential to fulfill what the early founders envisioned for the profession that was never fully achieved because of the prevailing dominance of the medical model and reduction of human illness to a cellular level or segregated body part after both World Wars. As the health care pendulum swings back toward a more holistic view of illness as having physical, cognitive, psychosocial, socioeconomic, and political factors, the occupational therapy profession may come full circle and be able to deliver the authentic, holistic intervention that was intended by the founders but never fully realized. The profession, however, must be ready with both a body of evidence and robust advocacy efforts that demonstrate the scope and effectiveness of occupational therapy services, as our professional competitors – physical therapy, nursing, social work, psychology – will also be vying for limited health care reimbursement funds and governance over legislation defining practice scope.

31.9 Summary

- Humans are occupational beings and are shaped by the occupations that are available in their environments, cultures, and families. Access to occupational participation is also influenced by race, ethnicity, educational level, socioeconomic status, ability level, gender, and gender orientation.
- Members of the larger society holding power also govern which occupational opportunities and roles are sanctioned or condemned based on such social constructs as race, educational level, socioeconomic level, gender, ableism, and gender orientation.
- The global COVID-19 pandemic heightened our awareness of societal problems embedded in Western society, including systemic racism, the high rate and stigmatization of mental health conditions among members of Western society, and the socially entrenched systems that maintain unequal pay and un/underemployment for women, individuals with disability, and Black and Brown communities.
- Armed with this increased understanding of the need to address diversity, equity, and inclusion in practice, future occupational therapy practitioners will be occupation-focused and community-based; strive to equalize access to and delivery of care for all service recipients, particularly diverse and marginalized populations; embrace service recipients as collaborators instead of passive receivers of care; promote interdependence instead of independence in recognition of the need for social connection; be aware of the issues related to intersectionality of a person's multiple identities, and its potential for cumulative impacts on a person's health and well-being; address mental health in all practice settings; and help service recipients distinguish between technology that enhances quality of life from technology that may disrupt occupational balance and social connection.

31.10 Review Questions

1. What social factors affect the occupations and occupational roles that humans have access to and opportunity to participate in?
2. What are examples of occupations and occupational roles that are sanctioned and condemned by the dominant group holding power in a society?

3. What are examples of the social conditions that came into public awareness during the global COVID-19 pandemic and how do these conditions affect occupational participation in Western society?
4. How will future occupational therapists respond to the social conditions of systemic racism, gender inequality, inaccessible and inequitable care, high rates of mental health challenges and stigmatization, and occupational imbalance?

Acknowledgments

We thank all co-editors (Tim Barlott, Bethan Collins, Diane Powers Dirette, Louise Gustafsson, and Stephen Isbel) and chapters authors for their contributions to this textbook.

References

Allam, L. (2020, July 13). 'Lack of money': 43% of Aboriginal people in remote communities have gone without food in past year. *The Guardian.* https://www.theguardian.com/australia-news/2020/jul/13/lack-of-money-43-of-aboriginal-people-in-remote-communities-have-gone-without-food-in-past-year

Baker, R. S., Brady, D., Parolin, Z., & Williams, D. T. (2021). The enduring significance of ethno-racial inequalities in poverty in the US, 1993–2017. *Population Research and Policy Review, 41,* 1049–1083. https://doi.org/10.1007/s11113-021-09679-y

Barroso, A., & Brown, A. (2022). *Gender pay gap in US held steady in 2020.* Pew Research Center. https://www.pewresearch.org/fact-tank/2021/05/25/gender-pay-gap-facts/

Boudreau, C., MacKenzie, S. A., & Simmons, D. J. (2022). Police violence and public opinion after George Floyd: How the Black Lives Matter Movement and endorsements affect support for reforms. *Political Research Quarterly, 75*(2), 10659129221081007. https://doi.org/10.1177/10659129221081007

Canadian Centre for Policy Alternatives. (2022). *Indigenous children face deplorable poverty.* https://policyalternatives.ca/newsroom/updates/indigenous-children-face-deplorable-poverty

Carli, L. L. (2020). Women, gender equality and COVID-19. *Gender in Management: An International Journal, 35*(7/8), 647–655. https://doi.org/10.1108/GM-07-2020-0236

Christian, M. (2019). A global critical race and racism framework: Racial entanglements and deep and malleable whiteness. *Sociology of Race and Ethnicity, 5*(2), 169–185. https://doi.org/10.1177/2332649218783220

Delgado, R., & Stefancic, J. (2017). *Critical race theory* (3rd ed.). New York University Press.

Emery-Whittington, I. G. (2021). Occupational justice: Colonial business as usual? Indigenous observations from Aotearoa New Zealand. *Canadian Journal of Occupational Therapy, 88*(2), 153–162. https://doi.org/10.1177/00084174211005891

Golestaneh, L., Neugarten, J., Fisher, M., Billett, H. H., Gil, M. R., Johns, T., Milagros, Y., Mokrzycki, M. H., Coco, M., Norris, K. C., Perez, H. R., Scott, S., Kim, R. S., & Bellin, E. (2020). The association of race and COVID-19 mortality. *eClinicalMedicine, 25,* 100455. https://doi.org/10.1016/j.eclinm.2020.100455

Gómez-Castillo, M. D., Escrivá-S, V., Tolosa-Pérez, M. T., Navarro-Bravo, B., Plateau, C. R., Ricarte, J. J., & Cuesta-Zamora, C. (2022). The link between non-suicidal self-injury (NSSI), body image and activity on social networking sites among female adolescents with an eating disorder. *Clinical Child Psychology and Psychiatry, 27*(3), 13591045221081191. https://doi.org/10.1177/13591045221081191

Gonzales, M. (2022). *Nearly 2 million fewer women in labor force.* Society for Human Resource Management. https://www.shrm.org/resourcesandtools/hr-topics/behavioral-competencies/global-and-cultural-effectiveness/pages/over-1-million-fewer-women-in-labor-force.aspx

Jones, S. E., Ethier, K. A., Hertz, M., DeGue, S., Le, D. V., Thorton, J., Lim, C., Dittus, P. J., & Geda, S. (2022). Mental health, suicidality, and connectedness among high school students during the COVID-19 pandemic: Adolescent Behaviors and Experiences Survey, United States, January–June 2021. *Morbidity and Mortality Weekly Report, 71*(Suppl. 3), 16–21. https://doi.org/10.15585/mmwr.su7103a3

Katayama, R., & Wadhwa, D. (2019). *Half the world's poor live in just 5 countries.* World Bank. https://blogs.worldbank.org/opendata/half-world-s-poor-live-just-5-countries

King, R. (2019). *Report: Wide disparity between mental and physical health coverage, payments.* https://www.fiercehealthcare.com/payer/report-wide-disparity-between-mental-and-physical-health-coverage-and-payments

Lavizzo-Mourey, R. J., Besser, R. E., & Williams, D. R. (2021). Understanding and mitigating health inequities: Past, current, and future directions. *New England Journal of Medicine, 384*(18), 1681–1684. https://doi.org/10.1056/NEJMp2008628

Morgan, R. E., & Thompson, A. (2020). *Criminal victimization, 2020.* US Department of Justice, Office of Justice Programs, Bureau of Justice Statistics. https://bjs.ojp.gov/sites/g/files/xyckuh236/files/media/document/cv20.pdf

Moss, E., McIntosh, K., Edelberg, W., & Broady, K. (2020). *The Black-White wealth gap left Black households more vulnerable.* Brookings Institute. https://www.brookings.edu/blog/up-front/2020/12/08/the-black-white-wealth-gap-left-black-households-more-vulnerable/

Northwestern University Institute for Policy Research. (2020). *What drives Native American poverty.* https://www.ipr.northwestern.edu/news/2020/redbird-what-drives-native-american-poverty.html#:~:text=Across%20the%20United%20States%2C%201,income%20of%20%202423%2C000%20a%20year

Panchal, N., Kamal, R., Cox, C., & Garfield, R. (2021). *The implications of COVID-19 for mental health and substance use.* Kaiser Family Foundation. https://www.kff.org/coronavirus-COVID-19/issue-brief/the-implications-of-COVID-19-for-mental-health-and-substance-use/#:~:text=Older%20adults%20are%20also%20more,to%20the%20current%20crisis

Proctor, S. L., Williams, B., Scherr, T., & Li, K. (2017). *Intersectionality and school psychology: Implications for practice.* National Association for School Psychologists. https://www.nasponline.org/resources-and-publications/resources-and-podcasts/diversity-and-social-justice/social-justice/intersectionality-and-school-psychology-implications-for-practice

Reinah, J. (2021). LGBTQIA+ public accommodation cases: The battle between religious freedom and civil rights. *Fordham Law Review, 90,* 261–277. https://heinonline.org/HOL/LandingPage?handle=hein.journals/flr90&div=11&id=&page=

Tanne, J. H. (2022). US abortion: Leaked document shows Supreme Court plans to overturn rights. *BMJ, 377,* o1122. https://doi.org/10.1136/bmj.o1122

Tausch, A., e Souza, R. O., Viciana, C. M., Cayetano, C., Barbosa, J., & Hennis, A. J. (2022). Strengthening mental health responses to COVID-19 in the Americas: A health policy analysis and recommendations. *Lancet Regional Health-Americas, 5,* 100118. https://doi.org/10.1016/j.lana.2021.100118

Totenberg, N. (2022). *Reproductive rights in America. Supreme Court overturns Roe v. Wade, ending right to abortion for decades.* National Public Radio. https://www.npr.org/2022/06/24/1102305878/supreme-court-abortion-roe-v-wade-decision-overturn

United Nations. (2021a). *Indigenous peoples have been disproportionately affected by COVID-19, Senior United Nations official tells Human Rights Council.* https://www.ohchr.org/en/press-releases/2021/09/indigenous-peoples-have-been-disproportionately-affected-COVID-19-senior

United Nations. (2021b). *COVID crisis to push global unemployment over 200 million mark in 2022.* UN News. https://news.un.org/en/story/2021/06/1093182

Index

Note: **Bold** page numbers refer to tables and *italic* page numbers refer to figures.

ableism 6, 23, 88, 195, **211**, 220–221, 224, 225, 241, 351, 361, 599, 654, 844
abstract thinking **488**
Acquisitional Frame of Reference **682**, 708
action **36**; activity 13, 757; body functions 394; cognition 381; collaborative 54; collective 237, 254, 258, 261; community 439–440; cultural 276; decoloniality 195; development of 132; direct 195; domains 89, 90, 91–93; experimental 290, 292; human 290–292; implementation of 133; knowledge to 586–587; legal 304; line of 153; mitigation 88; neutral 162; order 129; participatory 103, 243; performance skill 403; political 276; professional 273–274; social 261, 275, 276, 277, 329; space 132–133, **134**; structured 809; technical 276; territorial 439–440; for therapists 72; and thought 414–416, *417*, 418, 427; transformative 164, 261
action space 132–133, **134–135**
active recreation 758
activities of daily living (ADL) 13, 81, 223, 322, 610; assessment tools **614–619**, 620, 622–627; developmental trajectories 513; early adulthood **546**; of late adulthood 579–580; middle adulthood **558**, 561; occupations 13, **17**, 34, **326**, 459, 475, 489, 572, 610, 613, 620, 635, 670; of older adults 575; OTPF-4 definition and examples 16, **17**, **476**, 611; school-aged children approach **487–488**, 489–490, **495**; self-care 324, 610–613; of sexual activity 490, 836, 837, 845, 848; for Youth **522**
activity 321–322; analysis 387, 837, 845; component of HAAT Model 324; criminal 106, 180; defined 13, 37, 41; educational 672, 675, 703; examples 14; explicit 286; "Flying Squirrel" 724; fundraising 120; identified 38; illicit 236; learning 704; leisure as 747, 750, 755, 756, 774, 776; motor 385; and occupation 37–39; outputs 324; participation for school-aged children 474; physical 418, 421, 480, 481, 483, 491, 532–533, 563, 635, 640, 662, 719, 753, 786, 826; playful 738, 740; purposeful 37, 38, 231; recreation 774; and rest 808, 810; resultant 129; self-care 623, 626; sexual 490, 601, 837, 840, 846; social 532; use of 38; work 654
activity limitations 13, 595, 654, 757
Adam, J. 258
adaptation 21, 289, 467; function of 467; occupational *see* occupational adaptation; temporal 483; work 658–659, 660–661, 664
adaptive behavior 471, **689**, 844; skills 471
adaptive technology **320**
Addams, Jane 288
addiction to technology 603
ADL profile **614**, 623
adolescences 13, 454; awareness 485; case study 531–532; critical transitions to 475, 485, 490; defined 513; and

INDEX

health 518, **519–520**; leisure 751; Maslow's hierarchy of needs 520, *521*; middle-to-late adolescence (ages 15–19) 516–517, **517**; musculoskeletal strength 513, *514*; occupational profile 530–531; occupational range, basic and IADLs 521, **522–527**, '527, 530; occupations of 178–182; play in 722; virginity 840; Western Society Rites of Passage **528**; young-to-middle adolescence (ages 12–15) 514–515, *516*

adolescent development 512; changes during 517; goals **528–530**; theorists/theories 518, 520–521; trajectories 513

adult directed play 739

adult-learning 672, **678**

age 14, 149, 172, 294, 323, 425, 437, 503, 569, 594, 595, 598, 636, 653, 654, 746, 757, 780; categorization 513; celebrations 422; child's 489, 492, 493; chronological 554, 555, 675, 791, 799, 843; kindergarten 622; leisure participation 754; older 107, 454, 555, 674; school 13, 474, 480, 622; sexual participation 840; young 330

agency 343, 672; advertising 706–707; and belief 672–673; in daily life 577; health 325; human 160; individual 150; law enforcement 595; older adults 583–584; personal 358; sense of 672, 722, 738

aging: in place 574, 575, 577–580, 582; positive 146; process 568–569, 571, 579, 587

agism 151, 569, 573, 577–578, 587

Ahmed, K. A. 475

Ahmed-Landeryou, M. J. 9

Ainsworth, Mary 467

Aldrich, R. M. 149, 163

allies 202, 258–259, 306, 423, 609

alternative and augmentative communication (AAC) technology **320**

Amborski, A.M. 847

American Academy of Pediatrics (AAP) 325

Amores, Marcel Nazabal 230, 242–243

Anderson, D. M. 747

antiracism 193, 198, 202, 203

antiracist 197, 203, 205

arpilleras 258

art: and music 485, 752; of practice 64–65; and craft movement 37, 303, 433, 434

asexual 173, 241, 302, 839

Assessment of Leisure & Recreation **767**

Assessment of Motor and Process Skills (AMPS) 40, 55, 56, 81, 399, 620, 622

assistive products 52, 318–319, **319**, 329

assistive technology 20, 51, 132, 318–319, 321–324, 329, 391, 492, 661, 705, 776

associative play **456**, **728**, **732**

attachment 107, 467

attention deficit hyperactivity disorder (ADHD) 177, 179, 518, 725, **736**

augmentation 328

Ausman, C. 243

autism spectrum disorder (ASD) **462, 736**, 776

autonomy 85, 106, 252, 277, 455, 502, 538, 672, 839; of adulthood 540, 542, 549; and choice **214**, 223, 738; and control 422; financial 301, **539**; personal 626

Ayres Sensory Integration™ (ASI™) 738

Bandura, Albert 703

Barlott, T. 23

Barthel Index 223, **616**, 623, 625

Barton, George Edward 48

bathing **17**, 184, 223, 364, **476**, 483, 489, 521, **522, 546, 558**, 610–613, **614, 616, 617, 621**, 635, 839, 845

Bazyk, S. 480

Beagan, B.L. 201, 243, 305, 445

behaviorism 469–470, **677**, 702, 708

beliefs 7, 12–16, **19**, 20, 64, 66, 147, 153, 159, 173–174, 192, 251, 252, 324, 339, 370, 475, 502, 600, 787; cisnormativity 302; client factors of 578; colonial worldview's system 199–200; conscious and unconscious 68; cultural 5, 86, 812–813; defined 379–380; folk 197; personal 231; political 323; religious 167, 323, 595; societal 86, 220; spiritual 381, 394, 613, 838; values as 371, 434, 435, 844–845, 848

Benfield, A. 125, 126

Benjamin-Thomas, T.E. 151, 230, 243

Bentley, A. F. 291, 292

between-role balance 426

between-role conflict 426

between-role enrichment 426

biographical medicine 63

bisexual 173, 241, 302

Black Americans 174, 183, 184

Black and Indigenous People of Color (BIPOC) 204–205

Black Lives Matter Movement 6, 165, 596, 602

Blaise, D. 201

Boal, A. 257, 261

body function 13, 14, 51, 52, 322, 323, 382, 385, 403, 437, 655, 787, 845; cardiovascular 388; client factors **19–20**, 570, 662, 826; digestive functions 390; endocrine function 390; genitourinary function 390; hematological 388; immunological 388; internal 394; metabolic function 390; occupational performance 391; participants' 753; physiological 13; psychological 13;

reproductive functions 391; respiratory 388; of skin 391; voice and speech functions 390
body structure 13, 14, 52, 323, 382, 570, 655, 662, 686, 787, 845
Bolden, T. 723
Boone, M. E. 129–131
Borell, B. 199
bottom-up approach 371, 394, 686
Bourdieu, P. 161, 252, 254
Bowlby, John 467
Breines, E. 288, 289
Brennan, G. 307
Bronfenbrenner, U. 437, 439, 442, 478, 585; ecological theory 437, 439, 442, 478, 478, 585
Brooke, K. E. 612
Brown, Ted 21, 315
Bundy, A. C. 747, 748

Canadian Model of Occupational Participation (CanMOP) 39, 76, 91, 93–95, 104, 121, 442, 443; evidence 86–87; graphic representation of 85; occupation model 83–84; reasoning 84
Canadian Model of Occupational Performance and Engagement (CMOPE) 40, **42**, 442, 686, 758; in *Enabling Occupation II* 788; evaluation 686; integrated 445; occupational engagement 354–355; occupational therapy 39, 159, 324; sustainability initiatives 340–341
Canadian Occupational Performance Measure (COPM) 55, 56, 116, 620, 656, 758
Canadian Occupational Therapy Inter-relational Practice Process Framework (COTIPP) 83, 87, 88–89, 89, 91, 93, 95, 121
capitalism 105, 145, 220, 238, 241, 273, 288, 598–599
cardiovascular functions 387, 388, 572, 659
Cardoso da Silva, A. C. 104
career: advancement 303; CareerScope **499**; choice 557; development 542–543, 545; in occupational therapy 22; opportunities 173, 202; paths 557, 707; possibilities for 541; for women and people of color 172
career-and-care-crunch 542–543, **547–548**
caring role 556, 562, 644
Casson, Elizabeth 48
Castel, R. 274
casual leisure 752, 779, 780
child-centered 712, 715, 725
child directed play 725, 739, **739**
childhood: early 454, 455, 459, 475, 520, 674, 676, 737; home and caregivers 538–541, **546**, 549; illnesses 513; leisure occupations 747–749, 754; middle 454, 475, 485; occupations of 175–177, 179, 187, 304; play occupation 712–715, 723–724, 737, 739, 740; in United States 723–724
child-initiated play 738, **739**
child rearing 302, 307, **558**, 635
child's rights 241, 712, 722, 740
choice 149, 166, 194; career 303, 557; on health management 640–641; ideal 150; individual 149; and informed decisions 87, 88; leisure 754; life 425, 515; occupational 79, 93, 94, 106, 150, 161, 220–221, 241, 243, 302, 306, 307, 309, 339, 345, 354, 426, 475, 482, 601, 624, 837
chronic conditions 491, 574, 575, 579, 657, 660; clients with 389, 570, 572; and stigma 639–641
chronic disease 572, 576, 580, 640, 799
"chronotype" 421
Circles of Sexuality *838*, 838–839, **846**, 848; intimacy 838–839; reproduction 838, 840; sensuality 838, 839; sexual health 838, 840; sexual identity 838, 839; sexualization 838, 839; *see also* sexuality
cisgender: gap 303–304; identities 302–303; male privilege 303; occupational habits 325, 330; occupational identities 302–303; occupational issues 309; occupational roles 303, 309; occupational routines 309; privileges 302; roles 302–303
cisnormativity 302, 304
citizenship 6, 149, 193, 271, 361, **539**, 671
Clarke, Eleanor 288
"classical pragmatists" 286
client factors 16, 159, 322, 370–371, 664, 787, 843–845; and age-related change 570–572; assessment **372–378**; and chronic conditions 572–578; in OTPF-4 Domain **19–20**, 20; values, beliefs, spirituality 578–579
climate anxiety 338
climate change 336–337; on animals 478; environmental justice and human occupation 339; guidance from WFOT 338; and human occupation 337–339; human occupation and its contribution to 337; and its impact on human occupations 337–338; occupational justice and environmental sustainability 338–339
clinical reasoning 292
codesign 4, 9, 91, 243
cognition/cognitive 106, 125, 324, 370, 489, 502, 512–514, 541, 563; in aging 572; changes 570–571; client's 340; conditions 572; constructivism 704; defined 381–382; development 467–468, 720; functional 176, 342, 382, 436; nursing

609

INDEX

home placement 579; reframing 358, 360; science 114, 129; skills 13, 455, 521; specific mental functions 381–382
Cognitive Orientation to daily Occupational Performance (CO-OP) 55, 738, 775
cognitivism 703, 708
Cohn, E. 676
Coin Model of Privilege and Critical Allyship 4, *6*, *8*, 24
collaboration 124
collaborative action 54
collaborative relationship-focused occupational therapy 91, 93, 200
collaborative relationship-focused practice-approach 83, 87–89, 94, 95, 757
collecting 321, 752
collective action 237, 254, 258, 261
collective actors 252–254, 256, 259–262
collective occupations 32, 236, 254, 256, 261
collectives 84–88, 90, 94, 103, 149, 165, 204–206, 235, 238; self-care 628; social occupational therapy 277; through occupation 238–241
collectivist 121, 145, 197, 205, 354, 445, 788
Collins, Bethan 22–23
colonial beliefs and values 199
colonialism 105, 145, 148, 196–197, 199, 200, 205, 220, 235, 241, 361; historical 145; and occupation 192; reproductions of 198; settler 23, 193–194, 201
coloniality 194; decolonial academics 194; and decoloniality, relationship with 192–193; dominant practices of 162; and occupation, links between 198–199; of power 164; and racism 196, 198; value 206; without mitigations 204
colonial power 198, 200, 205
colonial worldview 193, 199; beliefs 199–200; characteristics 200–201, 203; goals 201; protections 201–203
colonization: British 173; forced 603; history of 173, 644, 645; impact of 597; of Indigenous peoples' doing and being 442; legacy of 105, 441; negative impacts 6; occupational stages 198–199, play in 416; practices 163; processes of 433; trauma of 644; White 597
colonized 151, 153, 164, 193, 203, 433
communities of practice **678**, 708
community(ies) 30–31, 87, 423; Black 490, 570, 596, 597, 598, 602, 604; Brown 596, 598, 602, 604; centers 179; children *178*; commitments 167; concepts of 222, 439; of concern 254; COVID-19 166; defined 440; disabilities 93; disadvantaged 180; doing 223; encountered 198; environment 480, 502, 518, 573, 575; excluded 198, 200–203; First Nation 597; green spaces 756; heteronormative 180, 186; history 85, 87, 90; identities 86; impoverished *175*; Indigenous 105, 145, 193, 200, 255, 435, 570, 625, 644–646; intervention 582–583; involvement 532, 787; knowledge 196, 224; leisure 582; LGTBQIA+ 22, 306, 556; local 81, 167; marginalized 6, 9, 203, 219, 532; matriarchal 638; mining 90; mobility 480, 487, 490, *523*, 575, 672; occupational engagement 354; to occupy time 33, 40; online 482; organizations 167, 583; of people 440; phase 120; play provision 723; post-colonial 198; of practitioners 244; programs 342, 364; refugee 220; religious 533; resources 86, 166; rural 77, 81; safety 84; and school systems 180, *180*, 342; sense of 343; settings 342, 723–725; social participation 575, 582; spaces 203, 277, 569; support 125; urban 93, 570; violence 243; voices 203; work 235, 492
community participation 241, 307, 388, 480, 575, 582, 787, 793
compensation 328
compensatory or recuperative leisure 752, 779, 780
competency: child's developmental 454; cultural 200–201, 203; occupational 483; social 786
concepts: CanMOP 84–86; contemporary 11; defined 466; of dignity 626–627; and events, relationships between 465; of IADLs 641; from MOHO 40, 77–82, 78–79, 94; normal and acceptable 220; occupational adaptation 358–361; occupational balance 355–358; occupational engagement 352–355; of participation 789; for person-centered care 65; of play date 475, 715–721; from Pragmatism 290–292; principal 11; of transaction and transactionalism 289
connection: between concepts 285, 483; between environment and well-being 435; between groups and communities of people 197; of ICF components 13; with individual or collective 89; inner 354; interpersonal 672; social 482, 515, 595, 600, 603, 758; between systemic racism and homelessness 184
Connell, R. W. 301
consolidation 358
construction: and negotiation of routines 420–421; of personal ethics and spirituality 513; of professional identities 152; of public sphere 273, 276; of self-efficacy and mastery 751; of social occupational therapy 275
constructive play **456**

INDEX

constructivism **677**; cognitive 704; social 468, 704
consumerist culture 337
consumer technology **320**
contemporary paradigm 31, 49
context(s) 13, 16, 132, 158, 160, 285, 291, 433, **464**, 489; of Brazilian social occupational therapy 275; of CanMOP 104; client 123–124; CMOP-E 788; of coloniality and racism 196; of complexity 128; cultural 478–482, 555; defined 443; educational 324; of habit formation 416; of human occupation 721–723, 791–792; of ICF 757; impact on IADLs and health management 636; of individual or collective 84; macro context 86, 89; meso context 86, 89; micro context 86, 87, 89; MOHO 758; in occupational therapy 114, 160–163; of OTPF-4 14; of overcoming problems 290; of people's lives 235; and person, occupation, interrelations of 159–160; of political repression 258; practice 121; of professional disciplines and sciences 285–286; of role theory 425; of sexuality 843; of social service institutions 269; sociocultural 40, 441, 721–723, 814; socio-historical context 149; of sustainable development 336; of total institutions 269
context modifications 419
contextualization 756–757
control: clients' 161; emotional 719; of goal setting 359; impulse 232, 515, 516, 776; internal 714; invasive 220; locus of 5; metabolism 389; motor 66, 576, 702, 725; over decision-making process 152, 359; postural 386; sense of 359, 627, 720; and shelter 270; social 162
co-occupation 16, 675
cooperative play **456, 728, 732**
Copley, J. A. 128
core values 14, 62, 64, 290
Correa Oliver, F. 104
Coster, W. 676
countertransference 68
COVID-19 pandemic: case study 317–318; food provisioning 165, 167; foreign invaders 387; home confinement 480; impacted economies and health care systems 9; impact on occupational function and participation 595–596; issues of inequity and marginalization 165–166; on occupational participation of school-aged children 502, 503; occupational performance 388; working from home 330, 661
crafts 37, 39, 251, 258, 303, 342, 433–434, 752

Crip **211**
Crip wisdom **211**
critical autism studies (CAS) **211**, 219
critical disability studies (CDS) 209–226, **212**; critical knowledges 217; engaging with, firmly situated, and belonging within 219–222
critically reflect 87–88, 90, 93, 239, 361
critical pedagogical theories 152
critical perspective: creating new framings 149–151; critical epistemology 145–147; to educational practice 151–153; problematizing individual solutions 147–149; social transformation 144, 145
critical race theory 145, 173, 175, 187, 595
critical reflexivity 145–147, 152, 164, 167, 203, 238, 241, 244
critical social theory 145, 164
critical theories 610
Cruz, D. 354
Csíkszentmihályi, M. 355
cue 127, 415, 418, 419
cue-contingent behavior 415, 421
culture/cultural 38, 41, 158, 271, 323, 337, 475, 503, 539, 544, 578, 585, 594, 595, 636, 664, 746, 788, 806, 812, 843, 847; Aboriginal 644; Anglophone 234; Asian, East 480; belief 5, 86, 812–813; Black and Brown 597; Caucasian, Western 813; Chinese 562; collectivist 354; competency 123, 200–204; and context 555; to cultural safety 203–205; disability 479, 481; environment 480–481; European, Western 433, 713; heteronormative 175, 602; Hispanic 829; Indigenous 435; integration of client 613; Latino 562; leisure 755–756; Mexican and Latin American 813; occupations 172, 440, 442; and practice cultural, intersectionality between 481; roles 16; safety 84, 203–205; sensitivity 21, 578; of systemic racism 186; therapist and client **117**, 122–123; traditional 7; Western 197, 222, 226, 426, 562; of workplace 54
Currie, C. 490

Dale, S. 130
dark-side of occupation 229–234, 243, 244
Davis, J. A. 353, 354
Davis, S. 841
decolonial 9, 164, 165, 192–198, 202–206; collectives 205, 206; curricula 195; praxis 9, 192, 194–196, 198, 203–206; profession 205
decoloniality 168, 192–196, 198, 202–206
decolonization 9, 21, 153, 165, 192, 196, 316, 595, 712
decolonized occupation 191, 206
decolonizing occupations 441, 442, 446

611

INDEX

Deleuze, G. 164
Denouement 259, 261, 262
dependence 222–224
determination of health 436, 437, 438
development: of action 132; adolescent *see* adolescent development; in adulthood 557; career 542–543, 545; cognition/cognitive 467–468, 720; of pragmatism 285; routines for **460–461**; sexual 515–516, **517**; sexuality **517**; sustainable 336, 343, 344, 544; technology 329–330; youth 513
Developmental Coordination Disorder 725, **736**
developmental milestones 455, 457, 458
developmental perspective 713, 812
developmental theories 518, **556**
Dewey, J. 160, 291, 292
dialectical 162
Dickie, V.A. 251, 291
Dieterle, C. 344
digestive functions 389
digital literacy 329–330
digital technology **320**
Dirette, D.P. 22
disability **212**; communities 93; culture 479, 481; language learners with 481; play 723; youth with 490
disability justice 212
disabled 23, 147, 148, **212**, 220–225, 251
disablism **213**, 219, 221, 225
disadvantage 12, 21, 145, 171–188, 219, 240, 310, 361, 537, 541, 544, 553, 556, 604, 708
discrimination 6, 305; banking 183; employment 186, 602; face 307; gendered 307; housing 183–184; racial 165, 307; societal 174; transphobic 173; workplace 308
discriminatory 88, 165, 173, 182, 200, 309, 640, 839
disease management 644
disruptive technology **320**
diversity: gender 6, 174, 181, 182, 187, 533, 595; hires 202; and inclusivity movement 303; racism 596–597
domain: action 89, 90, 91–93; OTPF-4 13, 16, **17**, **19–20**, 20, 322, 399, **560**
Donker-Cools, B. H. P. M. 664
Dos Santos, V. 249
Dowers, E. 305, 306
Doyle, S. 121
dressing 35, 128, 423, **476**, 489, 494, **522**, 558, 610–613, 623, 624, 629, 635, 642, 839
Du Bois, W. E. B. 288
Duckworth, S. 6
Dutta, A. 475

early adulthood: developmental tasks of **539**, 539–540; emerging adulthood 541–542, *542*; established adulthood 542–543, *543*; global perspective of 543–545; occupations of 545, **546–548**; stages of 540–541
early childhood, stages of 455
eating and swallowing **558**, 611
Ecological Systems Model of Occupational Therapy 437
ecological systems theory 437, 442, *478*, 585
ecological theories 442, 585
ecological validity 371
ecology 295, 437, 586
Ecology of Human Performance 437, 586
economic 6, 14, 16, 40, 75, 81, 102, 105–106, 161, 233, 268, 276, 277, 295, 303, 328, 336, 432, 433, 483, 576, 595, 599
education/educational: activity 672, 675, 703; application of theory 702–704; assessment of 686, **687–701**; contexts 324; critical perspective 151–153; defined 671; entry-level education 30; formal 6, 106, 335, **477**, 491, 541, 559, 670, 674, 702, 708; historical perspective 673–674; as human occupation throughout lifespan 675; informal 491, 559, 670, 674, 708; learner considerations 674; as occupation 705–707; participation **477**, 559, 671, 676, 684, 702, 708; sexuality 847–848; societal and learner perspectives 671–673
Einstein, A. 458
emancipatory experimentalism 253, 259–262, 295
emerging adolescence 513, 515
emerging adulthood 538, 540–544, 549
emerging technology **320**
Emerson, Ralph Waldo 455
Emery-Whittington, I. G. 151, 441
emotional: control 719; social-emotional 455, 471, 485, 489, 490, 495, 502, 748
employment: livable wage 172, *175*, 176, 183, 184, 187; occupational participation 183–184; paid 149, 235, 241, 487, 638, 662–663; services and support 149–151
end-in-view 291
endocrine functions 389
engrossing 780
enjoyment 10, 107, 385, 530, 672, **689**, 703, 705, 719, **734**, 747, 750, **772**, 780, 788, 838
entertainment 481, 540, 600, 752, 780
environment: communities 480, 502, 518, 573, 575; culture 480–481; history of 433–435; leisure 775–776; MOHO 78, 81; occupational *180*, 707; physical and social 158, 445, 489, 585, 721, 737, 740, 787; political 359; social 64, 158, 445, 489, 569,

585, 640, 716, 721, 737, 787, 788, 792;
  virtual 478, 481–482
environmental factors 14, 16, **18**, 24, 52,
  55, 72, 73, 77, 95, 159, 323, 325, 340,
  408, 437, 438, 443, 444, **444**, 446, 570,
  574–575, 587, 657, 686, 757, 775, 813, 843
environmental justice 339
environmentally sustainable health systems
  and policy 337
environmentally sustainable lifestyle 337
environmentally sustainable occupational
  engagement 340
Environmental Press Theory 585–586
Environmental Sustainability: and
  occupational therapy theory 339
environmental sustainability 240; climate
  change 337–339; community-based
  settings 342; hospitals and medical
  settings: inpatient, outpatient 341–342;
  Lifestyle Redesign® (LR) 343; nature-based
  occupations 342–343; and occupational
  justice 338–339; within occupational
  therapy education 343–344; occupational
  therapy practice 339–344; schools:
  primary, secondary, post-secondary 342
epistemic injustice **213**, 218–219, 222, 225
epistemic play **718**
epistemological pragmatism 295
epistemology(ies) 145–147, 286, 295,
  433–435, 441
equitable access to technology 328–329
equity: in access **684**; in outcomes **685**
Erikson, E. H. 466, 538, 556, 557, 563
escape 106, 424, 752
Eshin, K. 306
established adulthood 537, 538, 541–543,
  543
ethical reasoning 126
ethnicity 14, 22, 66, 122, 172, 307, 323, 493,
  541, 569, 594, 604, 633, 654, 713, 780,
  813, 843
Etowa, J. 361
Eurocentric 105, 163–165, 221
evaluation 20, 56, 121, 657–658, 660;
  functional capacity 657; and performance
  skills 407–408, *408*, **409**; sexuality
  843–845
Evans, K. L. 426
everyday technologies **320**
evidence-based practice 64, **118**, 121–122,
  125
exchange 277, 293, 344, 387, 444, 750, 752
exclusionary 147, 164, 236, 576
experiential knowledge **213**
ex-Permission, Limited Information, Specific
  Suggestions, and Intensive Therapy
  (ex-PLISSIT) model 837, 841–843, 848
explore 91, 92, 379, 380, 381, 458

express 235, 259, 837, 840
external support 354, 380

Farias, L. 163, 242
Fassin, D. 294
Favill, Henry B.
Fazio, L. 747
feeding 290, 386, 419, **476**, **486**, 494, **558**,
  573, 610, 613, 624, 629
Feeney, B. C. 748
female 301, 307
feminine 301, 305
figured world of occupation 231, 232, 243, 244
Fijal, D. 445
fine motor 150, **456**, 495, 513, *514*, 570, 576,
  580, 658, 661, 723, 725
First Nation peoples 21, 184, 187, 316, 597, 669
Fischl, C. 315
Fisher, A. G. 48–53, *50*, 161
Fleming, M. H. 125, 292
Flow Theory 355
Floyd, George 204, 596
"Flying Squirrel" activity 724
folk belief 197
Ford, E. 52, 53
form 423; of models 39; observations 131;
  occupational 131; of societal exclusion
  184, *185*
formal education 6, 106, 335, 477, 491, 541,
  559, 670, 674, 702, 708
formal operations 468, 520, 521
Foucault, Michel 164
4 Ps Model 308–309
Four Quadrant Model of Learning **681**
frames of reference (FoR) 65, 66, 72, 73, **118**,
  125, 466, 579, 675–686, 702, 708, 799
Francisco, B. R. 272
Frank, G. 249, 251–253, 292, 582
freedom of constraints from reality 714
freely chosen 470, **477**, 492, 714, 738
Frei, Eduardo 258
Freire, P. 152, 164, 257, 278
Frey, C. B. 330
Fridland, E. 809
frontal lobes 516
function 86, 416; of adaptation 467; body
  see body function; motor 342, 434, 455;
  recovery of 272
functional ability 318, 574, 587, 657
functional capacity evaluation 657
functional cognition 382
functional coordination 291
Functional Independence Measure 116, 223,
  495, **616**
functional mobility **476**, 489, 521, **522**, 558,
  573, 586, 610, 611, 613, 629
function-dysfunction continua/continuum 66,
  68, 466

613

INDEX

Gallagher, M. 307
Galvaan, R. 151, 161
games 327, 342, 458, 459, 471, 479, 481, 482, 485, **487**, **488**, 493, 494, 503, 531, 706, 714, **717**, **718**, 752, 756, 775; with rules 471, **487**, **488**, **717**, **718**; with rules play 471, 488
Ganz, M. 261
Garcia, J. 120
gardening 337, 342, 343, 486, 642, 755
Gard, G. 357
Gaztambide-Fernández, R. A. 193
gender: cisgender people 302–304; diverse communities 602; diversity 6, 174, 181, 182, 187, 533, 595; equality movement 6, 303; heteronormative binary standards 306–309; and human occupation 301–302; identity 14, **18**, 181, 302, 304, 305, 308–310, 485, 513, 515, 518, **529**, 569, 745, 780, 837, 839, 843, 846; inclusive services 308; inequality 599; norms 301, 304, 425; orientation 22, 172, 594, 595, 604; patriarchal oppression 600; role 302, 303, 305, 356, 425, 426, 839; and sexuality development 517; stereotypes 310; transgender and gender-non-conforming people 304–306
gendered discrimination 307
gender-non-conforming people 304–307, 309, 310
general systems theory 41
generativity 556, 557, 563
genitourinary system 390
gentrification 570
gerontechnology **321**
Gesell, Arnold 468
Ghul, R. 308
Gibson, C. 196, 198, 442
global mental functions 381, 383–384; body structures and function 383; example and application 384; interventions 384; occupational therapy practitioners 383–384
Global North 7, 8, 21, 32, 75, 102, 105, 109, 192–194, 200, 206, 209, 231, 434, 435, 439, 612, 625, 636, 637, 637, 639, 644, 646, 713, 715, 716, 722, 737
Global South 7, 102, 105, 109, 195, 205, 206, 236, 239, 241, 268, 435, 636, 713
Goldberg, Carole 250
Golledge, J. 37, 38
Golos, D. B. 479
Gramsci, A. 253
Grandner, M. A. 813
Green, H. 574
Grenier, M.-L. 201

grooming 223, 483, 521, **522**, 558, 610–613, 623, 629, 807
gross motor 150, 381, 386, **456**, 458, 485, 658
groups 11, 30, 36; age 107, 325, 421, 489, 518, 585, 754, 793; community 167, 480; cultural 38, 812; diagnostic 702, 725, **736**; Indigenous 106, 644; marginalized 9, 172, 174, 187, 578, 600, 624; minority 172, 174, 184, 518, 813; peer 179–181, 437, 787; privileged 146, 172, 594; social 51, 66, 81, 144, 145, 165, 220, 232, 236–238, 241, 361, 440, 485, 515, 517, 839
Guajardo, A. 235, 236
guided play 737–739
Guidetti, S. 642
Guitard, P. 747, 748
Gusfield, J.R. 251
Gustafsson, L. 21–22
Gutman, Sharon 22

Habermas, Jürgen 164
habit(s) 5, 194, 253, 291, 293, 415, 416, 418, 419, 422, 427, 482, 580, 844; defined 415–416; extinguishing and modifying existing habits 418–419; formation 415, 416, 418, 419, 422, 427, 580; occupational 325, 330; performance patterns 9, 13, 16, **18**, 159, 321–323, 325, 327, 328, 414–419, 454, 474, 482, 483, 577, 787; and routines 80, 257, 389; and social good 416–418, 417
habit stacking 419
habitual response 415
habituation 40, 70, 78, 79–81, 95, 339, 419, 758, 787, 788
Håkansson, C. 357
Hammell, K. W. 32, 33, 197, 200, 204, 309, 808
happenings 261
Harts, M. 200
Harvey, A. 35
Harvey, M. 438
Havighurst, R. J. 539, 548
health 6; crisis 165, 167; and illness 148; literacy 570, 580, 581; and occupation, relationship between 54; physical 80; professionals 90; promotion 129, 474, 482, **559**, 635, 655, 704, 753, 837, 846, **846**, 848; public 165, 167, 252, 271, 275, 325, 574, 597; and well-being 13, 76, 93, 94, 103, 107, 209, 234, 235, 302, 414, 421, 422, 424, 433, 440, 445, 475, 487, 504, 562, 569, 643, 653, 719, 723, 791, 799
health agency 325
Health and Work Performance Questionnaire 657

INDEX

health management 16, **17**, 322, 323, **326**, 475, **476**, **488**, 491, **546–547**, **636**; challenges and opportunities 638–639; defined 635; and IADL 634, 641; late adulthood 580; and maintenance **523**; older adults 576; OTPF-4 domain 16, 17; principals of recovery 642–644; school-aged children 491
hearing function 384
hegemonic 105, 145, 146, 255, 569, 612, 613
hematological functions 387
heteronormative 173–175, 180, 186, 187, 221, 306–310, 543, 549, 602, 623, 839; binary standards 306–309; standards 308, 310
heteronormativity 23, 220, 304
heterosexual 21, 23, 172, 181, 301, 302, 309, 542, 594, 600, 602
hierarchy of needs 466, *467*, 520, *521*, 637, *638*
high tech 318
Hinojosa, J. 125
historical context 41, 90, 94, 149, 162, 236, 432, 433, 434, 437, 439, 713
historical privilege 196, 199
historical trauma 159, 196, 645
history 270, 272; of colonization 173, 644, 645; communities 85, 87, 90; of environment 433–435; of occupational therapy 37, 288; of pragmatism 286–288; of profession 31; of technology 319
Hocking, C. 232, 527
Hoffmann, T. 122
homelessness 174, 177, 181–184, *185*, 187, 440, 613, 811
homosexual individual 302
Howard, J. 725
Human Activity Assistive Technology (HAAT) Model 323–324
human agency 160
human occupation 5, *11*; and climate change 337–339; contexts of 721–723, 791–792; issues and events impacting 5–9; lifespan education as 675; model of see Model of Human Occupation (MOHO); nature of 93, 342–343; occupational science on 93–94; occupational therapy on 93–94; play as 712–715, 724–725; situated nature see situated nature of occupation; social participation 791–792; and technology, relationship between 322–328, 330; types of 10–11
human occupational homeostasis 5, 9, 23
human rights 7, 109, 197, 237, 238, 276, 300, 303, 435, 438, 439, 652, 674, 713
Human Subsystems that Influence Occupation 41
Hurd, A. R. 747

identity 7, 65; categories 6; gender 14, **18**, 181, 302, 304, 305, 308–310, 485, 513, 515, 518, **529**, 569, 745, 780, 837, 839, 843, 846; occupational 40, 77–78, 82, 94, 95, 358–361, 363, 425–426, 483, 492, 493, 502, 585; sexual 75, 307, 309, 517, 542, 640, 836, 838–840, **846**, 848
Ikiugu, M. N. 289
illicit activity 236
immunological functions 387
implementation intentions 419
impulse control 232, 515, 516, 776
inaccessible and inequitable health and social care 602
incarceration 173, 175, 181–184, 186, 187, 596, 704
income 80, 149, 150, 165, 184, 235, 252, 258, 329, 339, 436, 545, 595, 597, 636, 642, 654, 672, 676, 683, 686, 746, 754, 755, 780
independence 104, 106, 145, 147, **214**, 251, 434, 480, 487, 517, 520, 539, 540, 542, 573, 582, 612
Indigenous: communities 105, 145, 193, 200, 255, 435, 570, 625, 644–646; culture 435; knowledge 167, 196, 198, 433, 436, 440–442; peoples' doing and being, colonization of 442; youth 416
individualism 160, 165, 203, 231, 291, 434, 556, 603
individuality 237, 517, 540
individuals 328, 360, 361, 364, 445, 490; and collectives 84–86, 88, 90–91, 94, 165, 235, 238–240, 244, 274, 277; disabled 221; health needs 65; memberships 361; survival of 84
inequity 6, 165, 172, 174–187, 203, 205, 303, 305, 329, 360, 596–598, 839
infant 107, 364, 454, 455, *457*, **460**, 468–471, **731**
informal education 491, **559**, 670, 674, 708
inquiry 195, 244, 256, 286. 287, 289, 290, 292, 747
instruction 70, 407, 479, 485, 487, 488, 490, 495, 658, 739
Instrumental Activities of Daily Living (IADL) 13, **17**, 34, 322, **326**, 356, 418, 459, 475, **476**, 490–491, **496**, 521, 539, 561, 572, 612, 633–646, 655, 839; and CADL Approach 641, 642; defined 635; Global North and Global South 636–638, 637; and health management 636, 641
integral 328
integrated approach 371, 382, 394
Integrated Canadian Model of Occupational Performance and Engagement 441, 445
intelligent technologies **321**

INDEX

intentional relationship approach 62, 67–68, 72, 73
interactional 66, 73, 433, 442–445, **444**
interactive reasoning 126
interdependence 64, 104, 162, **214**, 222–224, 254, 256, 434, 603, 604, 625, 628, 787, 789
interests 80, 107, 237, 410, 656, 657, 662, 792; children's 480, 495; client's 656; leisure 576–577, 746; personal **463**; social 532; work 481
Intergovernmental Panel on Climate Change 336
internal control 714
International Classification of Functioning, Disability and Health (ICF) 4, 12–14, 40, 318, 322, 323, 423, 436, 437, 642, 655, 686, 714, 757, 788
internet 6, 317, 318, 481, 482, 596, 600, 657, 707, 779
interpersonal connection 672
intersectional 6, 197, 351, 352, 361–362, 439, 713
intersectionality 174, 181–182, 188, 220, 307, 308, 365, 446, 481, 556, 576, 595, 602, 604, 654
intervention 20–21, 56, 121, 259, 702–705; to address leisure 774–776; challenges 625–626; child's functional performance 459, 462; communities 582–583; environmental and community 582–583; environmental sustainability-focused 343; gender-affirming 305; global mental functions 384; holistic 604; of late adulthood 579–582; methodologies 275, 278; neuromuscular and movement-related functions 387; occupational therapy 342–343, 371, 379, 380, 381, 383, 391, 392, 408–409, 826, **826–827**; with older adults 579; palliative and end-of-life care 389; performance pattern 583–584; and performance skills 408–410; play-based 725, 738–739; self care 613, 620, 625, 628; sensory functions 385; sexuality 843, 847–848; sleep and rest 826, **826–827**, 828–829; social occupational therapy 275; social participation 793; therapeutic 62–63, 63, 73; work 658–661
intimacy 466, 513, 538, 812, 836–840, 844, 845, **846**; *vs.* isolation 538
intimate relationship **529**, 538–541, 549
intrinsic motivation 354, 470, 580, **692**, 714, 719, 747
Isbel, S. 21
Iwama, M. K. 32, 114, 445

James, W. 286, 287, 292
Jehan, H. 813

Job Accommodation Network (JAN) 660–661, 664
job analysis 120, 656–658, 662, 664
Jones, S. 493
Josephsson, S. 292
Jungersen, K. 204
justice 64, 87, 90, 93, 94, 176–177, 179; environmental 339; occupational *see* occupational justice; play 722–723; social 8, 198, 231, 232, 316, 341

Kaepernik, Colin 426
Kantartzis, S. 32
Katz Index of Independence in Activities of Daily Living **617**
Katz, N. 625
Kawa model 121, 434, 445, 586
Kelly, J.R. 752
Kennedy-Behr, A. 725
Kennedy, J. 353, 354
Kielhofner, G. 31, 48, 77, 354, 361, 371
Kiepek, N. C. 229, 232, 233, 243
Kjellberg, A. 104, 643
Klein, S. 613
knowledge 146–147, 152, 163–167, 192, 271–273, 293, **402**; to action 586–587; client's 124; communities 196, 224; critical 217; decolonial approach 195–196; Eurocentric 105; experiential 213, 218, 222; implicit and explicit 121; Indigenous 167, 198, 433, 436, 440–442; medical-psychological 273–274; occupational therapist's 121; OTPF-4 15; valid 218–219
Kronenberg, F. 236, 256

laboratory-based medicine 63, 72, 73
Lachman, M. E. 556
Lancaster, Stephanie 315
language 6, 200, 235, 389, 455, **456**, 493; body 67, 67–68, 70, 72; colonizer's 198–199; English 33, 230; Latin American 231; learners with disabilities 481; occupational 56, 196; skills 776; Spanish 230, 231; speech 531; use 234
Lansdown, G. 722
late adulthood: agism 569; challenges 568–569; client factors 570–574, 578–579; environmental factors 574–575; intersectionality 570; intervention process 579–584; low educational attainment 570; misogyny 569; occupations of 568, 575–578; personal factors 569; racism 569–570; theories to support occupations 584–587
Latin America 103, 105–106, 234, 435, 544, 545; occupational therapy profession 105;

participation of older people 107; youth participation in 106
Latinx peoples 174, 184
Law, M. 613, 622, 624
laws of developmental direction 468
Lawton, M.P. 436
learning: activity 704; adult-learning 672, **678**; decolonial approach 195–196; defined 671; life-long **685**; online 329, 503; and play 720; play-centered 739; self-regulated **678**, 708; skills 672; social-cognitive **677**; style 673, **698, 699**
leisure: as activity 747, 750, 755, 756, 774, 776; addressing 774–776; adolescences 751; age participation 754; assessment of 758, **759–773**, 774; benefits of 750–752; case studies 776–779; casual 752, 779, 780; childhood 747–749, 754; choice 754; communities 582; compensatory or recuperative 752, 779, 780; culture 755–756; defined 747; environments 775–776; experiences 749–751, 774; exploration 418, **477**, **526**, 532, **560**, 747, 779, 780; meaning of 749–750; occupational performance 775; outcomes from 751; participation 754–756; play in 747–749, 748; profile and balance 774; and recreation 757–758; relational 752, 779, 780; role-determined 752, 779, 780; serious 752, 780; as state of mind 747; as time 747; tree of 746, 749, 749, 777, 779, 780; types of 752–754; unconditional 757, 779, 780
Leive, L. 809
Letts, L. 613, 622
Levin, K. A. 490
Levinson, D. J. 556, 557, 563
LGBTQQIA+ 839
life-long learning **685**
lifespan **548**; education as human occupation 675; leisure 751; life situations 791; participation across 235; sleep and rest 812; technology and occupation across 325, **326**, 327
lifestyle habits 14, 418, 704, 805
Lifestyle Redesign 343, 344
literacy 106, 166, 177, 184, 187, 234, 329–331, 483, 570, 580, 581, 674
lived body experience 80
low tech 318
Ludic play **718**

macro context 86, 96
madness 217, 220, 222, 225
Madsen, J. 292
mad studies **214**, 217–219
Magalhães, L. 232
male 301–303, 305, 307, 308, 839

male privilege 21, 303
Malfitano, A. P. S. 440
Malone, S. K. 813
marginalization 6, 151, 153, 165, 236, 240, 241, 284, 307, 318, 322, 541, 544, 569, 791
marginalized communities 6, 203, 532
Marterella, A. 50–52, 161
Martin, C. 585
Marx, K. 146, 279, 425
masculine 221, 299, 301, 304–306
Maslow, A.H. 466, 518, 520, 531, 637; hierarchy of needs 520, *521*
mastery play 716
materialist-historical occupational therapy 272
Matthews, J. L. 337
Mattingly, C. 125, 292
McCarthy, K., 305
McInnes, K. 725
meaning 84–86, 92, 94–95, 104, 203, 232, 237, 238, 342, 353
meaningful occupations 72, 107, 221, 305, 338, 357, 474, 569, 578, 579, 586, 714, 752, 788, 845
Mechanistic Paradigm 31, 49
meliorism 290, 295
mental capacities **78**
mental functions 13, 381–384; body structures and function 382; global *see* global mental functions; interventions 383; occupational performance example 382–383; occupational therapy practitioners 382; specific 381–382
meso context 86, 96
Mesquita Pinto, Jussara de 270
metabolic functions 389
methodological trends in occupational therapy 272
MeToo Movement 601
Meyer, A. 103, 288, 361, 808
Mezirow, J. 152
micro context 86, 87, 96
middle adulthood: activities of daily living 558, 561; caregiving of 561–563; defined 554–555; generativity *vs.* stagnation 556–557; midlife crisis or time of transition 557; occupational profile of 554, **558–561**, 561; psychosocial developmental tasks 556–557; Sandwich Generation 562–563; in 21st Century 555–556
middle childhood 454, 475, 485
middle-to-late adolescence 513, 516–517
midlife crisis 554–557
Mignolo, W. 164
Milan, S. 813
Mindell, J. A. 813
Mitcham, M. D. 671

INDEX

Model of Human Occupation (MOHO) 40, 42, 76, 77, 339–340, 355; concepts 78, 78–79; environment 78, 81; factors 78; habituation 78, 80, 419, 585; occupational competence 78; occupational identity 77; performance capacity 78, 80–81; in practice 81–82, 83; therapeutic reasoning 82; volition 78, 79–80
Model of Human Occupation Screening Tool 620
Model of Occupational Therapy Reasoning 114–116, *115*, 120, 121, 127, 133, 135
models of practice 39; action domains 91–93; CanMOP 83–87; collaborative relationship-focused practice 87–88; COTIPP 88–89; foundational processes 89–90; MOHO 77–83, **78–79**; practice scenario 76–77
modification 20, 52, 132, 133, 323, 380, 381, 389, 391, 410, 418, 419, 422, 655, 659, 664, 799, 826, 837, 842, 843, 845, 846, 848
Moen, E. 491
Molineux, M. 32, 33, 359
monitoring and modifying practice reasoning 133, **135**
Monzeli, G. A. 305
Moore, A. 422, 423
moral treatment 10, 433
Morrison, R. 809
Mosey, A. C. 610
motor 125, 398, 512, 574, 658; control 702, 725; fine **456**, 658; function 434, 455; gross **456**, 658; skills 13, 16, **19**, 381, 394, 398, **400**, 400–401, 436, 471, 485, 495, 706, 723, 776, 844
movement-related functions **374**, 383, 385–387, 661
Murray, A. 54
Mylopoulos, M. 809

Nahemow, L. 436
narrative: alignment 261; reasoning 126; studies 125–126, 259
nature: of human beings 256–257; of human occupation 93, 342–343; of occupational adaptation 359; of occupational disruption 130; of occupational dysfunction 130; of occupational therapy 433; of participation 105, 108; of reality 253; situated *see* situated nature of occupation
Nayar, S. 359
Need Ability Opportunity (NAO) Model of Sleep *810*, 810–811
neoliberal ideologies 220
neurodivergence **215**, 217, 220, 222, 223, 225
neurodivergent 217, 218–220, 222–225, 704

neurodiversity **215–216**; studies **216**
neuromuscular functions 385–387, 571; body structures and function 385–386; interventions 387; occupational performance example 387; occupational therapy practitioners 386–387
neutral position on racism 201
Newton, S. 673
Neysmith, S. M. 151
Nicholson, C. 293
Nixon, S. A. 6
non-linear dynamical system theory 716
non-play 725, 738
non-sanctioned occupations 12, 231, 232, 234, 237, 243, 244
normalcy/normality **216**
normative violence/the violence of normativity **216**
Nottingham Extended-Activities of Daily Living (NEADL) **617**

observational assessment/analysis 411, 494, 502, 625
occupational access 307, 594–595
occupational acquisition 521, 527, **547**
occupational adaptation 9, 13, 40, 77, 78; attributes 358–360; defined 358; theories/models 360, 361
occupational alienation 221
occupational apartheid 221, 307, 317
occupational balance 13, 16, 94, 151, 205, 561, 603, 704, 826; attributes 356; defined 355–356; and imbalance 420; theories/models 357–358
occupational behavior 353, 725
occupational choices 79, 106, 150, 161, 220, 221, 243, 339, 345, 426, 475, 482, 504, 601, 624, 705, 837
occupational competence 40, 78, 82, 94, 96, 359–361, 483, 485, 585
occupational consciousness 162, 198, 578
occupational disengagement 355
occupational dissonance 595
occupational engagement 13, 39, 77, 81–83, 95, 149, 165, 223, 225, 340, 364, 454; attributes 353–354; defined 352–353; theories/models 354–355
occupational environment *180*, 707
occupational equilibrium and occupational alignment 5
occupational identity 40, 77–78, 82, 94, 95, 358–361, 363, 425–426, 483, 492, 493, 502, 585
occupational imbalance 355–357, 361, 363, 365, 420, 598, 599, 603
occupational injustice 93, 94, 172–174, 184–185, 187, 188, 203, 220, 259, 302, 338, 339, 360, 599, 654, 839, 848

INDEX

occupational justice 21, 94, 104, 185, 204, 207, 578, 586, 664, 840; complex public health phenomenon 586; and environmental sustainability 338–339; issues of 722–723; sleep opportunity 811

occupational marginalization 151, 221

occupational opportunities 148, 345, 443, 594–595, 595, 604, 812, 829

occupational outcomes 21

occupational participation 40, 79, 91, 93, 319, 353, 443, 480, 483; in employment, home ownership, and transferring wealth intergenerationally 183–184; in families 182–183; inequity, disadvantage, and injustice 174–175; intersectionality and impact of gender diversity 181–182; in school-aged children 487, **487–489**, 489, 494–495, **495–502**; and well-being 502

occupational patterns 357, 603

occupational performance analysis 5, 11–13, 21, 36, 40, 51, 52, 56, 398, 399, 407, 408, 411, 775

Occupational Performance History Interview-II 80, 656

Occupational Performance Inventory of Sexuality and Intimacy (OPISI) 845, 848

Occupational Performance Model 436

occupational possibilities 87, 90, 145, 149, 151, 162, 220, 222, 358, 361, 416

occupational profile **462–465**, 530–531, 540; of early adulthood **546–548**; of middle adulthood 554, **558–561**, 561

occupational reconstructions 254, 258, 259–261

occupational reconstruction theory 249, 255; addressing social-structured problems 255–256; authority and power 258; collective actors and collective occupations 256; creativity and imaginative experimentation 257; denouement (post-experimentalism) 261; emancipatory experimentalism 260–261; mind-body engagement 256–257; narrative dimensions 259; overview and principles 254–259; philosophical influences of 252–254; as practice framework 259–261; pre-experimentalism 259–260; self-organizing desire 258–259

occupational rights 304, 338, 339, 438, 623, 627

occupational science: coloniality 192, 199, 205; defined 38; on human occupation 93–94; pragmatism 288–296; self care and ADL 610–611; theory 210, 808; and therapy, relationship between 9–10, *11*, 31–34, 39–41, 54, 153, 163–165, 192, 199, 221, 225, 285

occupational skills 78, 673

occupational therapy: coloniality 192, 199, 205; on human occupation 93–94; pragmatism 288–296; and science, relationship between 9–10, *11*, 31–34, 39–41, 54, 153, 163–165, 192, 199, 221, 225, 285; self care and ADL 610–611; of the South 105

Occupational Therapy Practice Framework - 4th edition (OTPF-4) 437, 787; activities of daily living 16, **17**, **476**, 611; client factors **19–20**, 20; contexts 14; domains 13, 16, **17**, **19–20**, 322, 399, **560**; health management 16, **17**; knowledge 15; performance skills 13, 16, **19–20**, 322, 399; work 16, **17**, **560**

occupational therapy theories 23, 54, 104, 121, 210, 309, 337, 339, 438, **677–682**, 788

occupation analysis 51, 52, 55, 56

occupation-based 51; practices 12, 143–153, 159, 160, 161, 165, 168; theory 579, 585, 587; therapeutic relationships 71

Occupation, Capability and Wellbeing Framework for Occupational Therapy 627

occupation-centered approach 31

occupation-centered practice 38, 50–51; complexity of 52–53; conversations about 56; defined 49–50; enacting 53–54; occupation and health 54; occupation and occupational therapy 48–49; prioritizing 55; strategies to support 54–56; tools that support 55; using occupational language 56

occupation-focused 48, 50–53, 56, 57, 83, 95, 120, 121, 127, 130, 135, 323, 594, 603, 604, 757

occupations of adolescents 512, **519–520**; basic and IADLs 521, **522–527**, 527, 530; case study 531–532; occupational profile 530–531; risk of **519–520**

occupations of early adulthood 537–549

ocupaciones colectivas 231, 235–238, 243

ocupaciones transgresoras 231, 237, 238, 243, 244

Oliver, M. 104

O*NET 656, 657, 664

Onlooker play **717**

ontology(ies) 164

oppression 6, 9, 84, 88, 145, 151, 159, 162, 175, 181, 187, 193, 195, 198, **216**, 232, 237, 238, 241, 253, 256, 257, 307, 361, 426, 603, 626; patriarchal 600; social **213**, 221, 295; systemic 173, 220, 225, 351, 365

Organisation for Economic Co-operation and Development 303, 544, 627

organization 6, 166, 167, 177, 301, 443, 445, 467, 490, 583, 752

orienting space 127–130, *128*, **134**

619

INDEX

Osborne, M. A. 330
Osler, William 64
outdoor play 480, 492, 719, 720
Overs, R. P. 752

Pacherie, E. 809
pansexual individual 302
Papini, G. 292
paradigm 31, 39, 48–50, 54, 72, 224, 252, 271, 289, 603, 641
Paradigm of Occupation 31, 48, 49
parallel play 471
parenting 174, 176, 186, 224, 304, 307, 362, 364, 426, 455, 542, 557
Parham, L. D. 747
Parten, M. 716
participation: across the lifespan 235; challenges 104–105; community 241, 307, 388, 480, 575, 582, 787, 793; concepts of 789; COVID-19 595–596; defined 103–104; educational 477, 559, 671, 676, 684, 702, 708; in Latin America 106; legacy of colonization 105; leisure 754; of older people 107; for school-aged children 474; of school-aged children 502, 503; sexual 840, 841, 845; sleep 547, 559, 807, 827; social *see* social participation; youth 502
patient-as-a-person movement 64
patient-reported measures 371
patriarchy 105, 145, 220, 235, 238, 241, 600, 602
patterns of daily occupation 78
Pavlov, Ivan 469, 702
Pediatric Evaluation of Disability Inventory 495, 622, 688
peers 179–181, 494; belonging 716; homophobic and transphobic 182; play activities 485; White 184–186
Peirce, Charles Sanders 286–287
Pentland, W. 35
Perales, F. 813
perceived competence 495, 747
performance analysis 398, 399, 407, 408, 411, 775
Performance Assessment of Self-care Skills 618
performance-based 494, 657, 686, 725
performance capacity 40, 78, 78–80, 339, 585, 629, 655, 758, 787, 788
performance patterns: habits 9, 13, 16, 18, 159, 321–323, 325, 327, 328, 414–419, 454, 474, 482, 483, 577, 787; rituals 9, 13, 16, 18, 159, 321–323, 325, 327, 328, 422–424, 454, 474, 482, 483, 577, 787; roles 9, 13, 16, 18, 159, 321–323, 325, 327, 328, 425–427, 454, 474, 482, 483, 577, 787; routines 9, 13, 16, 18, 159, 321–323, 325, 327, 328, 419–422, 454, 474, 482, 483, 577, 787
performance skills 399, 403; and evaluation 407–408, 408, 409; and intervention 408–410; monitoring, and outcomes 410; motor, process, or social interaction 398, 574; and occupational therapy process 406–407; OTPF-4 Domain is 13, 16, 19–20, 322, 399; universal 398, 399
person 42; clean and sober 362; factors 13, 40, 370–394, 653–654
personal activities of daily living (PADL) 610, 635
personal agency 358
personal causation 40, 655
personal factors 14, 16, 18, 24, 72, 73, 159, 322, 323, 340, 437, 443, 489, 569, 577, 578, 587, 686, 757, 787, 837, 843
personal hygiene and grooming 558, 611, 613
personalized medicine 62
person-centered care 61–73, 300, 371, 379, 568; art and science integration 64–65; defined 62; function-dysfunction continuum 68, 69; historical basis 63–64; intentional relationship approach 67–68; occupational goals in 71; occupational therapist 63; in occupational therapy 65–67; occupation as treatment in 72; philosophy in occupational therapy 64; postulates regarding change 70–71; theoretical base 68
person-centered theory 62, 65–67, 66, 67–68
person-environment fit 436, 439
Person-Environment-Occupation-Performance (PEOP) model 121
person factors 13, 40, 323, 369–394, 653–654
Phelan, S. K. 147
Phenix, A. 196
Philip, A. 723
philosophical assumptions 64
philosophy 54, 253, 255; person-centered 64; value and potential of 285–286
Phoenix, N. 308
physical activity 418, 421, 480, 481, 483, 491, 532–533, 563, 635, 640, 662, 719, 753, 786, 826
physical capacities 419
physical environment 42, 64, 86, 90, 158, 220, 340, 342, 436, 445, 489, 533, 572, 585, 716, 721, 737, 740, 756, 787
Piaget, J. 467, 468, 518, 520, 714
Pierce, D. 38, 39, 424
Pinto, J. M. 270, 272
Plage, S. 813
plan for transition 91, 93

620

INDEX

play 5, 11, 13, **17**, 34, 323, 425, 475; assessments **726–736**; attunement 470; body and movement 470; case study 723–724; categories 470; categorization of 716, **717–718**; characteristics of children based on different diagnostic groups **736**; and child's capabilities 719, 720; defined 714; deprivation 712, 722, 723, 738; disability and occupational therapy 723; engagement, participation, and social inclusion 719–720; health and well-being 719; health professionals 219; as human occupation 712–715, 724–725; imaginative 470; issues of occupational justice 722–723; and learning 720; in leisure occupations 747–749; meaning of 715–716; object 470; occupations of 176, **477**, **487**, **488**, 492–493, **499**, **548**, **560**; and playfulness 779, 780; purpose of 716, 719; reframing of 725, 737–739; and resilience 721; right to 722–723; routines 458; schemes 459, 470–471; social 471, 485; sociocultural and temporal situatedness 721–722; therapist-initiated to child-initiated **739**; transactions 714; typical 493

play-centered learning 739
playfulness 493, 713–716, 747–748, 774, 779; future 470; parental 493
playful work 725, 738–740
Plummer, T. 490
pluralism 163, 165, 168
pluralistic 167, 431–446
Pohlhaus, Jr., G. 218
Polatajko, H. J. 36, 37, 39, 353
political 14, 90, 93, 94, 101, 102, 105, 143, 145, 151, 253, 276, 294, 432, 439
political environment 359
politics 225, 242, 253, 273, 287, 585
positivism 163, 165, 168
post-colonial community 198
post-experimentalism 259, 261
postformal thought 541
postmodern 145, 163–165, 167, 168, 224
postmodernism 145, 165, 168
postpositivism 163
postulates 66, 70–71, 465, 466, 468
poverty 87, 106, 148, 174, 240, 256, 602; adolescents 179; adults of color 182, 187; affecting daily occupation 184; aging in 107; child 175, 176; escape 106; intergenerational 184
power: colonial 198, 200, 205; coloniality of 164; and privilege 6, 7, 194; sharing 198, 204; systems of 162–163
practice process 83–93, 115, 120, 121, 127, 136, 354, 408

practice reasoning: action space 132–133, **134–135**; aspects of 125–126; collaboration 124; EBP 121–122; Frames of Reference 125; guidelines and protocols 124; model of occupational therapy reasoning *115*, 115–116, **117–119**; monitoring and modifying 133, **135**; orienting space 127–130, *128*, **134**; process 120–122, 126–133, **134–135**; reasoning space 130–132, **134**; resources 125; role and scope 126; therapist and client 122–124

pragmatic method 287
pragmatic reasoning 126
pragmatic temperament 285, 293–296
pragmatism 12, 253; development of 285; future of 292; history of 286–288; influence on occupational therapy and science 288–290; philosophy 285–286; pragmatic temperament 293–295; situation 290; theory of inquiry 292; theory of transaction 291–292
pragmatist perspective 289, 299
pre-experimentalism 259–260
preschooler 453–471, 454, 480, 716, 739
pretend (dramatic) play 717
principles of development 468–469
privilege 197, 233; cisgender 302–303; coin model of 8; and power 6, 7, 194; social 145, 242, 595; white 6, 21, 199–200
problematic situations 250, 252–256, 292
problematization 145, 146, 154
process: aging 568–569, 571, 579, 587; colonization 433; decision-making 152, 359; foundational 89–91; practice 83–93, 115, 120, 121, 127, 136, 354, 408; practice reasoning 120–122, 126–133, **134–135**; skills 16, **19**, 40, 55, 81, 397–399, 401–403, 620, **687**, 844; therapeutic reasoning 81, 95
productivity 13, 34–36, **35**, 83, 84, 86, 94, 324, 610–611, 653, 655, 658, 664, 686, 788
protection 107, 180, 182, 199–203, 242, 244, 274, 276, 277, 307, 391, 573, 595, 600, 602, 652, 659, 676, 751
purposeful activity 37, 38, 231

quality of life 21, 106, 108, 177, 339, 343, 379, 385, 386, 491, 561, 580, 626, 791
quiet recreation 758

racialized targeting and trauma 200
racism 6, 9, 201, 221, 241, 361, 599; and coloniality 196–198; diversity, inequity, exclusion, injustice 596–597; neutral position on 201; personal factors 569–570;

621

INDEX

systemic 165, 173, 183–188, 184, 186, 351, 518, 596, 599; systems of 594–597, 599
Ramugondo, E. L. 194, 196, 198, 236, 256
reason 21, 31, 33, 90, 126, 130, 181, 195, 224, 295, 306, 319, 421, 521, 805, 806, 809
reasoning space 130–132, **134**
reciprocal relationships with local folk 197
recovery 133, 153, 272, 356, 379, 597, 603, 642–644, 807
recreation 13, 107, 179, 323, 494, 719; case studies 776–779; defined 747; within occupational therapy practice models and frameworks 757–758; playfulness 774; professionals in practice environments 756–757
Reed, K. L. 83
reflect 86–88, 90, 293, 361, 433
reflection 88, 408, 435; case study 777–779; critical 90, 203, 234, 235, 242, 279, 407; on relationship between technology and human occupation 330; therapists' 90
rehabilitation professionals 269
Reilly, M. 715, 720, 739
Reindal, S. M. 222
relational leisure 752, 779, 780
relational understandings 162–163
relationships: with coloniality and decoloniality 192–193; between concepts and events 465; family 182, 186, 603, 778; Intentional Relationship Approach 62, 67–68, 72–74; interpersonal 466, 541; intimate **529**, 538–541, 549; intimate partner 787, 793; with local folk, reciprocal 197; between occupation and health 48, 54; romantic 485, 517, 532, 549; social 235, 236, 274, 418, 485, 719; between technology and human occupation 322–328, 330; between technology and people with disabilities 289; therapeutic 35, 68, **69**, 71, 72, 121, 122
remediation 328
renaissance of occupation 49
reproduction 163, 197, 198, 301, 389, 425, 435, 703, 837, 838, 840, **847**, 848
reproductive rights 600, 601, *601*
resilience 5, 341, 344, 479, 480, 502, 503, 600, 719, 721, 723, 751, 780
respiratory functions 387–389
responsibility 181, 235, 483, 489, 538, 540–542, 549, 754; institutional 9; moral 345, 416; of occupational therapy students and practitioners 52; policymakers' 150; social 273; therapist's 71, 88
rest: and activity 808, 810; and sleep *see* sleep and rest

restoration 387, 424, 571, 575, 655, 659, 750, 751, 780, 808, 812, **821**, 846
restorative 16, 383, 435, 808, 810
retirement 91, 183, 186–188, 308, 358, 555, **560**, 569, 653, 656, 659, 661–662, *663*, 754, 812
Riggs, D. W. 301
rights-based approaches 88, 90, 93, 94, 436, 436, 438–439, 443, 712, 725
right to play 722–723, 725
Riquelme, P. L. 235
risk-taking behavior 532
rites of passage 521, 527, **528**
Rittel, H. W. J. 255
rituals: defined 16, 422, 844; everyday work of 424; examples **18–19**; performance patterns 9, 13, 16, 159, 321–323, 325, 327, 328, 454, 474, 482, 483, 577, 787; as re-working the everyday 422–423; as transformative 423–424
Rivermead Extended Activities of Daily Living Index **619**
Robertson, L. J. 114, 131
Rogers, J. C. 127
role(s) 35, **36**, 82; balance/imbalance 426; caregiving 556, 561; child's 482, 483; defined 16, 80, 425; examples **18**; gender 302, 303, 356; negotiating and renegotiating 554; occupational 66, 72, 73, 77, 148, 159, 182, 330, 358, 490, 586; performance patterns 9, 13, 16, 159, 321–323, 325, 327, 328, 454, 474, 482, 483, 577, 787; profession's 221–222; and scope **119**, 126, 128, 132, 133; social issues 426; social reproduction 425; therapist's 128, 223, 251
role-determined leisure 752, 779, 780
Romano, R. 455
romantic relationships 485, 517, 532, 549
Rosenfeld, M. S. 361
routines: changes in 421–422; construction and negotiation 420–421; defined 16, 482, 483; for development **460–461**; examples **18**; family 455, 462, 480; and habits 80, 257, 389; patterns 78, 80; performance patterns 9, 13, 16, 159, 321–323, 325, 327, 328, 454, 474, 482, 483, 577, 787; play 455, 458, *458*, 459, *459*; time use 420
Routine Task Inventory 625
Rudman, D. L. 10, 34, 146, 149, 231
rule-based play 716
Russell, E. 232
Ryan, A. 32

sacred texts 33
Sanderson, S. R. 83
sandwich generation 562–563

sanism 6, 23, **217**, 219, 224
Santos, B. d. S. 105
Santos, Boaventura 295
Santos, M. 293, 439
scaffolding 468, 513, 677, 704, 725, 812
Schell, B. A. B. 114, 125, 126
Schell, J. W 125
schema 467, 777, 810
Schkade, J. 359–361
Schneider, J. 304–306
school: activities of daily living **487–488**, 489–490, **495**; activity participation for 474; age 13, 474, 480, 622; and communities 180, *180*, 342; COVID-19 pandemic 502, 503; student 182, 184
school-aged children 473–504; assessment of occupational participation 482–494; case study 484–485; community environment 480; COVID-19 on occupational participation 503; cultural environment 480–481; developmental expectations for occupational participation 483, 485–487, **486**, **487–489**, 489; home environment 479; influence of environment and cultural context 478–482; occupational participation and well-being 502; occupation-centered assessments **495–502**; occupations of 475, **476–477**; performance patterns 482–483, *484*; school environment 479–480; virtual environment 481–482
School Assessment of Motor and Process Skills (School AMPS) **498**, **687**
Schultz, S. 359–361
Schwartz, I. S. 703
scientific reasoning 125
self-actualization 466, 520, 602, 637
self-care: activity 623, 626; ADL 324, 610–613; collectives 628
self-concept 516, 532, 533, **691**, 788
self-determination 13, 85, 87, 88, 495, **496**, 502–504, 533, 705
self determination theory (SDT) 85, 87, 672
self-directed 470, 471, 714, 738
self-efficacy 55, 339, 353, 471, 482, 493, 516, 580, 637, 672, 751
self-expression 716, 722, 837
self-management 13, 150, 389, 497, 635, 799
self-regulated learning **678**, 708
self-report **819**
sense of agency 672, 722, 738
sense of mastery 672, 719
sensory functions 382–385, 574
sensory play 716
sensuality 484, 836, 838–840, **846**
serious leisure 752, 780
settler colonialism 23, 193–195, 201
settler colonial legitimacy 204
sex 172, 223; adolescent 180; and gender 241, 754; for money 363; opposite 515; same 515; secondary 514, 516; survival 182; unprotected 180, 182, 532; work 233
sexual abuse 847–848
sexual activity **476**, 490, **522**, **558**, 601, 837, 840, 845, 846, 848
sexual development 515–516, **517**
sexual dysfunction 840, 841, 844
sexual expression 837, 845, 846
sexual health 836, 838, 840, 843, 845, **847**, 848
sexual identity 75, 307, 309, 517, 542, 640, 836, 838–840, **846**, 848
sexual issues 839, 841, 845–846
sexuality 6, 301–302, 391, 541, 554, 555, 636; addressing issues 845–846; and AOTA 837; circles of *see* Circles of Sexuality; defined 837, 848; education and interventions 847–848; evaluation 843–845; ex-PLISSIT Model *841*, 841–843; factors affecting 840–841; and gender **517**; human 13; as occupation 837
sexuality intervention 843
sexualization 836, 838, 839, 848
sexual orientation 14, **18**, 122, 485, 602, 837, 839, 843, 846, 847, 848
sexual participation 840, 841, 845
sexual reproduction 301, 837–838, 840, 848
sexual violence 847, 848
shared situations 252, 256, 259–261
sharing power 198, 204
Shordike, A. 424
Simaan, J. 196, 198
Simpson, Kristie 645
situated 160, 162; within CDS 219–222; occupation as 160–161; ontological and epistemological underpinnings 163–164; sociopolitical and cultural circumstances 146
situated nature of occupation 12, 159; defined 159–160; distinctions between people and environment 160–161; example 165–167; exemplifying 165; interrelations of person, occupation, and context 159–160; people, occupations, and contexts 161–162; systems of power 162–163
situation: clinical 71; complexity of 130–131; economic 108, 274, 421; person's 128; pragmatism 290; problematic 254–256, 259–260
skills: adaptive behavior 471; cognition/cognitive 13, 455, 521; social interaction 16, **20**, 322, 398, 403–406, **404–406**, 748, 787
skin functions 391, 392

INDEX

Skinner, B. F. 469, 703
Slagle, Eleanor Clarke 288, 671
sleep 11; ability 811; for adults **821–825**; assessment of s 815, **815–820**; defined 807–808; deprivation 807, 808, 814–815, 828; disruption 807, 808, 814; disturbance 806, 807, 808, **817**, **822**, 828, 829; duration 807, 813, 815; dysfunction 807; health 806, 813, **816**; need 810, 811, 828, 829; opportunity 810, 811, 828, 830; orchestration 810–811, 829; participation 547, **559**, 807, **827**; patterns 421, 491; preparation **476**, 547, 807, 809, 811, **826**; problems 6; quality of 491, 813, **821**, **825**; quantity of 491; safety 813
sleep and rest 13, **17**, 34, 322, 327, 384, 459, 475, **476**, **487**, **488**, 491, **497**, **525–526**, 547, 555, **559**, 561, 574, 576, 580, 635; case study 827–828; defined 807–808; levels of consciousness 809–810; lifespan and developmental perspective 812; occupational therapy interventions 826, **826–827**, 828–829; sociocultural implications 812–813, *814*; theoretical perspectives 808–809; theories of occupation 811–812
smartphones 318, 327
smell functions 384
Smith, A. B. 337
Smith, Emma M. 315
Smith, J. P. 813
Smith, M. 128, 132
Smith, Tuhiwai 164
Snowden, D. J. 129–131
social 6, 9, 13, 16, 39, 40, 81, 83, 90, 106–107, 143, 160–161, 239, 253, 277, 303, 324, 328, 336, 357, 359, 410, 440, 491, 493, 521, 595; action 261, 276, 277, 329; anthropology 252; constructivism 468
social-cognitive learning 677
social determinants 436–438, 586, 600, 671, 676, 683, 813
social determinants of health 197, 437–439, 474, 475, 504, 586, 600, 676, 812, 813; well-being 474, 475, 504
social-emotional 455, 471, 485, 489, 490, 495, 502, 748
social engagement 557, 787, 789, 846
social environment 64, 158, 445, 489, 569, 585, 640, 716, 721, 737, 740, 787, 788, 792
social good 269, 416–418
social inequities 75, 235, 241, 244
social injustice 172, 174, 195, 204
social interaction 327, 400, 719, 777, 787
social interaction skills 16, **20**, 322, 398, 403–406, **404–406**, 748, 787

socialization 148, 179–181, 481, 503, 577, 705, 758, 812
social justice 8, 198, 231, 232, 316, 341
socially transformative practices 145, 147, 149
social occupational therapy 12, 204, 244, 252, 439–440; articulation of resources in social field 278; Brazilian 275; dynamization of support network 278; historical perspective 269–273; individual territorial follow-ups 278; intervention methodologies 275; medical-psychological knowledge 273–274; political openness 273; propositions, actions, and dynamics 276–277; social problems 275; social vulnerability 274; workshops of activities, dynamics, and projects 277–278
social participation 13, **17**, 327, 439, 459, 475, 481–482; assessment selection 793; in context of human occupation 791–792; evaluating 792–793, **794–798**; interventions 793; multi-disciplinary definitions of 789, **790**, 791; occupational therapy's conceptualization 787–788; occupations 5, 323, **477**, **487**, **489**, 494, **501**, **502**, **527**, 548, **560–561**, 577, 582; peer interactions 494
social positioning 193, 196–197, 203, 205, 238, 244, 434
social question 252, 269–276, 279
social reconstructions 252
social relations 147, 235, 236, 254, 260, 274, 418, 485, 719
social relationships 235, 236, 274, 418, 485, 719
social responsibility 267, 273
social restrictions 221, 712
social sanctioning 229–244, 304
social transformation 144–145, 237, 238, 242, 243, 251, 253–254, 261, 272, 274
social transformation practice 261, 262
societally condemned activities 595
sociocultural and temporal situatedness 721–723
sociocultural-spatial occupation 721, *721*, 740
socio-cultural-spatial-political context 291, 713, 721
socioeconomic 144–145, 149, 151, 153, 177, 187, 307, 329, 339, 425, 436, 442, 479, 543, 602, 653, 713
socioeconomic status (SES) 5, 14, **18**, 22, 172–174, 323, 361, 554, 563, 570, 594, 595, 602, 604, 674, 713, 722, 746, 754, 756, 780, 843
socio-historical stigmatization 151
sociological theory 161

solitary play **733**, 753
specific mental functions 381–382
speech 80, 375, 383, 389–391, 404, 425, 531, 845
spiritual beliefs 381, 394, 613, 838
spirituality 13, 20, 84, 86, 322, 323, 340, 369–394, 490, 513, 578–579, 787, 844
sports 14, 103, 180, 181, 241, 277, 303, 355, 459, 479, 480, 482, 485, 488, 491, 493, 494, 513, *514*, 516, 532, 747, 752, 754, 757, 758, 776, 777, 780
stagnation 556–557, 563
Stanley, M. 359
Stebbins, R. A. 752
stigma 426, 562, 640–641, 756
stigmatization of mental illness 597
stigmatizing 200, 569, 640, 641
strengths-based approach 574, 579, 587
structured action 809
student 4, 9, 11; adolescent 179; BIPOC 205; critical reflexivity and awareness 152; entry-level education 30; high school student 182, 184; occupational therapy 12, 33, 52, 289, 302, 337, 671; postgraduate 12
Student Environment Tasks and Tools (SETT) Framework 324
Sturmberg, J. 585
subjectivity 277, 714
supremacy 165, 199–201, 220, 241
sustainability 595, 600; environmental 240, 293, 336–345; of Micheline's occupational participation 93
sustainable development 336, 343, 344, 544
Swenson, R. 305
Sy, M. P. 230, 243
systemic racism 165, 173, 183–188, 351, 518, 596, 599
systems of racism and agism 594–597, 599

task **36**, 757; activity 13; attention 382; complexity of 406; of early adulthood 545; environmental modifications 380; level 387; and occupation-based outcomes 371, 387, 393; performance of 386–387; remediation 383; work 660, *660*
task oriented approach 680
task-oriented measures 775
taste function 384
taxonomy 34–37, 39–41, 716, 727, 752, 789, 790
Taylor, B. 841
Taylor, R.R. 67, 68, 70, 72–74
teaching 9, 21, 23, 65, 65, 152, 203, 243, 271, 276, 323, 344, 480, 481, 531, 544, 556, 557, 671, 673, 676, 702, 738, 812
technical action 276

technology 600, 603; adaptive **320**; alternative and augmentative communication (AAC) **320**; assistive 20, 51, 132, 318, 321, 705; case study 317–318; consumer **320**; defined 317, 318; dependence or overreliance on 329; developments 329–330; digital **320**; disruptive **320**, 321–322; emerging **320**; equitable access to 328–329; and future of work 330; gerontechnology **321**; history of 319; and human occupation, relationships between 322–328, 330; information and communication **320**; intelligent **321**; interfacing with occupation 327–328; and occupation across lifespan 325, **326**, 327; in occupational therapy **320–321**; and people with disabilities, relationships between 289; within theoretical models and frameworks 322–325; welfare **321**
Technology Acceptance Model (TAM) 324–325
technology dependence or overreliance on technology 329
temperament 285, 293–296, 383, 456, 843
territorial action approach 439–440
territory 23, 249, 283, 284, 293, 431, 436, 439–440
theory(ies) 7, 33, 39, 276, 354–355, 357–358, 361; of adolescent development 518–521; analysis 465–466; application of 702–705; of cognitive development 467; critical pedagogical theories 152; critical race theory 145, 173, 175, 595; critical social theory 145, 164; on decision-making 114, 132; defined 676; of development in adulthood 557; ecological systems theory 437, 442, 478, 585; Environmental Press Theory 585–586; feminist 301; Flow Theory 355; general systems theory 41; of inquiry 292; masculine 301; of motivation 466; Occupational Reconstruction Theory 252–261, *255*; occupational science theory 210, 808; occupational therapy 23, 54, 104, 121, 210, 309, 337, 339, 438, **677–682**, 788; person-centered theory 62, 65–67, 66, 67–68; self-determination 85, 87, 672; sociological theory 161; to support occupations of late adulthood 584–587; transactional 291–292; transformative learning theory 152
therapeutic engagement 354
therapeutic reasoning 81, *82*, 95
therapist and client: context 123–124; culture **117**, 122–123; skills 122; values **118**, 122, 133, 152, 159, 628, 844–845; values and attitudes 122
therapist-reported measures 371

625

INDEX

Thomas, C. 221
time use 80, 355, 420, 427, 483
toddler 13, 386, 453–471, 454
toileting and toilet hygiene 476, 558, 611
Tolvett, M.P. 235, 236
top-down approach 370, 394
touch function 384
transaction(al) 160, 161, 162, 253, 289–292, 290–292, 357, 358, 359, 406, 415, 427, 433, 442–443, 446, 662, 714
transactionalism 289, 290, 442
transactional perspective 160, 291
transactional theory 291–292
transformative action 164, 261
transformative learning theory 152
transgender people 302, 304–310
transition 91, 93, 97, 151, 165, 178, 187, 289, 305, 306, 308, 358, 423, 458, 462, 474, 485, 490, 499, 512, 513, 520, 527, 531, 539–542, 549, 555–557, 562, 659–662, 692, 704, 754, 779, 810, 811
trauma 72, 85, 159, 182, 187, 196, 200, 242, 603, 644–646, 686, 708, 719, 839, 847–848
trauma-informed care 88, 836
Tree of Leisure 746, 749, 749, 777, 779, 780
Treharne, G. J. 301
Trentham, B. L. 151
Trujillo, Christopher 315
Tuck, E. 193
Turpin, M. 120
Tutton, R. 63
Twinley, R. 232–234

UN Climate Change Conference 341
unconditional leisure 757, 779, 780
Unger, R.M. 253, 295
universal availability 684
Universal Declaration of Human Rights 438, 652
unoccupied play **717**
Unsworth, C. A. 114, 125
unwarranted clinical variation 124

Valavaara, K. 196
Valderrama Núñez, C.M. 229, 235
values 16, 40, 62, 64–66, 73, 84, 85, 94, 121, 132, 192, 322, 324, 370, 394, 410, 538, 829, 837; client factors **19**, 20, **372–378**, 578, 612; core 5, 62; cultural 160; and decoloniality, link between 194; defined 371; family 479, 776, 829; MOHO 78, 80; moral 239; personal 5, 132, 370; privilege and supremacy 199; religious 239; of self-sufficiency and capitalist priorities 220; settler 151; shared 236–237, 252; social 240, 241, 273; therapist and client **118**, 122, 133, 152, 159, 628, 844–845

Van Vleet, M. 748
vestibular function 384
virtual environment 478, 481–482
visual function 384
voice 32, 66, 92, 200, 237, 238, 241, 327, 389–391, 415, 516, 576, 579, 595, 598, 645
volition 40, 78–82, 95, 161, 339, 455, 585, 655, 738, 787, 788
voluntary movements 36
volunteer 56, 257, 482, 492, 582, 653, 656, 659, 662, 664, 752
volunteering 13, 340, 364, 492, 651–664, 747
Vygotsky, L. S. 468

Wagman, P. 343
Walder, K., 358, 359
Walker, B. 845
Wang, Rosalie H. 315, 673
Watling, R. 703
Watson, A. 483
Watson, John 469
Webber, M. 255
welfare technology **321**
wellbeing 163, 200, 327, 379, 386, 627, 672
West, C. 295
Western Society Rites of Passage **528**
Whiteford, G. 54, 128
white privilege 6, 599, 669, 712, 745
white supremacy 165, 199, 220, 241
wicked problems 255
Wilcock, A.A. 103, 109, 231, 527, 808
Wilding, C. 54
women: Black 174, 183, 185–186, 599; Brown 174, 599; career options 172; cisgender 303–304; disorders 389; misogyny 569; in poverty 106; rights 6, 243, 301, 600, *601*; transgender 305, 308
work 9, 11, 34, 241, 277, 323, 542, 561, 603, 635, 787–788; activity 654; assessment 656–658; balance 356, 555–556; CanMOP 86–87; with clients and families 8, 53, 54, 123, 242, 418; community 235, 440, 492; conditioning 659; decolonial 195; future of 330; hardening 659–660; injuries 655; intervention 658–661; Late Adulthood 581–582; meaning of 653; in occupational therapy 221; older adults 576; opportunities 483; OTPF-4 Domain 16, **17**, 560; paid 151, 302; person factors and their influence on 653–654; and productivity 652–653; sex 233; social 220, 288; and volunteerism 475, 477, 487–489, 492, 499, 504
work adaptation 658–659, 660–661, 664; and compensation 660–661
work conditioning 659

worker role interview 80, 657
work hardening 659–660
work-like play 738, 740
work readiness 659
work remediation 659
World Federation of Occupational Therapists (WFOT) 33, 40, 103, 109, 302, 337, 338, 343, 344, 434, 623, 627
World Health Organization (WHO) 13, 14, 103, 318, 325, 329, 341, 381–385, 387–391, 436–438, 475, 561, 574, 575, 577, 582, 638, 655, 722, 757, 786, 789, 837, 845, 848

Yerxa, E. J. 31, 352, 353
young-to-middle adolescence 513, 514–515

youth 13; bullying 482; challenges for 512, 533; depression and suicidality among 598; development 513; diabled youth in Canada 147; with disabilities 490; homeless 181; impact of concussions 491; indigenous 416; mentorship programs 181; motivation 487; occupational participation 502; occupations for youth in young-middle and middle-late adolescence **522–527**; participation in Latin America 106; sexually diverse minority 181–182; transgender minority youth 181, 305

Ziviani, J. 672
zone of proximal development (ZPD) 468, 469